Trends in Andrology and Sexual Medicine

Series Editors

Emmanuele A. Jannini, Chair of Endocrinology & Medical Sexology (ENDOSEX), Department of Systems Medicine, University of Rome Tor Vergata, Roma, Italy

Carlo Foresta, Chair of Endocrinology, Department of Medicine, Unit of Andrology and Reproductive Medicine, University of Padua, Padova, Italy

Andrea Lenzi, Chair of Endocrinology, Department of Experimental Medicine, Section of Medical Pathophysiology, Food Science and Endocrinology Sapienza University of Rome, Rome, Italy

Mario Maggi, Chair of Endocrinology, Department of Experimental, Clinical and Biomedical Sciences, Andrology and Sexual Medicine Unit, University of Florence, Florence, Italy

This series will serve as a comprehensive and authoritative resource that presents state of the art knowledge and practice within the fields of Andrology and Sexual Medicine, covering basic science and clinical and psychological aspects. Each volume will focus on a specific topic relating to reproductive or sexual health, such as male and female sexual disorders (from erectile dysfunction to vaginismus, and from hypoactive desire to ejaculatory disturbances), diagnostic issues in infertility and sexual dysfunction, and current and emerging therapies (from assisted reproduction techniques to testosterone supplementation, and from PDE5i to SSRIs for premature ejaculation). In addition, selected new topics not previously covered in a single monograph will be addressed, examples including male osteoporosis and the approach of traditional Chinese medicine to sexual medicine. Against the background of rapid progress in Andrology and Sexual Medicine, the series will meet the need of readers for detailed updates on new discoveries in physiology and pathophysiology and in the therapy of human sexual and reproductive disorders.

Indexed in Scopus

This book series is published in partnership with the Italian Society of Andrology and Sexual Medicine SIAMS

Corresponding series editor and responsible for new book proposals:
Emmanuele A. Jannini eajannini@gmail.com

Camil Castelo-Branco • Sònia Anglès Acedo

Editors

Medical Disorders and Sexual Health

A Guide for Healthcare Providers

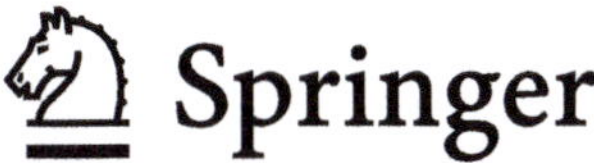 Springer

Editors
Camil Castelo-Branco
Hospital Clínic - University of Barcelona
IDIBAPS
Barcelona, Spain

Sònia Anglès Acedo
Hospital Clínic - University of Barcelona
IDIBAPS
Barcelona, Spain

ISSN 2367-0088   ISSN 2367-0096   (electronic)
Trends in Andrology and Sexual Medicine
ISBN 978-3-031-55082-9   ISBN 978-3-031-55080-5   (eBook)
https://doi.org/10.1007/978-3-031-55080-5

This Springer imprint is published by the registered company Springer Nature Switzerland AG
The registered company address is: Gewerbestrasse 11, 6330 Cham, Switzerland

If disposing of this product, please recycle the paper.

Contents

Contributors

Sònia Anglès Acedo Urogynecological Unit, Clinical Institute of Gynecology, Obstetrics and Neonatology, Hospital Clinic de Barcelona, Barcelona, Spain

Clinical Sexology Working Group, Hospital Clinic de Barcelona, Barcelona, Spain

Surgery and Medical-Surgical Specialties, Faculty of Medicine and Health Sciences, Universitat de Barcelona (UB), Barcelona, Spain

Institut d'Investigacions Biomèdiques August Pi i Sunyer, Barcelona, Spain

Alfonso Alias Hip Unit, Department of Orthopedic Surgery and Traumatology, Clinical Institute of Medical and Surgical Specialties, Hospital Clínic de Barcelona, Barcelona, Spain

Alicia Alpuente Headache Clinic, Neurology Department, Vall d'Hebron University Hospital, Barcelona, Spain

Isis Araujo Endoscopy and Gastrointestinal Motility Unit, Clinical Institute of Digestive and Metabolic Diseases, Hospital Clínic de Barcelona, Barcelona, Spain

José M. Balibrea Endocrine-Metabolic and Bariatric Surgery Unit, Germans Trias I Pujol University Hospital (Badalona), Barcelona, Spain

Department of Surgery, Autonomous University of Barcelona, Barcelona, Spain

Antoni Benabarre Hernández Bipolar and Depression Disorders Unit, Psychiatry and Psychology, Clinical Institute of Neurosciences, Hospital Clinic de Barcelona, Barcelona, Spain

Institut d'Investigacions Biomèdiques August Pi i Sunyer, Barcelona, Spain

Centro de Investigación Biomédica en Red de Salud Mental (CIBERSAM), Instituto de Salud Carlos III, Madrid, Spain

Medicine Department, Faculty of Medicine and Health Sciences, Universitat de Barcelona (UB), Barcelona, Spain

Laura Bertolasi Department of Neurology, University of Verona, Verona, Italy

Johannes Bitzer University Hospital Basel, Basel, Switzerland

Isabel Blanco Pulmonary Hypertension Unit, Hospital Clínic de Barcelona, Barcelona, Spain

Institut d'Investigacions Biomèdiques August Pi i Sunyer, Barcelona, Spain

Carla Box Clinical Institute of Medical and Surgical Specialties, Hospital Clinic de Barcelona, Barcelona, Spain

Clinical Sexology Working Group, Hospital Clinic de Barcelona, Barcelona, Spain

Albert Caballero Endocrine-Metabolic and Bariatric Surgery Unit, Germans Trias I Pujol University Hospital (Badalona), Barcelona, Spain

Department of Surgery, Autonomous University of Barcelona, Barcelona, Spain

Berta Caballol Inflammatory Bowel Disease Unit, Department of Gastroenterology, Clinical Institute of Digestive and Metabolic Diseases, Hospital Clínic de Barcelona, Barcelona, Spain

José Luis Callejas-Rubio Systemic Autoimmune Diseases Unit, Department of Internal Medicine, Hospital San Cecilio, Granada, Spain

Miquel Camafort Hypertension Unit, Department of Internal Medicine, Clinical Institute of Medicine and Dermatology, Hospital Clínic de Barcelona, Barcelona, Spain

Medicine Department, Faculty of Medicine and Health Sciences, Universitat de Barcelona (UB), Barcelona, Spain

Camil Castelo-Branco Gynecological Department, Clinical Institute of Gynecology, Obstetrics and Neonatology, Hospital Clinic de Barcelona, Barcelona, Spain

Clinical Sexology Working Group, Hospital Clinic de Barcelona, Barcelona, Spain

Surgery and Medical-Surgical Specialties, Faculty of Medicine and Health Sciences, Universitat de Barcelona (UB), Barcelona, Spain

Institut d'Investigacions Biomèdiques August Pi i Sunyer, Barcelona, Spain

Giovanni Corona Endocrinology Unit, Azienda AUSL, Bologna, Italy

Juan Manuel Corral Molina Urology Department, Clinical Institute of Nephrology and Urology, Hospital Clínic de Barcelona, Barcelona, Spain

Clinical Sexology Working Group, Hospital Clinic de Barcelona, Barcelona, Spain

Angela Cuccarollo School of Specialization in Obstetrics and Gynecology, University of Verona, Verona, Italy

Ob-Gyn Department, Alto Vicentino Hospital, Santorso, Vicenza, Italy

Maurizio D'Anna Urology Department, Clinical Institute of Nephrology and Urology, Hospital Clínic de Barcelona, Barcelona, Spain

Clinical Sexology Working Group, Hospital Clinic de Barcelona, Barcelona, Spain

Adelina Doltra Non-invasive Cardiac Imaging Section, Clinical Institute of Cardiovascular Medicine, Hospital Clínic de Barcelona, Barcelona, Spain

Clinical Sexology Working Group, Hospital Clinic de Barcelona, Barcelona, Spain

Gerard Espinosa Department of Autoimmune Diseases, Clinical Institute of Medicine and Dermatology, Hospital Clínic de Barcelona, Barcelona, Spain

Agnès Fernández-Clotet Inflammatory Bowel Disease Unit, Department of Gastroenterology, Clinical Institute of Digestive and Metabolic Diseases, Hospital Clínic de Barcelona, Barcelona, Spain

Jenaro A. Fernández-Valencia Hip Unit, Department of Orthopedic Surgery and Traumatology, Clinical Institute of Medical and Surgical Specialties, Hospital Clinic de Barcelona, Barcelona, Spain

Surgery and Medical-Surgical Specialties, Faculty of Medicine and Health Sciences, Universitat de Barcelona (UB), Barcelona, Spain

Ferran Fillat Hip Unit, Department of Orthopedic Surgery and Traumatology, Clinical Institute of Medical and Surgical Specialties, Hospital Clínic de Barcelona, Barcelona, Spain

Carme Font Clinical Sexology Working Group, Hospital Clinic de Barcelona, Barcelona, Spain

Irene Fuertes Dermatology and Venereology Unit, Clinical Institute of Medicine and Dermatology, Hospital Clínic de Barcelona, Barcelona, Spain

Clinical Sexology Working Group, Hospital Clinic de Barcelona, Barcelona, Spain

Pere Fusté Gynecological Department, Clinical Institute of Gynecology, Obstetrics and Neonatology, Hospital Clinic de Barcelona, Barcelona, Spain

Lydia Gaba Clinical Sexology Working Group, Hospital Clinic de Barcelona, Barcelona, Spain

Marta Gallego Inflammatory Bowel Disease Unit, Department of Gastroenterology, Clinical Institute of Digestive and Metabolic Diseases, Hospital Clínic de Barcelona, Barcelona, Spain

Inés García-Bouyssou Clinical Institute of Medical and Surgical Specialties, Hospital Clinic de Barcelona, Barcelona, Spain

Anna Giménez Palomo Bipolar and Depression Disorders Unit, Psychiatry and Psychology, Clinical Institute of Neurosciences, Hospital Clinic de Barcelona, Barcelona, Spain

Esther Gomez-Gil Clinical Sexology Working Group, Hospital Clinic de Barcelona, Barcelona, Spain

José Alfredo Gómez-Puerta Department of Rheumatology, Clinical Institute of Medical and Surgical Specialties, Hospital Clinic de Barcelona, Barcelona, Spain

Alessandra Graziottin Center of Gynecology and Medical Sexology, H. San Raffaele Resnati, Milan, Italy

Department of Obstetrics and Gynecology, University of Verona, Verona, Italy

Department of Endocrinology and Metabolic Diseases, Federico II University, Naples, Italy

Alessandra Graziottin Foundation for the Cure and Care of Pain in Women NPO, Milan, Italy

Fernando Gutiérrez Psychiatry and Psychology, Clinical Institute of Neurosciences, Hospital Clinic de Barcelona, Barcelona, Spain

Felicia A. Hanzu Endocrinology and Nutrition Department, Clinical Institute of Digestive and Metabolic Diseases, Hospital Clínic de Barcelona, Barcelona, Spain

Medicine Department, Faculty of Medicine and Health Sciences, Universitat de Barcelona (UB), Barcelona, Spain

Institut d'Investigacions Biomèdiques August Pi i Sunyer, Barcelona, Spain

Sara Laxe Rehabilitation Service, Clinical Institute of Medical and Surgical Specialties, Hospital Clinic de Barcelona, Barcelona, Spain

WHOFIC Academic Collaborating Center, Universitat de Barcelona, Barcelona, Spain

Clinical Sexology Working Group, Hospital Clinic de Barcelona, Barcelona, Spain

Lorena López Frías Urogynecological Unit, Clinical Institute of Gynecology, Obstetrics and Neonatology, Hospital Clinic de Barcelona, Barcelona, Spain

Clinical Sexology Working Group, Hospital Clinic de Barcelona, Barcelona, Spain

Mario Maggi Endocrinology Unit, Mario Serio Department of Experimental and Clinical Biomedical Sciences, University of Florence, Florence, Italy

Antoni Martin Moreno Sexology Clinic, Barcelona, Spain

Carmen Martínez Hematopoietic Stem Cell Transplantation Unit, Hematology Department, Clinical Institute of Hematology and Oncology, Hospital Clínic de Barcelona, Barcelona, Spain

Clinical Sexology Working Group, Hospital Clinic de Barcelona, Barcelona, Spain

Institut d'Investigacions Biomèdiques August Pi i Sunyer, Barcelona, Spain

Carmen Martinez Garcia Urology Department, Clinical Institute of Nephrology and Urology, Hospital Clínic de Barcelona, Barcelona, Spain

Roger Matheu Riviere Urology Department, Clinical Institute of Nephrology and Urology, Hospital Clínic de Barcelona, Barcelona, Spain

Eduard Mension Gynecological Department, Clinical Institute of Gynecology, Obstetrics and Neonatology, Hospital Clinic de Barcelona, Barcelona, Spain

Institut d'Investigacions Biomèdiques August Pi i Sunyer, Barcelona, Spain

Mireia Mora Porta Endocrinology and Nutrition Department, Clinical Institute of Digestive and Metabolic Diseases, Hospital Clínic de Barcelona, Barcelona, Spain

Institut d'Investigacions Biomèdiques August Pi i Sunyer, Barcelona, Spain

Pau Moreno Endocrine-Metabolic and Bariatric Surgery Unit, Germans Trias I Pujol University Hospital (Badalona), Barcelona, Spain

Department of Surgery, Autonomous University of Barcelona, Barcelona, Spain

Ernesto Muñoz-Mahamud Hip Unit, Department of Orthopedic Surgery and Traumatology, Clinical Institute of Medical and Surgical Specialties, Hospital Clinic de Barcelona, Barcelona, Spain

Surgery and Medical-Surgical Specialties, Faculty of Medicine and Health Sciences, Universitat de Barcelona (UB), Barcelona, Spain

Iuliia Naumova Department of Obstetrics and Gynecology, Faculty of Medicine, Saratov State Medical University n.a. V. I. Razumovsky of the Ministry of Health of Russia, Saratov, Russia

Aida Orois Añón Endocrinology and Nutrition Department, Clinical Institute of Digestive and Metabolic Diseases, Hospital Clínic de Barcelona, Barcelona, Spain

Sílvia Pastells Pujol Sexology Clinic, Barcelona, Spain

Esteban Poch Nephrology Department, Clinical Institute of Nephrology and Urology, Hospital Clinic de Barcelona, Barcelona, Spain

Surgery and Medical-Surgical Specialties, Faculty of Medicine and Health Sciences, Universitat de Barcelona (UB), Barcelona, Spain

Lara Quintas Marquès Gynecological Department, Clinical Institute of Gynecology, Obstetrics and Neonatology, Hospital Clinic de Barcelona, Barcelona, Spain

Clinical Sexology Working Group, Hospital Clinic de Barcelona, Barcelona, Spain

Ana M. Ramirez Pulmonary Hypertension Unit, Hospital Clínic de Barcelona, Barcelona, Spain

Institut d'Investigacions Biomèdiques August Pi i Sunyer, Barcelona, Spain

Luis J. Ramirez Núñez Hip Unit, Clinical Institute of Medical and Surgical Specialties, Hospital Clinic de Barcelona, Barcelona, Spain

Laura Ribera Torres Urogynecological Unit, Clinical Institute of Gynecology, Obstetrics and Neonatology, Hospital Clinic de Barcelona, Barcelona, Spain

Josep Riera Dermatology and Venereology Unit, Clinical Institute of Medicine and Dermatology, Barcelona, Spain

Cristina Ros Cerro Urogynecological Unit, Clinical Institute of Gynecology, Obstetrics and Neonatology, Hospital Clinic de Barcelona, Barcelona, Spain

Clinical Sexology Working Group, Hospital Clínic de Barcelona, Barcelona, Spain

Surgery and Medical-Surgical Specialties, Faculty of Medicine and Health Sciences, Universitat de Barcelona (UB), Barcelona, Spain

Institut d'Investigacions Biomèdiques August Pi i Sunyer, Barcelona, Spain

Raquel Salinas Rehabilitation Service, Clinical Institute of Medical and Surgical Specialties, Hospital Clinic de Barcelona, Barcelona, Spain

Maria Sepúlveda Gázquez Neuroimmunology and Multiple Sclerosis Unit, Neurology Department, Clinical Institute of Neurosciences, Hospital Clinic de Barcelona, Barcelona, Spain

Clinical Sexology Working Group, Hospital Clinic de Barcelona, Barcelona, Spain

Adria Serra Trullas Department of Orthopaedic Surgery, Clinical Institute of Medical and Surgical Specialties, Hospital Clínic de Barcelona, Barcelona, Spain

Mònica Serrano Clinical Institute of Neurosciences, Hospital Clínic de Barcelona, Barcelona, Spain

Jordi Tarascó Endocrine-Metabolic and Bariatric Surgery Unit, Germans Trias I Pujol University Hospital (Badalona), Barcelona, Spain

Department of Surgery, Autonomous University of Barcelona, Barcelona, Spain

Sara Tavares Nogueira General and Digestive Surgery, Clinical Institute of Digestive and Metabolic Diseases, Hospital Clínic de Barcelona, Barcelona, Spain

Josep Torremadé Barreda Urology Department, Clinical Institute of Nephrology and Urology, Hospital Clínic de Barcelona, Barcelona, Spain

Clinical Sexology Working Group, Hospital Clinic de Barcelona, Barcelona, Spain

Marta Torres-Ferrús Headache Clinic, Neurology Department, Vall d'Hebron University Hospital, Barcelona, Spain

Francisco Valdesoiro Psychiatry and Psychology, Clinical Institute of Neurosciences, Hospital Clinic de Barcelona, Barcelona, Spain

Irene Vinagre Endocrinology and Nutrition Department, Clinical Institute of Digestive and Metabolic Diseases, Hospital Clínic de Barcelona, Barcelona, Spain

How to Talk on Sexuality in a Medical Consultation

Camil Castelo-Branco

1 Introduction

A recent cohort study of patient data from the National Health and Nutrition Examination Survey found a significant association between lower sexual frequency and greater all-cause mortality among hypertense patients [1]. Similarly, it occurs with patients with coronary disease [2] and cancer [3]. Therefore, should physicians offer a sex prescription to patients living with chronic illness? How can healthcare providers help these patients access their capacity for sexual pleasure, a critical and life-affirming component of the human life?

According to the World Health Organization, sexual health is a state of physical, mental, and social well-being in relation to sexuality and not simply the absence of disease, dysfunction, or illness. Consequently, sexual health is a basic and fundamental part of general health and general well-being [4]. Therefore, sexual health can be described as the ability to have a pleasurable sex life and to adapt and self-manage it in the face of social, physical, and emotional challenges across the life span [5]. Medical conditions and its treatments, such as those described in this book as well as other chronic conditions [6], are such challenges. To offer the patients the necessary care for dealing with these conditions and therefore contribute to their general well-being, it is crucial that the discussion of sexuality and sexual health take part of the standard healthcare [5].

C. Castelo-Branco (✉)
Gynecological Department, Clinical Institute of Gynecology, Obstetrics and Neonatology, Hospital Clinic de Barcelona, Barcelona, Spain

Clinical Sexology Working Group, Hospital Clinic de Barcelona, Barcelona, Spain

Surgery and Medical-Surgical Specialties, Faculty of Medicine and Health Sciences, Universitat de Barcelona (UB), Barcelona, Spain

Institut d'Investigacions Biomèdiques August Pi i Sunyer, Barcelona, Spain
e-mail: ccastelo@clinic.cat

© The Author(s), under exclusive license to Springer Nature Switzerland AG 2024
C. Castelo-Branco, S. Anglès Acedo (eds.), *Medical Disorders and Sexual Health*, Trends in Andrology and Sexual Medicine,
https://doi.org/10.1007/978-3-031-55080-5_1

Many doctors recognize the importance of talking about sexuality and sexual issues with patients; however, discussing these topics can be problematic for them [7, 8]. Healthcare providers and patients cite barriers to discuss sexual issues. For example, patients attended by general practitioners in primary care referred that "embarrassment" and "nervousness" were the most common barriers to discussing sexual concerns, followed by "concern about keeping information private" and "concern about discrimination or being treated badly" as barriers [6], while for doctors, the concern about feeling limited in their ability to address sexual issues and the feeling that starting these conversations requires specialized knowledge and skills [9]. Healthcare givers dealing with patients complaining with chronic diseases referred that self-consciousness, lack of self-reliance, and patient characteristics such as ethnic, religion, and social values were important barriers in discussing sexual issues [10]. It should be noted that the ways in which such a sensitive topic is treated in the conversation can determine its development [8, 10]. Some authors have highlighted that the gap between provider and patient perspectives can negatively impact care when patients perceive that provider communication strategies reveal a lack of investment, caring, or knowledge [11]. Therefore, competent provider communication tailored to patient needs facilitates patient understanding and helps them achieve important goals that support quality of life [11]. In recent times, efforts were made to give tools for discussing sexual issues in medical settings and developing communication guidance interventions. Nevertheless, these proposals are frequently based on self-related feelings and experiences of patients and doctors concerning consultations [12, 13]. Such data do not explain how sexual issues were really managed in a medical office.

Several methods for discourse analysis are available; however, our focus is on those where the sequential analysis is a core element (e.g., the PLISSIT model, the five A model). This methodological approach gives discourse as action-oriented, meaning that people often perform a range of actions across the discourse. In addition, models such as PLISSIT or EX-PLISSIT that put consent at the center of the therapy can help healthcare givers to establish this conversation with patients. In partnered people, it is important to educate both the patient and their sexual partner about the possible consequences of the disease on their future sexuality and intimacy and to teach them to ask for help when they may need it. These conversations between physicians and their patients can also be constructed within this structure. To this date, systematic reviews of discourse analytic studies in healthcare settings on sexual issues are scarce [14]. These tools are especially useful for making recommendations on ways to carry out conversations on sexual issues in healthcare. With this holistic approach, in this chapter, we aim to detect how communication on sexual issues is put in motion in medical settings and the results of these talks, as well as to provide healthcare givers suggestions on how to communicate about topics related to sex, sexuality, and sexual health.

2 Clinical Interview

2.1 General Aspects to Take into Account

The clinical interview is the fundamental piece in the diagnosis and therapeutic approach to sexual problems and dysfunctions; it allows obtaining the necessary information to be able to make a correct diagnosis and becomes a first-order element in the therapeutic approach.

In this approach, firstly, we need to ask routinely about sexual well-being and pleasure; otherwise, we do not know the importance of sexuality in the patient's quality of life.

If healthcare professionals do not ask, they will not know what particular type of sexual activity is relevant for a person's pleasure, nor will they be able to suppose how they prioritize their sexual functioning in the context of their healthcare. Therefore, in an initial approach, three key questions should be considered: What are your goals? What does sex mean to you? What kinds of sexual play are important for your (and your partner's) pleasure?

There is no doubt that chronic diseases affect both general and genital physiology in a broad biopsychosocial spectrum including physical and psychological symptoms and relational and cultural elements. Diseases affecting neurovascular, neuroendocrine, or neuromusculoskeletal function have a significant effect on sexual function as a result of the disease process or its complications or the effect on identity and well-being. Furthermore, the treatments and its adverse events should be taken into account.

Managing the effects of chronic diseases on sexuality requires the ability to handle life's setbacks and is an overall representation of adaptability and flexibility. An acute or traumatic damage may need a comprehensive adjustment in sexual activity and function, but chronic diseases may require continuous adaptation to sexual changes.

It is to note also the role of the partner in cases of cancer and chronic diseases complaining with affected sexuality. The healthy partners have doubts on how to interact and have also their own sexual demands. Moreover, patients and mates may experience distress feeling the loss of something, sexual activity, which is not socially acceptable to complaint: the own/partner disease and the own/partner sexual pleasure.

Mounting evidence indicates that social support is associated with better outcomes of chronic diseases and reduced all-cause mortality; however, there is a significant lack of knowledge on the specific contribution of sexual functioning to these outcomes, and the potential prognostic significance of marital quality [15]. Sexual pleasure and satisfaction are important factors in relational satisfaction; therefore, asking on sexual issues, we help our patients to do better not only in their sexual health but also in their overall health.

## 2.2	Addressing Sexual Issues

In the management of sexual issues in a medical site, there are several unwritten guidelines that are crucial to consider when doctors try to introduce this topic in the conversation. Addressing sexual issues may be uncomfortable for both patients and healthcare providers. Introducing the PLISSIT model in regular medical care may be useful. First, P, permission. Let the patients express their experiences and complaints. Focus the talk on sexual pleasure better than in performance or activity. Performance is a bad-mannered expression when we are trying to start a conversation on sexual issues. It is important to highlight that pleasure, sensations, and satisfaction are the only "sexual expertise" that patients and partners look for and need.

Second, during conversation, it is also important to be compliant and take into mind that sex includes multiple experiences that change and occur throughout life [16]. Sex may encompass from a touch to the most bizarre acts imaginable. Thus, healthcare professionals need to be able to allow patients and partners to express their needs and facilitate them to think about the wide diversity of options to meet their sexual needs. For these reasons, it is especially important to give balanced information facilitating the acceptance of sexual changes due to the disease.

For a comprehensive management, it is necessary to record the effects of the disease on the patient's self-perception of their body. Many diseases, such as described in this book, not only affect body function but also impair self-esteem and body image. In many cases, a reorganization of self-concept occurs that induces patients to avoid sexual intimacy. Therefore, it is mandatory to assess these self-constructs to get changes in feelings, judgments, and behaviors and in this way to improve psychological and sexual well-being [17]. Doctors may also act as a sexual therapist encouraging patients to explore their body and detecting what feels good in it and what needs to be changed.

Finally, following a PLISSIT model, doctors at office can offer limited information and specific suggestions (Table 1). These first steps of the PLISSIT model P (permission), LI (limited information), and SS (specific suggestions) are affordable for every healthcare provider. The last step, intensive therapy, needs an expert on sexual medicine, and patients must be referred when sexual problems are not resolved with the initial intervention.

Table 1 Examples of sexual tips in a medical office

Allow open communication with partner(s)
Offer resources to facilitate communication
Consider physical and emotional needs for sexual play[a]
Explain patients and partners the need to allow adequate time for sexual play and encourage the ability to adjust or stop and start over
Use sexual aids and toys to enhance pleasure

[a]In many chapters of this book, specific counsels are given including adequate rest, pillows for comfort, aides for positioning, use of moisturizers and lubricants, etc.

2.3   Specific Considerations in a Talk on Sexuality

When dealing with issues related to sexual health and sexual medicine, different circumstances must be considered with added implications elsewhere of the information that the patient provides.

2.3.1   Healthcare Provider-Patient Interaction

There are many concerns in the patient's mind, including embarrassment when talking about sexual health. Often, patients complaining with sexual issues are anxious before and during the conversation with their doctors. Patients largely ruminate about the subject before coming, how to tell their complaints, and what words to use because they will explain something very intimate, and although they harbor the hope of a solution, they also doubt whether the doctor will pay attention to them or whether can really solve the problem. On the other hand, the healthcare provider needs knowledge and a good attitude towards sexuality, empathy, and to know how to establish an environment of confidence (Table 2).

Table 2 Difficulties to establish an environment of confidence

Healthcare professionals' beliefs and facts that impair good communication		
Few doctors ask about sexual health		
Many doctors believe that someone else will do it		
Some doctors referred fear of embarrassing themselves or their patients: I will offend them by asking		
Some doctors considered sexual dysfunction as an unavoidable consequence of aging: patient is too old, sick, young, etc.		
Patients never ask about it, so they must not care		
Lack of time/training: I do not know how to help or have time		
Doctors' social, cultural, and religious values: I do not agree with their lifestyle		
Some doctors neglected the importance of pleasant sex as an important part of quality of life: patient should be happy to be alive		

Patient beliefs and attitudes that impair good communication	
Ignorance about the etiology	A limited number of patients suffering from sexual dysfunction seek medical help
	Most patients are unaware that symptoms do not resolve over time
	Most patients are unaware that treatments are available
	Some patients discontinue treatments
Embarrassment, shame	Social, cultural, and religious values
	One of each three patients would not even tell the partner
	More than half of the patients fail to recognize the relationship between their main complaint and sexual dysfunction
Expect little healthcare provider help on sex	Most patients believe that doctor would be uncomfortable
	Most patients believe that doctor would dismiss the concerns
	Most patients believe that their family doctor does not know medical treatments for their sexual dysfunction

2.3.2 The Interview Management

The sexological talk is more than a medical structured history. The interaction of healthcare provider/patient needs to be lively, active, and adaptable depending on the established goals. Therefore, it is important to address the conversation in an operative and useful way. The conversation must focus on the specific issues that originate the patient's consultation separating the important from the anecdotal and maintaining the thread of conversation at all times.

2.3.3 Burden

Due to the nature of the problem, it is common that patients express nuisance and embarrassment to communicate sexual complaints or reply the questions related to it. The healthcare provider should avoid direct questions that may be embarrassing and distressing for patients. Another important issue is to be cautious with the interpretation of the patient complaint. An initial unfounded diagnosis by the healthcare provider about the process that affects the patient can produce a bias in the subsequent interview management aimed at confirming that diagnosis.

The health professional must know and put in practice some aspects of the medical interview to guarantee effective communication and avoid discomfort in the dialogue with their patients (Table 3).

Table 3 Points to take into account for an effective communication

Tips for an effective communication	
Allow the patient to express themselves freely Avoid structuring the comments and expressions, and ask questions following the initial diagnostic hypothesis Avoid confusing the target by confirming the diagnostic hypothesis	**Listen the patient discourse and pay attention on the patient talk**
Use easy-to-understand but technical language	**Vulgar language causes loss of authority and creates doubts in the patient about the doctor's skills**

3   How to Record a History of Sexual Dysfunction

There are different models to develop an effective interview on sexual issues: Masters and Johnson and Kolodny model [18], Lobitz and Lobitz [19], and Lopicolo and Heiman [20], and each of them dedicates a specific time to the anamnesis: Masters spends 7 h on several days. Kaplan spends 4 h [21], and Hawton dedicates a 45′ session to each member of the couple [22]. However, semi-structured interviews are the preferred model to assess sexual function, and the teaching, orienting, and permitting (TOP model as a part of the PLISSIT model) intervention model is useful for the management of sexual complaints in regular medical office. The use of protocols may facilitate the discussion of sexual issues in general, urology, or gynecological settings and has the potential to provide an effective approach to the complex aspects of sexual dysfunction. The TOP model has three phases: teaching the sexual response, in which the healthcare provider explains the physiology of the sexual response and focuses on the main phases (arousal, interest, orgasm); familiarizing patients with sexual issues, in which sexual education facilitates knowledge on the concept; and healthy and pleasurable experience of sexuality.

Before starting the sexual history, it is important to record a series of clinical and demographic data (Table 4). Once the previous history has been taken and the reason for the visit is known, the medical consultation may be focused on the sexual history. The goal of the sexual history is to identify the sexual problem, delineate possible contributing factors, and clarify the goals of treatment.

Table 4 Clinical and sociodemographic data to be recorded before starting a sexual talk with patient

Clinical and sociodemographic data
Reason for consultation
Age
Stable partner
Personal history of previous diseases
Present diseases and pharmacological treatments
Toxic habits including consumption of illegal drugs
Risk factors for sexually transmitted infections
Risk factors for unwanted motherhood
Risk factors for abuse
Risk factors for sexual dysfunction
The cognitive and affective state (anxiety, unhappiness, depression, adaptive disorder, etc.)

3.1   Identifying the Problem

To obtain an efficient sexual history, it is important to define the problem in as much detail as possible, also taking into account the couple's description, when it is possible. Therefore, the following circumstances should always be considered.

- Identify if the sexual problem is primary or secondary to another disorder. If the problem is purely sexual, information about masturbation experiences before the onset of the problem and finding out more about psychosocial factors or influences should be sought.
- The context in which it occurs: "general," if it occurs in all situations," and situational," if it only appears in certain circumstances. The sexual context, sexual stimuli, eroticism, and sensation of privacy and intimacy must be assessed. Examine the level of distress and performance anxiety. In general, when there is marked situational variation in a sexual problem occurrence (e.g., present in some situations but not others), psychological factors tend to predominate.
- The predominance of the etiological factors involved: organic (biological), psychological, social, or mixed factors, and whether these have great importance in the onset, severity, exacerbation, or maintenance of the sexual disorder.
- Address the area of sexuality affected: disorders of the sexual response cycle, disorders related to pain during sexual activity, disorders related to sexual identity, and disorders related to the orientation of desire and the pattern of sexual arousal (for a more detailed description and a comprehensive discussion on these issues, the reader is referred to next Chaps. 2–5).

3.2   Predisposing, Triggering, and Maintaining Factors

To detect the predisposing, triggering, and maintaining factors, a detailed sexual history including beliefs, sexual satisfaction and pleasure, and personal history of negative experiences must be recorded (Table 5).

It is essential, in the evaluation of a sexual complaint, to know if the affected subject has a partner and lives as a couple since the relationship between them is surely affected in some degree. Furthermore, if the couple's relationship was

Table 5 Actions to detect sexual problem-related factors

Evaluate sexual beliefs and cultural background in relation to sexuality issues
Ask about sexual activity and satisfaction before the first occurrence of the sexual problem
Ask about traumatic or humiliating negative sexual experiences
Evaluate the interpersonal relationship and the level of motivation and commitment of the couple
Explore and verbalize the expectations and objectives of the patient and their partner regarding what they want to achieve with therapy

previously deteriorated, it always ends up triggering a crisis, which often leads to a rupture.

It is of interest to record the detailed description of the patients' daily activities since these data can serve to identify the supporting conditions that maintain the dysfunction. In addition, it is important to include, in the sexual history, all the past attempts to solve the sexual problem. Knowing the procedures attempted to sort out the problem and the results achieved such as cognitive distraction, previous professional treatments, books, or other resources consulted may help the healthcare provider to consider the need of a sexual therapist or a sexual medicine specialist.

Finally, a key point in the initial approach is to get patients to verbalize their expectations and objectives and, when feasible, those of their partner regarding what they both want to achieve with sexual counseling.

3.3 Assess Psychosocial Problems

To complete a sexual history, it is mandatory to record psychosocial issues that may have a negative impact on the quality of life and sexual function. In this sense, the healthcare provider must ask about mood and daily fatigue and body image concerns, especially genital image, and rule out mental disorders or psychopathology (previous and current). Personality traits such as self-esteem, self-efficacy, sexual confidence, extroversion, and perfectionism, among others, modulate sexual functioning as well as interpersonal relationships; thus, personality traits and relationship-related problems need to be addressed since both have an important impact on sexual health [23]. Lifetime stressors, such as financial, work, or employment stress, cannot be neglected since evidence suggests that they have notable effects on health status and sexual function [24]. Moreover, psychosexual correlates should be investigated in patients consulting for sexual dysfunction because patients who had unwanted sexual experiences or sexual violence may require unique strategies to optimize the diagnostic and therapeutic workup of their sexual symptoms [25]. In the same way, social skills and sexual behavior are related and need to be discussed [26].

It is of importance to record the previous relationships with other persons and, in case the patient is at office with their present partner, both members feel treated equally. The attribution of responsibilities or the alignment with one of the members is always detrimental and should be avoided.

In conclusion, listen to the patient contextualize the complaint, do not rush into the diagnosis (the idea of process is essential; therefore, do not speed up), do not focus exclusively on the apparent symptom (it is important to distinguish between reason for consultation and diagnosis), do not start with prescriptions, and remember that each patient has their goals and their own story. Accompanying is the key; see, listen, communicate, and give additional adequate care for the couple.

References

1. Luo C, Xu S, Bao S, Zhang B, Zhong X, Huang Z, Li P, Liang J. Association between sexual frequency and all-cause mortality in young and middle-aged patients with hypertension: a cohort study of patient data from the National Health and nutrition examination survey 2005–2014. J Sex Med. 2023;20(8):1078–84. https://doi.org/10.1093/jsxmed/qdad079.
2. Brandis Kepler S, Hasin T, Benyamini Y, Goldbourt U, Gerber Y. Frequency of sexual activity and long-term survival after acute myocardial infarction. Am J Med. 2020;133(1):100–7. https://doi.org/10.1016/j.amjmed.2019.06.019. Epub 2019 Jul 8.
3. Chovanec M, Vasilkova L, Petrikova L, Obertova J, Palacka P, Rejlekova K, Sycova-Mila Z, Kalavska K, Svetlovska D, Mladosievicova B, Mardiak J, Mego M. Long-term sexual functioning in germ-cell tumor survivors. BMC Cancer. 2020;20(1):779. https://doi.org/10.1186/s12885-020-07301-6. PMID: 32819309; PMCID: PMC7439516.
4. World Health Organization. Defining sexual health: report of a technical consultation on sexual health, 28–31 January 2002, Geneva. Geneva: World Health Organization; 2006.
5. Van Lunsen RHW, Laan ETM. Sexual health. In: Steegers EAP, Fauser BC, Hilders CG, Jaddoe VW, Massuger LF, Schoenmakers S, van der Post JA, editors. Textbook of obstetrics and gynaecology: a life course approach Springer; 2019. p. 177–194
6. Basson R, Rees P, Wang R, Montejo AL, Incrocci L. Sexual function in chronic illness. J Sex Med. 2010;7:374–88. https://doi.org/10.1111/j.1743-6109.2009.01621.x.
7. Arring N, Barton DL, Reese JB. Clinical practice strategies to address sexual health in female cancer survivors. J Clin Oncol. 2023;41:JCO2300523. https://doi.org/10.1200/JCO.23.00523. Epub ahead of print.
8. Ryan KL, Arbuckle-Bernstein V, Smith G, Phillips J. Let's talk about sex: a survey of patients' preferences when addressing sexual health concerns in a family medicine residency program office. PRiMER. 2018;2:23. https://doi.org/10.22454/PRiMER.2018.728252. PMID: 32818195; PMCID: PMC7426112.
9. Gott M. "Opening a can of worms": GP and practice nurse barriers to talking about sexual health in primary care. Fam Pract. 2004;21:528–36. https://doi.org/10.1093/fampra/cmh509.
10. O'Connor SR, Connaghan J, Maguire R, Kotronoulas G, Flannagan C, Jain S, et al. Healthcare professional perceived barriers and facilitators to discussing sexual wellbeing with patients after diagnosis of chronic illness: a mixed-methods evidence synthesis. Patient Educ Couns. 2019;102:850–63. https://doi.org/10.1016/j.pec.2018.12.015.
11. Byrne M, Doherty S, McGee HM, Murphy AW. General practitioner views about discussing sexual issues with patients with coronary heart disease: a national survey in Ireland. BMC Fam Pract. 2010;11:40. https://doi.org/10.1186/1471-2296-11-40.
12. Canzona MR, Garcia D, Fisher CL, Raleigh M, Kalish V, Ledford CJW. Communication about sexual health with breast cancer survivors: variation among patient and provider perspectives. Patient Educ Couns. 2016;99:1814–20. https://doi.org/10.1016/j.pec.2016.06.019.
13. Benoot C, Enzlin P, Peremans L, Bilsen J. Addressing sexual issues in palliative care: a qualitative study on nurses' attitudes, roles and experiences. J Adv Nurs. 2018;74:1583–94. https://doi.org/10.1111/jan.13572.
14. Kelder I, Sneijder P, Klarenbeek A, Laan E. Communication practices in conversations about sexual health in medical healthcare settings: a systematic review. Patient Educ Couns. 2022;105(4):858–68. https://doi.org/10.1016/j.pec.2021.07.049. Epub 2021 Jul 29.
15. Coyne JC, Rohrbaugh MJ, Shoham V, Sonnega JS, Nicklas JM, Cranford JA. Prognostic importance of marital quality for survival of congestive heart failure. Am J Cardiol. 2001;88(5):526–9. https://doi.org/10.1016/s0002-9149(01)01731-3.
16. Joel S, Eastwick PW, Allison CJ, Arriaga XB, Baker ZG, Bar-Kalifa E, Bergeron S, et al. Machine learning uncovers the most robust self-report predictors of relationship quality across 43 longitudinal couples studies. Proc Natl Acad Sci U S A. 2020;117(32):19061–71. https://doi.org/10.1073/pnas.1917036117. Epub 2020 Jul 27. PMID: 32719123; PMCID: PMC7431040.

17. Barsky JL, Friedman MA, Rosen RC. Sexual dysfunction and chronic illness: the role of flexibility in coping. J Sex Marital Ther. 2006;32(3):235–53. https://doi.org/10.1080/00926230600575322.
18. Masters WH, Johnson VE, Kolodny RC. Human sexuality. Boston: Little, Brown and Company; 1982.
19. Lobitz WC, Lobitz GK. Clinical assessment in the treatment of sexual dysfunctions. In: LoPiccolo J, LoPiccolo L, editors. Handbook of sex therapy. Perspectives in sexuality. Boston: Springer; 1978. https://doi.org/10.1007/978-1-4613-3973-1_5.
20. LoPiccolo L, Heiman JR. Sexual assessment and history interview. In: LoPiccolo J, LoPiccolo L, editors. Handbook of sex therapy. Perspectives in sexuality. Boston: Springer; 1978. https://doi.org/10.1007/978-1-4613-3973-1_6.
21. Kaplan HS. The new sexual therapy. New York: Routledge (Taylor and Francis Group); 1975.
22. Hawton K. Sex therapy. Oxford: Oxford University Press; 1985.
23. Brotto L, Atallah S, Johnson-Agbakwu C, Rosenbaum T, Abdo C, Byers ES, Graham C, Nobre P, Wylie K. Psychological and interpersonal dimensions of sexual function and dysfunction. J Sex Med. 2016;13(4):538–71. https://doi.org/10.1016/j.jsxm.2016.01.019. Epub 2016 Mar 25.
24. Leserman J, Li Z, Hu YJ, Drossman DA. How multiple types of stressors impact on health. Psychosom Med. 1998;60(2):175–81. https://doi.org/10.1097/00006842-199803000-00012.
25. Maseroli E, Scavello I, Campone B, Di Stasi V, Cipriani S, Felciai F, Camartini V, Magini A, Castellini G, Ricca V, Maggi M, Vignozzi L. Psychosexual correlates of unwanted sexual experiences in women Consulting for Female Sexual Dysfunction according to their timing across the life span. J Sex Med. 2018;15(12):1739–51. https://doi.org/10.1016/j.jsxm.2018.10.004. Epub 2018 Nov 13.
26. Nangle DW, Hansen DJ. Relations between social skills and high-risk sexual interactions among adolescents. Current issues and future directions. Behav Modif. 1993;17(2):113–35. https://doi.org/10.1177/01454455930172002.

Gender and Orientation

Johannes Bitzer

1 Introduction

Human sexuality includes many different forms of behavior and expression. It is increasingly acknowledged that recognition of the diversity of sexual behavior and expression contributes to people's overall sense of well-being and health [1].

Understanding the related risks and vulnerabilities associated with the way sexual behavior and expression are perceived in society is also key to understanding barriers to health and how to address these.

Ill health related to sexuality represents a significant disease burden throughout the world. Sexual and gender minorities such as lesbian, gay, bisexual, transgender, and intersex people face both similar and different challenges in accessing health care services and ensuring that their health needs are met but, as a community, are more likely to experience human rights violations including violence, torture, criminalization, forced sterilization (often in the case of intersex persons), discrimination, and stigma because they are perceived to fall outside of socially constructed sex and gender norms [2].

2 Definitions

The definitions correspond to the broad variety of sexual expression and subjective sexual experiences. The basis for the various descriptions which overlap is the concept of sexuality and sexual health as summarized by the WHO [3].

J. Bitzer (✉)
University Hospital Basel, Basel, Switzerland
e-mail: Johannes.Bitzer@usb.ch

C. Castelo-Branco, S. Anglès Acedo (eds.), *Medical Disorders and Sexual Health*, Trends in Andrology and Sexual Medicine,
https://doi.org/10.1007/978-3-031-55080-5_2

- Sexuality is a central aspect of being human throughout life that encompasses sex, gender identities and roles, sexual orientation, eroticism, pleasure, intimacy, and reproduction. Sexuality is influenced by the intersection of biological, psychological, social, economic, political, cultural, legal, historical, religious, and spiritual factors.
- Sexual health is a state of physical, emotional, mental, and social well-being in relation to sexuality; it is not merely the absence of disease, dysfunction, or infirmity. Sexual health requires a positive and respectful approach to the possibility of having pleasurable and safe sexual experiences, free of coercion, discrimination, and violence. For sexual health to be attained and maintained, the sexual rights of all persons, at all ages and in all contexts, must be respected, protected, and fulfilled [3].

Human sexuality and the human sexual response have been viewed for a very long time basically as the sexual encounter between a man and a woman for the purpose of reproduction and experiencing sexual pleasure.

This concept of the heterosexual interaction between a biological man who feels being a male individual (cis man) and a biological woman who feels being a female (cis woman) is the predominant model lived by a large majority.

Human sexuality is however much broader and includes a large variety of sexual expression and sexual life.

People who did not follow the "classical model" in their sexual and their gender attributed behavior and did not correspond to the culturally assigned roles were either criminalized or pathologized, discriminated, and stigmatized.

In recent years, this sexual minority has become a name

LGBTQ+ is an acronym for "lesbian, gay, bisexual, transgender, and queer" with a "+" sign to recognize the limitless sexual orientations and gender identities used by members of this community.

To understand these minorities, it is important to learn about the different dimensions of sexual expression and know about the specific needs in sexual and reproductive health care [4–6].

3 Definitions

3.1 Biological Sex

3.1.1 Physical Dimension

This is covered by the term sex and describes the continuum between male and female bodies at birth including intersex individuals, which have biological features of both sexes based on the fact that the biological differentiation leading to male and female bodies is a process which is determined by different stages from chromosomes to gonads and to external genitalia and brain differentiation.

3.2 Sexual Orientation: Attraction

This dimension describes the sexual attraction felt by the individual. It is again along a continuum between being attracted by an individual of the same sex and/or gender identity as themselves (homosexual) and being attracted by an individual of the other sex and/or gender identity (heterosexual) or being attracted by both (bisexual) [4].

Lesbian women and gay men were once commonly grouped as homosexual, but this term is no longer used as it has a history in the wrongful pathologization of people with nonheterosexual orientations as a mental health disorder.

In a broader approach, the definition of sexual orientation is described as an inherent or immutable enduring emotional, romantic, or sexual attraction to other people. It is important to note that an individual's sexual orientation is independent of their gender identity.

3.3 Gender Identity

One's innermost concept of self as male, female, a blend of both, or neither—how individuals perceive themselves and what they call themselves. One's gender identity can be the same or different from their sex assigned at birth.

3.4 Gender Expression

External appearance of one's gender identity, usually expressed through behavior, clothing, body characteristics, or voice, and which may or may not conform to socially defined behaviors and characteristics typically associated with being either masculine or feminine.

3.5 Transgender

An umbrella term for people whose gender identity and/or expression is different from cultural expectations based on the sex they were assigned at birth. Being transgender does not imply any specific sexual orientation. Therefore, transgender people may identify as straight, gay, lesbian, bisexual, etc.

3.6 Gender Transition

The process by which some people strive to more closely align their internal knowledge of gender with its outward appearance. Some people practice a social transition, whereby they might begin dressing, using names and pronouns, and/or be socially recognized as another gender.

Others undergo physical transitions in which they modify their bodies through medical interventions.

3.7   Gender Dysphoria, Gender Incongruence

Clinically significant distress caused when a person's assigned birth gender is not the same as the one with which they identify.

3.8   Queer

A term people often use to express a spectrum of identities and orientations that are counter to the mainstream. Queer is often used as a catch-all to include many people, including those who do not identify as exclusively straight and/or folks who have non-binary or gender-expansive identities. This term was previously used as a slur, but has been reclaimed by many parts of the LGBTQ+ movement.

4   Determinants

The determinants of sexual orientation and identity are still debated.

There is evidence for genetic, biological, developmental, and environmental influences, which may interact with each other to form the individual orientation profile.

Taking into account that these manifestations are part of the normal variety of human sexual expressions, the questions about determinants are of lower importance compared to the gaps in adequate sexual and reproductive health care of this community [7].

5   Health Risks for Sexual Minorities

Many LGBTQIA+ individuals cannot easily and openly live the sexual life they would like to live [8–13].

The main threats to their sexual health and sexual well-being are the fear of social discrimination, loss of economic stability and position in the society, and violence.

These threats frequently contribute to an increase in risk behavior exposing the individual not only to STIs but also to sexual abuse and violence in a vicious circle.

An important part of care, which should be always included in the service, is the care for victims of sexual violence. The principles of intervention are the same as for non LGBTQIA+ individuals.

Gay, bisexual, and other men who have sex with men have the same health risks like other men.

Cardiovascular diseases and cancers are the leading causes of death.

They are additionally affected by the following factors:

- Higher rates of HIV and other sexually transmitted diseases (STDs)
  - Prevalence of HIV among sexual partners of gay, bisexual, and other men who have sex with men is 40 times higher, compared to that of sexual partners of heterosexual men
  - Receptive anal sex is 18 times more risky for HIV acquisition than receptive vaginal sex
  - Gay, bisexual, and other men who have sex with men on average have a greater number of lifetime sexual partners
  - Homophobia
  - Stigma (negative and usually unfair beliefs)
  - Discrimination (unfairly treating a person or a group of people differently)
  - Lack of access to culturally and orientation-appropriate medical and support services
  - Heightened concerns about confidentiality
  - Fear of losing one's job
  - Fear of talking about individual's sexual practices or orientation
- Tobacco and drug use
- Depression

Lesbian, bisexual, and other women who have sex with men and women have the same health risks like other women. They are additionally affected by:

- Homophobia
- Stigma (negative and usually unfair beliefs)
- Discrimination (unfairly treating a person or a group of people differently)
- Lack of access to culturally and orientation-appropriate medical and support services
- Heightened concerns about confidentiality
- Fear of losing one's job
- Fear of talking about individual's sexual practices or orientation

Transgender persons have the same health risks as non-transgender persons before the transition. They are additionally affected during and after transition by similar threats like the persons with a minority orientation like:

- Transphobia
- Stigma (negative and usually unfair beliefs)
- Discrimination (unfairly treating a person or a group of people differently)
- Lack of access to culturally and orientation-appropriate medical and support services
- Fear of losing one's job
- General violence
- Sexual violence
- Depression and suicide

During and after the transition, they have increased health risks related to the individual social, psychological, and medical interventions (see medical care below).

6 Special Needs of the LGBTQIA+ Community

Based on the understanding of the specific biological and psychosocial factors contributing to health in general and sexual health in particular, there is a need for specialized health care for this community [10, 11, 13, 14].

6.1 General Principles

The two main groups of minorities, namely, those persons with a nonexclusively heterosexual orientation and those persons belonging to the transgender community, share specific needs concerning the sexual health care.

Care should be provided in an environment in which the patients can feel safe and accepted with their sexual and gender expressions.

The HCP should be trained in communicating in a nonjudgmental, patient-centered way, which includes assessment of physical and psychosocial symptoms and concerns.

The basic approach is similar to the one practiced in sexual health care and is based on the biopsychosocial model including medical, psychosocial, and sexual history taking and medical examinations if needed.

These persons need services providing easy access to STI detection and treatment and sexual advice and counseling with respect to sexual dysfunctions (desire, arousal, orgasm, pain).

Due to the high prevalence of discrimination and victimization of persons belonging to sexual minorities, a central element is the availability of and access to professional psychological and mental health care.

This includes provision and access to care for victims of sexual violence.

6.2 Health Care for Persons with Various Forms of Nonexclusively Heterosexual Orientation

There are several instruments **to assess sexual orientation** to help the individual patient and the health care provider to better understand the needs and sexuality-related behaviors.

Starting from Kinsey's continuous scale, different diagnostic assessment questionnaires were developed [15, 16].

Coleman developed a model of sexual orientation for clinical assessment that included nine dimensions: current relationship status; self-identification identity; ideal self-identification identity; global acceptance of their current sexual orientation identity; physical identity; gender identity; sex-role identity and sexual orientation identity, as measured by behavior, fantasies, and emotional attachments; and, finally, the individual's past and present perception of their sexual identity compared to their idealized future [17].

The Klein Sexual Orientation Grid [18] is based on the response to the following questions:

Sexual attraction: To whom are you sexually attracted?

Sexual behavior: With whom have you had sex?

Sexual fantasies: About whom are your sexual fantasies?

Emotional preference: To whom do you feel more drawn or close to emotionally?

Social preference: With which gender do you socialize?

Lifestyle preference: In which community do you like to spend your time? In which do you feel most comfortable?

Self-identification: How do you label or identify yourself?

Specialized care by trained professionals is needed to help persons with their coming out and the integration of their sexual identity in their social environment including partners, family, work, etc.

HCPs should also be trained in principles and practice of behavioral medicine for those persons who show repetitive high-risk behavior (exposure to STI infections, violent encounters, etc.)

6.3 Health Care for Persons with Various Forms of Gender Incongruence

These persons need services and HCPs able to assess the individual expression of gender incongruence [14, 19–22].

This needs specific communication skills. HCPs should use a language which is nonjudgmental, based on respect and safety and adapted to the specific culture. It is important to discuss with transgender and gender-diverse people what language of terminology they prefer.

Assessing gender incongruence in children is based on questions regarding feelings and behaviors [19–21]:

- In boys (assigned gender), a strong preference for cross-dressing or simulating female attire, or in girls (assigned gender), a strong preference for wearing only typical masculine clothing and a strong resistance to the wearing of typical feminine clothing
- A strong preference for cross-gender roles in make-believe play or fantasy play
- A strong preference for the toys, games, or activities stereotypically used or engaged in by the other gender
- A strong preference for playmates of the other gender
- In boys (assigned gender), a strong rejection of typically masculine toys, games, and activities and a strong avoidance of rough-and-tumble play, or in girls

(assigned gender), a strong rejection of typically feminine toys, games, and activities
- A strong dislike of one's sexual anatomy
- A strong desire for the primary and/or secondary sex characteristics that match one's experienced gender

The condition is associated with clinically significant distress or impairment in social, school, or other important areas of functioning.

Assessing gender dysphoria and gender incongruence in adolescents and adults [19–21]

The definition refers to a marked incongruence between one's experienced/expressed gender and assigned gender, of at least 6 months' duration, as manifested by at least two of the following:

A marked incongruence between one's experienced/expressed gender and primary and/or secondary sex characteristics (or in young adolescents, the anticipated secondary sex characteristics)

A strong desire to be rid of one's primary and/or secondary sex characteristics because of a marked incongruence with one's experienced/expressed gender (or in young adolescents, a desire to prevent the development of the anticipated secondary sex characteristics)

A strong desire for the primary and/or secondary sex characteristics of the other gender

A strong desire to be of the other gender (or some alternative gender different from one's assigned gender)

A strong desire to be treated as the other gender (or some alternative gender different from one's assigned gender)

A strong conviction that one has the typical feelings and reactions of the other gender (or some alternative gender different from one's assigned gender)

The condition is associated with clinically significant distress or impairment in social, occupational, or other important areas of functioning.

7 The Therapeutic Approach [14]

After assessment, the persons need an individualized therapy which is based on the biopsychosocial model including interventions to modify the body and its functions like surgery and hormones on the one hand and mental health care to prepare and help the transsexual persons to cope with the desired changes.

This needs in general a multidisciplinary team including surgeons, endocrinologists, psychologists, and sexual therapists.

The general goal of combined psychotherapy, endocrine therapy, and surgical therapy (sometimes collectively referred to as "triadic" therapy) for persons with gender dysphoria is lasting personal comfort with the gendered self in order to maximize overall psychological well-being and self-fulfillment.

However, many adults with gender dysphoria find comfortable, effective ways of living that do not involve all the components of the triadic treatment sequence.

The duration and content of the treatment will depend upon the individual's needs. It will continue until the treatment goal of lasting personal comfort with the gendered self is achieved; agreement with the individual of a realistic and achievable goal of lasting personal comfort, rather than a much-desired but unachievable transformation into the desired gender, is a prerequisite.

Typically, the individual will spend at least two and sometimes several years in treatment before achieving their goal.

The three elements of treatment supported by psychotherapy, hormones, and surgery are as follows:

8 Experience in the Desired Gender Role

This refers to the social transition which includes formal steps and changes in the outer appearance like clothing and small change.

Before an individual can be referred for genital reassignment surgery, the WPATH SoC version sixth edition [22] recommends that they complete a period of no less than 12 months living exclusively in their desired gender role while under the supervision of a gender specialist health professional.

During this period, they are additionally advised to:

- Maintain full- or part-time employment, function as a student, function in community-based volunteer activity, or undertake some combination of these activities
- Acquire a legally recognized gender identity-appropriate first name
- Provide documentation that persons other than the therapist know that the patient functions in the desired gender role

These recommendations have been modified by the WHAT SoC version 9. The health care professional should discuss with the transgender person about the best way and the duration of this social transition.

9 The Achievement of an Endocrine Milieu Consistent with the Desired Gender (Hormone Therapy)

The endocrine treatment for trans women is based on the combination of estrogen and antiandrogen, and for trans men, it is the testosterone treatment [14, 23].

Potential side effects in trans women treated with estrogens include increased risk of venous thromboembolism, development of benign pituitary prolactinomas, temporary or permanent infertility, weight gain, reduction in size of the genitalia, emotional lability, liver disease, gallstone formation, somnolence, hypertension, and diabetes mellitus type 2.

Treatment might also increase cardiovascular risk; cigarette smoking, obesity, advanced age, heart disease, hypertension, thrombophilia, some cancers, and some endocrine abnormalities may increase side effects and risks of treatment.

Trans women treated with estrogens may become permanently infertile; all trans women offered cross-gender hormone therapies should be told about the potential impact on their fertility and, if requested, should be given information about gamete storage.

In trans women treated with estrogens, feminization is largely achieved by devirilization through the reduction of total testosterone, rather than by a direct effect of estrogens. Exogenous estrogens suppress the hypothalamic–pituitary–gonadal axis, resulting in reductions in LH and testosterone production. The endocrine goal is to provide a sex steroid milieu appropriate for a premenopausal woman.

The following are permanent changes: a deepening of the voice, clitoral enlargement, mild breast atrophy, increased facial and body hair, and male pattern baldness. Reversible changes include increased upper body strength; weight gain; increased social interest, sexual interest, and arousability; and decreased hip fat. Heredity limits the tissue response to hormones, and this cannot be overcome by increasing dosage. The degree of attainment varies from patient to patient. Menstrual bleeding usually ceases within 3 months of commencing testosterone therapy; this is also a reversible change.

10 Surgery and Other Physical Treatments to Change the Genitalia and Other Sex Characteristics

These interventions include breast surgery for trans men and trans women and genital reassignment surgery [14, 24, 25].

In trans women, genital reassignment surgery usually consists of penectomy and bilateral orchidectomy, with vulvo-vaginoplasty and construction of a sensate clitoris using penile and scrotal tissue as a single-stage procedure;

Those who undergo vaginoplasty will need to regularly use vaginal dilators for a prolonged period after surgery in order to maintain their neo-vagina. Orchidectomy only is a treatment option.

In trans men, there are several options like phalloplasty and penile prosthesis placed within their neo-phallus. Some trans men may elect to undergo less complex and demanding procedures, such as metoidioplasty; this involves the release of clitoral tissue and its forward repositioning to more closely approximate position of a penis.

11 Follow-Up Care

11.1 Specialized Medical Care [14, 26]

11.1.1 Safety in Follow-Up of Hormone Therapy
This includes possible effects of high-dose therapy with androgens or estrogens on polycythemia, liver failure, thrombosis, etc.; see above.

Cancer screening for present native organs (breast, prostate, uterus).

11.1.2 Follow-Up After Surgical Interventions

Follow-up after breast surgery and gender-affirming surgery of genitalia like removal of native gonads and uterus with the risk of iatrogenic nerve damage and loss of sensation and motor control in the pelvic floor and genital area, which can affect sexual functioning.

Trans women need to dilate their neo-vagina, and the shortening of the urethra and pelvic floor muscle tension may cause changes in their micturition patterns.

Surgical modification of urethra (neo-penis, metoidioplasty) can lead to urethral strictures and urethral fistulas.

Pelvic floor physiotherapy is an important part of follow-up care.

11.1.3 Endocrine Changes and Fertility

Trans and non-binary people who are taking gender-affirming hormone therapy may think that they no longer need birth control. **But hormone therapy alone will not protect trans and non-binary people from pregnancy**.

Periods stop for most trans men and non-binary people who were assigned female at birth (AFAB) after taking testosterone for a few months, but ovulation may still occur—even if they have never had a period.

For trans women and non-binary people who were assigned male at birth (AMAB) and are taking estrogen, the development of sperm in the testicles can still occur.

Gender-affirming hormone therapy does generally decrease fertility, but it cannot be relied upon as a form of contraception.

Regardless of gender identity, if two people are having unprotected penis-in-vagina sex, pregnancy can occur. Unplanned pregnancies do happen. Bisexual and lesbian-identified adolescents report significantly higher unintended pregnancy rates than do their heterosexual peers.

11.1.4 Contraception

For trans women and non-binary people who were assigned male at birth (AMAB) and are taking estrogen, the development of sperm in the testicles can still occur.

Internal and external condom:

- Effective (continuous use)
- Advantage: protection of STI including HIV

Permanent surgical options are available for patients who do not want to get pregnant at all:

- Orchidectomy
- Vasectomy

Transgender men have a small but nonetheless a persisting reproductive potential if they have intact uterus and ovaries until menopause or surgical sterilization.

Testosterone may not completely suppress ovarian function leading to irregular bleeding.

It is important to note that there is still a risk of pregnancy despite a lack of menstruation. Use of a contraceptive is still necessary even with testosterone therapy.

11.1.5 Combination Hormonal Contraceptives
Estrogen may or may not interfere with testosterone therapy:

- No medical contraindications
- Disadvantage: unwanted estrogen-related side effects (mental, female physical traits)

11.1.6 Progestin-Only Contraceptives
Progestin-only methods do not interfere with testosterone use:

- Advantages:
  - Inducing amenorrhea in trans men who still have bleeding under testosterone therapy
  - Additional masculinizing effect (hair growth)
  - Progestin-only injectable and long-acting reversible contraceptive devices (implant and IUDs) facilitating compliance and having a high rate of amenorrhea (Depot DMPA has the highest rate)

Copper IUD:

- Advantage:
  - Noninterference with hormonal treatment
  - Disadvantages:
  - Hypermenorrhea
  - First choice for women who are already amenorrheic

Condom:

- External and internal:
  - Less effective but essential for protection of STI

Permanent contraception:

- Permanent surgical options are available for patients who do not want to get pregnant at all.

12   Mental Health Care [8, 12]

Psychosocial health care should integrate the following elements and steps:

- Assess the client subjective experience and elucidate the effect of sexual stigma on psychological functioning.

- Apply an affirmative practice: assist in understanding and accepting the individual sexual orientation as a natural part of themselves, and do not aim for changes in the sexual orientation.
- Develop or strengthen strategies for coping and individual/group resources.
- Identify behaviors of self-stigmatization in attitudes, feelings, and beliefs and its impact on symptoms of distress.
  Assist in confronting and rejecting the negative conception.
  Cognitively restructure false self-attributions and self-blame:
- Foster self-acceptance and positively balance the different components of identity.
- Deal with the aftermath of the victimization.

13   Sexual Well-Being

As described above, the factors contributing to sexual well-being or sexual dysfunctions of transgender persons are frequently a combination of medical transition procedures and psychological and interpersonal distress.

The approach is based on the biopsychosocial model, which for these persons has the additional focus on the consequences of the transition therapy (see above).

14   Summary

The members of the LGBTQI* community represent the great variety of human sexual expressions. As a minority, they are still in many countries not integrated into health care and not included as equal to others in the society. They do however have the same rights including the right to have access to health services, which respond to their specific sexual and reproductive health needs:

Acceptance, respect, and understanding by health care professionals

Psychological support in overcoming social discrimination and help in building up their sexual identity

Psychosocial interventions for victims of sexual and general violence

Prevention, detection, and treatment of STIs

Specialized and targeted care (medical, endocrine, surgical, mental health interventions) in the various fields of reproductive and sexual health including contraception and sexual well-being

References

1. World Health Organization. Sexual health, human rights and law. Geneva: World Health Organization; 2015.
2. Winter S, Diamond M, Green J, et al. Transgender people: health at the margins of society. Lancet. 2016;388:390–400. https://doi.org/10.1016/S0140-6736(16)00683-8.
3. World Health Organization. Defining sexual health: report of a technical consultation on sexual health. Geneva: World Health Organization; 2006. p. 28–31.

4. UNAIDS. UNAIDS terminology guidelines. UNAIDS, 2015. http://www.unaids.org/sites/default/files/media_asset/2015_terminology_guidelines_en.pdf. Accessed 11 May 2016.

5. https://www.hrc.org/resources/sexual-orientation-and-gender-identity-terminology-and-definitions.

6. UCSF Transgender Care Navigation Program. "Terminology and definitions." UCSF Transgender Care Navigation Program. 2016. https://transcare.ucsf.edu/guidelines/terminology. Accessed 11 Sept 2019.

7. Graham R, Berkowitz B, Blum R, Bockting W, Bradford J, de Vries B, Makadon H. The health of lesbian, gay, bisexual, and transgender people: building a foundation for better understanding, vol. 10. Washington, DC: Institute of Medicine; 2011. p. 13128.

8. United Nations. Ending violence and discrimination against lesbian, gay, bisexual, transgender and intersex people, 2015. http://www.ohchr.org/Documents/Issues/Discrimination/Joint_LGBTI_Statement_ENG.PDF.

9. Blondeel K, et al. Evidence and knowledge gaps on the disease burden in sexual and gender minorities: a review of systematic reviews. Int J Equity Health. 2016;15:1. https://doi.org/10.1186/s12939-016-0304-1.

10. Campbell S. Sexual health needs and the LGBT community. Nurs Stand. 2013;32:35–8.

11. PAHO and WHO. Addressing the causes of disparities in health service access and utilization for lesbian, gay, bisexual and trans (LGBT) persons. World Health Organization; 2013.

12. Herek GM, Garnets LD. Sexual orientation and mental health. Annu Rev Clin Psychol. 2007;3:353–75.

13. Hashemi L, Weinreb J, Weimer AK, Weiss RL. Transgender care in the primary care setting: a review of guidelines and literature. Fed Pract. 2018;35(7):30.

14. Coleman E, Radix AE, Bouman WP, Brown GR, de Vries ALC, Deutsch MB, Ettner R, Fraser L, Goodman M, Green J, Hancock AB, Johnson TW, Karasic DH, Knudson GA, Leibowitz SF, Meyer-Bahlburg HFL, Monstrey SJ, Motmans J, Nahata L, Arcelus J, J. Standards of care for the health of transgender and gender diverse people, version 8. Int J Transgender Health. 2022;23(S1):S1–S260. https://doi.org/10.1080/26895269.2022.2100644.

15. Kinsey AC, Pomeroy WB, Martin CE. Sexual behavior in the human male. Philadelphia: Saunders WB & Co; 1948.

16. Sell RL. Defining and measuring sexual orientation: a review. Arch Sex Behav. 1997;26(6):643–58.

17. Coleman E. Assessment of sexual orientation. J Homosex. 1987;14(1–2):9.

18. Klein F. The bisexual option. 2nd ed. London: Routledge; 1993.

19. Jakob R. ICD update platform: gender identity alignment with ICD-11.

20. American Psychiatric Association. Diagnostic and statistical manual of mental disorders. 5th ed. Washington, DC: American Psychiatric Association; 2022.

21. World Health Organization. Gender, equity and human rights. World Health Organization; 2016.

22. The World Professional Association for Transgender Health's. Standards of care for the health of transsexual, transgender, and gender nonconforming people. 6th ed; 2011.

23. Hembree W, Cohen-Kettenis P, Delemarre-van de Waal H, et al. Endocrine treatment of transsexual persons: an Endocrine Society clinical practice guideline. J Clin Endocrinol Metab. 2009;94:3132–54.

24. Gooren LJ. Clinical practice. Care of transsexual persons. N Engl J Med. 2011;364(13):1251–7.

25. Service specification: Gender Identity Services for Adults (Surgical Interventions). https://www.england.nhs.uk/publication/service-specification-gender-identity-services-for-adults-surgical-interventions/.

26. Bockting WO, Goldberg JM. Guidelines for transgender care (special issue). Int J Transgenderism. 2006;9:3–4.

Sexuality Across Lifespan: Focus on Women's Vulnerabilities

Alessandra Graziottin and Angela Cuccarollo

1 Sexuality Across Lifespan I: Women's Vulnerabilities from Intrauterine Life to Adolescence

1.1 Introduction

Sexuality is a very dynamic dimension in human life. It is the expression of biological, psychodynamic, and context-dependent factors that act on the female (and male) body across lifespan, from conception to death.

Human sexuality is a multisystemic and multifactorial phenomenon. It comprises three main dimensions: sexual identity (Box 1), sexual function (Box 2), and couple relationship (Box 3). These dimensions are present in both sexes. Each recognizes biological, psychodynamic, relational, and context-related (affective, cultural, professional, and social) components.

A. Graziottin (✉)
Center of Gynecology and Medical Sexology, H. San Raffaele Resnati, Milan, Italy

Department of Obstetrics and Gynecology, University of Verona, Verona, Italy

Department of Endocrinology and Metabolic Diseases, Federico II University, Naples, Italy
e-mail: a.graziottin@studiograziottin.it

A. Cuccarollo
School of Specialization in Obstetrics and Gynecology, University of Verona, Verona, Italy

Ob-Gyn Department, Alto Vicentino Hospital, Santorso, Vicenza, Italy

From a biological point of view, sexuality depends on the harmonious coordination of the nervous, vascular, hormonal, metabolic, immunitary, and muscular systems [1]. In the shadow of clinical awareness, the intestinal and vulvovaginal microbiota are powerful modulators of psycho-immuno-neuro-endocrine health, which underlies general health and sexuality.

Box 1 Sexual Identity
Sexual identity encompasses four major dimensions:

- Biological sex
- Gender identity
- Role identity
- Sexual orientation

The reader is referred to the previous chapter, titled ***Gender and Orientation***, for a comprehensive discussion on sexual identity. In this chapter, potential disruptors of sexual identity from the fetal life to adolescence are briefly discussed.

Box 2 Sexual Function
Human **sexual function** can be divided into four main, dynamically interconnected, dimensions: sexual desire, sexual arousal (mental, systemic, and genital), orgasm, and resolution. The neuronal and vascular mechanisms underlying these phenomena appear to be similar between males and females; however, the sexual response is different between genders. These differences can partially be attributed to the anatomical dimorphism of the genitalia and the nervous system, as well as to different hormonal profiles [2]. Cultural and context-related factors further contribute to gender differences.

Sexual desire includes thoughts, fantasies, sexual day dreams, and motivation to initiate sexual activity in response to relevant internal or external stimuli. It is influenced by the attitude, mood, state of health, opportunities, and availability of a partner.

Sexual arousal is the set of physiological responses (cognitive-emotional and physical) that occur before and during sexual activity. It anticipates orgasm, when attainable. Sexual arousal includes:

- Mental arousal, which can be triggered by desire and erotic dreams, in rapid eye movement (REM) sleep, or with open eyes ("sexual day dreams").
- Systemic physical arousal: general, under the command of the parasympathetic system, characterized by superficial cutaneous vasodilatation ("a hot woman") with sexual flush; hardening of the nipples; increased salivation, heart rate, and blood pressure; breathing becoming deeper and diaphragmatic; and increased muscle tension, sweating, and pheromone production [2].

- Genital physical arousal, with vaginal lubrication and congestion/swelling/ turgor of the corpora cavernosa of the clitoral–urethral–vaginal complex [3]. The latter includes the equivalent of the corpus spongiosum of the urethra, which surrounds the outer third of the female urethra. Adequate congestion of the corpus spongiosum of the urethra is essential: when well congested, it increases vaginal arousal (corresponding to the former "G-spot"), while it behaves like an "airbag" which protects the urethra from the potential mechanical trauma of penetration, thus preventing post-coital cystitis. In men, genital arousal translates into erection, because the rigid tunica albuginea that surrounds the corpora cavernosa limits the distension of the penile cavernosal tissues, thus increasing the blood pressure within these specialized vessels. In women, the absence of albuginea causes the congestion of the cavernous bodies and genital tissues to result in greater vulvar and vaginal softness and better vaginal "habitability." Genital arousal depends on the anatomical and functional integrity of neural, endocrine, and vascular mechanisms which, following the release of vasodilatory neurotransmitters, primarily nitric oxide (NO) and vasoactive intestinal peptide (VIP), in response to the activation of the parasympathetic nervous system, lead to an increase in blood flow to the external genitalia and the vagina.

The **orgasmic response** begins when the excitation with genital congestion reaches its peak, thanks to the growth of mental, somatic, and genital sensations and emotions of pleasure, with parallel and rapid increase in heart rate, blood pressure, rhythm, and depth of the breath. After a few suspended moments of intense and exquisite pleasure, the involuntary contractions of the levator ani muscle and of the superficial trigone of the perineum begin, accompanied by a further increase in heart rate and a sensation of pleasant euphoria [2]. In clinical practice, many women report reaching orgasm with clitoral stimulation, others with penetration or both, and still others with nipple stimulation or anal penetration or with just erotic wording.

Orgasm is a sensory-motor reflex, with a short arc at the medullary level, on which descending corticomedullary fibers can modulate the time and intensity of the orgasmic reflex, accelerating or delaying it. Genital stimulation reaches the spinal cord via the pudendal (clitoris, vulvar, and anal regions), pelvic, and hypogastric (vagina and uterus) nerves and is transmitted via the spinothalamic and spinoreticular pathways to the CNS. Recent MR imaging studies have shown that the brain areas activated during orgasm are sensory, motor, reward, frontal cortex, and brainstem areas [4].

In men, contraction of the smooth muscles of the vas deferens, seminal vesicles, prostate, and urethra results in ejaculation. In women, the emission of liquid during orgasm can have different causes. If limited to a few drops, it can be an expression of the production of liquid by embryonic residues of the prostate. When examined, this fluid has the characteristics of prostatic fluid, including the presence of prostate-specific antigen (PSA). When the liquid is more abundant, it is urine. This orgasmic leakage is more frequent in women who suffer from detrusor muscle instability, urgency, or frank urge incontinence.

Orgasm is accompanied by an increase in the secretion of oxytocin, a neurohormone with multiple functions. Its increase modulates both the reward system and the level of emotional attachment, as it "writes" in the brain the face and name of the person who is making us happy at that moment [5].

The **resolution** indicates the return to the baseline situation in nervous (cerebral and peripheral), vascular, endocrine, pressure, muscular, respiratory, and genital congestion terms. From an emotional and sexual point of view, erotic satisfaction is the first factor in relaunching desire and excitement.

The physiological development of the sexual function requires good physical and psycho-emotional health, so that the mind and the body can both allow a high biological response and concentrate on fully savoring the range of emotions and multisensory pleasure that a desired intercourse can give to both partners.

The activation of the parasympathetic system, the "commander of peace times," guarantees the harmonious involvement of the endocrine, cardiovascular, respiratory, muscular, nervous, and genital tissue components, up to experiencing "memorable" excitements and orgasms when an intense sexual drive and an adequate and well-tuned partner reach extraordinary heights of pleasure.

Conversely, the activation of the sympathetic system, the "wartime commander," due to inhibitions and fears, acute or chronic stress, genital and sexual pain, chronic lack of sleep, performance anxiety, and aggressive or violent contexts, can alter all phases of sexual function with different destructiveness.

For the classification of female sexual dysfunctions (FSDs), the reader is referred to the following chapter, titled *Sexuality Across Lifespan II: FSD Classification and Women's Vulnerabilities in the Reproductive Age*.

Box 3 Couple Relationship

Passionate desire and rapid excitement, excellent male and female genital arousal/congestion, refined capacity for erotic expression, intuition of the partner's needs and desires, skin feelings, sharing of loving and emotional language, and intense chemical attraction (primarily from pheromones) contribute to the achievement of a profound erotic, sensual, and sexual intimacy with a gift of deep satisfaction by and for both members of the couple, defined as *eupareunia*. This description applies to any type of couple relationship.

The magic state of intense erotic attraction lasts, on average, from a few months to 2 years. It can then evolve toward a more stable sexual and emotional relationship, with a good erotic understanding and a couple planning that can last for life. Or it can end with a variably smooth or painful breakup of the couple, if the search for the ignited passion of the nascent state of erotic desire is considered essential to feel alive, from one or both partners.

Male sexual dysfunctions, primarily erectile dysfunction, can be one of the predisposing, precipitating, and/or maintenance factors for female sexual dysfunctions [6, 7]. Conversely, female sexual dysfunctions can lead to sexual dysfunctions in the partner. In these cases, the carrier of the symptom (symptom carrier) and the inducer of the symptom (symptom inducer/co-inducer) deserve a careful and balanced evaluation [7]. For more insights into these aspects, please refer to the chapter *Sexuality Across Lifespan IV: Focus on Men Vulnerabilities*.

In summary, biological, psychosexual, relational, and context-related factors can negatively affect the couple's erotic intimacy, with a disruptive effect.

The prevalence of sexual dysfunctions is extremely high in women. In the United States, the prevalence of sexual dysfunctions ranges from 10 to 52% for men and from 25 to 63% for women, depending on the disorder considered [8].

In a landmark study by Laumann et al. the overall prevalence of sexual dysfunction in women aged between 18 and 59 was 43%. Out of these, 22% reported low sexual desire, 14% difficulty reaching orgasm, and 7% pain during intercourse [9].

A 2007 European study, carried out by Graziottin on 2467 women aged between 20 and 70, found a prevalence of 29% for sexual desire disorders, 22% for arousal disorders, 19% for of orgasm, and 14% for sexual pain disorders [10].

Female sexual dysfunctions (FSDs) are distributed in a continuum from dissatisfaction (with integrity of the physiological response, but emotional-affective frustration) to dysfunction (with or without pathological modifications) up to pathology rooted in the biological domain first [1]. FSDs can cause varying degrees of personal and interpersonal distress. Furthermore, female sexual dysfunctions can be interdependent, leading to FSD comorbidity [7].

Sociocultural factors can influence both the personal perception and the modality of verbal expression that women (but also men) have of their sexual problems [7].

General practitioners, pediatricians, and gynecologists play a leading role in the prevention and care of women's health throughout their lives, also in terms of sexuality, on the biological and clinical front first. Healthcare professionals should encourage their patients to openly discuss problems concerning sexuality, thus being able to:

- Establish whether the patient's sexual problem is of organic, psychological, or mixed nature.

- Provide scientifically rigorous answers, in simple and easily understandable language for women.
- Base the doctor-patient relationship on mutual respect and esteem, essential for a solid therapeutic alliance, a prerequisite for an appropriate diagnosis and effective treatment.
- Propose a multimodal therapeutic strategy, since the factors involved can be multiple (which often makes it appropriate to involve other professional figures).

A competent analysis of sexual problems must begin with a detailed sexual history (Box 4). For a more comprehensive discussion on how to talk about sexuality during a medical consultation, the reader should refer to Chap. 1 (***How to Talk on Sexuality in a Medical Consultation***).

Box 4 Sexual History
The sexual history is essential in the clinical evaluation. It includes:

(a) The general anamnesis, which the gynecologist should have already in the medical record, integrated with a few questions s about the woman's sexuality and sexual complaints, if any.
(b) An accurate objective examination, in particular of the vulva, pelvic floor, and internal genital organs, which cannot be surrogated with instrumental examinations.
(c) The diagnosis of comorbidity between different sexual disorders.
(d) The diagnosis of comorbidity between sexual dysfunctions and other gynecological and/or systemic pathologies.

In the clinical examination, the woman's posture is a neglected, yet very important factor, as it modulates the diaphragmatic breathing. This is essential to maintain a parasympathetic dominance during intercourse and an appropriate tonus of the pelvic floor. When adequate, the tonus is an underappreciated factor contributing to quality of arousal and orgasm, not to mention the active role the woman has with the voluntary sensual movements of the pelvic floor that can further increase both her and her partner arousal. Opposite to that, the hypertonic pelvic floor is the leading biomechanical component of sexual pain disorders.

The most important difficulties in the sexual history taking include, but are not limited to, the following:

- The lack of formal training in sexual medicine during the medical school and the resident training in different specialties.
- The difficulty of communication between doctor and patient, given the intimate and confidential subject involved in sexual issues.

Many women still present their sexual request to the gynecologist through pain, which is the symptom that the patient perceives as more easy to communicate in the medical field. On the other hand, many doctors find it embarrassing and inconvenient to discuss sexual problems with their patients, because they perceive the inadequacy of their clinical training in this area and because they fear both "wasting time" and not being able to give adequate therapeutic answers.

The absence of adequate and open communication between doctor and patient contributes to the diagnostic omission and to the worsening, up to the chronicity, of sexual disorders that could be well resolved if promptly addressed, hence the importance of investigating these issues in order to finally be able to offer qualified diagnoses and therapies to the patient and the couple.

Human sexuality is a vast topic. For this reason, sexuality across the lifespan will be treated in four chapters, including this one and the following, titled respectively:

- *Women's Vulnerabilities I: From Intrauterine Life to Adolescence*
- *Women's Vulnerabilities II: FSD Classification and the Reproductive Age*
- *Women's Vulnerabilities III: From Early Menopause to Senescence*
- *Men's Vulnerabilities IV: Sexuality Across Lifespan*

The aim of these four chapters is to give general practitioners, pediatricians, and other medical specialists the cultural basis to understand the fundamental aspects of human sexuality, through the various stages of life.

1.2 Intrauterine Life

The intrauterine life is emerging as a critical period for human health and specifically for human sexuality. The quality of maternal attachment (secure, avoidant, or anxious) is overdetermined by the migration of fetal stem cells to the mother brain and specifically to the limbic system, where they determine a major rearrangement of neuronal connections. This discovery shows the unexpected role of the fetus as a "love shaper" of his/her mother's caring attitudes. It raises as well many questions on how premature deliveries, pathologies in pregnancy, or surrogate pregnancy can affect this process and impact the emotional and sexual well-being of the newborn [11].

The **ontogeny of gender identity** begins in utero, due to the influence of fetal genetic and biological factors (chromosomal sex, adequate development of the gonads and consequent hormone secretion, adequate or less expression of hormone receptors in fetal tissues). Furthermore, the effect of maternal biological factors must be considered (among which the plasma levels of the mother's sex hormones, physiological or pathological, of endogenous or exogenous origin stand out), as well as psychosexual and behavioral factors (including diet, alcohol, and drug abuse) related to the woman's life context. All of these elements influence the development of primary sex characteristics as well as the prenatal brain endocrine imprinting [12, 13]. For example, persistently elevated androgen levels in congenital adrenogenital syndrome contribute to a masculinizing imprinting of the brain of the female fetus. Or, again, the persistent biological and/or psychic stress in the mother can lead to an increase of weak androgens of adrenal and ovarian production, which can determine the androgenization of the brain of the female fetus and reduce the androgenization of the brain of the male fetus, as they compete with fetal androgens for binding to brain receptors.

The quality and intensity of prenatal endocrine imprinting are already a first factor of solidity or vulnerability in the construction of sexual identity from a psychodynamic point of view, making intrauterine life a pivotal moment in the development of **gender dysphoria**, a condition that becomes evident during childhood and especially adolescence.

See the previous chapter (***Gender and Orientation***) for a more comprehensive discussion on gender identity and gender dysphoria.

Gestational diabetes and **obesity** are risk factors not only for the pregnant woman, but also for her offspring. In fact, gestational diabetes and obesity increase the risk of fetal macrosomia and consequent shoulder dystocia, which can lead to permanent disabilities. On the other hand, these conditions also increase the risk of intrauterine growth restriction.

Looking to the long-term consequences, gestational diabetes exerts a dysmetabolic priming on the offspring, increasing the risk of childhood and adolescent obesity, a potential disruptor of self-confidence, self-esteem, and sexual well-being [14].

Iron deficiency (ID) and **iron-deficiency anemia** (IDA) during pregnancy are frequently neglected causes of fetal vulnerability during intrauterine development.

Significant anemia in pregnancy (hemoglobin concentration <11 g/dL in the first trimester or <10 g/dL in the second and third trimesters) has a widely variable prevalence considering different studies, ranging from 2% up to 26% in low-income populations. ID is the most common cause of significant anemia during pregnancy and postpartum [15].

Two are the most relevant consequences among the many: impairment of the child neurocognitive development on the one side and a doubled risk of maternal depression after delivery. The latter may impact the quality of mother-child attachment and self-confidence and emotional balance of the newborn, which can deeply impact his/her future sexual well-being.

Obstetricians should therefore be aware of the long-lasting consequences that anemia in pregnancy and postpartum can have on the emotional and sexual health of the newborn and be more proactive in diagnosing and treating iron-deficiency anemia in pregnancy.

There is an emerging need to point out the importance of a ***pregnancy ecology***, paying attention to poor and low cultural strata of the population above all.

Alcohol, cigarettes, and drugs poison the fetus, with increasing toxic effects with increasing doses, leading to long-term consequences, general and sexual, in the lifespan. There is not a minimum safe dose for each of the three. The key recommendation is therefore to avoid completely alcohol, cigarettes, and drugs for the sake of fetal general and sexual health.

In addition, the diet of the mother during pregnancy has an impact on the health and intestinal microbiota of the offspring. This relates not only to an adequate increase of maternal weight during pregnancy and an adequate dietary income or supplementation of macro- and micronutrients (like iron), but also to pollutants in the food and/or in the environment. For example, the presence of microplastic has been recently demonstrated in the placenta. The potential impact of environmental pollutant and endocrine disruptors on the fetal sexual development is still under investigation [16]. It deserves a much proactive attention and obstetric care.

1.3 Childhood

During childhood, the perception of **gender sexual identity** is believed to be structured with two fundamental dynamics: identification with the parent of the same sex, or a stable substitute, and complementation with the parent of the opposite sex, or a stable substitute [17]. Additional factors that modulate the formation and perception of sexual identity in childhood include social cues, from the color of the ribbon at birth to the colors and types of clothes, as well as the games given or encouraged; educational styles, even in the extended family, with grandparents and new partners of the father and/or mother; rewarded and stigmatized behaviors; type of interactions between adults and children; effect of psycho-emotional traumas, primarily abandonment and/or separation of parents; and neglect and/or sexual abuse. These factors contribute to the progressive structuring of gender identity, to the wounds that can harm it, and to the mechanisms, conscious and unconscious, with which difficulties and traumas disturb the experience of identity when they are not adequately understood.

Childhood sexual abuse is a powerful cause of sexual problems later in life, of which the pediatrician as well as the gynecologist, but also the general practitioner and the psychiatrist, must be aware. The diagnosis of genital or perianal condylomatosis or other sexually transmitted diseases in a child should immediately question a potential sexual abuse.

Vulvar pain during childhood is a diagnostic dilemma, and it is usually difficult for the little girl to express her symptoms verbally. Vulvar pain can be triggered by accidental factors (for example, injuries in the playground or straddle injuries) or can be voluntarily provoked to the child by female genital mutilations or sexual abuse [18].

The differential diagnosis is between:

- Vulvovaginitis.
- Genital trauma.

- Genital masses.
- Dermatologic pathologies.
- Musculoskeletal dysfunctions.

The evaluation of vulvar pain in children deserves a competent short- and long-term perspective, as it may have an extremely negative impact on many aspects of the girl future sexuality.

1.4 Adolescence

Adolescence is one of the most critical periods in human sexuality. Here, we will focus on a few emerging factors of vulnerability.

Body and **genital image** self-perception is powerfully modulated by social media and pornography (Box 5). On the other hand, the perception we have of our body and genitals is a key aspect in sexual life, potentially contributing to sexual dysfunctions.

Box 5 Social Media, *Influencers*, and Pornography: The Effects on Body and Genital Image

Social media use impacts **body image**, with different effects depending on the platforms used. Visual platforms, such as Instagram or Pinterest, are more dysfunctional for body image than textual platforms, such as Facebook or Twitter [19].

Taking and editing selfies, but not *posting* them because "you do not like yourself," can have negative effects on body image. On the contrary, positive comments and *likes*, through the activation of the reward system, can increase the impact of exposure to idealized content, such as those usually *posted* by celebrities and *influencers*.

The influence of social media is of particular relevance in adolescents, and it can contribute to eating disorders, due to the so-called *pathoplasticity*. The continuous self-comparison with what is *posted* by *influencers* and celebrities is one of the elements of contemporary vulnerability in adolescents [20]. Contents of *thinspiration*, deliberately created to enhance thinness, but also contents of *fitspiration*, theoretically created to promote a healthy lifestyle, are characterized in the same way by: sexual suggestiveness, body comparison, and messages inciting restrictive food intake and exercise as a method of compensation [21, 22]. On the other hand, there are also *influencers* and *divulgers* that create contents of real body positivity.

In 2010, Herbenik and Reece created the **Female Genital Self-Image Scale (FGSIS)**. The score at the FGSIS relates to the score in every domain of the Female Sexual Function Index (FSFI), including the total score, with the only exception of the desire domain. A positive perception of one's own genitals reduces sexual distress [23]. A Swedish cross-sectional study from 2022 collected anonymous data from 3503 men and women: 3.6% of women and 5.5% of men reported very low self-esteem regarding their external genitalia; 13.7% of women and 11.3% of men considered genital plastic surgery [24]. In this study, a better perception of genitals was related to a bigger penis for men and to small labia minora in women.

Usually, the vulva is represented by mass media, Internet, and pornography as a flat line between legs, without hair and protrusion, in a prepubertal aesthetic. This representation leads to a perceptive bias. Educational initiatives, both directed to general population (such as *The Labia Library* by Women's Health Victoria) and to healthcare providers, pointing out the vast range of normality in the look of female external genitalia, would have a massive impact on genital self-esteem, reducing the recourse to female genital cosmetic surgery to selected patients.

The most common female genital cosmetic surgery is labiaplasty. This procedure should be limited to women with persistent symptoms of genital discomfort after educational and psychological interventions and to women with significant labia minora asymmetry after complete development of external genitalia.

Body image and genital image have a profound relationship: women unsatisfied of their body appearance have a higher risk to be dissatisfied with their external genitalia.

Sexual fluidity (variable sexual orientation in different moments of life, associated with a lack of need to define one's sexual orientation) and **gender fluidity** (variable identification of oneself as belonging to a certain gender or the refusal to label oneself binary) are new coined definitions, describing apparently growing phenomena among young people [25, 26].

However, we do not currently have the elements to determine if the phenomenon is actually increasing or if there is a bias due to the fact that only in recent years it has become common to define oneself as gender fluid (*bigender*, *trigender*, *gender fluid*, *pangender*). Epidemiological studies have been initiated [25].

Further studies are needed to understand the biological and psychological factors that determine the phenomena of sexual and gender fluidity and the possible causes of their real or apparent increase among adolescents.

Gender dysphoria is a condition in which gender identity does not coincide with biological sex, with persistent psychological distress. Subjects with gender dysphoria show psychological distress with relationship difficulties, anxiety, depression, and sometimes suicidal tendencies. The psychological consequences are linked to the incongruence between assigned sex and gender identity and to traumatic experiences, lack of acceptance, and/or variable stigmatization by society [27].

A neglected aspect of gender dysphoria concerns the enormous energy expenditure dedicated to understanding and defining one's gender identity and to living with the depressive state, even severe, that derives from it, with consequent less energy to invest in cultivating talents and life projects. This becomes particularly evident during the peripubertal phase, when the appearance of secondary sexual characteristics forces the very young adolescent to get out of the illusion of gender neutrality and to seek help from the family and health professionals. Psychological support remains of primary importance, but in case of marked symptoms, the current orientation is to suspend the flow of pubertal events, using gonadotrophin-releasing hormone (GnRH) analogues. The goal is to maintain a relative physical neutrality, so as to give the psychotherapist time to understand the deep perception of sexual identity, accompanying the adolescent up to 16 years of age, when it is believed that he/she is more able to choose in which direction to evolve. Withdrawal of GnRH analogue therapy allows for the resumption of normal pubertal development. If, on the other hand, the diagnosis of gender dysphoria is confirmed, therapy with feminizing or virilizing hormones can be undertaken in specific cases.

Adolescents nowadays are generally less used to control their impulses. This leads to impulsive behaviors toward food, sex, alcohol, and drugs. **Eating disorders** are particularly frequent in adolescent girls (even though the prevalence is increasing in adolescent boys).

Eating disorders, especially related to impulsiveness like bulimia, show frequent pathoplasticity with **sexual impulsivity**. On the other hand, anorexia, characterized by a restrictive eating behavior, is frequently associated with a "freezing" in sexual interest and sexual life. The low sexual hormone levels in underweight girls can only partially explain this sexual silence. A careful clinical investigation should evaluate in parallel biological and psychosexual etiologies of the "sexual freezing."

Excessive dietary income associated with overweight and obesity and low physical activity in childhood and adolescence are risk factors for the development of **insulin resistance** and **polycystic ovary syndrome (PCOS)**, which can impact self-perception and self-confidence, increasing the risk of perceived sexual inadequacy, besides causing infertility.

Pediatricians, general practitioners, and gynecologists should pay great attention to diet and physical activity of adolescent girls, to promote healthier lifestyles. Physical activity is fundamental in the lifespan for biological, psychological, and emotional reasons and also to protect sexuality. Sports, and in particular team sports, release negative emotions, improve emotional and social intelligence, and increase the ability to relate and cooperate with others. They train therefore the basic emotional skills that may also enhance more positive intimate relationships.

On the other hand, some kind of sports can have detrimental effects of sexuality, leading to genital trauma, pudendal neuropathy, or pelvic floor hypertonicity (Box 6).

Box 6 Sports and Sexuality: The Dark Side

Cycling is a physical activity that helps to prevent cardiovascular disease, diabetes, cancer, hypertension, obesity, depression, and osteoporosis. But cycling carries (in both men and women) the risk to report genital straddle injuries or saddle genital lesions in the long term.

There is a proven association between agonist cycling and reduced genital sensations. In particular, cycling is associated with pudendal neuropathy, which usually manifests itself with unilateral numbness and/or burning pain, due to the entrapment of the pudendal nerve between the pubic bones and the saddle.

In a survey published in 2019, female cyclists reported a prevalence of female sexual dysfunction, genital numbness, and genital pain of 53.9%, 58.1%, and 69.1%, respectively [28]. There was a statistically significant association between genital numbness/genital pain and sexual dysfunction in the participants. More studies are needed to understand how to alleviate these symptoms and if the resolutions of symptoms correlate with better sexual function [28].

Moreover, the saddle can cause skin lesions like edema, friction injuries, bruises, sores, ulcers, folliculitis, and abscesses, but also a condition called "bicyclist vulva," characterized by vulvar unilateral lymphedema [29, 30].

Horse-riding is another, usually ignored, possible cause of genital trauma and pudendal neuropathy.

Pilates and **yoga** are considered sports with a low impact on pelvic floor, but they both have an important isomeric component that can lead to higher intra-abdominal pressure. If the instructor and/or the woman are not aware of the importance of coordinating the contraction of the abdominal muscles with the contraction of the pelvic floor muscle, these sports can lead to pelvic floor dysfunction. In particular in young nulliparous women, attention must be paid to pelvic floor hyperactivity, balancing abdominal breathing and adduction exercises with abduction ones.

Adolescents engage in sexual activity earlier than before 1960. **Sexual impulsivity** increases the risk of adolescents to have intercourses with people they scarcely know, frequently under the effect of alcohol and/or drugs, and without using barrier contraceptives. These behaviors can lead to **adolescent unwanted pregnancies** and **sexually transmitted diseases** with long-term consequences. Among sexually transmitted diseases, chlamydia and gonorrhea can lead to **pelvic inflammatory disease** (PID), a common cause of deep dyspareunia, chronic pelvic pain, and infertility later in life.

1.5   Conclusion

Vulnerabilities affecting women's sexuality can stem from intrauterine life, across childhood, to adolescence. Different pathologies and toxics from inappropriate behavioral habits during pregnancy can make the early phases of sexual identity and sexual function fragile. Sexual dysfunctions, in women and men, can have their roots in childhood or adolescent problems. A more careful clinical vision is needed when considering the early phases of sexuality, with a lifespan perspective.

2   Sexuality Across Lifespan II: FSD Classification and Women's Vulnerabilities in the Reproductive Age

Alessandra Graziottin

a.graziottin@studiograziottin.it and Angela Cuccarollo

2.1   Introduction

Knowledge of **female sexual dysfunctions (FSDs)** and their classifications is key for every physician, to set the appropriate clinical conversation frame.

From adolescence to senescence, women and men can develop different sexual dysfunctions [1]. A diagnosis of sexual dysfunction is established only if the symptoms cause personal distress.

The most important **FSDs**, according to the ISSWSH classification, include [31]:

- Hypoactive sexual desire disorder (HSDD).
- Female arousal disorder (FAD).
- Persistent genital arousal disorder (PGAD).
- Female orgasm disorder (FOD).
- Sexual pain-penetration disorders (SPPDs).

In this chapter, the classification used will be consistent with DSM-IV-TR. The DSM-5 eliminated the classic definitions of desire and arousal disorders, creating a single category of female sexual interest/arousal disorder (FSIAD). This position has been widely contested. The ISSWSH nomenclature committee and the ICD have therefore reintroduced the label hypoactive sexual desire disorder (HSDD).

For the discussion on sexual pain-penetration disorders, the reader is referred to the chapters titled *Chronic Pain and Female Sexual Dysfunction* and *Sexual Pain and Pelvic Floor Disorders*. In this chapter, we will focus on all the other female sexual dysfunctions, with a pragmatic approach useful in the physician's daily clinical practice.

Special attention will be devoted to **women's sexuality in the reproductive age**, with focus on the most neglected phases of pregnancy and puerperium.

2.2   Prevalence and Diagnosis of FSDs

The cumulative prevalence of FSD is around 40–50%, with great heterogeneity among different studies [10, 32]. The prevalence increases with age, especially after menopause, if the woman is not receiving an adequate hormone replacement therapy (HRT). Physical inactivity, inappropriate eating choices and habits, smoking, alcohol, drug abuse, and excess of virtual life are among the most destructive factors of female sexuality.

Each sexual dysfunction has clinically different characteristics depending on whether it is:

- Present from the beginning of sexual life (**primary** or **lifelong**) or appearing after months or years of normal function (**secondary** or **acquired**).
- Present in any situation and, potentially, with any partner (**generalized**) or limited to the current partner or specific situations (**situational**).
- Of **biological**, **psychological**, or **mixed** etiology.

The diagnosis of female sexual dysfunctions requires [1]:

- **An accurate clinical history**, with attention to the woman's words and to predisposing, precipitating, and maintenance factors of physical, psychosexual, and relational type. A respectful overture could include questions such as the following: "Women would often like to have more information about sexuality. If you are interested, a few more questions could be included in our clinical conversation. Are you currently sexually active? Are you satisfied with your sexuality, or are there questions or problems you would like to discuss?" In the context of a well-taken clinical history, key first-line biological factors contributing to FSD could be well addressed. Confidence increases when this part of the clinical history and first-line therapeutic suggestions are routinely considered. If the sexual problem appears to be significant, with complex etiology, a second appointment to focus on FSD should be arranged. Alternatively, referral to a colleague competent in sexual medicine would be appropriate.
- **A rigorous physical examination**, paying attention to postural factors and genital conditions that can cause pain and/or negative feedbacks, progressively inhibiting desire and arousal. These include pelvic floor hypertonicity, vulvodynia, outcome of perineal lesions during childbirth, vulvar lichen sclerosus, and genitourinary syndrome of menopause [1, 18, 33]. Genital physical examination is necessary to evaluate tissue trophism, modulated by an appropriate hormonal milieu and the integrity of vascular, nerve, and muscle structures. Vulvoscopy, Q-tip test, and vaginal swab smear are useful tests for diagnosing dermatological, inflammatory, and infectious vulvar and vaginal pathologies, which can interfere with the peripheral sexual response. The gynecologist has an essential role in the diagnosis and treatment of the biological genital causes of FSD. Only a multimodal therapy can address FSDs and release desire, arousal, and orgasm that will otherwise be trapped by negative genital feedbacks.
- **Screening tools**, including the Brief Profile of Female Sexual Function (B-PFSF), which can be easily used by doctors who are not experts in FSD.

- **Specific questionnaires**, including the Female Sexual Function Index (FSFI) and the Female Sexual Distress Scale (FSDS), the most used also for clinical research purposes.
- **Hormonal dosages**, when the clinical history suggests a dysendocrine component as a possible cause of the disorder (hypoandrogenism, hypoestrogenism, hyperprolactinemia, and hyper/hypothyroidism), before and after the menopause.
- **Second-level instrumental examinations** for selected cases, which include neurophysiological tests, magnetic resonance imaging of the spinal cord, vulvar and/or clitoral echo-color Doppler, and vulvar and/or clitoral thermography.

2.3 Hypoactive Sexual Desire Disorder (HSDD)

Hypoactive, or reduced, sexual desire disorder (HSDD) is the most common female sexual dysfunction, with a prevalence ranging from 17 to over 50% [6]. In the PRESIDE study, a population-based study of over 50,000 American women, 37.7% of participants reported low sexual desire and 10% reported a frank hypoactive sexual desire disorder [34]. In Europe, the estimated prevalence of women with desire disorders is 29% [10].

HSDD is defined, according to the ICD-11 and the ISSWSH, as:

1. Reduced or absent spontaneous sexual desire (sexual fantasies or thoughts).
2. Reduced or absent desire responsive to erotic stimulation or stimulation.
3. Inability to maintain desire or interest in sexual activity once it has begun.

Listening carefully to the exact words of the woman (Box 7) is the first diagnostic element, more effective than classifications and questionnaires. Loss of sexual desire, pain during intercourse, and vaginal dryness are the sexual complaints usually reported by women, while sexual arousal disorder and orgasmic disorder usually emerge during an accurate clinical interview.

The exact biological mechanisms that determine HSDD are not known, and no biochemical or neuroimaging alterations have been described so far to specifically identify women affected [1].

Box 7 HSDD in Women's Words

"I have no sexual desire." "I no longer have desire." "Since I gave birth I no longer feel any sex drive." "After menopause desire is dead and buried." "How can I have desire with this dryness here?!"

"Since I have pain in intercourse I no longer have desire." "Now I get cystitis after every intercourse: I'm so scared that I don't try anymore." "I see myself fat and ugly, I can't even bear being touched." "If it were up to me I wouldn't do it, but my husband insists ...."

"He has always suffered from precocity and I was always blank. He never went to the doctor. Now I'm fed up and I don't want to anymore."

The leading risk factors for reduction or loss of sexual desire are briefly summarized here, "to open active windows in the physician brains" while taking a general and focused clinical history.

Systemic Factors [1]:

- **Iron deficiency and iron-deficiency anemia (IDA)**: Iron is essential for the synthesis of dopamine, the main neurotransmitter of the appetitive, seeking, and pleasure system (seeking-appetitive-lust system) [35]. IDA is one of the most neglected biological etiologies of low desire in women in the fertile age. If heavy menstrual bleeding is present (more than five tampons or pads/day), it must be treated with a progesterone or contraceptive pill with a short hormone-free interval.
- **Chronic lack of sleep and/or chronic stress**: They alter the biological basis of biorhythms and neurovegetative balance, which feeds the energy and instinctual basis of desire.
- **Age**: The reduction of testosterone and DHEA, biological engines of desire, from the age of 20 onwards, and the age-related increase in systemic inflammation and neuroinflammation consume vital energy and instinctual drive.
- **Sex hormone deficiencies**, particularly androgens. Etiologies include:
  - Hypothalamic amenorrhea.
  - Puerperium and breastfeeding.
  - Hyperprolactinemia.
  - Menopause (see the following chapter).
  - Premature ovarian failure (see chapter ***Endocrine Disorders and Sexuality II: Ovary***).
- **High levels of sex hormone binding globulin (SHBG)**: This protein binds testosterone, reducing the levels of free, biologically active testosterone. Increased levels are common in women taking hormonal contraceptive therapy.
- **Hypothyroidism**.
- **Obesity**.
- **Chronic medical conditions**, including endometriosis, heavy and/or painful periods, fibromyalgia, chronic fatigue syndrome, and autoimmune diseases, in young women, as well as diabetes, dysmetabolic diseases, hypertension, and cardiovascular and neurological diseases, more relevant with increasing age. In all chronic pathologies, the underlying systemic inflammation and the associated neuroinflammation are persistent killers of sexual desire.
- **Psychiatric diseases**, such as depression. The relationship between depression and HSDD is bidirectional: depression increases the risk of suffering from HSDD by 50–70%, and the diagnosis of HSDD is associated with a 130–210% increased risk of suffering from depressive symptoms [6, 36].
- **Psychoactive and non-psychoactive drugs**, including benzodiazepines, lithium, SSRIs, tricyclic antidepressants, antihypertensive drugs, GnRH agonists and analogues, hormonal contraceptives, antiandrogens, tamoxifen, aromatase inhibitors, and chemotherapy agents.
- **Substance abuse**.

Negative Feedback from the Genitals [1]:

- Vaginal dryness, from biological or psychosexual factors.
- Vulvovaginal atrophy (VVA)/genitourinary syndrome of the menopause (GSM).
- Sexual pain on penetration (introital and/or deep dyspareunia).
- Vulvar pain.
- Postcoital cystitis, which appears 24–72 h after the intercourse.
- Hyperactive pelvic floor, which contributes to the biomechanical component of sexual pain and associated comorbidities. Rehabilitation with a competent physiotherapist or midwife is key.
- Difficulty or absence of orgasm.

Psychosexual Factors [1, 6]:

- Self-imposed repressions derived from religious, cultural, and family context, beliefs, and taboos.
- Low self-esteem and dissatisfaction with one's body image.
- Restrictive eating disorders.
- Past or current domestic violence and abuse.

Partner Sexual Dysfunctions [1, 6]:

- Premature ejaculation.
- Erectile dysfunction.
- Absence of desire.

In these cases, the partner is the *symptom inducer* and the woman, who complains of the fall of desire from persistent sexual dissatisfaction and frustration, is the *symptom carrier*. It is therefore the partner that should be looked after (see chapter *Sexuality Across the Lifespan IV: Men's Vulnerabilities*).

2.3.1 Treatment Strategies

It is important to favor lifestyles that are friends of desire (Box 8) and discourage those that are its enemies (Box 9).

Box 8 Green Light: Lifestyle Friends of Desire and Happy Sexuality (*modified from Graziottin e Cuccarollo* [37])
- Forty-five minutes of daily morning walk outdoor, to optimize biorhythms.
- Thirty minutes of toning exercises twice a week.
- Healthy diet.
- Regular sleep (at least 7 h/night).
- Limited or no alcohol consumption (maximum two units of alcohol/week).
- Avoidance of smoking and drugs.
- Protection from sexually transmitted diseases with the constant use of a condom in any type of intercourse (vaginal, anal, oral) and from the beginning of sexual life.
- Tailored hormonal contraception.

> **Box 9 Red Light: Lifestyle Enemy of Desire and Happy Sexuality (*modified from Graziottin e Cuccarollo* [37])**
>
> - Alcohol: sexual dysfunctions in alcohol abusers have a prevalence of 61% [38].
> - Active/passive cigarette smoking: it is the most important modifiable cause of sexual dysfunction [39].
> - Drugs: sexual dysfunction in opioid users has a prevalence of 75% [38].
> - Chronic lack of sleep.
> - Physical inactivity.
> - Obesity.
> - Lack of outdoor life.
> - Excessive indoor life, with overexposure to artificial light from electronic devices:
>   - Alteration of the circadian rhythm of melatonin, with:
>   - (a) Low-quality sleep.
>   - (b) Impaired hypothalamic master-clock activity.
>   - (c) Alteration of neurovegetative and endocrine biorhythms.
>   - Vitamin D deficiency.
>   - Increased oxidative stress.
>   - Low levels of oxytocin, with high risk of social isolation and depression.
> - Sexual promiscuity and discontinuous or absent use of condoms, with high vulnerability to sexually transmitted diseases.
> - Long-distance cycling (see previous chapter).

Consistently with the etiological diagnosis, the physician should focus the first-line therapy on:

- **Iron-deficiency anemia** (IDA), by correcting the causes, including heavy periods and low dietary intake.
- **Estrogenic, androgenic, or mixed deficiency** (see the following chapter).
- **Pelvic floor hyperactivity**, more frequent in nulliparous women or women who have given birth only by caesarean section, and who complain of sexual pain and comorbidities.
- **Genital conditions**, primarily the genitourinary syndrome of menopause (GSM) (see the following chapter), which contribute to the onset of vaginal and vulvar dryness, pain, cystitis, and anorgasmia.

Therapy can be integrated with centrally acting drugs (currently not approved in many countries), such as flibanserin or bremelanotide.

The help of qualified professionals is required for psychotherapy and/or sexual therapy and/or uro-andrological therapy of the partner's sexual disorders. However, a parallel evaluation of biological, besides psychosexual, factors is mandatory. The psychotherapeutic treatment of female sexual dysfunctions alone, without adequate correction of the biological cofactors, **has a high risk of being ineffective**. For example, a woman can complain of persistent loss of sexual desire and persistent sexual pain after having being sexually abused. Besides giving words to her emotional fear, anguish, and pain with a competent psychotherapy, she needs to be well evaluated from the medical point of view, with a specific attention to a hyperactive defensive pelvic floor. If present, a competent physiotherapy should be offered and carried out. Otherwise, the sole psychotherapy cannot resolve the biomechanical component of pain and the secondary loss of sex drive because of the persistent pain, besides the negative effects of having been abused, as Ellen Laan and coworkers have well proven in a paradigmatic study [40].

The integration of medical, rehabilitative, and psychosexual therapy is decisive in many cases.

2.4 Female Sexual Arousal Disorder (FSAD)

Sexual arousal disorder has a significant prevalence among women. The PRESIDE study showed that the prevalence of low female sexual arousal, without associated distress, is 26.1%, while the pathological form, with associated distress, has a prevalence of 5.4%, which rises to 7.5% among middle-aged patients (45–64 years) [34]. The estimated prevalence of arousal disorders for European women is 22% [10].

In the **DSM-V**, arousal disorder is not described as a separate entity, but combined with HSDD, in the diagnosis of female sexual interest/arousal disorder (FSIAD). However, desire and arousal can be disconnected. Great interpersonal variability is reported between "subjective arousal" (subjective mental engagement during sexual activity) and "physiological arousal" (vaginal lubrication and other genital and non-genital sensations) [41].

The nomenclature proposed by the **ISSWSH** differentiates between [42]:

- **Female genital arousal disorder (FGAD)**, characterized by the difficulty or inability to achieve or maintain an adequate genital response.
- **Female cognitive arousal disorder (FCAD)**, characterized by the difficulty or inability to achieve or maintain an adequate mental arousal in association with sexual activity.

To make a diagnosis, symptoms must be present for at least 6 months and be associated with personal distress.

Arousal disorders in the clinical practice overlap with lack of lubrication or frank vaginal dryness and poor vulvar/clitoral congestion.

The most frequent risk factors can be biological and/or psycho-relational.

Biological factors include, but are not limited to [1]:

- **Biobehavioral**, leading to biological damage (Box 9):
  - Cigarette smoking, with vascular disease and neuropathy.
  - Frequent and long-distance cycling, with pudendal neuropathy.
- **Hormonal**: low levels of sex steroids (estrogens and androgens), which can contribute to poor vaginal lubrication and poor congestion of the corpora cavernosa.
- **Dysmetabolic and cardiovascular**:
  - Diabetes mellitus: the sexual domains most involved are arousal and lubrication.
  - Obesity, metabolic syndrome, dyslipidemia, and hypertension, with endothelial dysfunction.
- **Muscular**:
  - Pelvic floor hyperactivity, primary or acquired in response to inflammation and/or pain. It narrows the vaginal opening, causing pain associated with penetration attempts. This can induce a reflex inhibition of both mental and genital arousal, contributing to poor or absent lubrication and pain at the onset of penetration (**introital, or superficial dyspareunia**).
  - Pelvic floor hypotonus from birth injuries with genital hyposensitivity or pain.
  - Fibromyalgia.
- **Neurological**:
  - Pudendal neuropathy.
  - Iatrogenic neuropathy after chemoradiotherapy for anorectal, cervical, or bladder cancer.
  - Iatrogenic damage from pelvic surgery.
  - Multiple sclerosis or spinal cord injuries.

Psycho-Relational Factors [1, 43]:

- **Psychological with biological correlates**:
  - Anxiety and depression.
  - Body image disturbances.
  - Eating disorders.
  - History of sexual abuse.
- **Relational**:
  - Unsatisfactory couple relationship and communication.
  - Partner's sexual dysfunction.
  - Inadequate stimulation and/or erotic competence of the partner.
- **Contextual**:
  - Environmental stressors.
  - Cultural attitudes.

2.4.1 Treatment Strategies

Women in fertile age, with normal hormonal levels, experience beneficial effects with physiotherapy reducing pelvic floor hyperactivity and/or with psychosexual therapy. Behavioral causes, such as smoking, should be reduced. Compression of the nervous terminations on the bicycle saddle should be addressed in cyclist women.

During breastfeeding, vaginal dryness can be relieved by nonhormonal treatments such as lubricants, vitamin E, PEA gel, vaginal probiotics (containing *Lactobacillus crispatus* and other *Lactobacillus*), and oxygen therapy. Minimal doses of promestriene or estriol can be considered when dryness is severe and does not respond to nonhormonal treatments.

The different therapies of vaginal dryness after menopause will be discussed in the following chapter.

2.5 Persistent Genital Arousal Disorder/Genito-Pelvic Dysesthesia (PGAD/GPD)

The existence of an entity termed **persistent genital arousal disorder (PGAD)** was postulated in the early 2000s [1, 44]. It is defined by the ISSWSH as a persistent or recurrent, unwanted, and intrusive feeling of genital arousal lasting at least 3 months and resulting in personal distress [45].

There are also other types of **genito-pelvic dysesthesia (GPD)**, such as vibration, tingling, burning, contractions, itching, and pain.

PGAD/GPD is usually felt at the clitoral level, but may involve other genito-pelvic regions. Sensations include being on the verge of orgasm, experiencing uncontrollable orgasms, and/or having an excessive number of orgasms, which are not followed by genital decongestion, resolution, and satisfaction [1]. The woman is very disturbed by this state of involuntary and persistent arousal, disabling for its pervading intrusiveness and the waste of vital energy. Furthermore, the symptoms are not associated with sexual desire or fantasies, which differentiates this diagnosis from that of hypersexuality [46].

The estimated prevalence is 0.6–3% [47]. Sensory hyperactivity originating from the genitals, the spinal cord, and/or the brain has been proposed as the cause of the disorder; however, there are no conclusive data.

Major biological risk factors for PGAD/GPD include [1, 45]:

- Clitoral, vestibular, vulvar, and vaginal pathologies.
- Pelvic floor hyperactivity.
- Pudendal neuropathy.
- Lumbar disc disease.
- Organic disorders of the central nervous system, like epilepsy and transient ischemic attack.
- Spontaneous or iatrogenic hyperandrogenisms.

Associated psychosocial factors should also be investigated [46].

A correct diagnosis is essential, avoiding inappropriate labels of *nymphomania*. No treatment protocol for PGAD is currently recommended. If this diagnosis is suspected, the patient should be referred to a center with specific clinical experience in this disease.

2.6   Female Orgasm Disorder (FOD)

Female orgasmic disorders are common: a study on a sample of 1500 American patients found that 24% had not reached orgasm for several months in the previous year [47]. In Europe, the estimated prevalence is 19% [10].

The ISSWSH defines **female orgasm disorder (FOD)** as a condition characterized by persistent or recurrent impairment in the frequency, intensity, and/or timing of orgasm, and/or associated pleasure, lasting for a minimum of 6 months and associated with personal distress [48]. In particular [48]:

- Frequency alterations: orgasm occurs with reduced frequency or is absent (**anorgasmia**).
- Alterations in intensity: orgasm occurs with reduced intensity (**muted orgasm**).
- Timing alterations: orgasm occurs too late (**delayed orgasm**) or too soon (**spontaneous or premature orgasm**).
- Alterations of pleasure: orgasm occurs with absent or reduced pleasure (**anhedonic orgasm**, or **pleasure-dissociative orgasmic disorder**, PDOD).

A distinct entity is the **female orgasmic illness syndrome (FOIS)**, characterized by the appearance of peripheral and/or central adverse symptoms (headache, confusion, impaired verbal memory, clonus, gastrointestinal symptoms, muscle pain, asthenia) preceding, accompanying, or following orgasm, with no impairment of orgasm quality [1, 48].

Also in the case of FOD, the most common predisposing factors can be biological or psycho-relational.

Biological Factors [1]:

- Age-dependent involution of about 50% of the clitoral cavernous bodies, well proven by Tarcan back in 1999 [49], is the most neglected biological etiology of blunted orgasm. It can be associated with significant vulvar dystrophy and/or vulvar lichen sclerosus.
- Alterations of the genital vessels, resulting from cardiovascular diseases and/or metabolic syndrome and smoking.
- Hypoandrogenism and/or hypoestrogenism, particularly postmenopausal (see the following chapter).
- Dysfunctions of neuronal transmission, peripheral or central, afferent or efferent:
  - Peripheral neuropathies (diabetic, actinic, chemotherapy-induced).
  - Pudendal neuropathy.
- Pelvic floor dysfunctions: hypo- or hyperactivity.
- Inflammatory, infectious, and immunological disorders causing dyspareunia.

Psycho-Relational Factors [1]:

- Poor body and/or genital image.
- Negative emotions associated with sexual activity.
- Shame or embarrassment, due to religious beliefs, familiar or cultural inhibitions.
- Inadequate communication with the partner.
- Partner's sexual dysfunctions.

2.6.1 Therapeutic Strategies

There are currently no approved therapies for FOD. In clinical practice, reducing modifiable risk factors, primarily smoking and obesity, is the first step.

Rehabilitation of the pelvic floor plays a central role, when hypotonicity or hypertonicity of the levator muscle is a relevant etiological cofactor, as occurs, for example, in marked postpartum hypotonia.

Psychosexual therapy maintains a specific role when pertinent factors emerge.

After the menopause, the positive role of testosterone will be discussed in the next chapter.

2.7 Pregnancy and Puerperium

In healthy women, with a **physiological pregnancy**, a desired sexual intercourse has no contraindications. The good frequency of intercourses seems to correlate with the physiological progress of the gestation itself and with better maternal-fetal outcomes, although data are not conclusive [50]. On the other hand, a serene woman, with a desired pregnancy and a good couple relationship, can enjoy an even more satisfying sexuality and more intense orgasms, given the greater genital congestion typical of pregnancy, particularly in the second trimester.

In general, the frequency of intercourse decreases during the first trimester (mostly for psychological reasons), may increase in the second trimester (probably due to increased genital congestion), and decrease again in the third trimester due to the increased uterine size, sensation of the child as an active "listening" presence, and/or physical discomfort [1]. The vast majority of women would like to have more information on sexuality during pregnancy from their healthcare providers.

In the **postpartum period**, the presence of the newborn, sleep shortage, iron-deficiency anemia (IDA), depression and fatigue, hormonal changes, episiotomy scar, and any perineal damage can reduce desire and frequency of intercourses. Breastfeeding women report lower sexual desire and satisfaction than non-breastfeeding women [51].

The failure to diagnose postpartum sexual difficulties, in particular intercourse pain, remains a transversal problem in all countries. A 2015 Australian study found that 43% of women suffered from severe sexual pain at 6 months postpartum, 28% at 12 months, and 23% at 18 months, with a devastating effect on the couple (Box 10) [52].

In comorbidity with intercourse pain, the woman can experience vulvodynia, urinary incontinence, and fecal incontinence, which in turn are factors that worsen sexual function.

Box 10 Sexual Pain After Delivery

The passage of the fetal head into the birth canal involves the levator ani muscle. In the expulsive phase, this leads to a lengthening of about three times the fibers of the puborectalis muscle, essential for continence. The expulsive phase of labor is a moment of extreme vulnerability for the perineum and the pelvic floor, with important implications in subsequent sexual life. However, based on the data available to date in relation to the risk of maternal and neonatal complications, the execution of caesarean section with the indication of prevention of perineal trauma alone is not justifiable [53].

The most important obstetric risk factors for damage to the pudendal nerve, the levator ani muscle, the endopelvic fascia, and the anal sphincter are [53]:

- An operative vaginal delivery.
- The duration of the expulsive period: the prolonged compression of the pudendal nerve can provoke a partial and transient denervation.
- An excessively short expulsion period: it does not allow the pelvic floor muscles to adapt progressively to the passage of the fetal head.
- Use of Kristeller's maneuver: it increases the trauma of the elevator complex and can determine its detachment from the anchorage on the tendon arch, with an increased risk of genital prolapse and cystocele.
- Fetal macrosomia.

Sexual pain, associated with perineal tears, episiorrhaphy, and occult perineal damage, can then be exacerbated by [54]:

- Hypoestrogenism in lactation, with fall of desire and vaginal dryness.
- Iron-deficiency anemia, which reduces sexual desire and doubles the risk of depression.
- Neuroinflammation, caused by the peak of pro-inflammatory cytokines resulting from the involution of the myometrial mass, which from 1200–1500 g at the end of pregnancy returns to 80–100 g at the end of the lochia.
- Postpartum depression, which reduces the ability to cope with pain and kills sexual desire.

The negative consequences of perineal trauma can probably be avoided by [53, 54]:

- Antepartum prevention:
  - Good pregnancy monitoring, avoiding excessive weight gain and adequately managing gestational diabetes if present, to reduce the risk of fetal macrosomia.
  - Adequate preparation for childbirth by the midwife, including perineal massages, aimed at optimizing pelvic floor relaxation, and teaching of diaphragmatic breathing.
- Intrapartum prevention:
  - Relaxation: a serene environment and adequate information allow the pregnant woman to face the birth with less stress and consequently less muscle contraction.

- Hot compresses during the expulsive period.
- Distanced and paused expulsive thrusts and slow descent of the head.
- Selective and reasoned use of vaginal operative delivery, with respect for the physiological times of birth, and abstention from unnecessary medical interventions.
- Minimization of the use of episiotomy: as per the WHO and the ACOG recommendations, it is indicated in less than 5% of vaginal deliveries and only in case of signs of fetal distress in the advanced expulsive period, and usually in association with the application of an obstetric cup.
- Postpartum prevention:
  - Appropriate recognition and treatment of perineal lesions, according to the indications provided in 2018 by the ACOG Practice Bulletin No. 198, based on the available literature.

Six months after delivery, 46.4% of women who had a perineal suture complained of dyspareunia, compared with 31.2% of women with intact genitalia at delivery [52]. The percentage of women who complain of dyspareunia rises to 59.5% in case of use of an obstetric cup [52]. The fact that even women with intact genitalia complain of postpartum dyspareunia suggests the presence of occult pelvic floor lesions with long-term and often unrecognized neuropathies.

In the event that an episiotomy and the consequent episiorrhaphy have become necessary or that there has been a spontaneous perineal laceration requiring suture, the woman must be instructed to adequate care of the wound [53, 54]:

- Use, in the first few days, of pain-killers as needed, such as paracetamol and NSAIDs, which are not contraindicated in breastfeeding.
- Application of ice to the perineal region, taking care not to cause cold burns.
- Exposure of the wound to the air to facilitate healing.
- Use of donut cushions, if useful for maintaining the sitting position without pain.

For all women who present sexual pain after childbirth, even in the absence of macroscopically evident perineal lesions, it is necessary to [53, 54]:

- Prevent constipation, with adequate hydration and nutrition and with moderate physical activity.
- Maintain adequate perineal hygiene.
- Perform a competent rehabilitation of the pelvic floor muscles, possibly associated with the off-label use of vaginal diazepam, as early as 1–2 months after delivery, if the woman is not breastfeeding.
- Use lubricants (without petroleum jelly, which can irritate the vaginal lining), estriol, promestriene, hyaluronic acid, and vitamin E to correct vaginal dryness.

All the attention necessary to bring the woman back to optimal psycho-physical conditions must be undertaken, since good general health is a necessary prerequisite for any sexual therapy. Among these interventions, the correction of iron-deficiency anemia, particularly frequent in postpartum women, is mandatory.

2.8 Factors of Sexual Vulnerability in Reproductive Age

2.8.1 Endometriosis

Endometriosis is a powerful disruptor of female sexual function in young women. It is a progressive, chronic pathology, which affects one or two out of ten women. Despite the high prevalence, the diagnostic delay ranges between 4 and 12 years.

The natural history of endometriosis (and, in general, of all chronic pathologies) can be read as a two-stage film. In the first stage of the disease movie, symptoms and signs are present, while small endometriosis lesions are still below the visibility threshold; in the second stage of the film, the endometriotic lesions become visible with current imaging methods and diagnostic laparoscopy (Fig. 1).

Regarding the relationship between endometriosis and female sexual dysfunction, it should be emphasized that pain on penetration (**dyspareunia**) is a predictive symptom of endometriosis (OR of 9.4) [55].

For a complete discussion on endometriosis, we refer the reader to the pertinent chapter.

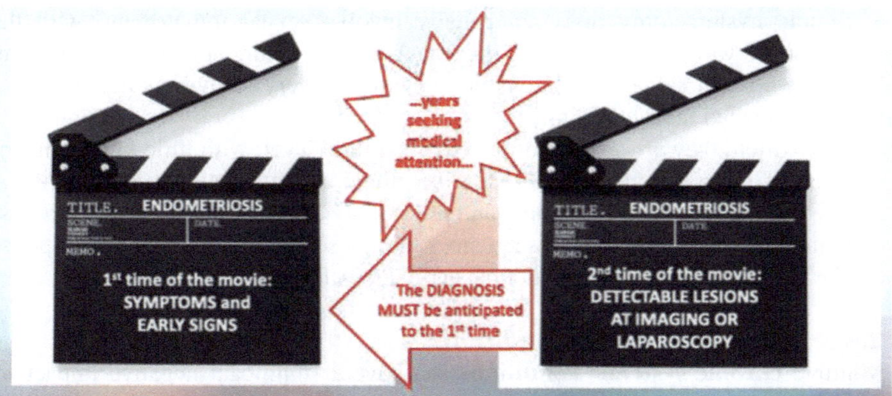

Fig. 1 Endometriosis: a two-times movie. [In this figure, endometriosis is represented as a movie in two times, as presented by the authors during the Endometriosis Consensus in Strasbourg (September 15–17, 2022)]

2.8.2 Infertility

Infertility and the use of **medically assisted reproductive techniques** can have a negative effect on one's body image and the couple's relationship. They can therefore induce or exacerbate sexual dysfunctions.

2.8.3 Sexual Abuse

Current or previous **sexual abuse** is an element of vulnerability in sexual function across the lifespan. A worrying spike of sexual abuse during pregnancy is reported. On the other hand, women who were victims of childhood sexual abuse are at higher risk of having an adverse experience with pregnancy, childbirth, and child care [56].

2.8.4 Cancer

Women diagnosed with **cancer**, especially gynecological and breast cancer, and treated for it, frequently experience considerable anxiety about their sexual future. However, they rarely find clinical availability for competent advice on this topic in the oncological field, with rare exceptions.

For a discussion about these topics, we refer the reader to the next chapter and to the subsequent pertinent chapters (***Lower Gastrointestinal Cancer and Sexual Function***; ***Sexuality in Adult Cancer Survivors in the Era of Precision Oncology***; ***Breast Cancer and Sexual Health***).

2.8.5 Gynecological Surgery

The main gynecological surgery a woman can undergo during reproductive age is **hysterectomy**. Adnexectomy must be avoided if possible, to preserve hormonal function. This is usually not possible if the indication to surgery is a gynecological cancer.

Simple hysterectomy does not usually involve sexual impairment, with the exception of women who had an important uterine component in their orgasm. Women who complain of sexual dysfunction after surgery often think that hysterectomy diminished their femininity.

More often, they are women of low sociocultural level, with little knowledge of the type of intervention that is proposed to them and of what it really entails. A detailed explanation of the anatomy and physiology of the genital system, their possible modifications, and the consequences that these may have on sexual response can be very useful in dispelling doubts and fears before surgery is carried out.

2.8.6 Chronic Systemic Conditions

Multiple **chronic systemic conditions** can have a significant negative impact on sexual desire and function [37]. It can be direct or due to side effects of medications. Some of these diseases, for example neurological and autoimmune pathologies, have a strong negative effect on the self-image women have, besides affecting the physiological basis of the sexual response itself.

For a comprehensive dissertation about these topics, the reader should refer to the pertinent chapters in this book.

2.9   Conclusion

Female sexual dysfunctions (FSDs) are common in adolescence, reproductive age, and menopause. In reproductive age, greater attention should be paid to sexual vulnerabilities that can occur during pregnancy and puerperium. Every physician, top of the list family physicians and gynecologists, should routinely include a few sexual questions in their general clinical history, to give the woman patient the solid feeling that a respectful listening, a competent diagnosis, and first-line therapeutic advice will be offered if indicated.

3   Sexuality Across Lifespan III: Women's Vulnerabilities from Early Menopause to Senescence

Alessandra Graziottin and Angela Cuccarollo

3.1   Introduction

Key vulnerabilities affecting women during perimenopause, menopause, and senescence will be the focus of this chapter. Premature ovarian insufficiency and associated female sexual dysfunctions (FSDs) are discussed in the chapter ***Endocrine Disorders and Sexuality II: Ovary***.

The **diagnosis of menopause** is based on the absence of menstrual periods for 12 consecutive months and on specific menopausal symptoms in hysterectomized women [57–59]. The average age at menopause is 51 years. *Perimenopause* is a vulnerable period of life, usually lasting several years, that begins with the appearance of the first symptoms and ends 1 year after the final menstrual period [57]. Both the diagnosis of menopause and perimenopause can be made without hormonal test in healthy women aged over 45 years [57]. It is appropriate to use FSH test to diagnose menopause in women aged 40–45 years complaining of menopausal symptoms, including a change in their menstrual cycle, and in women aged under 40 years in whom premature menopause is suspected [57].

Menopause is defined as *premature* when it is complained of before age 40; *early* when it happens before age 45; and *late onset* when the last period is reported after age 55 [59].

3.2   Symptoms of Perimenopause and Menopause

Women in perimenopause usually experience a change in the pattern of their menstrual cycle (oligomenorrhea, polymenorrhea, polymenorrhagia, menometrorrhagia, or a mixed pattern of these conditions). Women in menopause are by definition in amenorrhea.

Heavy menstrual bleeding is frequent in perimenopause, causing iron-deficiency anemia (IDA), fatigue, depression, memory difficulties, poor work productivity, and loss of sex drive with impaired sexual response.

Besides changes in menstrual pattern, women in perimenopause and menopause can present with a variety of symptoms, as summarized in Table 1.

Table 1 Symptoms of perimenopause and menopause

Brain-driven symptoms	Sexual and urogenital symptoms	Musculoskeletal symptoms
Neurovegetative disorders • Insomnia • Night tachycardia • Hot flushes	**Sexual symptoms** • Loss of sexual drive, sexual interest, and desire • Reduced central and peripheral arousal • Vaginal dryness • Introital or superficial dyspareunia/sexual pain • Orgasmic difficulties, with fading of the intensity of orgasmic pleasure • Decreased frequency of sexual activity • Decreased overall sexual response	**Joint symptoms** • Pain • Stiffness • Swelling • Morning rigidity – Early osteoarthritis
Affective disorders • Mood swings • Perimenstrual syndrome • Irritability • Depression • Anxiety	**Body image and body feelings concerns** • Reduced metabolism • Increase in body weight and white abdominal fat • Poor body image and frustrating body feelings • Skin aging; changes in hair and nail • Breast loss of shape and texture	**Muscle symptoms** • Myalgia • Reduced strength • Early sarcopenia
Cognitive and motor disorders • Concentration difficulties • Memory difficulties • Reduced verbal fluency • Loss of fine motor skills		**Bone/disc symptoms** • Reduced height • Back pain (of mixed origin)

Gastrointestinal symptoms	Urinary symptoms	Worsening of menstrual symptoms in perimenopause
• Irritable bowel syndrome (IBS) worsening • Bloating/swelling • Digestive difficulties • Constipation	• Nycturia • Urgency/urge incontinence • Stress incontinence • Mixed incontinence • Postcoital cystitis • Recurrent cystitis	• Dysmenorrhea • PMS • Sleep disorders • Binge eating • Headache • Chronic pelvic pain • Water retention/swelling • Menstrual asthma

3.3 Female Sexual Dysfunctions in Menopause and Senescence

Female sexual dysfunctions (FSDs) increase across **menopause** and **senescence** in sexually active women, due to hormonal changes per se and through their impact on all organs and tissues involved in the physiology of women's sexual function [7, 60, 61]. Aging, concurrent pelvic and systemic pathologies, and partner's sexual dysfunctions further contribute. Contextual factors, economic difficulties, low educational level, difficulties to obtain an appropriate medical diagnosis and treatment of FSDs, and work-associated and family-related issues further complicate the clinical scenario. The prevalence of FSDs increases with age and especially after menopause, if:

1. The woman is not receiving adequate lifestyle's information and does not commit herself to better daily habits
2. Appropriate assessment of comorbid dysfunctions/pathologies is not carried out
3. A well-tailored menopausal hormone therapy (MHT) is not timely started, when not contraindicated

The sexual and urogenital disorders most frequently complained of with advancing age, and especially after the menopause, when not treated with at least topical MHT, contribute to the genitourinary syndrome of menopause (GSM). They are listed in Table 1. For a comprehensive discussion on FSDs across the lifespan, please refer to the previous chapter.

Sexual symptoms may anticipate the last menstrual period of several years: they can be the first alerting symptom of an impending early menopause.

Key biological changes that contribute to the increase of FSDs from perimenopause to senescence include low sexual hormone levels, involution of clitoral cavernous bodies, and systemic low-level inflammation and neuroinflammation.

- **Low sexual hormone levels**
- Variations in the levels of sexual hormones can reduce sexual desire/interest/drive, with worsening of the whole sexual response and reduced frequency of sexual activity [7, 60, 61]. Main changes in the sexual system determined by hormonal variations include:
- Genito-pelvic and urinary changes [18]
  - Vulvar aging/dystrophy
  - Reduction in the production of vaginal lubricating fluid
  - Loss of vaginal elasticity, associated with a reduction in the mucosa thickness with progressive atrophy of the vaginal wall
  - Involution of cavernous bodies and vaginal vascular system
  - Involution of the pelvic floor muscles, with increasing connective component
  - Nerves aging
  - Involution of the urethral and bladder architecture with thinning of the urethral wall

All these contribute to the genitourinary syndrome of the menopause (GSM).

- Systemic changes
  - Skin and cutaneous adnexal changes, with increasing wrinkles, skin thinning, whitening and loss of hair, and nail fragility
  - Weight gain and fat accumulation around the abdomen and hips
  - Breast loss of shape and texture
  - Postural changes and loss of muscular and bone trophism

All these changes in body appearance affect body self-image and body feelings, with variable effects on psychological well-being and sexual function, according to the esthetic values and priorities of the woman's cultural background.

In addition, some of them have general health and sexual consequences:

- The increase of white abdominal fat is a predictor of metabolic and cardiovascular diseases (also contributing to FSD due to genital vessel and nerve damage) [62].
- Loss of muscular and bone trophism, together with poor posture and body balance, increases the risk of falls and fractures, with reduced mobility and autonomy in daily activities and progressive decline in neurological functioning.

Plasmatic levels of testosterone and dehydroepiandrosterone (DHEA), the biological fuels of sex drive and arousal, peak around 20 years of age and then progressively decline [63, 64]. Testosterone and its active metabolite dihydrotestosterone (DHT) are the most potent endogenous ligands of androgen receptors. Testosterone can be considered as a prohormone, acting through the three main mechanisms represented in Fig. 2. Testosterone is produced in women, in their reproductive age,

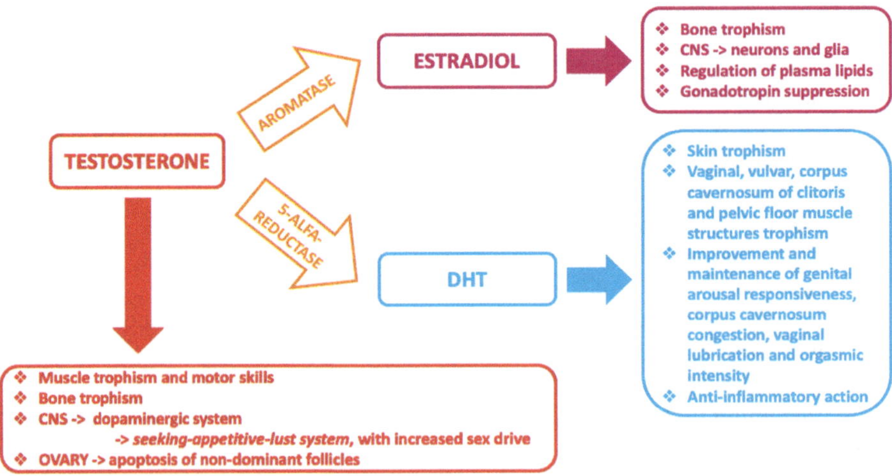

Fig. 2 Testosterone as a prohormone *(courtesy of S. Bhasin, modified by the authors)*

for about a quarter in the ovaries, a quarter in the adrenal glands, and the remaining in peripheral fat tissues [65]. The decreased ovarian activity in menopause also involves Leydig cells that are responsible for the secretion of testosterone. A woman in her 50 s has lost about 50% of testosterone and 60–70% of DHEA, mainly of adrenal production.

A dramatic drop in estrogens and progesterone levels is the leading endocrinological feature of menopause, with the final stop of menstrual periods. In parallel, the gradual age-related decline of androgens contributes to systemic and urogenital aging and to a low-grade systemic inflammation, typical of postmenopause (Box 11) [66]. Androgen deficiency is related to specific signs and symptoms (**androgen insufficiency syndrome—AIS**) (Box 12) [67].

Box 11 Sexual Hormone Levels in Women

In 1999, Rogerio Arnaldo Lobo compared the levels of different hormones in the various ages of a woman's life, using the picograms/milliliter as the only unit of measurement (Table 2) [68]. With this simple equivalence, it emerged that androgens in childbearing age are much more represented in the female body than estrogens, with the exception of pregnancy, and that iatrogenic menopause, with surgical removal or radio-chemotherapeutic destruction of the ovarian tissue, reduces testosterone levels far more than physiological menopause.

Box 12 Androgen Insufficiency Syndrome (AIS)

The most frequently reported systemic, urogenital, and sexual symptoms and signs of androgen deficiency include the following:

Systemic

- Asthenia
- Reduced energy and vitality
- Reduced assertiveness
- Hypotonic ("slumped") posture
- Anxiety and depression
- Loss of strength, muscle mass, and competence; underlying inflammation; and destruction of muscle tissue (sarcopenia)
- Inflammation and pain

Urogenital

- Urgency/urge incontinence
- Stress incontinence
- Mixed incontinence
- Recurrent cystitis

- Hypoactive pelvic floor (worsening of postdelivery outcomes)
- Hyperactive pelvic floor, in nulliparous and women who had only cesarean deliveries
- Vulvovaginal dystrophy/atrophy: pale color, reduced mucosal thickness, petechiae
- High vaginal pH (6.5–7)
- Clitoral and/or vulvar hypotrophy
- Loss and/or whitening of vulvar hair
- Labia conglutination, if lichen sclerosus is comorbid

Sexual

- Generalized hypoactive sexual desire disorder
- Reduced central and peripheral arousal
- Reduced excitability/sexual responsiveness
- Vaginal dryness
- Orgasmic disorders, with longer congestion time and reduced orgasmic intensity ("my clitoris is dead")
- Coital pain/superficial dyspareunia/sexual pain
- Cystitis after intercourse ("postcoital cystitis," 24–72 h after intercourse)

Table 2 Levels of sexual hormones in women, in picograms/milliliters

	Healthy woman in reproductive age	Menopause	Iatrogenic menopause
Estrogens	100–150	10–15	10
Testosterone	400	290	110
Androstenedione	1.900	1.000	700
DHEA	5.000	2.000	1800
DHEA-S	3.000.000	1.000.000	1.000.00

The drop in sex hormone's levels is even more sudden and destructive if it is associated with **iatrogenic menopause** [69, 70]. In particular, bilateral oophorectomy reduces not only estrogen and progesterone levels, but also testosterone's plasma levels up to 80%.

Iatrogenic menopause is the consequence of *surgical removal* of the ovaries or of their functional destruction due to *chemotherapy* and/or *radiotherapy*. In adjunct, radiotherapy, used in the treatment of genital, bladder, and anorectal cancer, induces important changes at the level of the genital system (atrophy, loss of elasticity, reduction in the caliber and length of the vagina up to the conglutination of its walls), which can have dramatic repercussions on sexual function [71]. Vaginal dilators used daily, possibly associated with local creams based on estrogen and/or plant-derived testosterone, can maintain vaginal "habitability." Moreover, **chemotherapy**, besides premature iatrogenic menopause, can cause hair loss and consequent poor self-image, asthenia, and atrophic changes in the vagina. All these factors contribute to the biological basis of FSDs.

MHT, if promptly initiated, can reduce most of the systemic and sexual complications resulting from iatrogenic menopause [72]. Therefore, MHT should be proposed to all women undergoing iatrogenic menopause, in line with law number 1 and law number 2 of world endocrinology (Box 14), with the exception of women affected by hormone-dependent tumors (breast, endometrium, and ovaries) or by high thrombotic risk. MHT has no contraindications in case of HPV-related squamous cell carcinomas [73].

- **Age-dependent involution of clitoral cavernous bodies**
  Back in 1999, Tarcan demonstrated that the clitoral cavernous bodies undergo an age-dependent involution of about 50% from the second to fifth decades of life [49]. It is often associated with significant vulvar dystrophy and/or vulvar lichen sclerosus. This involution correlates linearly with the decrease of testosterone levels since the 20s onwards and the parallel reduced orgasmic capacity. It can be limited and delayed by a timely topical treatment with testosterone cream.
- **Cortisol, low-grade systemic inflammation and neuroinflammation**
- Aging is usually associated with two major biological features [74]:
  1. A progressive increase of cortisol levels (the only hormone that increases with age).
  2. A parallel worsening of low-grade systemic inflammation and neuroinflammation.
  3. Low-grade systemic inflammation and neuroinflammation are also inversely correlated to the decline in androgen levels: the lower the androgen levels, the higher the inflammation (Fig. 2) [60].
- Hot flashes do not simply means "feeling hot." Every hot flash causes a threefold increase in the plasmatic cortisol levels, which can last for 3 h on average. This means that if a woman has eight hot flashes a day, she will persistently have significantly higher cortisol level, further contributing to her systemic inflammation, deterioration of health conditions, and vitality loss. In addition, symptoms such as insomnia, mood swings, and joint and muscle pain have direct pro-inflammatory effects on the central nervous system and indirect effects, through the stress-induced dysbiosis of intestinal microbiota and its effects on the gut brain [75].
- All these neglected biological mechanisms translate into a progressive erosion of the vital energy and loss of the instinctual sex drive, contributing to the disruption of women's sexuality during perimenopause, menopause, and senescence.

3.4   Treatment of Perimenopausal and Menopausal Symptoms

Appropriate lifestyle interventions, menopausal hormone therapy (MHT) (systemic and topical), and rehabilitation of the pelvic floor offer, if synergically used, can significantly improve perimenopausal and menopausal symptoms and FSDs. To address concomitant male sexual dysfunctions, if present, is mandatory. Please see the chapter **Medical Disorders and Sexual Health: Sexual Vulnerabilities in Men**.

Selective estrogen receptor modulators (SERMs) are another important option available to treat GSM and a few menopausal symptoms (Box 13).

> **Box 13 SERMs in the Treatment of GSM and Menopausal Symptoms**
> SERMs used to treat menopausal symptoms are ospemifene and bazedoxifene.
>
> **Ospemifene** is administered orally to treat moderate to severe GSM, with specific benefits on genital and sexual symptoms. It can be prescribed to women with a history of breast cancer, after they have completed all hormonal therapies, including tamoxifen, and to healthy women who are afraid of or do not want MHT. Most frequent side effects complained by patients taking this drug include recurrent vulvovaginal mycotic infections and mild worsening of vasomotor symptoms.
>
> **Bazedoxifene** is an alternative to progestogens to prevent endometrial hyperplasia or cancer during estrogen assumption (*see below*) [58].

- **Lifestyle interventions**
- A healthy lifestyle is the first intervention to be recommended to perimenopausal and menopausal women, including [37]:
  - 45 min of brisk walk outdoor in the morning, to reset the pineal gland ("the solar sensor") and melatonin circadian biorhythm, improve the sleep patterns, and (re)synchronize the hypothalamic master clock and associated circadian biorhythms
  - No cigarette smoke and no drug abuse
  - Zero/very limited alcohol intake
  - Healthy diet and physical activity, to maintain normal weight and healthy intestinal microbiota
  - Care of appropriate posture and body balance
  - Integration with vitamin D and B, iron and folic acid, if necessary
- **Systemic Hormonal Therapy**
- Menopausal hormone therapy (MHT) consists of the administration, systemic and/or topical, of estrogens, progestogens, and androgens (Box 14). Systemic MHT will be discussed here, and the topical in the next paragraph.

During the *perimenopausal transition*, MHT is not indicated and contraception is mandatory in sexually active women to prevent unwanted pregnancies [76]. For these reasons, oral contraceptives (both estro-progestin combined therapy and oral progestogens) or levonorgestrel medicated IUS can be useful both to treat perimenopausal symptoms (including heavy menstrual bleeding) and to guarantee adequate contraception [61].

Box 14 Why to Prescribe MHT: Follow the Two Main Laws in Endocrinology
The cornerstones at the base of the prescription of MHT are the two fundamental laws of endocrinology, according to the first author (AR) lifelong perspective and clinical practice:

1. If a gland is removed for benign reasons, the deficient hormone/hormones must be replaced.
2. If a gland is not working enough, the deficient hormone/hormones must be integrated.

Coherently with these two laws of the world endocrinology, valid and applied to all gland deficiencies (hypophysis, thyroid, parathyroid, adrenals, pancreas, testicles), MHT for menopause is biologically and endocrinologically appropriate. In the authors' opinion, **to deny a woman the right to and the fair information for a tailored MHT is a serious medical omission**.

Treatment is even more compelling after premature ovarian insufficiency, where rigorous data indicate a significant increase of serious comorbidities and risk of earlier death if left untreated, in comparison with age-matched women with normal ovarian function.

The vast majority of women can assume MHT during menopause. Eighty-seven percent of menopausal patients followed by the first author (AG) are on lifelong MHT, with a consistent cluster of patients now well above their 80s. Type of estrogens and progestogens, doses of hormones, route of administration, and regimen are tailored according to leading symptoms and signs, age, comorbidities, and woman's preferences. The remaining 13% do not receive standard MHT because of main contraindications.

Absolute **contraindications** to MHT include [58]:

– Uninvestigated abnormal uterine bleeding (AUB)
– Breast cancer
– Hormone-dependent endometrial cancer type I/untreated endometrial hyperplasia
– Uterine sarcoma
– Granulosa cell tumors and low-grade serous ovarian tumors (especially endometrioid type)
– Coronary and cerebrovascular pathology (e.g., angina, heart attack, stroke)
– Venous thromboembolism (VTE)
– Liver disease, until functional markers return within normal range
– Cutaneous porphyria
– Otosclerosis
– Hypersensitivity to the active drug or to some excipient
– Refusal of the woman

General principles in the prescription of MHT are [58]:

- Start therapy early after menopause, and in any case before age 60 or within 10 years from the last menstrual cycle.
- Personalize the therapy in terms of active principle, dose (start with low doses and increase progressively to the minimum effective dose), and way of administration. In case of very early premature ovarian insufficiency, i.e., before the age of 20, the dose should be appropriate to guarantee the reach of peak bone mass density and all the anatomic and functional systemic benefits.
- Reduce dose with aging.

There are no mandatory indications to stop MHT at a certain age or after a certain number of years of therapy [58]. MHT can be continued until benefits overcome risks. Therefore, it can be continued, according to the woman's wishes, until she enjoys general well-being and has healthy lifestyles and no new contraindications emerge.

Systemic MHT could be administered as [58]:

- Estrogens: estradiol and estriol, and in the next future estetrol. The route of administration includes oral drugs, transdermal patches, spray and gel, and vaginal rings.
- Progestogens: oral drugs, vaginal micronized progesterone, IUD containing levonorgestrel (*off-label*).
- Testosterone and DHEA: oral, injectable, or transdermal drugs.

Systemic MHT, with *estrogens and progestogens* in women with uterus (to prevent endometrial hyperplasia or cancer) and with *estrogens alone* in previously hysterectomized women, is indicated to treat vasomotor symptoms, insomnia, psychological symptoms, and joint and muscular pain [57, 58]. It is also indicated to maintain trophism of urogenital tissues, skin and skin appendages, breast, vertebral disc, muscles, and bones [58].

The role of *androgens* in MHT in menopausal women is controversial, and the main indication is hypoactive sexual desire disorder (HSDD).

The use of *systemic testosterone* is not currently approved in most countries, despite a recent meta-analysis demonstrating its impressive efficacy in improving all sexual domains, and its limpid safety in postmenopausal women [77]. It is therefore still an *off-label* prescription which must be carried out with written informed consent [78].

Dehydroepiandrosterone (DHEA) is an endogenous steroid hormone. It acts as a weak androgen, a weak estrogen, and a neuro-steroid. It is the progenitor of all sexual hormones. As it launches all the pubertal events ("adrenarche"), reaching its peak around 20 years of age, it is considered as "the hormone of youth." It is available in different countries, even as an over-the-counter drug, but systemic therapy is currently banned in Italy.

Before prescribing MHT, women should undergo:

- General blood tests (blood count, liver and kidney function indices, lipids, and glucose) for a comprehensive metabolic assessment
- Weight and height measure to check the body mass index (BMI) and the abdominal circumference (when visceral obesity is present)
- Blood pressure
- Breast and gynecological examination
- Pelvic ultrasound
- Mammography
- Pap test or HPV test
- Bone densitometry: before the age of 50 in selected cases of POI and/or when osteopenia/osteoporosis are suspected on the clinical basis (celiac women, long amenorrhea periods, persisting restrictive eating disorders, low vitamin D and calcium intake); after the age of 50 according to national guidelines

After the beginning of MHT, the woman must be re-evaluated at 3 months and then every year to assess the efficacy and tolerability [57]. If symptoms persist, the woman should be referred to a menopause expert [57].

The risk of venous thromboembolism (VTE) is slightly increased by oral but not transdermal MHT. Therefore, transdermal therapy should be considered in women at higher risk of VTE, such as obese, elderly (especially aged more than 65 years), and known thrombophilic women [57, 58, 79, 80]. In case of a strong family history of VTE or hereditary thrombophilia, the woman should be referred to a hematologist for assessment before prescribing MHT [57].

Systemic MHT, started before age 60 or within 10 years from the last menstrual cycle, does not increase (and probably diminish) the risk to develop cardiovascular disease (CVD) or diabetes mellitus type 2 (DM2) [57, 58, 81]. On the other hand, well-compensated CVD and DM2 are no absolute contraindications to MHT [57, 58].

Patients with uterine myomas, hypercholesterolemia and hypertriglyceridemia, active gallbladder disease, hypertension, and obesity and smokers do not have absolute contraindications to MHT, especially if low doses and transdermal administration are considered. In patients affected by migraine with aura, transdermal administration should be cautiously preferred as well.

MHT is not associated with an increased risk to die due to breast cancer. MHT with estrogens alone is associated with little or no change in the risk to develop breast cancer. Moreover, if estradiol is associated with micronized progesterone (MP that is identical to the progesterone produced by the corpus luteum) or dydrogesterone, there is no increase in the risk of breast cancer.

A familiar history of breast cancer does not contraindicate MHT.

In women with BRCA mutation after oophorectomy, MHT should be taken into account until 51 years (average age of natural menopause) [58]. Prolonged therapy should otherwise be individualized.

MHT is contraindicated in case of previous breast cancer. Systemic MHT could be considered in selected case of severe, invalidating vasomotor symptoms; low-dose vaginal estrogens or DHEA (*see below*) could be considered in case of severe GSM symptoms, in both cases sharing the decision with the oncologist and after a written consensus by the woman.

There is an increasing interest in so-called **compounded bioidentical hormones** for MHT. Both physicians and women must be aware that efficacy and safety, quality, purity, and constituents of such unregulated galenic compounds are not demonstrated [58]. For this reason, "unless an authorized equivalent preparation is not available," the prescription of compounded bioidentical hormones should be avoided (*see below for the discussion on galenic testosterone*) [58, 78].

On the sidelines, **herbal medicine**, and especially isoflavones and black cohosh, as an alternative to MHT, has demonstrated efficacy in relieving vasomotor symptoms. However, the woman must be aware that the multiple preparations available have different efficacy and uncertain safety and may interact with other drugs [58].

- **Rehabilitation of the pelvic floor**
- In case of **comorbidity with pelvic floor hypertonicity**, more frequent in nulliparous women or women who have given birth only by cesarean section, **physiotherapy** is essential to relax the over-contracted muscles, thus reducing the biomechanical components of sexual pain, vestibulodynia, and comorbid postcoital cystitis. The use of vaginal dilators can complement the rehabilitation therapy.

3.5 Genitourinary Syndrome of the Menopause and Topical Hormone Therapy

Genitourinary syndrome of the menopause is characterized by vulvovaginal, sexual, and urinary symptoms (Table 3) [33]. These symptoms underlie a chronic and destructive inflammatory process that involves full-thickness genitourinary anatomical structures, leading to vulvovaginal atrophy (VVA) and parallel involution of urethral, bladder, and corpora cavernosa structures, as well as muscle-connective structures of the pelvic floor [82].

These genital biological impairments are important etiological factors both in the decline of postmenopausal sex drive (HSDD) and in the reduction of genital arousal, pleasure, and orgasmic intensity.

Table 3 Symptoms of GSM

Vulvovaginal	Sexual	Urinary
• Vaginal dryness	• Lack of vaginal lubrication	• Urgency
• Burning	• Coital pain/dyspareunia	• Dysuria
• Itching	• Orgasmic difficulties	• Cystitis
• Leucorrhoea	• Sexual dysfunctions	

Vulvovaginal and sexual symptoms of GSM can be effectively treated with **local therapy**, like:

- Vulvar and vaginal lubricants and moisturizers
- Laser treatments
- Estrogen cream or ovules
- Testosterone cream
- Prasterone ovules

Local therapy can lead to more significant results if used in synergy with systemic MHT and pelvic floor rehabilitation.

- **Lubricants and moisturizers**
- Vulvar and vaginal lubricants and moisturizers are the first-line therapeutic to GSM, but they have limited efficacy.
- **Laser treatments**
- Vaginal laser therapy (especially Er:YAG and microablative CO_2) demonstrated effectiveness in restoring vaginal health, improving VVA symptoms and sexual function. The data suggest that both Er:YAG and CO_2 vaginal lasers are safe energy-based therapeutic options for the management of GSM symptoms in postmenopausal women and breast cancer survivors [83].
- **Estrogen creams and ovules**
- Estrogen creams and ovules are the first hormonal option to be considered. Topical low-dose estrogens do not seem to have proliferative effects on the endometrium; thus, progestogen association is not required in non-hysterectomized women.
- Concerns exist about local estrogen therapy in breast and other hormone-dependent cancer survivors. However, topical estrogens can be considered in case of unresponsiveness to nonhormonal therapies.
- **Testosterone cream**
- All tissues in the genitourinary tract are rich in androgen receptors (ARs) that mediate a powerful trophic role. Therefore, **topical testosterone therapy** is an effective treatment of GSM. Testosterone exerts trophic, anti-inflammatory, sexual, and reconstructive effects on vulva, vestibule, vagina, urethra, corpus cavernosum of clitoris, and pelvic floor muscles [82].
- Maseroli et al. demonstrated in vitro the anti-inflammatory and immunomodulatory effects of DHT, testosterone's metabolite, on human vaginal smooth muscle cells [82]. This scientific evidence supports the clinical experience of over 40 years of the first author (AG), with the use of topical testosterone to treat VVA and related symptoms in menopause. Anecdotally, after 2–3 months of application of testosterone cream on the vulva, many partners report the return of genital sexual perfume lost with menopause. Observation correlates with the well-known effect induced by testosterone on the secretion of sebum and pheromones at the vulvar level, with consequent increase in the olfactory and gustatory allure in oral genital sex.

The experts in the Global Consensus in 2014 sided against testosterone therapy and even more against compounding preparations. In 2019, there was an important turning point, with the experts stating that therapy with "bioidentical" testosterone compounds cannot be recommended for the therapy of HSDD, due to the lack of data on safety and efficacy, "unless an authorized equivalent preparation is not available" [78]. The compounding drug must be prepared according to the Good Manufacturing Practices (GMP), and dosages "should be limited to reaching plasma levels within physiological values for premenopause" [78].

According to the Global Consensus 2019, the main indication for systemic testosterone therapy remains hypoactive sexual desire disorder (HSDD) [78]. However, GSM is the anatomical factor that most contributes to the suppression of desire, due to negative genital feedback and the disappointing sexual response. Given these biological evidences, according to the authors, it is appropriate to consider GSM as the main indication for topical genital therapy. Compounding preparations based on testosterone can therefore be indicated for the treatment of GSM, especially when the patient complains mainly of genital sexual symptoms.

In addition, the vulvovaginal administration of testosterone leads to a variable amount of systemic absorption of the drug, depending on dose and anatomical conditions that favor absorption, such as large contact surface with the drug, rich network of vessels, and high mucosal permeability more frequent at the beginning of treatment in case of severe atrophy.

The systemic absorption of testosterone has dual effects:

- Positive, in case of loss of sexual desire, which can be improved in its biological component by testosterone.
- Negative, in case of sensitivity of skin and hair appendages to the androgenic effects of testosterone, with seborrhea, acne, hypertrichosis, hirsutism, and alopecia.

Due to these potential negative effects, it is advisable to dose testosterone both before and during treatment, to exclude supraphysiological levels [78].

To date, there is no medicinal specialty in testosterone cream, for vulvovaginal use, approved by the AIFA and the EMA. The only testosterone-based drug approved for women is AndroFeme®1, a cream registered in 2020 in Australia and used to treat postmenopausal women with HSDD. Therefore, in the absence of authorized testosterone vaginal creams for the treatment of vulvovaginal and sexual symptoms in postmenopausal women, the use of testosterone-based compounding preparations is consistent with the 2019 Global Consensus and has demonstrated efficacy and safety (Box 15).

> **Box 15 Efficacy and Safety of Testosterone Therapy**
> Evidence on the beneficial effects of androgen, particularly testosterone, therapy on postmenopausal women has been available since 1946 [84]. A recent systematic review and meta-analysis demonstrated that testosterone administered non-orally (e.g., via transdermal patches or cream) improves sexual function in postmenopausal women with low sex drive [77].
>
> In 2019, the Global Consensus stated that **systemic therapy with testosterone** (at doses close to premenopausal physiological doses), up to 24 months, **does not** (level 1, grade A) [78]:
>
> – Increase mammographic density.
> – Impact the risk of breast cancer.
> – Associate with major adverse events.
>
> Therefore, it is reasonable to assume that local therapy at low doses is at least as safe as systemic administration.

Testosterone is administered for therapeutic purposes as [84]:

– **Esters**: synthetic prodrugs that differ from testosterone in chemical and pharmacokinetic characteristics, especially a longer half-life, with reduced frequency of administration.
– **Bioidentical**: semisynthetic testosterone, obtained from a plant matrix containing steroid-based molecules, with a plasmatic half-life of less than 12 h and complete elimination within 24 h.

The two currently most prescribed compounding preparations of testosterone for vulvovaginal use are the following [84]:

1. **Testosterone propionate**

   It is a testosterone ester. The compounding formulation, in stringy Vaseline, at 1% or 2%, has been used in gynecology for more than 50 years. Given the testosterone propionate long half-life, this ointment should usually be applied in "minimal amounts" (the ointment should be taken with the fingertip of the index finger, in the amount of about 1 cm wide by a millimeter thick, and then applied to the vulva and vestibule) to minimize negative systemic effects. After about 2 weeks of attack therapy, a vulvovaginal application twice a week is recommended. However, since the estimate of the "minimum amount" is subjective, the variability on the amount of ointment actually administered per day and absorbed is very wide.

2. **Vegetal origin testosterone**

   It is commonly formulated in Pentravan® transdermal cream and administered thanks to Topi-Click® pharmaceutical dispensers at maximum dosage of 2.8 mg/day. Due to the elimination time of 24 h, daily administration is possible without the risk of negative systemic effects.

The plasma concentration of testosterone in women presents a single acrophase in the very early hours of the morning and then maintains a baseline level throughout the rest of the day [85]. Therefore, the morning administration is optimal.

The patient should test the drug, applying a click of cream at the level of the pubis, once a day, for a week. If no adverse reactions appear, the patient can continue by applying a first click on the labia, half by side (not on the clitoris, unless in case of severe atrophy, to avoid unwanted increases in volume), and a second click at the vaginal entrance and, with the finger, on the anterior vaginal wall, to optimize the effectiveness also on urinary symptoms. After 3 months of treatment, the patient should be re-examined for the optimal maintenance dose.

Women with early, spontaneous or iatrogenic, menopause can benefit even more from treatment with topical testosterone, possibly associated with systemic MHT [72]. Testosterone therapy is contraindicated in women who have had hormone-dependent breast, endometrial, or ovarian cancer.

- **Prasterone**
  Prasterone is the synthetic analogue of DHEA that is available for prescription in vaginal ovules. In this formulation, it is indicated for the treatment of GSM. DHEA is absorbed into epithelial cells of the vagina and here is converted into androgens and estrogens, exerting its effects according to the principles of intracrinology.

3.6 Conclusion

Perimenopause, menopause, and senescence can cause, worsen, or precipitate FSDs, with a multifactorial etiology. A more comprehensive attention to women in perimenopausal and menopausal ages should be guaranteed by all practitioners. Adequate interventions (healthy lifestyles, MHT, and rehabilitation of pelvic floor) should be promoted if indicated to effectively address the leading biological etiologies of FSDs.

References

1. Graziottin A, Maseroli E, Vignozzi L. Female sexual dysfunctions: a clinical perspective on HSDD, FAD, PGAD, and FOD. In: Bettocchi C, Carrieri G, Cormio L, Busetto GM, editors. Practical clinical andrology. Springer; 2022.
2. Calabrò RS, Cacciola A, Bruschetta D, Milardi D, Quattrini F, Sciarrone F, la Rosa G, Bramanti P, Anastasi G. Neuroanatomy and function of human sexual behavior: a neglected or unknown issue? Brain Behav. 2019;9:e01389. https://doi.org/10.1002/brb3.1389. PMID: 31568703; PMCID: PMC6908863.
3. Jannini EA, Buisson O, Rubio-Casillas A. Beyond the G-spot: clitourethrovaginal complex anatomy in female orgasm. Nat Rev Urol. 2014;11:531. https://doi.org/10.1038/nrurol.2014.193.

4. Wise NJ, Frangos E, Komisaruk BR. Brain activity unique to orgasm in women: an fMRI analysis. J Sex Med. 2017;14:1380. https://doi.org/10.1016/j.jsxm.2017.08.014. PMID: 28986148; PMCID: PMC5675825.

5. Carter CS. Sex, love and oxytocin: two metaphors and a molecule. Neurosci Biobehav Rev. 2022;143:104948. https://doi.org/10.1016/j.neubiorev.2022.104948. PMID: 36347382; PMCID: PMC9759207.

6. Clayton AH, Goldstein I, Kim NN, Althof SE, Faubion SS, Faught BM, Parish SJ, Simon JA, Vignozzi L, Christiansen K, Davis SR, Freedman MA, Kingsberg SA, Kirana PS, Larkin L, McCabe M, Sadovsky R. The International Society for the Study of Women's Sexual Health Process of care for management of hypoactive sexual desire disorder in women. Mayo Clin Proc. 2018;93:467.

7. Graziottin A, Maseroli E. Sexual pain disorders, vestibulodynia, and recurrent cystitis: the evil trio. In: Bettocchi C, Carrieri G, Cormio L, Busetto GM, editors. Practical clinical andrology. Springer; 2022.

8. Okobi OE. A systemic review on the association between infertility and sexual dysfunction among women utilizing female sexual function index as a measuring tool. Cureus. 2021;13:e16006. https://doi.org/10.7759/cureus.16006. PMID: 34336497; PMCID: PMC8319583.

9. Laumann EO, Paik A, Rosen RC. Sexual dysfunction in the United States: prevalence and predictors. JAMA. 1999;281:537. https://doi.org/10.1001/jama.281.6.537.

10. Graziottin A. Prevalence and evaluation of sexual health problems—HSDD in Europe. J Sex Med. 2007;4:211–9. https://doi.org/10.1111/j.1743-6109.2007.00447.x.

11. Tartagni MV, Graziottin A. The love-shaper: role of the foetus in modulating mother-child attachment through stem cell migration to the maternal brain. Eur J Contracept Reprod Health Care. 2023;28:216. https://doi.org/10.1080/13625187.2023.2216326.

12. Bakker J. The role of steroid hormones in the sexual differentiation of the human brain. J Neuroendocrinol. 2022;34:e13050. https://doi.org/10.1111/jne.13050. Epub 2021 Oct 27.

13. Brann DW, Lu Y, Wang J, Zhang Q, Thakkar R, Sareddy GR, Pratap UP, Tekmal RR, Vadlamudi RK. Brain-derived estrogen and neural function. Neurosci Biobehav Rev. 2022;132:793. https://doi.org/10.1016/j.neubiorev.2021.11.014. PMID: 34823913; PMCID: PMC8816863.

14. Catalano PM, Kirwan JP, Haugel-de Mouzon S, King J. Gestational diabetes and insulin resistance: role in short- and long-term implications for mother and fetus. J Nutr. 2003;133:1674S. https://doi.org/10.1093/jn/133.5.1674S.

15. Means RT. Iron deficiency and iron deficiency anemia: implications and impact in pregnancy, fetal development, and early childhood parameters. Nutrients. 2020;12:20447. https://doi.org/10.3390/nu12020447. PMID: 32053933; PMCID: PMC7071168.

16. Ragusa A, Svelato A, Santacroce C, Catalano P, Notarstefano V, Carnevali O, Papa F, Rongioletti MCA, Baiocco F, Draghi S, D'Amore E, Rinaldo D, Matta M, Giorgini E. Plasticenta: first evidence of microplastics in human placenta. Environ Int. 2021;146:106274. https://doi.org/10.1016/j.envint.2020.106274.

17. Baldaro Verde J, Graziottin A. L'enigma dell'identità. Il transessualismo. Torino: EGA-Edizioni Gruppo Abele; 1991.

18. Graziottin A, Murina F. Vulvar pain: from childhood to old age. Springer; 2017.

19. Vandenbosch L, Fardouly J, Tiggemann M. Social media and body image: recent trends and future directions. Curr Opin Psychol. 2022;45:101289. https://doi.org/10.1016/j.copsyc.2021.12.002.

20. Nesi J. The impact of social media on youth mental health: challenges and opportunities. NC Med J. 2020;81:116. https://doi.org/10.18043/ncm.81.2.116.

21. Alberga AS, Withnell SJ, von Ranson KM. Fitspiration and thinspiration: a comparison across three social networking sites. J Eat Disord. 2018;6:39. https://doi.org/10.1186/s40337-018-0227-x. PMID: 30534376; PMCID: PMC6260773.

22. Jerónimo F, Carraça EV. Effects of fitspiration content on body image: a systematic review. Eat Weight Disord. 2022;27:3017. https://doi.org/10.1007/s40519-022-01505-4. PMID: 36401082; PMCID: PMC9676749.

23. Benabe E, Fuentes Y, Roldan G, Ramos M, Pastrana M, Romaguera J. The perceptions of female genital self-image and its associations with female sexual distress. Int J Gynaecol Obstet. 2022;157:90. https://doi.org/10.1002/ijgo.13827.

24. Hustad IB, Malmqvist K, Ivanova E, Rück C, Enander J. Does size matter? Genital self-image, genital size, pornography use and openness toward cosmetic genital surgery in 3503 Swedish men and women. J Sex Med. 2022;19:1378. https://doi.org/10.1016/j.jsxm.2022.06.006.

25. Richards C, Bouman WP, Seal L, Barker MJ, Nieder TO, T'Sjoen G. Non-binary or genderqueer genders. Int Rev Psychiatry. 2016;28:95. https://doi.org/10.3109/09540261.2015.1106446.

26. Ventriglio A, Bhugra D. Sexuality in the 21st century: sexual fluidity, vol. 29. East Asian Arch Psychiatry; 2019. p. 30.

27. Lavorato E, Rampino A, Giorgielli V (2022) Gender dysphoria: overview and psychological interventions. In: Bettocchi C, Carrieri G, Cormio L, Busetto GM (ed.) Practical clinical andrology, Springer

28. Greenberg DR, Khandwala YS, Breyer BN, Minkow R, Eisenberg ML. Genital pain and numbness and female sexual dysfunction in adult bicyclists. J Sex Med. 2019;16:1381. https://doi.org/10.1016/j.jsxm.2019.06.017.

29. Baeyens L, Vermeersch E, Bourgeois P. Bicyclist's vulva: observational study. BMJ. PMID: 12130610; PMCID: PMC117232. 2002;325:138.

30. Trofaier ML, Schneidinger C, Marschalek J, Hanzal E, Umek W. Pelvic floor symptoms in female cyclists and possible remedies: a narrative review. Int Urogynecol J. 2016;27:513. https://doi.org/10.1007/s00192-015-2803-9.

31. Parish SJ, Cottler-Casanova S, Clayton AH, McCabe MP, Coleman E, Reed GM. The evolution of the female sexual disorder/dysfunction definitions, nomenclature, and classifications: a review of DSM, ICSM, ISSWSH, and ICD. Sex Med Rev. 2021;9:36.

32. Imprialos KP, Koutsampasopoulos K, Katsimardou A, Bouloukou S, Theodoulidis I, Themistoklis M, Doumas M. Female sexual dysfunction: a problem hidden in the shadows. Curr Pharm Des. 2021;27:3762. https://doi.org/10.2174/1381612827666210719104950.

33. Portman DJ, Gass ML, Vulvovaginal Atrophy Terminology Consensus Conference Panel. Genitourinary syndrome of menopause: new terminology for vulvovaginal atrophy from the International Society for the Study of Women's Sexual Health and the North American Menopause Society Menopause. 2014;21:1063. https://doi.org/10.1097/GME.0000000000000329.

34. Shifren JL, Monz BU, Russo PA, Segreti A, Johannes CB. Sexual problems and distress in United States women: prevalence and correlates. Obstet Gynecol. 2008;112:970. https://doi.org/10.1097/AOG.0b013e3181898cdb.

35. Toxqui L, Vaquero MP. Chronic iron deficiency as an emerging risk factor for osteoporosis: a hypothesis. Nutrients. 2015;7:2324.

36. Atlantis E, Sullivan T. Bidirectional association between depression and sexual dysfunction: a systematic review and meta-analysis. J Sex Med. 2012;9:1497. https://doi.org/10.1111/j.1743-6109.2012.02709.x.

37. Graziottin A, Cuccarollo A. La sessualità nella donna: implicazioni cliniche in ginecologia e ostetricia. In: Pescetto G. De Cecco L. (curatori Pecorari D. Ragni N.), Ginecologia e ostetricia. Nuova edizione a cura di Simone Ferrero. In press.

38. Ghosh A, Kathiravan S, Sharma K, Mattoo SK. A scoping review of the prevalence and correlates of sexual dysfunction in adults with substance use disorders. J Sex Med. 2022;19:216. https://doi.org/10.1016/j.jsxm.2021.11.018.ù.

39. Harte CB, Meston CM. The inhibitory effects of nicotine on physiological sexual arousal in nonsmoking women: results from a randomized, double-blind, placebo-controlled, cross-over trial. J Sex Med. 2008;5:1184. https://doi.org/10.1111/j.1743-6109.2008.00778.x.

40. Postma R, Bicanic I, van der Vaart H, Laan E. Pelvic floor muscle problems mediate sexual problems in young adult rape victims. J Sex Med. 2013;10:1978. https://doi.org/10.1111/jsm.12196.

41. Handy AB, Freihart BK, Meston CM. The relationship between subjective and physiological sexual arousal in women with and without arousal concerns. J Sex Marital Ther. 2020;46:447.

42. Parish SJ, Meston CM, Althof SE, Clayton AH, Goldstein I, Goldstein SW, Heiman JR, McCabe MP, Segraves RT, Simon JA. Toward a more evidence-based nosology and nomenclature for female sexual dysfunctions—part III. J Sex Med. 2019;16:452. https://doi.org/10.1016/j.jsxm.2019.01.010.
43. Segnini I, Kukkonen TM. Psychological management of arousal disorders. In: Goldstein I, Clayton AH, Goldstein AT, Kim NN, Kingsberg SA, editors. Textbook of female sexual function and dysfunction: diagnosis and treatment. 1st ed. Wiley; 2018.
44. Basson R. Women's sexual desire—disordered or misunderstood? J Sex Marital Ther. 2002;28:17–28. https://doi.org/10.1080/009262302252851168.
45. Goldstein I, Komisaruk BR, Pukall CF, Kim NN, Goldstein AT, Goldstein SW, Hartzell-Cushanick R, Kellogg-Spadt S, Kim CW, Jackowich RA, Parish SJ, Patterson A, Peters KM, Pfaus JG. International Society for the Study of Women's sexual health (ISSWSH) review of epidemiology and pathophysiology, and a consensus nomenclature and process of care for the management of persistent genital arousal disorder/genito-pelvic dysesthesia (PGAD/GPD). J Sex Med. 2021;18:665.
46. Pease ER, Ziegelmann M, Vencill JA, Kok SN, Collins CS, Betcher HK. Persistent genital arousal disorder (PGAD): a clinical review and case series in support of multidisciplinary management. Sex Med Rev. 2022;10:53.
47. Simons JS, Carey MP. Prevalence of sexual dysfunctions: results from a decade of research. Arch Sex Behav. 2001;30:177. https://doi.org/10.1023/a:1002729318254.
48. Parish SJ, Goldstein AT, Goldstein SW, Goldstein I, Pfaus J, Clayton AH, Giraldi A, Simon JA, Althof SE, Bachmann G, Komisaruk B, Levin R, Spadt SK, Kingsberg SA, Perelman MA, Waldinger MD, Whipple B. Toward a more evidence-based nosology and nomenclature for female sexual dysfunctions—part II. J Sex Med. 2016;13:1888.
49. Tarcan T, Park K, Goldstein I, Maio G, Fassina A, Krane RJ, Azadzoi KM. Histomorphometric analysis of age-related structural changes in human clitoral cavernosal tissue. J Urol. 1999;161:940.
50. Kong L, Li T, Li L. The impact of sexual intercourse during pregnancy on obstetric and neonatal outcomes: a cohort study in China. J Obstet Gynaecol. 2019;39:455. https://doi.org/10.1080/01443615.2018.1533930.
51. Ghasemi V, Beheshti Nasab M, Saei Ghare Naz M, Shahsavari S, Banaei M. Estimating the prevalence of dyspareunia according to mode of delivery: a systematic review and meta-analysis. J Obstet Gynaecol. 2022;42:2867. https://doi.org/10.1080/01443615.2022.2110461.
52. McDonald EA, Gartland D, Small R, Brown SJ. Dyspareunia and childbirth: a prospective cohort study. BJOG. 2015;122:672. https://doi.org/10.1111/1471-0528.13263.
53. Crescini C. Prevenzione dei traumi perineali e del dolore correlato nel post parto. In: Colao A. Graziottin A. Uccella S. (a cura di), Atti e approfondimenti di farmacologia del corso ECM su "Dolore, infiammazione e comorbilità in ginecologia e ostetricia", organizzato dalla Fondazione Alessandra Graziottin per la cura del dolore nella donna Onlus, Milano, 23 novembre 2022, p. 95–99.
54. Graziottin A, Cuccarollo A, Donini M. Diagnosi e cura del dolore sessuale dopo il parto. In: Colao A. Graziottin A. Uccella S. (a cura di), Atti e approfondimenti di farmacologia del corso ECM su "Dolore, infiammazione e comorbilità in ginecologia e ostetricia", organizzato dalla Fondazione Alessandra Graziottin per la cura del dolore nella donna Onlus, Milano, 23 novembre 2022, p. 100–109.
55. Ballard KD, Seaman HE, de Vries CS, Wright JT. Can symptomatology help in the diagnosis of endometriosis? Findings from a national case-control study—Part 1. BJOG. 2008;115(11):1382–91. https://doi.org/10.1111/j.1471-0528.2008.01878.x.
56. Brunton R, Dryer R. Child sexual abuse and pregnancy: a systematic review of the literature. Child Abuse Negl. 2021;111:104802. https://doi.org/10.1016/j.chiabu.2020.104802.
57. NICE guideline [NG23] Menopause: diagnosis and management. 2015. https://www.nice.org.uk/guidance/ng23. Accessed 5 Dec 2019.

58. The 2022 Hormone Therapy Position Statement of the North American Menopause Society Advisory Panel. The 2022 hormone therapy position statement of the North American Menopause Society. Menopause. 2022;29:767. https://doi.org/10.1097/GME.0000000000002028.

59. Rees M, Abernethy K, Bachmann G, Bretz S, Ceausu I, Durmusoglu F, Erkkola R, Fistonic I, Gambacciani M, Geukes M, Goulis DG, Griffiths A, Hamoda H, Hardy C, Hartley C, Hirschberg AL, Kydd A, Marshall S, Meczekalski B, Mendoza N, Mueck A, Persand E, Riach K, Smetnik A, Stute P, van Trotsenburg M, Yuksel N, Weiss R, Lambrinoudaki I. The essential menopause curriculum for healthcare professionals: a European Menopause and Andropause Society (EMAS) position statement. Maturitas. 2022;158:70. https://doi.org/10.1016/j.maturitas.2021.12.001.

60. Graziottin A, Cuccarollo A, Uccella S, Franchi MP. Estrogeni e infiammazione. L'Endocrinologo. 2022;23:281. https://doi.org/10.1007/s40619-022-01073-w.

61. Graziottin A, Cuccarollo A, Franchi MP, Uccella S. Patologie mestruali e contraccezione: principi di personalizzazione della scelta terapeutica. L'Endocrinologo. 2022;23:503. https://doi.org/10.1007/s40619-022-01155-9.

62. Anagnostis P, Paschou SA, Katsiki N, Krikidis D, Lambrinoudaki I, Goulis DG. Menopausal hormone therapy and cardiovascular risk: where are we now? Curr Vasc Pharmacol. 2019;17:564. https://doi.org/10.2174/1570161116666180709095348.

63. Harper AJ, Buster JE, Casson PR. Changes in adrenocortical function with aging and therapeutic implications. Semin Reprod Endocrinol. 1999;17:327. https://doi.org/10.1055/s-2007-1016242.

64. Davison SL, Bell R, Donath S, Montalto JG, Davis SR. Androgen levels in adult females: changes with age, menopause, and oophorectomy. J Clin Endocrinol Metab. 2005;90:3847. https://doi.org/10.1210/jc.2005-0212.

65. Ostrowska Z, Zwirska-Korczala K, Pardela M, Drozdz M, Kos-Kudla B, Buntner B. Circadian variations of androstenedione, dehydroepiandrosterone sulfate and free testosterone in obese women with menstrual disturbances. Endocr Regul. 1998;32:177.

66. Castelán F, Cuevas-Romero E, Martínez-Gómez M. The expression of hormone receptors as a gateway toward understanding endocrine actions in female pelvic floor muscles. Endocr Metab Immune Disord Drug Targets. 2020;20:305. https://doi.org/10.217 4/1871530319666191009154751.

67. Bachmann G, Bancroft J, Braunstein G, Burger H, Davis S, Dennerstein L, Goldstein I, Guay A, Leiblum S, Lobo R, Notelovitz M, Rosen R, Sarrel P, Sherwin B, Simon J, Simpson E, Shifren J, Spark R, Traish A. Female androgen insufficiency: the Princeton consensus statement on definition, classification, and assessment. Fertil Steril. 2002;77:660. https://doi.org/10.1016/s0015-0282(02)02969-2.

68. Lobo RA. Treatment of menopausal women. Boston: Lippincott, Williams & Wilkins; 1999.

69. Graziottin A, Koochaki PE, Rodenberg CA, Dennerstein L. The prevalence of hypoactive sexual desire disorder in surgically menopausal women: an epidemiological study of women in four European countries. J Sex Med. 2009;6(8):2143–53.

70. Pillay OC, Manyonda I. The surgical menopause. Best Pract Res Clin Obstet Gynaecol. 2022;81:111. https://doi.org/10.1016/j.bpobgyn.2022.03.001.

71. Tramacere F, Lancellotta V, Casà C, Fionda B, Cornacchione P, Mazzarella C, De Vincenzo RP, Macchia G, Ferioli M, Rovirosa A, Gambacorta MA, Colosimo C, Valentini V, Iezzi R, Tagliaferri L. Assessment of sexual dysfunction in cervical cancer patients after different treatment modality: a systematic review. Medicina (Kaunas). 2022;58:91223. https://doi.org/10.3390/medicina58091223. PMID: 36143900; PMCID: PMC9504584.

72. Graziottin A, Lukasiewicz M, Serafini A. Sexual rehabilitation after gynecological cancers. In: Reisman Y, Gianotten WL, editors. Cancer, intimacy and sexuality. Springer; 2017.

73. Deli T, Orosz M, Jakab A. Hormone replacement therapy in cancer survivors—review of the literature. Pathol Oncol Res. 2020;26:63. https://doi.org/10.1007/s12253-018-00569-x. PMID: 30617760; PMCID: PMC7109141.

74. Martocchia A, Gallucci M, Noale M, Maggi S, Cassol M, Stefanelli M, Postacchini D, Proietti A, Barbagallo M, Dominguez LJ, Ferri C, Desideri G, Toussan L, Pastore F, Falaschi GM,

Paolisso G, Falaschi P, AGICO Investigators. The increased cortisol levels with preserved rhythmicity in aging and its relationship with dementia and metabolic syndrome. Aging Clin Exp Res. 2022;34:2733. https://doi.org/10.1007/s40520-022-02262-1.

75. Malesza IJ, Malesza M, Walkowiak J, Mussin N, Walkowiak D, Aringazina R, Bartkowiak-Wieczorek J, Mądry E. High-fat, western-style diet, systemic inflammation, and gut microbiota: a narrative review. Cells. 2021;10:113164. https://doi.org/10.3390/cells10113164. PMID: 34831387; PMCID: PMC8619527.

76. FSRH. Clinical guideline: contraception for women aged over 40 years (August 2017, amended July 2023). https://www.fsrh.org/documents/fsrh-guidance-contraception-for-women-aged-over-40-years-2017/.

77. Islam RM, Bell RJ, Green S, Page MJ, Davis SR. Safety and efficacy of testosterone for women: a systematic review and meta-analysis of randomised controlled trial data. Lancet Diabetes Endocrinol. 2019;7:754. https://doi.org/10.1016/S2213-8587(19)30189-5.

78. Davis SR, Baber R, Panay N, Bitzer J, Perez SC, Islam RM, Kaunitz AM, Kingsberg SA, Lambrinoudaki I, Liu J, Parish SJ, Pinkerton J, Rymer J, Simon JA, Vignozzi L, Wierman ME. Global consensus position statement on the use of testosterone therapy for women. J Clin Endocrinol Metab. 2019;104:4660. https://doi.org/10.1210/jc.2019-01603. PMID: 31498871; PMCID: PMC6821450.

79. Lambrinoudaki I, Brincat M, Erel CT, Gambacciani M, Moen MH, Schenck-Gustafsson K, Tremollieres F, Vujovic S, Rees M, Rozenberg S. EMAS position statement: managing obese postmenopausal women. Maturitas. 2010;66:323. https://doi.org/10.1016/j.maturitas.2010.03.025.

80. Tremollieres F, Brincat M, Erel CT, Gambacciani M, Lambrinoudaki I, Moen MH, Schenck-Gustafsson K, Vujovic S, Rozenberg S, Rees M, European Menopause and Andropause Society. EMAS position statement: managing menopausal women with a personal or family history of VTE. Maturitas. 2011;69:195. https://doi.org/10.1016/j.maturitas.2011.03.011.

81. Schenck-Gustafsson K, Brincat M, Erel CT, Gambacciani M, Lambrinoudaki I, Moen MH, Tremollieres F, Vujovic S, Rozenberg S, Rees M, EMAS. EMAS position statement: managing the menopause in the context of coronary heart disease. Maturitas. 2011;68:94. https://doi.org/10.1016/j.maturitas.2010.10.005.

82. Maseroli E, Cellai I, Filippi S, Comeglio P, Cipriani S, Rastrelli G, Rosi M, Sorbi F, Fambrini M, Petraglia F, Amoriello R, Ballerini C, Lombardelli L, Piccinni MP, Sarchielli E, Guarnieri G, Morelli A, Maggi M, Vignozzi L. Anti-inflammatory effects of androgens in the human vagina. J Mol Endocrinol. 2020;65:109. https://doi.org/10.1530/JME-20-0147.

83. Salvatore S, Ruffolo AF, Phillips C, Athanasiou S, Cardozo L, Serati M, EUGA Working Group. Vaginal laser therapy for GSM/VVA: where we stand now—a review by the EUGA Working Group on Laser. Climacteric. 2023;26:336. https://doi.org/10.1080/13697137.2023.2225766. Epub 2023 Jul 3.

84. Graziottin A. Topical testosterone cream: dosing, safety, efficacy and rationale of use. J Plast Pathol Dermatol. 2022;18:193–203.

85. Traish AM, Kim N, Min K, Munarriz R, Goldstein I. Role of androgens in female genital sexual arousal: receptor expression, structure, and function. Fertil Steril. 2002;77:11. https://doi.org/10.1016/s0015-0282(02)02978-3.

Sexuality Across Lifespan IV: Focus on Men's Vulnerabilities

Giovanni Corona, Mario Maggi, and Alessandra Graziottin

1 Introduction

Male sexuality faces old and new vulnerabilities in the lifespan. Biological factors, endocrinological first, may increase the boy's vulnerability to self-identity crisis during the adolescent years. Gynecomastia, defined as benign proliferation of glandular tissue of the breast in men, is a paradigmatic event (Box 1). It is a very frequent, usually transient, pubertal event that may trigger major sexual concerns in the most fragile boys. In spite of its high prevalence, it is still under-recognized and underdiagnosed in the clinical setting. It is therefore the first highlight of this concise review, with the aim of raising physicians' awareness on its subtle and yet potentially disrupting role in adolescents. Of note, gynecomastia, prevalent in adolescent boys, has a second wave in the elderly, with a slightly different pathogenetic pathway. However, its impact on male sexual identity is mainly limited to young adolescents.

G. Corona (✉)
Endocrinology Unit, Azienda AUSL, Bologna, Italy

M. Maggi
Endocrinology Unit, Mario Serio Department of Experimental and Clinical Biomedical Sciences, University of Florence, Florence, Italy

A. Graziottin
Center of Gynecology and Medical Sexology, H. San Raffaele Resnati, Milan, Italy

Department of Obstetrics and Gynecology, University of Verona, Verona, Italy

Department of Endocrinology and Metabolic Diseases, Federico II University, Naples, Italy
e-mail: a.graziottin@studiograziottin.it

© The Author(s), under exclusive license to Springer Nature Switzerland AG 2024
C. Castelo-Branco, S. Anglès Acedo (eds.), *Medical Disorders and Sexual Health*, Trends in Andrology and Sexual Medicine,
https://doi.org/10.1007/978-3-031-55080-5_4

A second major vulnerability factor is alcohol and drug abuse, dramatically increasing among adolescents in all the Western world [1]. Indeed, young adult males are more likely to demonstrate health risk behaviors than other individuals. Key emerging problematic links between alcohol and adolescents' sexuality are summarized in Box 2. Early diagnosis of health risk behaviors within this population is vital to promote effective focused educational programs and timely therapeutic interventions.

Focusing on the longer lifespan perspective, a large body of evidence has clearly documented that life expectancy has progressively increased during the last two centuries as a result of medical, social, and economic advances over disease [2–4]. Despite a little opposite trend observed during COVID-19 pandemia [5], further increase in life expectancy is supposed to occur in the following years. In particular, it has been estimated that by 2050, nearly one in five people will be over the age of 60. In the same years, the world's population of people aged 60 years and older will reach around 2.1 billion [2]. Successful aging represents the new challenge for all high-income countries [2]. In line to what is reported by Marcus Tullius Cicero, at the age of 62 years in the "*Cato Maior de Senectute*," the combination of adequate physical and mental lifestyle behavior still represents the main sources of youth: "... *habenda ratio valetudinis, utendum exercitationibus modicis, tantum cibi et potionis adhibendum ut reficiantur vires, non opprimantur.*"

A complex interaction between general health, psychological well-being, and a good couple fitness, all supported by an adequate endocrine milieu, is the cornerstone for a satisfactory human sexuality [6–9] in the lifespan. This chapter focuses more on male sexual disorders that increase with age.

Aging can affect all the aforementioned components resulting in sexual impairment and vulnerabilities. Despite this evidence, however, several population-based studies have clarified that a large proportion of older adults are still interested in sexual activities, with men usually being more frequently sexually active when compared to women [10–12]. Interestingly, based on the combination of two large cross-sectional surveys of aging populations in the United States, Lindau and Gavrilova [11] previously reported that although sexually active life expectancy is longer for men, men are used to lose more years of sexually active life as a result of poor health than women. Accordingly, life expectancy at birth is lower in men when compared to women in all Western countries [13]. The analysis of the specific reasons supporting the latter observation is out of scope of this chapter, but several data have demonstrated that many traditional cardiovascular (CV) risk factors and comorbidities, including obesity, type 2 diabetes mellitus (T2DM), arterial hypertension, and dyslipidemia, are more often observed in males when compared to females [11]. Wrong lifestyle behaviors such as smoking, alcohol consumption, reduced physical activity, and a diet rich in fat and carbohydrates and poor in vegetables and fruits can all explain the observed differences. In addition, men are used to consult medical care more often for an acute problem and less frequently for a preventive care, contributing to a delay in identifying and modifying potential risk factors [14].

The development and the commercialization of phosphodiesterase type 5 inhibitors (PDE5is) in the global market in the late 1990s and early 2000s have initially promised to overcome all erectile problems, particularly those related to aging men, mainly supported by vascular problems [3, 7, 8, 15]. Data derived from the last 30 years have clarified that erectile dysfunction (ED) should be considered a symptom related to the perturbation of three main domains, including organic, relational, and intrapsychic components [16]. While the association between ED and CV risk factors [17] as well as with reduced testosterone (T) levels [18] is well recognized and investigated, the impact of relational and psychological aspects on ED is often neglected. The modification of social and familiar conditions occurring with aging, such as death of the partner, worsening of social status, deterioration of support networks, and health- and finance-related family problems, might all contribute to sexual difficulties. Furthermore, the development or worsening of depressive and anxiety symptoms due to sexual difficulties or generated by the aforementioned physiological changes can, in turn, contribute to the CV risk profile [19].

The "she" partner aging, specifically when the woman suffers from untreated menopausal symptoms and/or untreated genitourinary syndrome of the menopause (GSM), with its cluster of vulvovaginal, sexual, and urinary symptoms, can be the inducer and/or the precipitating factor of male sexual dysfunctions (MSDs), in the shadow of clinical awareness (Box 3). See also Women' vulnerabilities in the life span [Chaps. 2 and 3 (Menopause and Senescence)].

The aim of this chapter is to summarize and critically analyze the main changes occurring in male sexual response across lifespan, providing some practical suggestions on how to manage them to guarantee, or at least improve, a satisfying sexuality even at older age.

2 Age-Related Physiological Modification of Male Sexual Response

Several physiological modifications occur at penile level as a consequence of normal aging. A progressive reduction in smooth muscle content and an increase in connective tissue have been reported in the corpora cavernosa [20]. These changes, along with a decline in the number of β-adrenergic and cholinergic receptors, support the development of an increased α-adrenergic activity and lead to a reduced corpora cavernosa elasticity, impairing normal response for achieving and maintaining an erection [20]. A reduction of penile sensitivity has also been described along with a gradual decline in penile rigidity [20]. Hence, whereas at younger age visual stimulation represents the most important factor for triggering male sexual response [21], achieving and maintaining an erection in aging men are mainly dependent on direct physical stimulation. Accordingly, a more intense stimulation (very often associating manual and oral activity) is required before penile vaginal intromission [20]. The plateau stage of sexual response is also prolonged with age, whereas the duration of orgasm declines progressively. Finally, the length of the refractory period is particularly increased [20] (see also Fig. 1 and Table 1). Besides penile structure modifications, several other body changes can represent possible source of sexual impairment in aging men. In particular, gynecomastia frequently occurs in adulthood and particularly in the elderly people (up to 60%) [22]. An underlining

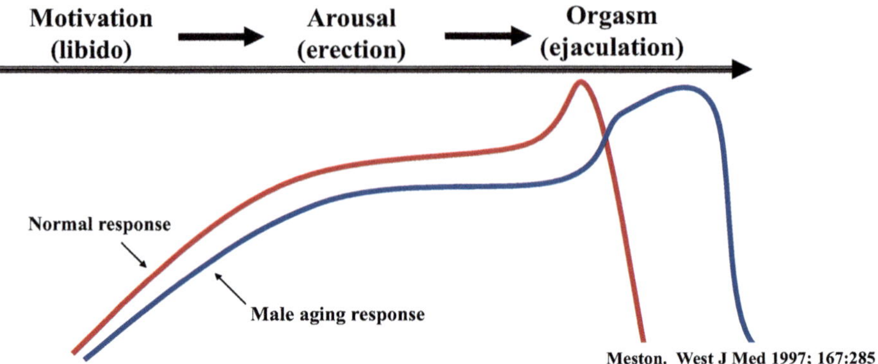

Fig. 1 Modification of the sexual response cycle: men. [Based on data from Meston CM. Aging and sexuality. West J Med. 1997 Oct;167(4):285–90]

Table 1 Modification of the sexual response cycle: men

↓ Corpora cavernosa elasticity (↓ β-adrenergic and cholinergic receptors; ↑deposition of connective tissue), ↓ penile sensitivity. *Achieving and maintaining an erection more dependent on direct physical stimulation.* Partners may facilitate the erectile response by providing a more intense stimulation

↓ The plateau stage is also prolonged with age

↓ Duration of orgasm: fewer muscle contractions and decreased expulsive ejaculatory force

↑ Length of the refractory increased

breast cancer is a quite rare condition (0.1%), whereas other specific underlying conditions (including systemic diseases, drugs, and endocrinopathies) can be found in around 45–50% [22]. This unexpected growth can as well cause a fastidious and worrisome sense of tension. In addition, it can create an underdiagnosed consequence on men's emotional well-being and sense of masculinity, which can, in turn, have negative consequences on sexual performance [22]. The sexual vulnerability is higher in younger men and adolescents, and in men of any age, with a less solid sexual identity and/or anxiety-depressive disorders. Similar considerations can be done for all other body changes including fat accumulation as well as hair graying and loss, which can be a variable source of emotional distress and anxiety [23].

3 Sexual Function/Dysfunction Across Lifespan

3.1 Epidemiological Data

A large body of evidence has documented an age-dependent decline of sexual performance as a function of age. Accordingly, the number of men reporting frequent desire, erection, orgasm, and intercourse, all decrease as a function of age [16, 24].

Interestingly, however, the same data have often emphasized that the observed age-related decrease in erectile function is not always associated with bothering symptoms and an increased concern about it [12, 25, 26]. Accordingly, the Krimpen study, a population-based study involving 1688 men (aged 50–78 years), enrolled in a Dutch municipality near Rotterdam, reported that, although the prevalence of sexually active men declined as a function of aging, up to 30% of the subjects who declared to be sexually active did not have normal erection [25]. Hence, what we can derive from the critical analysis of the available data is that normal erections are not an absolute requisite to remain sexually active in aging couples. In fact, similar considerations can be derived from women perspectives [27]. In line with these findings, data derived from the European Male Aging Study (EMAS), involving more than 3300 community-dwelling men (mean age: 60 ± 11 years), randomly selected from eight European centers, showed that although more than 50% of the subjects, older than 70 years, declared an ED problem, 47% reported at least one instance of sexual intercourse, 24% masturbation, 58% petting, and 75% thinking about sex in the previous 4 weeks [12]. Similar results were derived from the Health in Men study, a longitudinal population-based survey including 3274 men aged 75–95, from Perth, Western Australia [28], and the Men in Australia Telephone Survey (MATeS) including representative sample population (n = 5990) of Australian men older than 40 years [29].

Although, as previously reported, the prevalence of several sexual dysfunctions increases with age, an opposite trend has been reported for self-reported premature ejaculation (PE) [11, 29–31]. However, despite the different epidemiological distribution, the same negative trend as a function of aging was reported also for PE-related concern [30].

Interestingly, data derived from the National Social Life, Health, and Aging Project (NSHAP), a nationally representative sample of older community-dwelling US adults, showed that the prevalence of sexual problems among sexual minority men defined as those who have sex with men or with both women and men was similar to that observed in heterosexual men [32, 33].

3.2 Main Determinants

3.2.1 Organic Conditions

As previously reported, associated chronic conditions, which prevalence increases with aging, represent one of the most important determinants of sexual impairment observed in elderly people. Accordingly, using a previously validated sexual history tool—SIEDY, a 13-item structured interview [34]—a direct linear relationship between the impact of organic domain (as evaluated by Scale 1 score) and aging-related ED has been observed [16] (see also Fig. 2). In line with this observation, several factors can specifically contribute to the deterioration of male sexual function in elderly people. The following sections will briefly summarize the most important conditions (Fig. 3).

Modification of the sexual response cycle: men

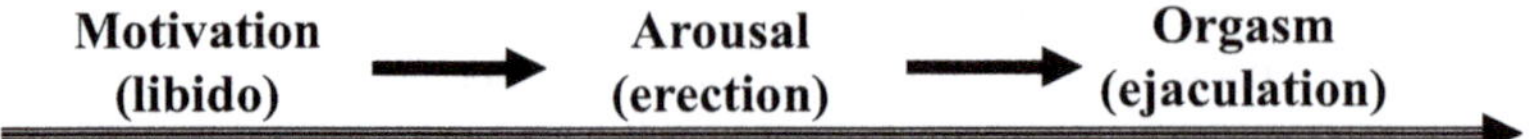

- ↓ Corpora carvernosa elasticity (↓ β-adrenergic and cholinergic receptors; ↑deposition of connective tissue), ↓ penile sensitivity. *Achieving and maintaining an erection more dependent on direct physical stimulation.* Partners may facilitate the erectile response by providing a more intense stimulation

- ↓ The plateau stage is also prolonged with age.

- ↓ duration of orgasm: fewer muscle contractions, and decreased expulsive ejaculatory force.

- ↑ length of the refractory increased

Fig. 2 Modification of the sexual response cycle: men. [Based on data from Meston CM. Aging and sexuality. West J Med. 1997 Oct;167(4):285-90]

Variation in SIEDY scale score as a function of the aging process

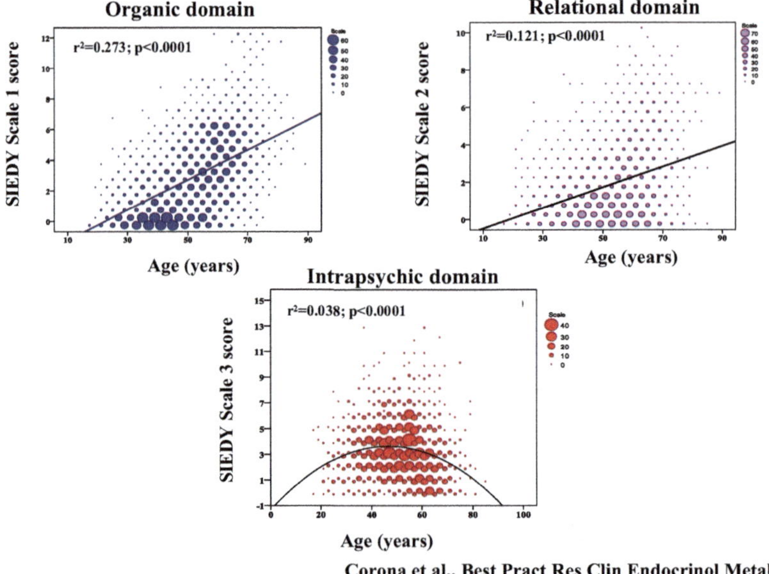

Fig. 3 Variation in SIEDY scale score as a function of the aging process

- *Obesity*: Available data have documented that obesity, and in particular central obesity, is associated with either arteriogenic ED or reduced T levels [35]. Accordingly, weight loss can improve erectile function and ameliorate circulating T levels [36]. In addition, obesity-related complications such as T2DM, arterial hypertension, and dyslipidemia can further complicate the figure [35].
- *Diabetes mellitus*: ED is a frequent multifactorial complication of DM with an overall prevalence ranging from 37.5 to 66.3% in type 1 and type 2 DM [37].

Age, presence of associated DM complications such as peripheral neuropathy, nephropathy, and atherosclerosis, as well as disease duration and metabolic control, represent the major factors in determining the prevalence and severity of ED in DM [37].

- *Arterial hypertension*: Subjects with arterial hypertension have sevenfold increased risk of ED when compared to normotensive individuals [38]. Although with limited evidence due to the lack of placebo-controlled studies, several classes of antihypertensive drugs have been associated with a higher risk of ED, particularly β-blockers and thiazide diuretics [39]. Conversely, angiotensin-converting enzyme inhibitors, angiotensin receptor, alpha-blockers, or calcium channel blockers showed no effect or even a positive role in erectile function [39].

- *Dyslipidemia*: Several observational studies have documented a strong association between ED and elevated total (TC) and low-density lipoprotein (LDL) cholesterol or reduced high-density lipoprotein (HDL) cholesterol [40, 41]. In particular, TC higher than 240 mg/dL or HDL-C lower than 30 mg/dL is related to twofold increased risk of ED [42]. In line with these data, the use of statin therapy can improve erectile function [7].

- *Cardiovascular diseases*: A large body of evidence documented that ED and CV diseases (CVDs) should be considered **different manifestations of a common underlying vascular pathology**. Furthermore, data derived from the last 20 years have clearly documented that ED can represent the first sign of a forthcoming CVD [17]. Interestingly, available data support the concept that ED represents a better predictor of CV events particularly in younger and uncomplicated subjects, since the accumulation of the associated morbidities in the elderly population can reduce the role of ED in the stratification of CV risk [17]. In this population, an impaired penile vascular flow, detected through penile Doppler ultrasound, can further increase the risk of CV events [43].

- *Hormonal factors*: Current evidence indicates that total T decreases naturally as a function of age. This phenomenon is particularly enhanced according to the increase of the associated comorbidities. The term "late-onset hypogonadism" (LOH) has been introduced to describe this phenomenon [44]. T plays a crucial role in regulating male sexual function acting at central and peripheral levels [45]. Accordingly, the EMAS study has clarified that sexual symptoms and low libido reduced spontaneous and sex-related erections [12]. In particular, they are the most specific determinants of LOH [3]. In line with these data, T replacement therapy in hypogonadal men (total T < 12 nmol) is associated with the improvement of all aspects of sexual function, although less evident effects are observed in more complicated patients such as those with more severe form of ED [46]. In line to what is observed for total T, current data have documented an age-dependent decline of dehydroepiandrosterone (DHEA) and its sulfate (DHEAS) [47]. However, the role of DHEA and DHEAS in male sexual function is limited [47]. Similarly, whereas hyperprolactinemia plays a clear negative role in sexual desire, its contribution in the pathogenesis of ED is more conflicting [45]. Finally, quite strong evidence supports the role of thyroid hormones in the regulation of ejaculatory reflex. Hyper- or hypothyroidism has been associated with PE or delayed ejaculation (DE), respectively [31]. Conversely, the role of thyroid hormones in the regulation of erectile function and sexual desire is more limited [7, 45].

- *Urological conditions*: ED is a common side effect of pelvic surgery performed due to several malignancies. The prevalence of ED as a consequence of radical prostatectomy ranges from 90 to 94% at 24 months [7]. High ED rates are also reported after surgical interventions for bladder and colorectal cancers [7]. Low urinary tract symptoms (LUTSs) represent other well-known risk factors for ED, **since the two conditions share similar risk factors** including metabolic disorders and hormonal imbalance [48]. In addition, some medications commonly used for the treatment of benign prostate hyperplasia (BPH)-related LUTS, such as 5-alpha-reductase inhibitors, can further worsen the figure [49].

3.2.2 Marital and Couple Fitness Determinants

In line to what is reported for males, the presence of sexual dysfunction in the female partner could amplify the patient's sexual problem. Accordingly, menopausal related complaints, such as vaginal dryness and dyspareunia, hot flashes, night sweats, sleep problems, as well as mood changes, can all negatively influence female sexual function and potentially worsen male sexual dysfunction [50]. On the other side, increasing data have documented that female partners of men with ED frequently report an impaired sexual function, including a decrease in sexual desire and level of arousal, as well as a reduced frequency of orgasm and satisfaction with sexual activity [51, 52]. Considering the aforementioned evidence, it is not surprising that data derived from a large sample of patients seeking medical care for ED showed that the weight relational domain, as derived from SIEDY Scale 2 score, progressively increased as a function of age as observed for the organic domain (Fig. 2) [16]. Accordingly, marital conflicts and tensions, relationship perturbation, poor intimacy and communication problems, as well as mismatches in sexual desire and sexual activities might be amplified in elderly people after a long unsatisfactory relationship [16, 53]. Epidemiological data have shown that men report a higher frequency of sexual activities and a more positive and permissive attitude toward sex when compared to women at all ages [10, 11, 16]. The latter discordant behavior might cause harmful consequences leading to an impairment of couple fitness or extramarital affairs.

It should be clarified that an optimal couple intimacy and a satisfactory relationship can have not only positive outcomes on sexual function. In fact, several data have clarified that social interaction and, in particular, marital sustainment can also play a protective role in the stratification of CV risk by supporting the successful cure of sexual problems and by stimulating emotions, affection, and health-related and coping behaviors [54].

3.2.3 Intrapsychic Determinants

The impact of intrapsychic component on ED, including the presence of anxiety and depressive symptoms, has been frequently considered to play a major role in younger individuals. Accordingly, the analysis of the distribution of SIEDY Scale 3 score (dealing with the intrapsychic domain of ED) as a function of age showed that the best fitting model was obtained through a quadratic regression (Fig. 2). The latter observation suggests that the psychological factors mainly affect younger and middle-age subjects [16]. Performance anxiety in younger individual or life stressors derived from work activity or from other conditions which can affect the more active period of life can explain, at least partially, this association. However, it is important to recognize that several stressful conditions can affect elderly people contributing to the impairment of sexual function by increasing the likelihood of depression and/or anxiety. Accordingly, the death of the partner, the loss of a job, or the worsening of social status due to health- and/or finance-related problems can often occur during the lifespan. In addition, the resumption of sexual interactions after a period of inactivity due to a divorce or a death of a spouse is frequently associated with sexual difficulties due to feelings of misery, guilt, and anger [20]. Finally, social stereotypes and cultural aspects which support active sexuality only in younger people can further exacerbate anxiety and depressive symptoms, inducing a sense of shame due to the persistent sexual interest discouraging people from seeking medical care for solving the problem.

4 Conclusion

Male sexuality, and specifically male sexual function, can be impaired or frankly damaged by biological, behavioral, or contextual factors. Every physician, family physicians first, should routinely include a few questions on their male patients' sexuality and the leading potential disruptors, health-related factors first, but also behavioral, such as substance or pornography abuse. Such a simple and constant overture, with a short, accurate medical history along with few biochemical examinations, could prove to be a really "revolutionary behavior." It would prevent the "collusion of silence" between a physician who still does not ask, and keeps sexuality out of reach in his/her clinical setting, and a male patient who does not dare to ask for help.

Box 1 Pubertal Gynecomastia: "Am I Becoming a Woman?"
The Clinical Features

The transient pubertal growth of the mammary gland ("pubertal gynecomastia") is a frequent, disturbing, and yet very underappreciated event. It is more frequent at 13–14 years of age. It may hurt the inner sense of sexual identity and increase gender anxiety in vulnerable boys. The word "gynecomastia" is derived from the Greek terms "gyné" (woman) and "mastós" (breast).

Up to 50% of male adolescents present with a variable gynecomastia, when the small mammary gland is stimulated by the powerful action of increasing waves of pubertal hormones. In particular, the transient excess of estradiol (E2)-to-testosterone (T) ratio, within the breast tissue, is credited to triggering the gland proliferation.

The resulting transient breast growth is variable, from a minimal tumescence of the gland beneath the nipple to an important growth, symmetric or asymmetric, of the two breasts. Overweight and obesity can further complicate the condition by increasing E2 conversion from T in the adipose tissue or by increasing the adipose tissue to the glandular component ("pseudogynecomastia").

This unexpected growth can as well cause a fastidious and worrisome sense of tension. Usually, the breast growth undergoes a spontaneous regression in a 6–8, max 24, months' time. However, these months can seem eternal to a worrying boy, with underdiagnosed consequences on his emotional well-being and his sense of masculinity, more so if this growing breast becomes the target of ironic and/or aggressive comments, bullying, and stigmatization, usually reported as more frequent against obese boys.

The Inner Perception

"What is happening to me?" "Am I becoming a woman?": These inner thoughts, so anguishing that cannot be confessed to parents or closer friends, can trigger deep fears and anxiety, and depressive and/or defensive behaviors, that should be intercepted, recognized, understood, and addressed by parents and caring physicians.

The Alerting Signals

Many boys with gynecomastia give up practicing sports and refuse to go on holidays to seaside or lake resorts. They become suddenly shy of undressing, also in front of parents or siblings. As nobody raises the subject, they think to be the "only" abnormal boy in the world, with a problem that is perceived as the most anguishing a boy can have.

Action

Gynecomastia should be introduced in every school conversation about pubertal events, as a physiological ("normal") and short-lasting phenomenon, that will spontaneously regress in the majority of cases.

The family physician, or the pediatrician, should reassure the boy that the temporary swelling is just an expression of high waves of hormones, responsible for his general growth, beard, voice changes, hairs, strength, erotic dreams, and nocturnal sperm emission. He should be told that it is a very frequent event that does not touch or change his sense of being a boy in the transition of becoming a man.

The boy should as well be reassured that he will be well looked after and cured, if the gynecomastia is persisting beyond 6–8 months, if it is very asymmetric between the left and right breasts, if it is perceived as excessive and/or triggers aggressive behaviors, or if it is the tip of the iceberg of other rare health problems. When indicated, a specific endocrinological consultation should be suggested in order to exclude pathological forms of gynecomastia (more frequently observed in adulthood), including the use of interfering drugs, endocrinological problems, liver and kidney failure, or rare neoplasms.

Controlled data on pharmacologic treatment are limited. Tamoxifen, a selective estrogen receptor modulator (SERM) with antiestrogenic action on the breast, has been used in a limited series of patients.

The accurate surgical, cosmetic removal of the hypertrophic mammary gland can be considered in selected cases and particularly when the problem is lasting for more than 1 year.

A qualified psychosexual support should be offered to boys who are mostly vulnerable to the negative impact of gynecomastia. The opportunity for the boy to give words to his deepest "unspeakable" fears and thoughts to a listening and competent physician and or/psychotherapist can usually prove to be the most effective therapy in the majority of cases. Meanwhile, the mammary tumescence spontaneously regresses, with a final relief.

Box 2 Substance Use and Sexual Vulnerabilities in Boys

Young people are more prone to experience and exhibit health risk behaviors than older individuals. Young adult males have higher prevalence of health risk behaviors than their female counterparts. This male vulnerability increases both self-morbidity and mortality, with a parallel increased risk of aggressive and offending behaviors against others.

Substance-related risk behaviors, such as alcohol, drug abuse, and cigarette smoking, are dramatically on the rise. The use of one substance usually co-occurs with other substances, potentiating the damaging effect on the general health. They are more dangerous in adolescents, due to the higher brain vulnerability to the disrupting and long-lasting effect of different toxic substances.

Sexuality is as well vulnerable to substances use. On the one side, they increase the risk of earlier sexual debut, unprotected promiscuity, sexually transmitted diseases, and unwanted pregnancies. On the other, they may be a predisposing or precipitating factor for specific sexual dysfunctions, either maintenance erectile difficulties or premature ejaculation.

A more proactive action on the physician's side, in terms of preventing interventions, actively asking about substance at every medical consultation, and timely therapeutic commitment, when indicated, could prevent many young boys from initiating or maintaining substance use and abuse while protecting their health and sexuality.

Box 3 Symptom Inducer and Symptom Carrier

The boy, or the man, with a sexual problem usually consults the family physician or the specialist alone. Less frequently, he consults along with a partner. In real life, human beings usually make love or have sex with someone else (in virtual life, the situation is different, almost the opposite, as loneliness is the hallmark of virtual sex). In the shadow of clinical awareness, and of the clinical conversation, this someone may have a say or be the predisposing, precipitating, or maintaining cofactor of male sexual problems (and vice versa for women).

To unveil the potential role of the partner in the etiology of the current complaint, a simple set of questions should be included in the clinical history:

- *Is your sex problem present with every partner and in every situation, say, is it generalized?*
- *Or is it limited to a specific partner or to a specific situation, say, is it "situational," for example, when you are too stressed with a demanding job* vs. *when you are happily relaxed on holidays?*
- *Do you have a stable partner?*
- *If yes, does he or she have a normal sexual response? Or does he or she have any sexual difficulty or problem?*

In case of a heterosexual stable relationship, the dyadic interplay in the onset and maintenance of male sexual problem is more frequently diagnosed in case of unconsummated marriages or relationships and erectile deficits in adult or elderly men.

Unconsummated Marriage or Relationship

The young man may mainly consult the physician complaining of either:

- **Maintenance erectile deficit**, i.e., he has the erection but he cannot maintain it, usually because of peaks of anxiety triggering a hyperadrenergic tone, with vasoconstriction and loss of erection
- **Extremely rapid premature ejaculation** at vulvar level

In both cases, he could be the "symptom carrier," while she could be the (involuntary!) "symptom inducer" when:

- She suffers from lifelong sexual pain disorders, with a variable phobia of penetration (formerly "vaginismus") and a tightened defensive pelvic floor that prevents penetration at all
- By her own anxiety and fear, she contributes to such a pervading anxiety that he cannot control the ejaculatory reflex any further, more so when she is terrified at the only idea of feeling pain and he is afraid of hurting her.

Myriam de Senarclens (1921–1993), a Swiss psychoanalyst, used to say (personal communication): "For a mysterious attraction, men who are afraid of penetrating usually fell in love with a woman who is afraid of being penetrated."

It is therefore appropriate to encourage a couple consultation. If the diagnosis is confirmed, and the partner really suffers from severe sexual pain disorders (either vaginismus or severe dyspareunia), to plan a parallel medical and psychosexual therapy with physicians, usually gynecologists or physician, well trained in female sexual medicine, is mandatory for a successful outcome.

Erectile Deficits in Adult or Elderly Men

The maintenance erectile deficit can be induced or precipitated by severe vulvovaginal atrophy, now defined as "genitourinary syndrome of the menopause," with poor or no lubrication at all. Penetration becomes more difficult when her genital situation is complicated by a tightened pelvic floor (more frequent in menopausal women who are nulliparous or who delivered only by cesarean section). So she could be the "symptom inducer" or the precipitating factor, and he the "symptom carrier" (with a variable degree of vascular or neuroendocrine etiology of his ED).

A simple set of questions help to clarify the situation:

- *Do you have a stable relationship?*
- *How old is your wife/partner?*
- *Are you aware if she is menopausal?*
- *Does she suffer from vaginal dryness or sexual pain, more so in recent months or years?*
- *If yes, do you think she would be willing to receive help for her dryness and pain, at least with a local (genital) treatment?*
- *And to participate in a simple, medically focused, couple therapy?*

If the answers describe a "she" co-problem, it is appropriate to recommend a couple evaluation. If both partners agree, a parallel treatment should be proposed (see the chapter on women's vulnerabilities in the lifespan), besides treating the ED accordingly.

For her, vaginal estrogens or prasterone and short-term vaginal diazepam (5 mg) to relax the pelvic floor, when tightened, in synergy with a competent physiotherapy are the first-line therapy to address postmenopausal vaginal dryness and sexual pain, more so in case of premature menopause. A vulvar and vaginal treatment with a cream of testosterone of vegetal origin may well enhance women's physical sexual response and sexual pleasure.

In the clinical setting, both partners confirm a well-enjoyed "plus" in terms of significant improvement of genital arousal/congestion and intensity of orgasm. Anecdotally, many partners refer (to AG) that the improved scent and genital taste (due to the refreshed pheromone secretion) further boost their sexual attraction/drive and pleasure in having sex with their lifelong companion.

In both cases, with a competent and well-tailored medical treatment, each partner could enjoy feeling the protagonist of a refreshed and more satisfying sexual relationship.

References

1. Flesia L, Cavalieri F, Angelini S, Bottesi G, Ghisi M, Tonon E, et al. Health-related lifestyles, substance-related behaviors, and sexual habits among Italian young adult males: an epidemiologic study. Sex Med. 2020;8(3):361–9.
2. Kontis V, Bennett JE, Mathers CD, Li G, Foreman K, Ezzati M. Future life expectancy in 35 industrialised countries: projections with a Bayesian model ensemble. Lancet. 2017;389(10076):1323–35.
3. Corona G, Maggi M. The role of testosterone in male sexual function. Rev Endocr Metab Disord. 2022;23(6):1159–72.
4. Corona G, Guaraldi F, Rastrelli G, Sforza A, Maggi M. Testosterone deficiency and risk of cognitive disorders in aging males. World J Mens Health. 2021;39(1):9–18.
5. Corona G, Pizzocaro A, Vena W, Rastrelli G, Semeraro F, Isidori AM, et al. Diabetes is most important cause for mortality in COVID-19 hospitalized patients: systematic review and meta-analysis. Rev Endocr Metab Disord. 2021;22(2):275–96.
6. Boddi V, Corona G, Fisher AD, Mannucci E, Ricca V, Sforza A, et al. "It takes two to tango": the relational domain in a cohort of subjects with erectile dysfunction (ED). J Sex Med. 2012;9(12):3126–36.
7. Corona G, Cucinotta D, Di Lorenzo G, Ferlin A, Giagulli VA, Gnessi L, et al. The Italian Society of Andrology and Sexual Medicine (SIAMS), along with ten other Italian Scientific Societies, guidelines on the diagnosis and management of erectile dysfunction. J Endocrinol Investig. 2023;46:1241.
8. Salonia A, Bettocchi C, Boeri L, Capogrosso P, Carvalho J, Cilesiz NC, et al. European Association of Urology guidelines on sexual and reproductive Health-2021 update: male sexual dysfunction. Eur Urol. 2021;80(3):333–57.
9. Dewitte M, Bettocchi C, Carvalho J, Corona G, Flink I, Limoncin E, et al. A Psychosocial Approach to Erectile Dysfunction: position statements from the European Society of Sexual Medicine (ESSM). Sex Med. 2021;9(6):100434.
10. Nicolosi A, Laumann EO, Glasser DB, Moreira ED Jr, Paik A, Gingell C. Sexual behavior and sexual dysfunctions after age 40: the global study of sexual attitudes and behaviors. Urology. 2004;64(5):991–7.
11. Lindau ST, Schumm LP, Laumann EO, Levinson W, O'Muircheartaigh CA, Waite LJ. A study of sexuality and health among older adults in the United States. N Engl J Med. 2007;357(8):762–74.
12. Corona G, Lee DM, Forti G, O'Connor DB, Maggi M, O'Neill TW, et al. Age-related changes in general and sexual health in middle-aged and older men: results from the European Male Ageing Study (EMAS). J Sex Med. 2010;7(4 Pt 1):1362–80.
13. Liou L, Joe W, Kumar A, Subramanian SV. Inequalities in life expectancy: an analysis of 201 countries, 1950–2015. Soc Sci Med. 2020;253:112964.
14. Wang Y, Hunt K, Nazareth I, Freemantle N, Petersen I. Do men consult less than women? An analysis of routinely collected UK general practice data. BMJ Open. 2013;3(8):e003320.
15. Corona G, Razzoli E, Forti G, Maggi M. The use of phosphodiesterase 5 inhibitors with concomitant medications. J Endocrinol Investig. 2008;31(9):799–808.
16. Corona G, Rastrelli G, Maseroli E, Forti G, Maggi M. Sexual function of the ageing male. Best Pract Res Clin Endocrinol Metab. 2013;27(4):581–601.
17. Corona G, Rastrelli G, Isidori AM, Pivonello R, Bettocchi C, Reisman Y, et al. Erectile dysfunction and cardiovascular risk: a review of current findings. Expert Rev Cardiovasc Ther. 2020;18(3):155–64.
18. Rastrelli G, Corona G, Maggi M. Testosterone and sexual function in men. Maturitas. 2018;112:46–52.
19. Rastrelli G, Corona G, Fisher AD, Silverii A, Mannucci E, Maggi M. Two unconventional risk factors for major adverse cardiovascular events in subjects with sexual dysfunction: low

education and reported partner's hypoactive sexual desire in comparison with conventional risk factors. J Sex Med. 2012;9(12):3227–38.

20. Echeverri Tirado LC, Ferrer JE, Herrera AM. Aging and erectile dysfunction. Sex Med Rev. 2016;4(1):63–73.

21. Georgiadis JR, Kringelbach ML. The human sexual response cycle: brain imaging evidence linking sex to other pleasures. Prog Neurobiol. 2012;98(1):49–81.

22. Kanakis GA, Nordkap L, Bang AK, Calogero AE, Bártfai G, Corona G, et al. EAA clinical practice guidelines-gynecomastia evaluation and management. Andrology. 2019;7(6):778–93.

23. Mirmirani P. Age-related hair changes in men: mechanisms and management of alopecia and graying. Maturitas. 2015;80(1):58–62.

24. Kessler A, Sollie S, Challacombe B, Briggs K, Van Hemelrijck M. The global prevalence of erectile dysfunction: a review. BJU Int. 2019;124(4):587–99.

25. Blanker MH, Bohnen AM, Groeneveld FP, Bernsen RM, Prins A, Thomas S, et al. Correlates for erectile and ejaculatory dysfunction in older Dutch men: a community-based study. J Am Geriatr Soc. 2001;49(4):436–42.

26. Perelman M, Shabsigh R, Seftel A, Althof S, Lockhart D. Attitudes of men with erectile dysfunction: a cross-national survey. J Sex Med. 2005;2(3):397–406.

27. Mitchell KR, Mercer CH, Ploubidis GB, Jones KG, Datta J, Field N, et al. Sexual function in Britain: findings from the third National Survey of Sexual Attitudes and Lifestyles (Natsal-3). Lancet. 2013;382(9907):1817–29.

28. Hyde Z, Flicker L, Hankey GJ, Almeida OP, McCaul KA, Chubb SA, et al. Prevalence and predictors of sexual problems in men aged 75–95 years: a population-based study. J Sex Med. 2012;9(2):442–53.

29. Holden CA, McLachlan RI, Pitts M, Cumming R, Wittert G, Agius PA, et al. Men in Australia Telephone Survey (MATeS): a national survey of the reproductive health and concerns of middle-aged and older Australian men. Lancet. 2005;366(9481):218–24.

30. Corona G, Rastrelli G, Bartfai G, Casanueva FF, Giwercman A, Antonio L, et al. Self-reported shorter than desired ejaculation latency and related distress-prevalence and clinical correlates: results from the European Male Ageing Study. J Sex Med. 2021;18(5):908–19.

31. Sansone A, Aversa A, Corona G, Fisher AD, Isidori AM, La Vignera S, et al. Management of premature ejaculation: a clinical guideline from the Italian Society of Andrology and Sexual Medicine (SIAMS). J Endocrinol Investig. 2021;44(5):1103–18.

32. Obedin-Maliver J, Lisha N, Breyer BN, Subak LL, Huang AJ. More similarities than differences? An exploratory analysis comparing the sexual complaints, sexual experiences, and genitourinary health of older sexual minority and sexual majority adults. J Sex Med. 2019;16(3):347–50.

33. Fredriksen-Goldsen KI, Kim HJ. The science of conducting research with LGBT older adults—an introduction to aging with pride: National Health, Aging, and Sexuality/Gender Study (NHAS). Gerontologist. 2017;57(suppl 1):S1–s14.

34. Petrone L, Mannucci E, Corona G, Bartolini M, Forti G, Giommi R, et al. Structured interview on erectile dysfunction (SIEDY): a new, multidimensional instrument for quantification of pathogenetic issues on erectile dysfunction. Int J Impot Res. 2003;15(3):210–20.

35. Corona G, Rastrelli G, Filippi S, Vignozzi L, Mannucci E, Maggi M. Erectile dysfunction and central obesity: an Italian perspective. Asian J Androl. 2014;16(4):581–91.

36. Allen MS, Walter EE. Health-related lifestyle factors and sexual dysfunction: a meta-analysis of population-based research. J Sex Med. 2018;15(4):458–75.

37. Kouidrat Y, Pizzol D, Cosco T, Thompson T, Carnaghi M, Bertoldo A, et al. High prevalence of erectile dysfunction in diabetes: a systematic review and meta-analysis of 145 studies. Diabet Med. 2017;34(9):1185–92.

38. Wang XY, Huang W, Zhang Y. Relation between hypertension and erectile dysfunction: a meta-analysis of cross-section studies. Int J Impot Res. 2018;30(3):141–6.

39. Farmakis IT, Pyrgidis N, Doundoulakis I, Mykoniatis I, Akrivos E, Giannakoulas G. Effects of major antihypertensive drug classes on erectile function: a network meta-analysis. Cardiovasc Drugs Ther. 2022;36(5):903–14.

40. Feldman HA, Goldstein I, Hatzichristou DG, Krane RJ, McKinlay JB. Impotence and its medical and psychosocial correlates: results of the Massachusetts Male Aging Study. J Urol. 1994;151(1):54–61.

41. Corona G, Cipriani S, Rastrelli G, Sforza A, Mannucci E, Maggi M. High triglycerides predicts arteriogenic erectile dysfunction and major adverse cardiovascular events in subjects with sexual dysfunction. J Sex Med. 2016;13(9):1347–58.

42. Wei M, Macera CA, Davis DR, Hornung CA, Nankin HR, Blair SN. Total cholesterol and high density lipoprotein cholesterol as important predictors of erectile dysfunction. Am J Epidemiol. 1994;140(10):930–7.

43. Rastrelli G, Corona G, Lotti F, Aversa A, Bartolini M, Mancini M, et al. Flaccid penile acceleration as a marker of cardiovascular risk in men without classical risk factors. J Sex Med. 2014;11(1):173–86.

44. Isidori AM, Aversa A, Calogero A, Ferlin A, Francavilla S, Lanfranco F, et al. Adult- and late-onset male hypogonadism: the clinical practice guidelines of the Italian Society of Andrology and Sexual Medicine (SIAMS) and the Italian Society of Endocrinology (SIE). J Endocrinol Investig. 2022;45(12):2385–403.

45. Corona G, Isidori AM, Aversa A, Burnett AL, Maggi M. Endocrinologic control of men's sexual desire and arousal/erection. J Sex Med. 2016;13(3):317–37.

46. Corona G, Rastrelli G, Vignozzi L, Maggi M. Androgens and male sexual function. Best Pract Res Clin Endocrinol Metab. 2022;36(4):101615.

47. Corona G, Rastrelli G, Giagulli VA, Sila A, Sforza A, Forti G, et al. Dehydroepiandrosterone supplementation in elderly men: a meta-analysis study of placebo-controlled trials. J Clin Endocrinol Metab. 2013;98(9):3615–26.

48. Corona G, Vignozzi L, Rastrelli G, Lotti F, Cipriani S, Maggi M. Benign prostatic hyperplasia: a new metabolic disease of the aging male and its correlation with sexual dysfunctions. Int J Endocrinol. 2014;2014:329456.

49. Corona G, Tirabassi G, Santi D, Maseroli E, Gacci M, Dicuio M, et al. Sexual dysfunction in subjects treated with inhibitors of 5α-reductase for benign prostatic hyperplasia: a comprehensive review and meta-analysis. Andrology. 2017;5(4):671–8.

50. Graziottin A. Vaginal biological and sexual health—the unmet needs. Climacteric. 2015;18(Suppl 1):9–12.

51. Fisher WA, Rosen RC, Mollen M, Brock G, Karlin G, Pommerville P, et al. Improving the sexual quality of life of couples affected by erectile dysfunction: a double-blind, randomized, placebo-controlled trial of vardenafil. J Sex Med. 2005;2(5):699–708.

52. Fisher WA, Rosen RC, Eardley I, Sand M, Goldstein I. Sexual experience of female partners of men with erectile dysfunction: the female experience of men's attitudes to life events and sexuality (FEMALES) study. J Sex Med. 2005;2(5):675–84.

53. Marieke D, Joana C, Giovanni C, Erika L, Patricia P, Yacov R, et al. Sexual desire discrepancy: a position statement of the European Society for Sexual Medicine. Sex Med. 2020;8(2):121–31.

54. Robles TF, Kiecolt-Glaser JK. The physiology of marriage: pathways to health. Physiol Behav. 2003;79(3):409–16.

Chronic Pelvic Pain, Sexual Pain, and Female Sexual Dysfunction

Johannes Bitzer, Camil Castelo-Branco,
and Lara Quintas Marquès

1 Introduction

Chronic pelvic pain, sexual pain, and female sexual dysfunctions are prevalent diseases. It is well known that sexual pain has a direct impact on patients' quality of life and significantly affects their relationships [1]. Numerous and different factors, including physical and psychological pathologies, are known to provoke chronic pelvic pain and sexual pain.

In this chapter, we will try to find out the factors that can cause pain; we will perform the diagnostic approach and discuss about the treatment options available to treat these diseases.

Johannes Bitzer and Camil Castelo-Branco contributed equally with all other contributors.

J. Bitzer (✉)
University Hospital Basel, Basel, Switzerland
e-mail: jbitzer@uhbs.ch

C. Castelo-Branco
Gynecological Department, Clinical Institute of Gynecology, Obstetrics and Neonatology, Hospital Clinic de Barcelona, Barcelona, Spain

Clinical Sexology Working Group, Hospital Clinic de Barcelona, Barcelona, Spain

Surgery and Medical-Surgical Specialties, Faculty of Medicine and Health Sciences, Universitat de Barcelona (UB), Barcelona, Spain

Institut d'Investigacions Biomèdiques August Pi i Sunyer, Barcelona, Spain
e-mail: ccastelo@clinic.cat

L. Quintas Marquès
Gynecological Department, Clinical Institute of Gynecology, Obstetrics and Neonatology, Hospital Clinic de Barcelona, Barcelona, Spain

Clinical Sexology Working Group, Hospital Clinic de Barcelona, Barcelona, Spain
e-mail: lquintas@clinic.cat

© The Author(s), under exclusive license to Springer Nature Switzerland AG 2024   93
C. Castelo-Branco, S. Anglès Acedo (eds.), *Medical Disorders and Sexual Health*, Trends in Andrology and Sexual Medicine,
https://doi.org/10.1007/978-3-031-55080-5_5

1.1 The Impact of Chronic Pain and Pain During Sexual Intercourse on Sexual Health

Chronic pain conditions, such as fibromyalgia, or pelvic pain disorders, such as endometriosis, can also interfere with sexual functioning. Chronic pain can affect sexual health through decreasing libido or provoking difficulties with arousal. It is important to note that the psychological impact of chronic pain, including anxiety, depression, and body image concerns, can also exacerbate sexual health issues. Experiencing pain during such an intimate act as sexual intercourse can lead to fear and avoidance of sexual activities and provoke a dissatisfaction for both partners.

There are two clinical scenarios in which chronic pelvic pain, pelvic floor pathology, and sexuality present together:

- Scenario I: *The patient presents with sexual pain as the leading symptom.*
- Scenario II: *The patient suffers from a specific disease leading to chronic pelvic pain and other symptoms.*

Before delving into the subject, it would be convenient to understand the definition of chronic pain and the types of pain that exist. The disease has a negative impact on the patient's quality of life and sexual function. Often, these patients do not spontaneously report their sexual health distress, but only after the physician proactively addresses the problem. In both cases, patient care should be based on a biopsychosocial model for understanding pain and sexual function and have a holistic approach to health and disease.

Chronic pelvic pain (CPP) is defined as pain originating from pelvic organs or structures and lasting for more than 6 months [2]. Chronic pelvic pain can either be a symptom of an underlying disease, which led to tissue or nerve damage, or become a disease in itself without being caused by another pathology [3]. This ambiguity or double face of CPP is the main clinical challenge of this disorder. The experience of pain is complex and involves many mechanisms and interactions between the periphery and the central nervous system [4].

1.2 Pathogenesis of Pelvic Pain

To understand the complexity of the patient's pain experience, the physician should be aware of the different organ and functional systems involved in the pathogenesis of pelvic pain [5–7].

Three pathways of pain formation can be distinguished:

(a) Nociceptive pain: Chronic pelvic pain arises from the damage of nonneural tissue and is due to the activation of nociceptors (activated fiber C will transmit pain signals to the brain centers) (pathology of pelvic organs).

   For example: endometriosis, chronic pelvic inflammatory disease, musculoskeletal diseases, and chronic urological disorders.

(b) Neuropathic pain: Chronic pain is caused by a lesion or a disease of the somatosensory nervous system (neuropathic disorder).

For example: lesions or compression of the pelvic plexus or pelvic nerves (hypogastric nerves, pudendal nerve, etc.).

(c) Nociplastic pain: Chronic pelvic pain is due to abnormal processing of pain signals without any clear evidence of tissue damage or discrete pathology involving somatosensory system. This enhancement in the function of central nervous system results in an increased sensation of pain (hyperalgesia) or a sensation of non-painful stimulus (allodynia) [8].

For example: fibromyalgia.

Cross sensitization occurs when a pathologically painful organ can lead to a non-painful organ becoming painful [9, 10].

For example: irritable bowel syndrome, bladder pain syndrome, and myofascial pelvic pain [11].

## 2	Scenario I: The Patient Presents with Sexual Pain as the Leading Symptom

### 2.1	Sexual Dysfunction

Female sexual dysfunction is a continuum of psychosexual disorders centered on sexual desire with interrelated problems of arousal, orgasm, and sexual pain that impairs the quality of life for many women [12].

Sexual dysfunction is described in DSM IV as "disturbances in sexual desire and/or the psychophysiological changes that characterize the sexual response cycle and cause marked distress and interpersonal difficulties" [13].

The classification of dysfunctions follows, until now, more the linear model and comprises the following entities:

- Sexual desire disorder (hypoactive sexual desire disorder, sexual aversion disorder)
- Sexual arousal disorder
- Orgasmic disorder
- Sexual pain disorder (vaginismus, dyspareunia)
- Other sexual pain disorders (noncoital)

DSM V tries to integrate the sexual pain disorders into one category: genito-pelvic pain/penetration disorder (GPPPD) [14]. The DSM V diagnostic criteria for GPPPD include difficulty with at least one of the following: (1) experiencing vaginal penetration, (2) pain with vaginal penetration, (3) fear of vaginal penetration or of pain during vaginal penetration, and (4) pelvic floor muscle dysfunction.

The current DSM V includes vaginismus and dyspareunia in the new category of GPPPD:

- Dyspareunia is a persistent or recurrent pain with attempted or complete vaginal entry and/or vaginal sexual intercourse.
- Vaginismus is a persistent or recurrent difficulty to allow vaginal entry of a penis/finger/any object despite the woman's expressed wish to do so.

2.2   The Sexual Experience

A sexual experience refers to any physical or psychological activity that involves sexual arousal and leads to sexual satisfaction. It is the result of a process occurring on different levels. This is described by the biopsychosocial model, which summarizes the interaction of 4-dimensional processes or axes [14]:

- Axis 1: Biological factors
- Pathophysiological processes (diseases and drugs)
- Almost all physical diseases can impact sexual function, either by direct damage to the structure of the genital organs or by indirect effects on the neurovascular and neuromuscular elements of the physiological sexual response. A large number of drugs interfere with sexual function through neurotransmitters in central and peripheral sexual response patterns.
- For example: endocrine factors like hypothyroidism, diabetes, hyperprolactinemia, postpartum period, menopause, or oral contraceptives that may interfere with sexual function
- Axis 2: Individual psychological factors
- Dysfunctional sexual learning (sexual script) trauma, specific personality traits
- For example: sexuality-aversive education, early-life experiences like neglect or abuse, events during adolescents, and performance anxiety abuse
- Axis 3: Interpersonal relationship factors
- Communication deficits, conflicts about needs
- For example: routine and habituation, conflicts, discrepancy of needs among the partners, noncommunication, emotional dissatisfaction, third-party involvement, etc.
- Axis 4: Sociocultural factors
- For example: norms and social role definitions, sexual myths, and misconceptions

2.3   The Interaction of Chronic Pain and Sexual Dysfunction

Different types of interaction can be distinguished:

(a) There is a shared psychophysiological pathway which contributes to pain syndrome and sexual dysfunction at the same time.

In these patients, the predominant feature is that signals from the body are strongly modified by central nervous processing patterns involving sympathetic and parasympathetic pathways leading to altered perception and/or efferent pathways. These patients suffer from combined psychophysiological dysregulation that manifests in dysfunctional syndromes of bowel, bladder, and sexual physiology.

Clinical examples are:

- Somatoform disorder
- Irritable bowel syndrome (IBS)
- Bladder pain syndrome
- Depression/anxiety with predominant physical symptoms

(b) The sexual dysfunction is a main contributing factor to chronic pelvic pain. Previous traumatic and painful sexual experiences induce neurovascular and neuromuscular reactions that result in increased inhibitory and defensive pathways from the brain to the pelvic sympathetic and parasympathetic plexus involved in sexual physiology. These factors contribute to pelvic floor pathology with dysfunctions of the pelvic floor ability to maintain stability, on the one hand, and to open the vaginal inlet and outlet, on the other hand. This is the musculoskeletal component in the pathogenesis of chronic pelvic and vulvar pain [15–17].
Clinical examples are:

- Sexual traumatization and sexual violence leading to lifelong vaginism based on pelvic floor dysfunction [18]
- Performance anxiety and sexual phobic reactions leading to pelvic floor dysfunction contributing to chronic vestibulodynia

(c) Chronic pelvic pain is the main contributing factor to sexual dysfunction. Structural defects interfere with the physiological pathways of the sexual response cycle.
Clinical examples are:

- Endometriosis [19]
- PID
- Tumors, etc.

(d) Chronic pelvic pain is one of the factors of a multifactorial pathogenesis of sexual dysfunction. In these patients, it is not the direct impact of the pelvic pathology, but other conditioning factors play an important role.
Clinical examples are:

- Couple conflicts or partner behavior
- Coexisting affective disorder
- Metabolic disorders
- Body image disturbances

(e) Comorbidities of CPP and sexual dysfunction as independent clinical entities: Patients with preexisting sexual dysfunction independent of their chronic pelvic pain syndrome with little interaction between the different clinical conditions.

2.3.1 Evaluation and Diagnostic: The Biopsychosocial Approach

Considering the complexity of chronic pain and sexual dysfunction on their own and the possible interaction of both systems, it is important that the healthcare professional develops a comprehensive and structured approach with a detailed clinical history [20, 21].

In this approach, we have two parts:

Part 1 refers to the establishment of a **descriptive diagnosis**.

Part 2 describes the way to an **explanatory diagnosis** (including understanding the pathogenesis of the problem):

- Step 1: Open the book, and encourage patients to talk [15]
- Patients often have trouble communicating their sexual problems, including pain during sexual activity, in the *physician's office. Therefore, it is* necessary to proactively ask about sexual health.
- A good introducing question could be:
- "Are you sexually active?" "Are there any problems or complaints you would like to talk about?"
- The patient may say: "It hurts (sometimes) when we have sex." "It feels uncomfortable. We have to stop."
- Step 2: *The pain history*
- It is important to ask the patient about the details of its symptoms.
- For example: "When does the pain occur, and where is it located?" "Are there situations and moments when it does not hurt?" "When and how did the pain start?"
- *Sexual problem-centered questions*
- *For example:* "What about your interest and desire to have sex?" "Do you feel mentally and physically aroused … Is your vagina sufficiently wet?" "Can you achieve orgasm?" "Was this different before?" "Was there a time when you had a satisfying sex life?"
- Step 3: *The descriptive diagnosis*
- Description of the patient's signs and symptoms:
  - Location on the genitals, whether it is superficial or deep or mixed
  - Duration, in terms of lifetime (primary/secondary) and in terms of the episode itself (at what time or with what activity it appears during the sexual encounter). Abrupt beginning or slowly developing
  - Single pain disorder or combined
  - Factors that increase and decrease the pain
  - Associated symptoms (itching, stinging, increased vaginal discharge, urinary leakage, LUTS, etc.)
  - Characteristics of the pain: stabbing, burning, intermittent, intense, or aching
  - Whether or not it is affected by postures and/or situations and/or sexual partners
  - Previous treatments that have been used and whether or not they have been successful

In this way, the physician will be able to evaluate the main clinical features that may already guide further diagnostic steps or the development of a diagnostic working hypothesis.

Examples:

- *Deep pain:* endometriosis, PID, Crohn's disease, IBS
- *Superficial (introital) pain: vulvovaginal atrophy, vulvovaginal infection, vulvar* dermatoses, vulvodynia
- *Mixed forms*: lower urinary tract infection, radiation

Long-standing, generalized, and slowly developing pain syndromes are usually more complex and multifactorial than those where the beginning is associated with specific event or change.

The next part of the diagnostic process focuses on understanding of the pathogenesis of the symptom. The goals are to establish an explanatory diagnosis, which allows the clinician to set up a therapeutic plan.

Step 4: *Sexual and short biographic history*
- "Let us go back a moment and have a look at your previous sexual experiences."
- The main questions relate to sex education, including affective and sexual experiences related to family, adolescence, relationships, and relationship with the family.
- Including a short biographic history: "I would like to get to know you better":
  • Major life events
  • Life phases
- Step 5: *Medical history (including gynecological history):*
- We should perform an exhaustive exploration of the most common gynecological and non-gynecological medical causes related to sexual dysfunction with or without pain.
- For example: dermatological problems, psychological problems, irritable bowel syndrome, malignant or premalignant diseases, endometriosis, myomas, etc.
- Step 6: *Clinical examination, imaging, and laboratory exams*
- The physical examination is of vital importance. We must keep in mind that the examination may be painful for the patient, so we must be extremely careful.
- The general physical examination will include body weight with tissue distribution, skin and hair, and vital signs.
- The gynecological examination should include a careful investigation of the vulva and vagina, assessment of the pelvic floor muscles (presence of muscular trigger points, evaluate the muscular tone [22]), signs of infection, form and mobility of the cervix, uterus, and adnexa.
- The physician should also attempt to establish a pain map. This includes a cotton swab testing of the vulva and the vestibulum used to localize painful areas and to classify the areas as painless or having mild, moderate, or severe pain [23].

- Regarding pelvic pain, it is important to note the location of pain, irradiation, and intensity of pain.
- Microscopic examination (wet mount) of vaginal discharge should be routine. Further microbiologic examination should be done if indicated.
- Ultrasound is indicated in case of suspected pelvic pathology.
- This second part of the diagnostic process (steps 4–6) will result in the explanatory diagnosis that can be summarized in a table based on the concept of the biopsychosocial model.
- In this model, the findings of the interview and the examination are organized in a two-dimensional way:
- Dimension 1 refers to biological, psychological, and social factors
- Dimension 2 refers to the phase of life or the time of life during which these factors have become relevant. We can distinguish predisposing factors (usually in the first phase of life), precipitating factors (factors that have a temporal relationship with the onset of symptoms), and maintaining factors (factors that contribute to the maintenance and chronicity of symptoms)

Factor matrix	Biological	Psychological		Social
		Individual	Relationship	
Predisposing	Family risks, pregnancy, and birth-related risks	Early trauma Abuse Neglect	Traumatic separation Humiliation	Broken family Early separation Migration
Precipitating	Disease, drugs, biological transition	Loss Life transition Separation	Distancing Third party New experience SexDysfPart	Migration, cultural norms, social changes
Maintaining	Pelvic floor dysfunction Musculoskeletal dysfunction	Anxiety False beliefs, stress responses	Conflicts Reproach circles Lack of skills to talk	Secondary reinforcement in the environment

The explanatory diagnosis will make it possible to distinguish three groups of patients presenting with sexual pain.

Group 1:

- Sexual pain coincides with the onset of a disease process and may be predominantly attributed to a specific disease and/or its treatment.
- Psychosocial factors (individual and personal) contribute to a lesser extent to the experience of pain and the chronicity.
- No significant impact of drugs and the environment.

For example: malignant diseases, endometriosis, VVA, urogenital syndrome of menopause

Group 2:

- There is an association between the sexual pain and a specific disease or treatment.
- In addition, there are non-disease-specific psychosocial factors (individual and interpersonal) that contribute greatly to the experience of pain and chronicity.
- Emotional and behavioral responses often intensify symptoms.

For example. recurrent infections, endometriosis, lack of sufficient arousal, increased anxiety, depression, pelvic floor disorder, vaginism

Group 3:

- Without punctual association with specific disease or treatment, but with a history of chronic recurrent disease (LUTs, infections)
- No major psychosocial contributing factors

For example: disorder of nerve transmission and central nervous signal processing, neuropathic pain

There is often overlap between the groups, especially in cases of long-term pain.

2.3.2 The Individualized Treatment Plan

An individualized treatment plan should be established that integrates the different therapeutic options by addressing all the causal factors that have been detected during the diagnostic procedure. Treatment should have a multidisciplinary framework.

General supportive interventions:

(A) *Psychoeducation and Counseling (Individual and Couple)*
   (a) Empowerment of patients, explanation
   (b) Elements of cognitive behavioral therapy
      These interventions focus on the psychotherapeutic principles of reorganization and correction of thought patterns and reframing of experience; self-induced relaxation and imagination, including breathing; and mindfulness training.

(B) *Physiotherapy:*
   (a) *Pelvic floor therapy*
      Different studies have shown the presence of pelvic floor muscular dysfunction in women with chronic pelvic pain and sexual dysfunction. These women present hypertonicity in their pelvic floor muscles and have a poorer pelvic floor muscle strength and control. The goal of pelvic floor therapy is to restore the proper function to the pelvic floor muscles and tissues, decrease neural tension and pain, and try to improve sexual function and, at the same time, make patients aware that the pelvic floor is an important organ with passive and active functions.

      Different treatments are described at musculoskeletal level: myofascial release and trigger-point release, joint mobilization, neural mobilization, scar tissue mobilization, visceral manipulation, vestibule desensitization, bowel and bladder retraining, exercise training, breathing practices, biofeedback, vaginal dilator, and electrical stimulation [24].

In addition to physiotherapy treatment, the use of infiltrations of local anesthetics and/or botulinum toxin may be useful [25].

(b) *General body awareness therapy*

These interventions are intended to help patients become aware of their body, especially the pelvic floor, as an organ and a unity. They can learn to be aware of their own interpretation of the sensory perception and thus learn to modify the cognitive response, which will impact the emotional element of the pain reaction.

Relaxation exercises focus on the visceral and emotional components of chronic pain.

Disease-specific interventions:

(A) Treatment of the underlying disorder
  (a) Surgical procedure, drug treatment, hormonal treatment
  (b) This treatment follows the guidelines given for the specific disease diagnosed to the patient (caution with possible side effects on sexual function)
(B) Modification of existing treatment to improve sexual health:
  (a) Change of analgesics (*adding anticonvulsants with a focus on the neuropathic component of pain*)
  (b) Change of antidepressants (*use of tricyclics to modify the emotional component of pain*)
  (c) Change of hormonal treatment (*use of progestogens instead of GnRH agonists in endometriotic pain, use of combined hormonal contraceptives in a long-cycle mode*)
(C) Rehabilitation:
  (a) Dilatation after radiotherapy

Targeting pain

(D) Pain treatment:
  (a) Pharmacological options: The use of various antinociceptive, anti-inflammatory, and neuromodulating agents comes from the evidence that women with chronic pelvic pain and sexual dysfunction might have increased innervation and/or sensitivity of nociceptors in pelvic region, as well as an abnormal processing of pain signals in the central nervous system [26, 27].

Antinociceptive agents: topical lidocaine, capsaicin

Anti-inflammatory agents: corticosteroids

Neuromodulating agents: anticonvulsants (gabapentin) and/or antidepressants (amitriptyline, duloxetine). Antidepressant medications are thought to exert their pain-mediating effects by increasing the release of inhibitory neurotransmitters (noradrenalin and serotonin), which play a role in modulating signaling from peripheral nociceptors.

(b) Analgesic interventions (blockade of afferent nerves)

(E) Psychological interventions including sex therapy:

(a) Counseling

(b) Individual and couple sex therapy

These interventions focus, on the one hand, on possible underlying factors of sexual pain arising from trauma and life events and, on the other hand, on maintenance factors coming from individual responses or couple interaction. The treatment aims to reduce pain and its associated distress and improve sexual function and satisfaction for both partners.

3   Scenario II: Patient with Specific Disease Leading to Chronic Pelvic Pain and Other Symptoms

In this scenario, the patient has previously been diagnosed with pelvic pathology.

The focus of care is primarily on the disease and its treatment. Early in the care process, sexual health is often not a priority concern of patients and physicians and is frequently not addressed. However, it is well known that diseases of the genital organs are closely related to sexual function and dysfunction.

We can distinguish different levels of interaction [20, 21]:

- The biological impact:
  (a) Destruction of tissues involved in sexual response, such as nerves and vascular supply to the vulva, vagina, and pelvic floor resulting in arousal and sexual pain disorders

    For example: vulvar and vaginal malignancies, cervical carcinoma

  (b) Morphological changes in the pelvic anatomy leading to symptoms and dysfunctions such as pain, bleeding, and infertility, with a negative impact on sexual desire, arousal, and pain

    For example: endometriosis, fibroma

  (c) Alteration and dysregulation of endocrine actions that modulate the human sexual response, leading to decreased desire, arousal, and, ultimately, painful sexual intercourse

    For example: hypoestrogenism in the context of cancer treatment, endometriosis, perimenopause

  (d) The dysregulating impact on central nervous neurotransmitter actions due to drug treatments leading to low desire, partner distress, and eventually secondary pain disorder

- The psychological impact:
  (a) The general threat of the disease, which can create anxiety and a depressive mood that negatively impacts sexual interest and sexual arousal, thus increasing the risk of painful sexual intercourse.

(b) Relationship distress leading to conflict, discrepancy of needs, etc. The disease often requires adaptation of both partners and, frequently, new definitions of roles and interactions.

3.1 The Diagnostic Workup for Patients with Pelvic Pathology Leading to Sexual Dysfunction

In many patients with organic disease, the threat of the disease and the respective anxiety and concerns occupy the center of the patient's and the healthcare professional's attention. Therefore, it is important to make the sexual history part of the overall diagnosis and to proceed according to the steps described above.

In establishing a comprehensive diagnosis, the focus is on the impact of the disease on sexual health. To understand the impact, the physician would evaluate the sexual life prior to diagnosis to understand the changes caused by the disease and its treatment:

- How important was sexuality in his day life?
- How satisfied was the patient with his sexual life, and how satisfied was he with his body and his relationship?
- Where there any problem regarding sexual function?

The physician will then assess the impact of the disease according to the different levels.

We have described this as the eight Ds [20]:

1. **Danger** to life leading to anxiety and depression
2. **Destruction** of organs and tissues involved in the sexual response
3. **Disruption of endocrine regulation** of the sexual response
4. **Dysregulation of neurotransmitters** involved in the sexual response
5. **Disfigurement** with negative impact on body image
6. **Disability and pain**
7. **Disease load with comorbidities (incontinence, etc.)**
8. **Drugs** especially antihormones and chemotherapeutics

3.1.1 The Treatment Plan

The treatment plan consists of two components:

Sexual Rehabilitation

In patients with pelvic pathology, treatment may lead to permanent loss of several components of the sexual function of the healthy individual (see above).

For these patients, it is important to work with them in several steps:

(a) Assess permanent losses or changes, and help patients learn to accept these limitations.

(b) Evaluate the components of the sexual life that the patient can experience and live.

(c) To help the patient develop a new concept of sexual life based on these resources.

For example:

- Shift of focus from intercourse as the dominant sexual practice to other practices including the use of sex toys.
- Keep intimacy alive with kissing, caressing, touching, and being emotionally close to each other.
- From passionate sex and love to recreational sex and intimacy.
- For these patients, elements of sensate focus therapy can be very helpful.

Chronic Pain and Sexual Therapy

The elements described above constructed the individualized treatment plan for the different symptoms and levels of dysfunction.

The multidisciplinary approach includes:

Mental health interventions

(a) Psychotherapy and/or pharmacotherapy to help patients cope with the anxiety or depression

(b) Couple therapy to help couples and patients understand and discuss the changes they are experiencing

Chronic pain therapy

(a) Drugs
(b) Targeted local nerve blocks

Physiotherapy

(a) Pelvic floor rehabilitation
(b) Vaginal dilatation after radiation therapy

Local hormonal and drug treatments with estrogens or SERMS or DHEA

4   Conclusion

In this chapter, we have talked about the existing interconnections between chronic pelvic pain and sexual pain and how they have an impact on sexual health. Many different causes can provoke pelvic pain and sexual pain, which can lead to sexual dysfunction. These causes include physical and/or psychological factors (Fig. 1). Any discomfort or pain reported during sexual activity needs to be taken into account, as well as the underlying causes of this pain need to be identified in order to establish a correct and effective therapeutic plan.

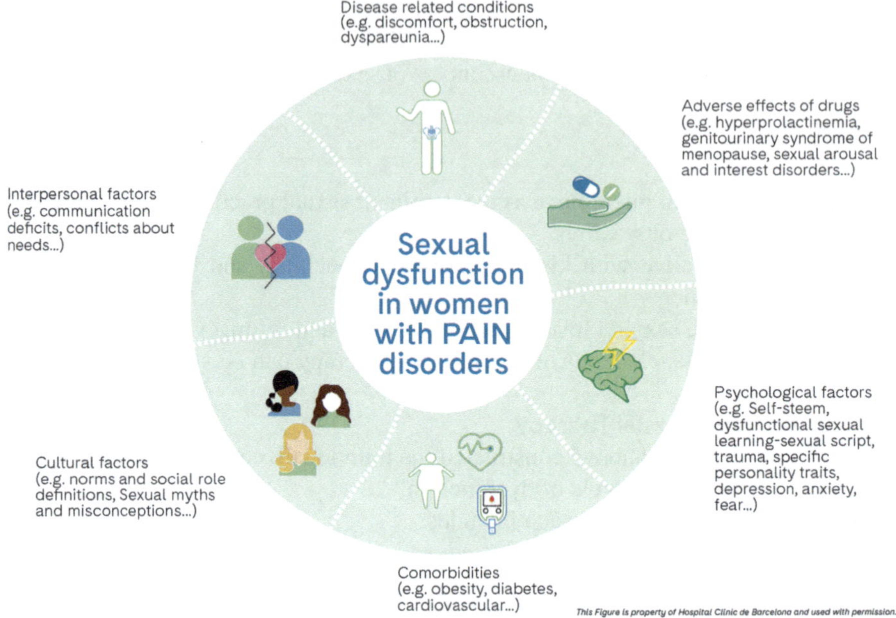

Fig. 1 Sexual dysfunction in women with PAIN disorders

In these patients, a multidisciplinary care program addressing all the aspects causing pain and affecting their sexual health should be considered and taken into account, including pelvic floor physiotherapy, psychological interventions, pain education, and pharmaceutical or interventional treatments. Patients should be empowered so that they can participate in the improvement of their sexual health.

References

1. Gandhi J, Khan SA. Letters to the Editors A vicious cycle of causes and consequences of dyspareunia: rethinking the approach to management of genitourinary syndrome of menopause. Am J Obstet Gynecol. 2017;217(5):625. https://doi.org/10.1016/j.ajog.2017.07.030.
2. www.acog.org/Patients/FAQs/Chronic-Pelvic-Pain.
3. Clauw DJ, Essex MN, Pitman V, Jones KD. Reframing chronic pain as a disease, not a symptom: rationale and implications for pain management. Postgrad Med. 2019;131(3):185–98. https://doi.org/10.1080/00325481.2019.1574403.
4. Stratton P, Berkley KJ. Chronic pelvic pain and endometriosis: translational evidence of the relationship and implications. Hum Reprod Update. 2011;17(3):327–46.
5. Loeser JD. A new way of thinking about pains. Pain. 2022;163(9):1670–4.
6. Speer LM, Mushkbar S, Erbele T, College T, Sciences L. Chronic pelvic pain in women. Am Fam Physician. 2016;93:380–7.
7. Cohen SP, Vase L, Hooten WM. Chronic pain: an update on burden, best practices, and new advances. Lancet. 2021;397(10289):2082–97. https://doi.org/10.1016/S0140-6736(21)00393-7.
8. Woolf CJ. Central sensitization: implications for the diagnosis and treatment of pain. Pain. 2011;152(Suppl 3):S2–15. https://doi.org/10.1016/j.pain.2010.09.030.

9. Lamvu G, Carrillo J, Ouyang C, Rapkin A. Chronic pelvic pain in women: a review. JAMA J Am Med Assoc. 2021;325(23):2381–91.

10. Giamberardino MA, Costantini R, Affaitati G, Fabrizio A, Lapenna D, Tafuri E, et al. Viscero-visceral hyperalgesia: characterization in different clinical models. Pain. 2010;151(2):307–22. https://doi.org/10.1016/j.pain.2010.06.023.

11. Giamberardino MA, Affaitati G, Fabrizio A, Costantini R. Myofascial pain syndromes and their evaluation. Best Pract Res Clin Rheumatol. 2011;25(2):185–98. https://doi.org/10.1016/j.berh.2011.01.002.

12. Buster JE. Managing female sexual dysfunction. Fertil Steril. 2013;100(4):905–15. https://doi.org/10.1016/j.fertnstert.2013.08.026.

13. American Psychiatric Association. DSM IV: Diagnostic and statistical manual of mental disorders. 4th ed; 1994.

14. American Psychiatric Association. DSM V: Diagnostic and statistical manual of mental disorders. 5th ed; 2013.

15. Brandenburg U, Bitzer J. The challenge of talking about sex: the importance of patient—physician interaction. Maturitas. 2009;63:124–7.

16. Yong PJ, Mui J, Allaire C, Williams C. Pelvic floor tenderness in the etiology of superficial dyspareunia. J Obstet Gynaecol Can. 2014;36(11):1002–9. https://doi.org/10.1016/S1701-2163(15)30414-X.

17. Parish SJ, Bitzer J. Sexual medicine education and training. In: Goldstein I, Claytoon AH, Goldstein AT, Kim NN, Kingsberg SA, editors. Textbook of female sexual function and dysfunction: diagnosis and treatment. Wiley Blackwell; 2016. p. 7–16.

18. Karsten MDA, Wekker V, Bakker A, Groen H, Olff M, Hoek A, et al. Sexual function and pelvic floor activity in women: the role of traumatic events and PTSD symptoms. Eur J Psychotraumatol. 2020;11(1):1–9. https://doi.org/10.1080/20008198.2020.1764246.

19. Barbara G, Facchin F, Meschia M, Berlanda N, Frattaruolo MP, Vercellini P. When love hurts. A systematic review on the effects of surgical and pharmacological treatments for endometriosis on female sexual functioning. Acta Obstet Gynecol Scand. 2017;96(6):668–87.

20. Bitzer J, Platano G, Tschudin S, Alder J. Sexual counseling for women in the context of physical diseases. J Sex Med. 2007;4(1):29–37. https://doi.org/10.1111/j.1743-6109.2006.00395.x.

21. Farmer MA Anatomy and physiology of sexual pain. In: Goldstein I, Claytoon AH. Goldstein AT, Kim NN Kingsberg SA, editor. Textbook of female sexual function and dysfunction. Wiley Blackwell; 2018. p. 257–280.

22. Meister MR, Sutcliffe S, Ghetti C, Chu CM, Spitznagle T, Warren DK, et al. Development of a standardized, reproducible screening examination for assessment of pelvic floor myofascial pain. Obstet Gynecol Surv. 2019;74(6):338.

23. Haefner HK, Collins ME, Davis GD, Edwards L, Foster DC, Hartmann ED, Kaufman RH, Lynch PJ, Margesson LJ, Moyal-Barracco M, Piper CK. The vulvodynia guideline. J Low Genit Tract Dis. 2005;9(1):40–51.

24. Morin M, Carroll MS, Bergeron S. Systematic review of the effectiveness of physical therapy modalities in women with provoked vestibulodynia. Sex Med Rev. 2017;5(3):295–322. https://doi.org/10.1016/j.sxmr.2017.02.003.

25. Zoorob D, South M, Karram M, Sroga J, Maxwell R, Shah A, et al. A pilot randomized trial of levator injections versus physical therapy for treatment of pelvic floor myalgia and sexual pain. Int Urogynecol J. 2015;26:845–52.

26. Rosen NO, Dawson SJ, Brooks M, Kellogg S. Treatment of vulvodynia: pharmacological and non-pharmacological approaches. Drugs. 2019;79:483. https://doi.org/10.1007/s40265-019-01085-1.

27. Vogel JJ. Pain specialist management of sexual pain—IV. Pharmacological. Sex Med Rev. 2023;11:98–105.

Pelvic Floor Disorders and Sexuality 1: Urinary Incontinence

Sònia Anglès Acedo, Lorena López Frías,
and Cristina Ros Cerro

1   Introduction

Sexual health is a state of physical, emotional, mental, and social well-being in relation to sexuality, which requires the possibility of having pleasurable and safe sexual experiences [1].

The real impact of urinary incontinence (UI) and its treatments on women's sexual health remains a complicated issue, as most of the publications in this field do not intend to identify the proportion of problems which are directly related to UI. Therefore, the aspects of female sexuality which become affected by UI itself remain unclear. Good-quality studies on sexual health in women with UI are mandatory to improve their sexual management focused on a multidisciplinary and bio-psychosocial approach.

The original version of the chapter has been revised. A correction to this chapter can be found at
https://doi.org/10.1007/978-3-031-55080-5_35

S. Anglès Acedo (✉) · C. Ros Cerro
Urogynecological Unit, Clinical Institute of Gynecology, Obstetrics and Neonatology, Hospital Clinic de Barcelona, Barcelona, Spain

Clinical Sexology Working Group, Hospital Clinic de Barcelona, Barcelona, Spain

Surgery and Medical-Surgical Specialties, Faculty of Medicine and Health Sciences, Universitat de Barcelona (UB), Barcelona, Spain

Institut d'Investigacions Biomèdiques August Pi i Sunyer, Barcelona, Spain
e-mail: sangles@clinic.cat; cros@clinic.cat

L. López Frías
Urogynecological Unit, Clinical Institute of Gynecology, Obstetrics and Neonatology, Hospital Clinic de Barcelona, Barcelona, Spain

Clinical Sexology Working Group, Hospital Clinic de Barcelona, Barcelona, Spain
e-mail: llopez3@clinic.cat

As one of the most prevalent pelvic floor dysfunctions, UI is defined by involuntary loss of urine. According to the type of UI, the most prevalent are:

- Stress UI (SUI): involuntary leakage of urine on effort, physical exertion, sneezing, or coughing
- Urgency UI (UUI): involuntary loss of urine associated with urgency (complaint of sudden, compelling desire to pass urine which is difficult to defer)
- Mixed UI (MUI): the association between SUI and UUI

It is estimated that the prevalence of overall UI ranges from 25 to 45% [2], being 10–39% for SUI, 1–7% for UUI, and 7–25% for MUI.

Quality of life of women with UI is negatively affected, although it is not a life-threatening condition. Moreover, quality-of-life impairment may be related to its multiple dimensions, thus altering the physical, social, emotional, and sexual well-being of those women.

1.1 Urinary Incontinence During Sexual Activity

According to the International Continence Society (ICS)/International Urogynecological Association (IUGA) consensus on the terminology for assessment of female sexual health [3], there are two new definitions for UI during sexual activity:

- Penetration UI: loss of urine with vaginal stimulation (penile, manual, or with a sexual toy)
- Orgasmic UI: loss of urine occurring at orgasm, regardless of the sexual behavior that has triggered it

These more accurate definitions allow us to evaluate all women, regardless of their sexual orientation and the existence or not of a partnership.

However, most of the studies in this field were performed according to the previous terminology "coital UI" defined as the complaint of involuntary loss of urine occurring during or after vaginal intercourse [3].

The rate of coital incontinence is 2–60% [4–6]; however, it is an underreported symptom by patients and an understudied symptom by health care professionals, and some study bias may also affect the real rate. Published literature is mainly performed in heterosexual female population [7, 8]. This symptom is based frequently on self-perception of women about being *sexually active* without a clear terminology for that concept, which unfortunately is still linked to partnered sexuality and/or intercourse, which may lead out of the collected data those women with different sexual behaviors (e.g., solo-sex participants, women without vaginal activity). Moreover, most of the studies focused on coital incontinence among women who attend urogynecological units (coital incontinence rate 10–66%) [4, 5, 7, 9], and only few studies included women among overall population (coital incontinence rate 2%) [10].

The physiopathological mechanism underlying coital UI is not yet elucidated, although some studies focused on the correlation of that symptom and the urodynamic diagnosis. Classically, penetration UI has been associated with urodynamic SUI, and orgasmic UI has been associated with urodynamic detrusor overactivity. Nevertheless, more recent studies have suggested the association between orgasmic UI and urodynamic SUI by intrinsic urethral sphincter deficiency [4, 11, 12].

In addition, in an unknown proportion of female population, during the female sexual response, different vaginal fluids may be expelled (vaginal lubrication, squirting, female ejaculation), so an appropriate differential diagnosis will be needed to avoid mix-up with an episode of UI during sexual activity. These physiological processes may be isolated or coexist in the same women. All of them are self-considered a positive phenomenon, which improves women and partner's sexual life. Therefore, vaginal lubrication, squirting, female ejaculation, and UI during sexual activity are different phenomena with various mechanisms and could be differentiated according to source, quantity, expulsion mechanism, and subjective feelings during sexual activities [13, 14]. However, to date, knowledge on vaginal sexual fluids is controversial, and further studies in that field are needed. Contrary to the lack of scientific evidence information, there is increasing exposure of general population to inaccurate or incomplete information about sexual vaginal fluids as squirting or female ejaculation through porn, erotic movies, or different social channels. Frequently focused on specific sexual response with specific sexual behaviors, which can be the origin of unrealistic sexual expectations for both women and their partners, it should not be assumed as "sexual standards." Therefore, from health care professional point of view, it is important to be aware that some of our patients may present any kind of sexual fluid expulsion or a combination of them, and we should reassure them as a physiological phenomenon. However, the absence of these symptoms during sexual activity and orgasm is also considered as a normal sexual response, and women should also be aware of that to avoid frustration.

2 The Impact of Urinary Incontinence on Female Sexual Health

2.1 Sexual Activity Among Women with UI

Among women with UI, the rate of sexual inactivity is estimated at around 5–38% [6]. Any type of UI, even if not occurring during sexual activity, can alter sexual behavior and well-being, leading women to decide to stop any kind of sexual activity (solo sex and partnered sex).

In addition, sexually active women with UI may also report an impairment of their sexual activity such as more avoidance behaviors, less sexual frequency, or restriction of some specific sexual activity. It is estimated that 25–38% sexually active women would restrict their sexual activity due to UI [6].

Unfortunately, most of the studies exclude sexually inactive women, missing the opportunity to understand whether women might be inactive because of the impact of their UI. However, some studies have examined the factors associated with sexual inactivity or decreased sexual activity in female UI population, underlying the lack of a partner and UI during sexual activity as the most important ones. However, none of the studies compared sexually inactive with active women; therefore, the role of UI in being single is still unknown, although it probably causes difficulties to achieve stable or sporadic emotional and/or sexual relationships. Of note, women should be specifically asked for UI during sexual activity in the gynecologic visits due to the strongly negative impact on women's sexuality [4]. Other factors as dyspareunia, wetness at night, embarrassment, depression, and need for a separate bed were also related to sexual inactivity in women with UI [6].

2.2 Sexual Function Among Women with UI

It is broadly accepted that UI has a negative impact on sexual function. However, the way this influence occurs, directly or indirectly, remains unclear, especially when we seek to understand the mechanisms involved in this outcome [15].

Among women with UI, the rate of sexual dysfunction is estimated at around 23–56%. Common across nearly all studies, all UI types were associated with higher rate of sexual dysfunction compared to women without UI. Multiple studies suggest that MUI has the greatest impact, followed by UUI, which is found to be more bothersome than SUI regarding sexual life [6]. Moreover, UI during sexual activity is reported as one of the most relevant factors of sexual function impairment. A cross-sectional multicentric Spanish study [5] conducted in sexually active women who attended the gynecologist seeking treatment for UI and/or overactive bladder tried to identify factors associated with quality of life and measured by a specific questionnaire (King's Health Questionnaire). Focused on the items about the impact on couple and sexual life comprised in the personal relations dimension, it is possible to verify that women with coital UI have greater impairment than those without it. Furthermore, in the multiple regression model, coital UI was the only independent variable associated with a worse quality of life (adjusted by all types of UI, body mass index, age, and other variables).

UI symptoms may cause clinically relevant psychological and physical consequences, which impair sexual life. Therefore, multiple domains of sexual function may be affected in women with UI. All types of UI may alter different aspects of sexual response, and different studies found association with lack of interest or arousal or lubrication, orgasmic disorder, lower sexual satisfaction, and poorer self-image and self-esteem, with dyspareunia being the more prevalent (8–44%) sexual dysfunction in UI female population [5, 6, 16, 17]. In that line, Salonia et al. [9] conducted a cross-sectional study comparing 227 women with UI and/or lower urinary tract symptoms to 102 control women. They were assessed with a comprehensive history that included validated questionnaires, a physical examination, a urodynamic test, and the Female Sexual Function Index (FSFI). Sexual dysfunction was diagnosed in 46% of these patients with UI, and the most frequent sexual dysfunctions were dyspareunia (44%), lack of interest (34%), arousal disorder (23%), and orgasmic disorder (11%).

3 The Impact of Urinary Incontinence Treatments on Female Sexuality

Management of UI should be tailored to each woman according to type, severity, and bother of UI symptoms; associated pelvic floor disorders; health status and comorbidities; age; and frailty. In addition, it is important to consider current sexual life and the presence of sexual dysfunction, as well as future sexual expectations. There are different options to manage UI symptoms: conservative treatment, pharmacological treatment, or surgical treatment. All of them may impact female sexuality of women with UI, and health care professionals should be aware of its role to provide proper counseling to each patient, considering both positive and negative effects on sexual activity and function.

3.1 Coping Strategies

Coping strategies are defined as those measures aimed at helping users to live with their condition in the best possible way, adapting lifestyles to regain a sense of control and a more positive experience [18].

Most of the women with UI reported coping strategies regarding their sexuality, both those who experience UI during sexual activity and those who do not. It can affect partnered sex on intimacy, proximity, and partner dynamics, but also solo sex due to the frustration of loss of control. Bidzan et al. [19] classified women with SUI during intercourse in separate categories according to the severity of coping strategies. The aim of these strategies may be different:

- Complete avoidance of sexual activity: e.g., women who are not allowed to enjoy sexual experience due to the presence (or fear) of UI during sexual activity or due to the smell (self-esteem impairment)
- Changes that minimize the risk of urine leaks during sex but at the same time limit sexual satisfaction for women and also their partner: e.g., to reduce sexual activity frequency
- Changes that minimize the risk of urine leaks during sex but at the same time limit sexual satisfaction for women, preserving sexual partner's satisfaction: e.g., to reduce the time of sexual intercourse by adjusting to the minimum to guarantee the partner climax, fake orgasm to shorten the sexual time, or avoid orgasm in women with orgasmic UI
- Changes that minimize the risk of urine leaks during sex but permit women and partner sexual satisfaction: e.g., less restrictive strategies such as urinating before sexual activity, fluid intake restriction, or restricting some sexual behaviors linked to UI
- Changes that minimize the impact on sexuality of urine leaks during sex, allowing women and partner sexual satisfaction: e.g., to use towels to protect the bed, to engage in sexual activity in the shower or bath, or to wash before sexual activity

Health care professionals should investigate deeply into that kind of coping strategies to better understand the real impact of UI on women's sexuality.

3.2   Conservative Treatment

3.2.1   Pelvic Floor Muscle Training

Pelvic floor muscle training (PFMT) is the first-line treatment for women with UI [20].

The PFMT consists of exercise to improve PFM strength, endurance, power, relaxation, or a combination of these parameters. It should be individualized and personalized and may be performed at home with periodic supervision by the therapist. Before starting the program, an assessment of the state and strength of the muscles must be carried out (by means of a vaginal examination). Sometimes, it can be helpful to use a biofeedback device (a device that offers an acoustic or visual signal that monitors the performance of the exercises) facilitating the woman to observe a better proprioception, both in contraction and relaxation.

Women with any type of UI after carrying out a PFMT program improve their sexual function [21]. The UI symptom improvement after treatment may reduce anxiety and fear of women during sexual activity, decreasing dyspareunia. In addition, probably the improvement in sexual function is also produced by improving muscle function. A multicenter study [22] of women with pelvic floor disorders from the USA and the UK concluded that a strong pelvic floor is associated with higher rates of sexual activity as well as higher sexual function scores on the condition impact domain of the PISQ-IR and the orgasm domain of the FSFI. In that line, a secondary analysis of a randomized trial in women with UI after PFMT studied on predictors of improvement in sexual function. It was found that greater adherence to PFMT, improvement in PFM strength, and decreased frequency of urine loss are predictors of improved sexual quotient. It also suggests that PFMT was more beneficial with respect to sexual function in those women who presented sexual dysfunction at the beginning of the study [23].

PFMT is not only important for improving muscle strength. The rate of dyspareunia in women with UI is high. In some cases, the pain is caused by increased muscle tone, hypertonia, myofascial syndrome, or muscle spasm.

In these cases, pain and consequently sexual function can be improved through proprioception exercises of the pelvic floor muscles (learning to coordinate this muscle, knowing how to relax). A useful technique for that may be the progressive muscular relaxation (also known as Jacobson's technique): control the tension in each muscle group, paying attention to the contrast when contracting and relaxing [18].

Finally, learning to coordinate PFM, knowing how to relax and contract, getting control of duration (resistance), and even reaching a specific rhythm allow women with UI to rule over a part of their body. It permits women to achieve power over their sexuality and can often be a gateway to work on self-efficacy and self-esteem [24].

3.2.2   Intravaginal Devices for SUI

Intravaginal devices for UI are intended to provide some support to the bladder neck and possibly some compression to the urethra to correct SUI [18].

Some of the most commonly used devices for SUI are specific pessaries and tampons. Both devices are recommended to be removed for sexual intercourse, although some vaginal continence pessary users decide to keep it during sexual activity.

In contrast to the extensive literature on prolapse pessaries, there are scarce publications regarding sexual activity and function among users of continence pessaries.

A randomized study [25] on conservative treatment of SUI included three groups: continence pessary, behavioral therapy (PFMT and continence strategies), or combination therapy. The authors did not find sexual improvement among those women who did not improve their SUI symptoms, neither comparing different groups. Among women successfully treated for SUI, participants were more likely to experience improvement in continence during sexual activity after treatment with behavioral therapy or combination therapy than with the pessary alone. A limitation of that study was that the rate of women who removed their continence pessary during sexual activity was not recorded. Additionally, study participants did not receive specific instructions regarding whether they should remove the pessary for sexual activity. The authors speculate that removal of the pessary for sexual activity, even among those successfully treated, could have prevented these women from experiencing improvements in continence during sexual intercourse.

In a multicentered randomized trial [26] comparing continence pessary (CP) with a disposable intravaginal continence device (DICD) for SUI, sexual function was evaluated with a generic sexual questionnaire. Female Sexual Function Index (FSFI) scores went down in the CP group and increased in the DICD group over the treatment period (4 weeks). However, these results should be considered with caution due to the small sample size and high rate of dropout and because sexual function was not the primary outcome. Therefore, the authors concluded that these sexual findings need further exploration in future studies to examine the impact of continence devices and SUI on sexual function.

3.3 Pharmacological Treatment

The use of local hormonal treatment (estrogen or androgen) to manage genitourinary syndrome of menopause frequently associated with UUI in menopausal women is broadly accepted and recommended in all international guidelines. These treatments act on the vaginal mucosa increasing its thickness, re-vascularizing the epithelium, increasing the number of superficial cells and vaginal pH, and restoring the vaginal flora, leading to both UUI symptom and sexual symptom improvement [27]. A similar effect seems to be observed with ospemifene [27, 28].

In a systematic review and meta-analysis [28], a significant improvement of female sexual function was described after antimuscarinic and beta-adrenergic administration in women with UUI and/or overactive bladder, but only in those women whose UI symptoms improved. Serati et al. [7] found that orgasmic UI is curable by antimuscarinic treatment in about 60% of women with UUI and urodynamic detrusor overactivity.

3.4 Surgical Treatment

3.4.1 Bulking Agents

Urethral bulking agents have emerged in recent years as a minimally invasive surgical management for SUI. Despite an increasing literature on this topic, the impact of bulking agents on female sexuality is absent in most of the recent systematic reviews and meta-analyses [29–31].

According to a narrative review [32] and a systematic review/meta-analysis [33], dyspareunia was a complication reported among 3.8–10% of women after treatment with Urolastic®, but 0% with other bulking agents as Bulkamid®, Macroplastique®, Durasphere®, and Coaptite®. However, the adverse effects after bulking agent procedure have not been properly reported in all the studies, so possible negative impact on sexuality is understudied.

On the other hand, the positive impact on sexuality associated with improvement of SUI symptoms after injection seems to be demonstrated in few studies [34, 35]; however, it seems to be lower compared to other surgical options. In a randomized trial conducted in Finland by Itkonen Freitas et al. [36], 224 women suffering from SUI in whom PFMT had failed were included (111 mid-urethral sling vs. 113 bulking agent). Sexual function through the Pelvic Organ Prolapse/Urinary Incontinence Sexual Questionnaire-12 improved in both groups ($p < 0.001$ for mid-urethral sling and $p = 0.01$ for bulking agent), with higher scores ($p < 0.001$) for mid-urethral sling, at 1-year follow-up.

3.4.2 Mid-Urethral Sling

Mid-urethral sling has been, and currently is, the preferred method for primary surgical management of SUI for more than 20 years around the world, due to the high cure rates at mid- and long term, confirming a significant improvement of the sexual function after stress UI surgical treatments.

A recent meta-analysis [37] focused on sexual function after mid-urethral slings for SUI, based on 22 trials which used validated sexual questionnaires. A significant sexual function improvement was found at mid-term follow-up (12–24 months after surgery). Moreover, desire, arousal, orgasm, lubrication, satisfaction, and dyspareunia were significantly better postoperatively. Only seven studies assessed coital UI before and after surgery, highlighting a significant decrease after surgery. A prospective observational study [38] in 82 women with urodynamic SUI and coital UI (58% penetration UI, 15% orgasmic UI, and 25% both) found that 86% of participants were very much or much better after mid-urethral sling procedure (91% among women with penetration UI, 69% women with orgasmic UI, and 85% women with both). Therefore, most of the women with SUI and any type of UI during sexual activity will improve their sexuality after surgery.

However, mid-urethral sling intervention may cause side effects, which can impair female sexuality due to anatomic, physiological, vascular, neurological, and hormonal alterations in the anterior vaginal wall. It is important to identify the subgroup of women with de novo or persistent pain after surgery (e.g., fibrosis, mesh exposure, mesh tension, etc.), decreased sensitivity associated with lubrication, and arousal and/or orgasm disorder. In order to detect possible complications in the sexual sphere, it is key to perform a postoperative sexual assessment among all women.

3.4.3 Other Surgical Treatments

Traditional surgeries for SUI as autologous fascia sling or Burch colposuspension are more complex interventions associated with higher complication rates. Sexual impact after these surgeries has been poorly studied, and controversial results were found, which may not allow us to provide clear recommendations.

The use of energy-based therapies, as laser or radiofrequency, to treat SUI has increased in last years, frequently with a double advertising: to improve SUI symptoms but also female sexual function. However, there is no evidence for recommendation of energy-based therapy to improve SUI when compared to placebo or other treatments according to high-quality studies [39], so the positive improvement of sexual function related to the improvement of SUI symptoms should not be expected. In that line, a recent meta-analysis based on four RCT and two non-RCT studies did not confirm that energy-based treatments improved the sexual function of women with SUI [40].

Botulinum toxin injection is an alternative for refractory UUI. In the previously mentioned systematic review and meta-analysis by Balzarro et al. [28], the impact of that treatment in female sexual function has been analyzed in two studies. A significant improvement of the global sexual function was found, as well as an improvement of UUI symptoms. Focused on sexual dimensions, lubrication did not improve, whereas arousal, orgasm, and satisfaction were significantly better after treatment. Data on desire and pain were controversial, as they only improved in one of the two studies.

Another option for refractory UUI is the sacral neuromodulation. Most of the studies which have investigated female sexual function were retrospective and secondary analysis. A systematic review and meta-analysis of 13 studies [41] showed a significant improvement of global sexual function after this treatment. The nine studies in which sacral neuromodulation was done primarily for urinary indications retained a positive effect on sexual function when analyzed separately. There was a significant improvement in pain, arousal, and satisfaction, whereas lubrication or orgasm dimension did not change. A strong trend toward improvement in desire after sacral neuromodulation was observed. However, the authors highlight that the issue of whether the improvement in sexual function is entirely due to the resolution of a functional bladder disorder or due to a direct effect of sacral neuromodulation on sexual function needs further examination.

An RCT [42] comparing botulinum toxin ($n = 190$) to sacral neuromodulation ($n = 174$) found a significant improvement of sexual function after both treatments, without differences between groups.

4   Cognitive and Behavioral Therapy in Women with Urinary Incontinence

As mentioned previously, UI may impact physical, emotional, mental, and social aspects of female sexual well-being (Fig. 1). Despite conservative, pharmacological, and/or surgical management, women with UI should struggle with sexual challenges explained above in this chapter, with the emotional and behavioral factors playing an important role in coping with the disease.

According to that, offering a combination of cognitive and behavioral approaches through cognitive behavioral therapy (CBT) may help women with UI to recognize their distorted attitudes and dysfunctional behaviors, connecting thoughts, feelings, physical sensations, and actions. To change some thoughts and behaviors, regular discussions and organized behavioral tasks are used. The main goal is to modify patterns and to get beneficial changes in the patient's mood, sexual attitude, and sexual self-confidence [43–45].

In that line, an RCT [46] conducted on 84 reproductive-aged women (18–45 years old) with UI tried to investigate the effect of CBT on sexual self-esteem and sexual function through sexual validated questionnaires. After 8 weekly sessions of CBT, a statistically significant difference ($p < 0.001$) in sexual self-esteem, both mean score and its domains (skill/experience, attractiveness, control, moral judgment, and adaptiveness), was found. In the control group, only significant changes in skill/experience, control, and moral judgment dimensions were observed, but these

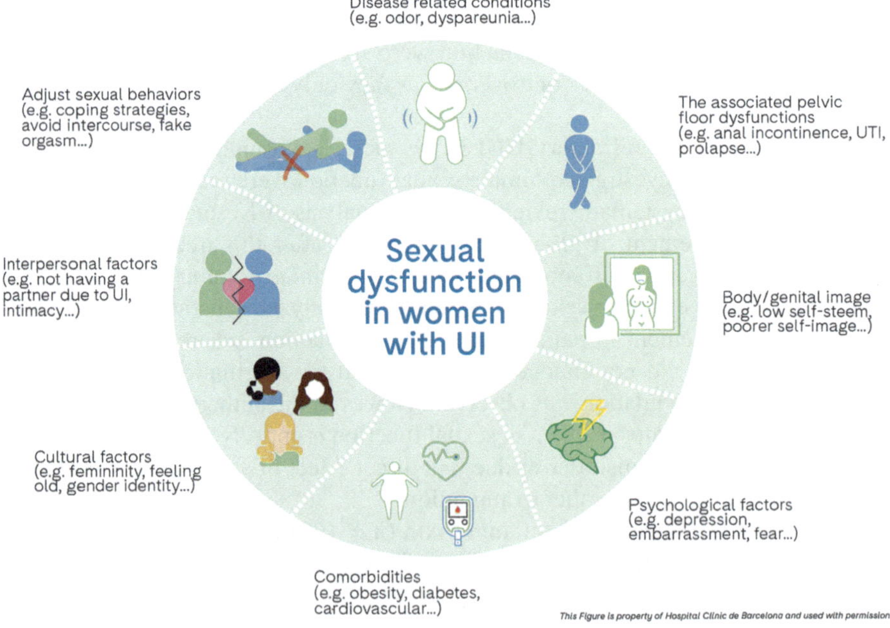

Fig. 1 Sexual dysfunction in women with UI

changes were downward and slight compared to the intervention group. Moreover, a statistically significant difference ($p < 0.001$) in sexual function, both mean score and its domains (behavioral-emotional, physical, and partner related), was found in the CBT group. In the control group, only significant change in physical dimension was observed, but this change was downward and slight compared to the intervention group. Both changes in self-esteem and sexual function were maintained 4 weeks after the intervention. The authors also found a positive correlation between the sexual self-esteem/self-confidence and sexual function.

Therefore, CBT should be recommended as a noninvasive, low-cost, and effective way to improve female sexuality in women with UI. It should be considered as an adjuvant alternative to any conservative, pharmacological, and surgical treatment selected by the patient to treat her UI, to achieve a biopsychological approach, and to provide a comprehensive management of the complex sexual issues presented by those women. Of note, this therapeutic option should be offered within a multidisciplinary team and may be provided by any trained health care professional as specialized nurses, physiotherapists, gynecologists, urologists, or general practitioners.

5   Conclusion

Sexual activity and function may be affected in women with any type of UI, with the presence of UI during sexual activity being one of the most relevant factors. Physical, psychological, emotional, and sociocultural factors may play a role in sexual impairment in those women. Conservative, pharmacological, and surgical treatments for UI usually have a positive impact on female sexuality, although it is important to highlight that a subgroup of women can maintain, worsen, or develop a sexual dysfunction after these treatments. A multidisciplinary biopsychosocial approach within the shared decision-making process to treat UI should be offered considering the current sexual life and sexual expectations for the future of each patient.

Further high-quality studies among sexually inactive women, women who only engage in solo-sex behaviors, and gender minority population are needed to understand the real impact of UI and its treatments on female sexual health.

References

1. World Health Organization. Defining sexual health. Report of a technical consultation on sexual health, 28–31 January 2002, Geneva. Geneva: World Health Organization; 2006.
2. Milsom I, Altman D, Cartwright R, Lapitan MC, Nelson R, Sjöström S, Tikkinen K. Epidemiology of urinary incontinence (UI) and other lower urinary tract symptoms (LUTS), pelvic organ prolapse (POP) and anal (AI) incontinence. In: Cardozo L, Rovner E, Wagg A, Wein A, Abrams P, editors. Incontinence. International consultation on incontinence. 7th ed; 2023. p. 13–130.
3. Rogers RG, Pauls RN, Thakar R, Morin M, Kuhn A, Petri E, et al. An International Urogynecological Association (IUGA)/International Continence Society (ICS) joint report on

the terminology for the assessment of sexual health of women with pelvic floor dysfunction. Neurourol Urodyn. 2018;37:1220–40.

4. Illiano E, Mahfouz W, Giannitsas K, Kocjancic E, Vittorio B, Athanasopoulos A, et al. Coital incontinence in women with urinary incontinence: an international study. J Sex Med. 2018;15:1456–62.

5. Espuña Pons M, Puig Clota M. Coital urinary incontinence: impact on quality of life as measured by the King's Health Questionnaire. Int Urogynecol J Pelvic Floor Dysfunct. 2008;19:621–5.

6. Duralde ER, Rowen TS. Urinary incontinence and associated female sexual dysfunction. Sex Med Rev. 2017;5:470–85.

7. Serati M, Salvatore S, Uccella S, Nappi RE, Bolis P. Female urinary incontinence during intercourse: a review on an understudied problem for women's sexuality. J Sex Med. 2009;6:40–8.

8. Jha S, Strelley K, Radley S. Incontinence during intercourse: myths unravelled. Int Urogynecol J. 2012;23:633–7.

9. Salonia A, Zanni G, Nappi RE, Briganti A, Dehò F, Fabbri F, Colombo R, Guazzoni G, Di Girolamo V, Rigatti P, Montorsi F. Sexual dysfunction is common in women with lower urinary tract symptoms and urinary incontinence: results of a cross-sectional study. Eur Urol. 2004;45(5):642–8. https://doi.org/10.1016/j.eururo.2003.11.023.

10. Shaw C. A systematic review of the literature on the prevalence of sexual impairment in women with urinary incontinence and the prevalence of urinary leakage during sexual activity. Eur Urol. 2002;42(5):432–40. https://doi.org/10.1016/s0302-2838(02)00401-3.

11. Lau H, Huang W, Su T. Urinary leakage during sexual intercourse among women with incontinence: incidence and risk factors. PLoS One. 2017;12:e0177075.

12. El-Azab AS, Yousef HA, Seifeldein GS. Coital incontinence: relation to detrusor overactivity and stress incontinence. Neurourol Urodyn. 2011;30:520–4.

13. Pastor Z, Chmel R. Differential diagnostics of female "sexual" fluids: a narrative review. Int Urogynecol J. 2018;29:621–9.

14. Pastor Z, Chmel R. Female ejaculation and squirting as similar but completely different phenomena: a narrative review of current research. Clin Anat. 2022;35(5):616–25. https://doi.org/10.1002/ca.23879. Epub 2022 Apr 16.

15. Pinheiro Sobreira Bezerra LR, Britto DF, Ribeiro Frota IP, Lira do Nascimento S, Morais Brilhante AV, Lucena SV, et al. The impact of urinary incontinence on sexual function: a systematic review. Sex Med Rev. 2020;8:393–402.

16. Escura Sancho S, Ribera-Torres L, Castelo-Branco C, Anglès-Acedo S. Impact of urinary incontinence on women's sexuality. Clin Exp Obstet Gynecol. 2022;49(2):49.

17. Roos A, Thakar R, Sultan AH, Burger CW, Paulus ATG. Pelvic floor dysfunction: women's sexual concerns unraveled. J Sex Med. 2014;11:743–52.

18. Bo K, Frawley HC, Haylen BT, Abramov Y, Almeida FG, Berghmans B, Bortolini M, Dumoulin C, Gomes M, McClurg D, Meijlink J, Shelly E, Trabuco E, Walker C, Wells A. An International Urogynecological Association (IUGA)/International Continence Society (ICS) joint report on the terminology for the conservative and nonpharmacological management of female pelvic floor dysfunction. Int Urogynecol J. 2017;28(2):191–213. https://doi.org/10.1007/s00192-016-3123-4. Epub 2016 Dec 5.

19. Bidzan M, Smutek J, Bidzan L. Psychosexual biography and the strategies used by women afflicted with stress urinary incontinence during intercourse: two case studies. Med Sci Monit. 2010;16(1):CS6–10.

20. Imamura M, Williams K, Wells M, McGrother C. Lifestyle interventions for the treatment of urinary incontinence in adults. Cochrane Database of Syst Rev. 2015;2015(12):CD003505.

21. Dumoulin C, Hay-Smith J. Pelvic floor muscle training versus no treatment, or inactive control treatments, for urinary incontinence in women. Cochrane Database Syst Rev. 2018;10:CD005654.

22. Kanter G, Rogers RG, Pauls RN, Kammerer-Doak D, Thakar R. A strong pelvic floor is associated with higher rates of sexual activity in women with pelvic floor disorders. Int Urogynecol J. 2015;26:991–6.

23. Sacomori C, Cardoso FL. Predictors of improvement in sexual function of women with urinary incontinence after treatment with pelvic floor exercises: a secondary analysis. J Sex Med. 2015;12:746–55.

24. Bø K, Talseth T, Vinsnes A. Randomized controlled trial on the effect of pelvic floor muscle training on quality of life and sexual problems in genuine stress incontinent women. Acta Obstet Gynecol Scand. 2000;79:598–603.

25. Handa VL, Whitcomb E, Weidner AC, Nygaard I, Brubaker L, Bradley CS, Paraiso MF, Schaffer J, Zyczynski HM, Zhang M, Richter HE. Sexual function before and after non-surgical treatment for stress urinary incontinence. Female Pelvic Med Reconstr Surg. 2011;17(1):30–5. https://doi.org/10.1097/SPV.0b013e318205e263. PMID: 21572534; PMCID: PMC3092501.

26. Nekkanti S, Wu JM, Hundley AF, Hudson C, Pandya LK, Dieter AA. A randomized trial comparing continence pessary to continence device (Poise Impressa®) for stress incontinence. Int Urogynecol J. 2022;33(4):861–8. https://doi.org/10.1007/s00192-021-04967-9. Epub 2021 Sep 9.

27. Cardozo L, Chermansky C, Igawa Y, Lee K, Michel M, Sahai A, Wein A. Pharmacological treatment of urinary incontinence. In: Cardozo L, Rovner E, Wagg A, Wein A, Abrams P, editors. Incontinence. International consultation on incontinence. 7th ed. Plymouth: Plymbridge Distributors; 2023. p. 13–130.

28. Balzarro M, Rubilotta E, Mancini V, Trabacchin N, Oppezzi L, Li Marzi V, et al. Impact of overactive bladder-wet syndrome on female sexual function: a systematic review and meta-analysis. Sex Med Rev. 2019;7:565–74.

29. Siddiqui ZA, Abboudi H, Crawford R, Shah S. Intraurethral bulking agents for the management of female stress urinary incontinence: a systematic review. Int Urogynecol J. 2017;28(9):1275–84. https://doi.org/10.1007/s00192-017-3278-7. Epub 2017 Feb 21.

30. Capobianco G, Saderi L, Dessole F, Petrillo M, Dessole M, Piana A, Cherchi PL, Dessole S, Sotgiu G. Efficacy and effectiveness of bulking agents in the treatment of stress and mixed urinary incontinence: a systematic review and meta-analysis. Maturitas. 2020;133:13–31. https://doi.org/10.1016/j.maturitas.2019.12.007. Epub 2019 Dec 11.

31. Braga A, Caccia G, Papadia A, Treglia G, Castronovo F, Salvatore S, Torella M, Ghezzi F, Serati M. Urethral bulking agents for the treatment of recurrent stress urinary incontinence: a systematic review and meta-analysis. Maturitas. 2022;163:28–37. https://doi.org/10.1016/j.maturitas.2022.05.007. Epub 2022 May 26.

32. Serati M, Braga A, Salvatore S, Torella M, Di Dedda MC, Scancarello C, Cimmino C, De Rosa A, Frigerio M, Candiani M, Ruffolo AF. Up-to-date procedures in female stress urinary incontinence surgery: a concise review on bulking agents procedures. Medicina (Kaunas). 2022;58(6):775. https://doi.org/10.3390/medicina58060775. PMID: 35744038; PMCID: PMC9227870.

33. Hoe V, Haller B, Yao HH, O'Connell HE. Urethral bulking agents for the treatment of stress urinary incontinence in women: a systematic review. Neurourol Urodyn. 2021;40(6):1349–88. https://doi.org/10.1002/nau.24696. Epub 2021 May 20.

34. Leone Roberti Maggiore U, Alessandri F, Medica M, Gabelli M, Venturini PL, Ferrero S. Periurethral injection of polyacrylamide hydrogel for the treatment of stress urinary incontinence: the impact on female sexual function. J Sex Med. 2012;9(12):3255–63. https://doi.org/10.1111/j.1743-6109.2012.02955.x.

35. Latul YP, Casteleijn FM, Zwolsman SE, Roovers JWR. Sexual function following treatment for stress urinary incontinence with bulk injection therapy and mid-urethral sling surgery. J Sex Med. 2022;19(7):1116–23. https://doi.org/10.1016/j.jsxm.2022.03.620.

36. Itkonen Freitas AM, Mikkola TS, Rahkola-Soisalo P, Tulokas S, Mentula M. Quality of life and sexual function after TVT surgery versus Bulkamid injection for primary stress urinary incontinence: 1 year results from a randomized clinical trial. Int Urogynecol J. 2021;32(3):595–601. https://doi.org/10.1007/s00192-020-04618-5.

37. Lai S, Diao T, Zhang W, Seery S, Zhang Z, Hu M, et al. Sexual functions in women with stress urinary incontinence after mid-urethral sling surgery: a systematic review and meta-analysis of prospective randomized and non-randomized studies. J Sex Med. 2020;17:1956–70.

38. Atılgan AE, Eren EC. The effect of tension-free vaginal tape on coital incontinence concomitant with stress urinary incontinence. Low Urin Tract Symptoms. 2021;13:118–22.

39. Zhang C, Chen Y, Liu S, Chen J, Shen H, Luo D. Effect of vaginal energy-based treatment on female stress urinary incontinence: a systematic review and meta-analysis of randomized controlled trials. World J Urol. 2023;41(2):405–11.

40. Pavarini N, Valadares ALR, Varella GM, Brito LGO, Juliato CRT, Costa-Paiva L. Sexual function after energy-based treatments of women with urinary incontinence. A systematic review and meta-analysis. Int Urogynecol J. 2023;34(6):1139–52. https://doi.org/10.1007/s00192-022-05419-8. Epub ahead of print.

41. Khunda A, McCormick C, Ballard P. Sacral neuromodulation and sexual function: a systematic review and meta-analysis of the literature. Int Urogynecol J. 2019;30(3):339–52. https://doi.org/10.1007/s00192-018-3841-x. Epub 2018 Dec 7.

42. Andy UU, Amundsen CL, Honeycutt E, et al. Sacral neuromodulation versus onabotulinumtoxinA for refractory urgency urinary incontinence: impact on fecal incontinence symptoms and sexual function. Am J Obstet Gynecol. 2019;221:513.e1–e15.

43. Sarabi P, Parvizi F, Kakabaraee K. The effectiveness of cognitive behavioral sexual therapy on sexual function, dysfunctional beliefs, knowledge and sexual self-confidence of women with sexual dysfunction. J Anal Cogn Psychol. 2019;10(3):9–27.

44. Rostamkhani F, Ghamari M, Babakhani V, Effat-al-Sadat Merghati Khoei E. The effectiveness of "cognitive-behavioral therapy" on the sexual function and schema of postmenopausal women. J Health Promot Manag. 2020;9(6):96–107.

45. Nezamnia M, Iravani M, Bargard MS, Latify M. Effectiveness of cognitive-behavioral therapy on sexual function and sexual self-efficacy in pregnant women: an RCT. Int J Reprod Biomed. 2020;18(8):625.

46. Moradinasab S, Iravani M, Mousavi P, Cheraghian B, Molavi S. Effect of cognitive-behavioral therapy on sexual self-esteem and sexual function of reproductive-aged women suffering from urinary incontinence. Int Urogynecol J. 2023;34:1753–63. https://doi.org/10.1007/s00192-023-05460-1. Epub ahead of print. PMID: 36715741; PMCID: PMC9885913.

Pelvic Floor Disorders and Female Sexuality II: Pelvic Organ Prolapse

Sònia Anglès Acedo, Laura Ribera Torres,
and Cristina Ros Cerro

1   Introduction

Pelvic organ prolapse (POP) is the descent of different pelvic organs from their usual anatomical position, secondary to the failure of the supporting structures. So, it is the definition of an anatomical change. However, these anatomical changes could be considered within the normal range in some women. Therefore, the diagnosis of POP ideally requires clear clinical evidence, which implies that the woman reports symptoms of genital lump. It is estimated that the prevalence of any degree of POP oscillates around 30% of the female population, being symptomatic in a 5–10% of the cases [1], a fact which mainly occurs when the POP reaches or exceeds the hymen (stage II) [2]. The prevalence of POP among female transgender population after a gender-affirmation surgery has been reported to be about 2–10% [3], being the use of sacrospinous ligament fixation associated with a significantly decreased risk of prolapse of the neovagina [4].

S. Anglès Acedo (✉) · C. Ros Cerro
Urogynecological Unit, Clinical Institute of Gynecology, Obstetrics and Neonatology, Hospital Clinic de Barcelona, Barcelona, Spain

Clinical Sexology Working Group, Hospital Clinic de Barcelona, Barcelona, Spain

Surgery and Medical-Surgical Specialties, Faculty of Medicine and Health Sciences, Universitat de Barcelona (UB), Barcelona, Spain

Institut d'Investigacions Biomèdiques August Pi i Sunyer, Barcelona, Spain
e-mail: sangles@clinic.cat; cros@clinic.cat

L. Ribera Torres
Urogynecological Unit, Clinical Institute of Gynecology, Obstetrics and Neonatology, Hospital Clinic de Barcelona, Barcelona, Spain
e-mail: laribera@clinic.cat

© The Author(s), under exclusive license to Springer Nature Switzerland AG 2024
C. Castelo-Branco, S. Anglès Acedo (eds.), *Medical Disorders and Sexual Health*, Trends in Andrology and Sexual Medicine,
https://doi.org/10.1007/978-3-031-55080-5_7

POP is frequently associated with other pelvic floor dysfunctions, such as an impairment of the urinary, anorectal, or sexual function. However, understanding sexuality is far more challenging than inquiring about POP symptoms.

2   Sexuality Assessment in Women with POP

Among women with POP, sexual life is not systematically evaluated in the routine clinical practice. Likewise, no robust data are available regarding the impact of POP and the treatment options for POP on sexual activity and function.

Terminology in this field has been heterogeneous until recent years, a fact that hardens the comparison between scientific studies. At present, consensus documents which provide us with standardized terminology to evaluate the sexuality of women with urogynecological pathology are available [5]. Their objective is to improve both our routine clinical practice and the analysis of results in research projects.

On the other hand, the methodology used to evaluate the sexuality of women with POP has been highly variable among different studies, another fact that hinders the interpretation of results. In relation to the measuring instruments employed, it should be noted that:

- Many studies exclusively focus on dyspareunia (persistent or recurrent pain or discomfort with vaginal penetration or its attempt) [6–9].
- Other studies use non-validated questionnaires [7, 8]
- Some studies use generic validated questionnaires (e.g., Female Sexual Function Index—FSFI), which do not take into consideration the impact of POP on sexuality [10–13].
- Some studies use condition-specific validated questionnaires (e.g., Pelvic organ prolapse/urinary Incontinence Sexual Questionnaire IUGA Revised—PISQ-IR), which include questions to evaluate the impact of POP on sexual life [9–11, 14–23].

Considering the study population, most studies are solely focused on the evaluation of sexually active women [7, 10–13, 23, 24]. Therefore, studies which report sexual inactivity among women with POP and its relation to the pathology and its treatment remain scarce. Moreover, data of POP (and treatments) impact on female sexuality among women who engage on solo sex or sexual diversity population (LGBTQIA+) are scarce or not available in the literature. With reference to the time of data collection, in longitudinal studies, it is common for sexual life to be evaluated only after treatment, meaning that its preoperative (or prior to conservative treatments) information is not well documented, a fact that may limit the conclusions of the study results [6]. Finally, regarding statistical power, most studies which investigate the impact of POP or its surgical treatment on sexuality are based on the analysis of secondary variables [6, 25].

In order to give counseling to women with POP regarding their sexual life and future expectations, it is recommended to include a systematic evaluation of the sexual activity and function, according to the standardized terminology and by means of condition-specific validated questionnaires, in the baseline clinical interview. Likewise, after treatments for POP, especially the surgical ones, sexuality must be reevaluated to determine both positive and negative effects of the range of therapeutic options currently available [2, 6].

3 The Impact of POP on Sexual Activity

Among women with symptomatic POP, the rate of sexual inactivity is estimated around 47% [26]. Half of women with advanced POP and indication for surgical treatment are sexually inactive [16, 17]. The impact of POP on the decision to be sexually inactive differs between both studies (20% vs. 45%), with it being the third cause of inactivity for the population with native tissue vaginal surgery indication (after the "lack of interest" and "absence of partner") while it was the main reason for inactivity in the population with POP and indication for mesh surgery [17]. Probably, the higher the stage and/or the more symptomatic the POP, the bigger the effect on sexual inactivity. However, these discrepancies may also be explained by the different study populations (non-sexually active women pending of mesh surgery were younger and had a partner in a higher proportion and greater POP stage than those pending of native tissue surgery).

Different studies have examined the factors associated with sexual inactivity by comparing sexually inactive with active women. A multicenter, cross-sectional study of women with POP stage ≥ 2 [18] reported that marital status was independently associated with sexual activity. Moreover, in that study, age, hypertension, and body image score were also independently associated with sexual activity, whereas prior urogynecological surgery, menopause, POPDI score, and POP-Q stage were not. Similarly, Anglès et al. [19] found "absence of partner" as the only independent factor associated with sexual inactivity in women with POP stage ≥ 3 (after adjusting for other factors such as age, time since menopause, total vaginal length, or presence of dyspareunia).

Therefore, sexual activity among women with POP is mainly affected by "not having a partner"; however, the role of POP in being single has not been deeply explored in the literature although POP may cause difficulties to achieve stable or sporadic sexual and/or emotional relationships.

On the other hand, not only sexually inactive women may experience an alteration in their sexual activity because of POP, but also sexually active women may restrict their sexual activity due to fear of the lump sensation during intercourse, which could result in a decrease in their usual sexual frequency and affect their quality of life. Again, a difference in the proportion of women in the general population is observed in the previously mentioned articles, affecting four out of ten sexually active women [16] vs. six out of ten [17]. According to Barber et al. [14], one-third of the patients with POP reported that their pelvic floor condition significantly affected "moderately" or "greatly" their ability to have sexual relations.

4   The Impact of POP on Sexual Function

POP may cause, among women who suffer from it, clinically relevant psychological and physical consequences which impair sexual life.

According to Hawton's biopsychosocial model, body image and self-esteem deterioration represent maintenance factors for sexual dysfunctions [27]. There is evidence that women who seek medical attention because of a POP problem perceive an alteration of their body image, femininity, and attraction capacity due to the sensation of "lump in the genitals," which impairs their quality of life and female sexuality [24, 28]. Insecurity about partner's sexual satisfaction and worries for negative image of their vagina, discomfort or obstruction for POP, and loss of general attractiveness (feeling old, less feminine, not sexy) are the most common concerns about sexual life in these populations [24]. Those women perceive body image issues as the most important factor altering their sexuality; moreover, sexual desire, arousal, satisfaction, and orgasm may also be affected [24].

On the other hand, women with POP may relate dyspareunia for mechanical reasons because the presence of a genital lump can complicate coital activity and be a cause of pain. Sobhgol et al. [7] evaluated gynecological factors associated with dyspareunia and found an association between dyspareunia and the symptom (p-value <0.0001) and sign (p-value <0.04) of POP.

5   The Impact of Conservative Treatment for POP on Female Sexuality

Pelvic floor muscle training (PFMT) is recommended as a first-line treatment for symptomatic POP. There is Level 2 evidence supporting an improvement of women's sexual function after PFMT for POP according to the findings of a systematic review [29], although literature on this topic is scarce.

A recent literature review [25] was published about PFMT in women with POP based on RCT studies between 1996 and 2021. None of the studies had sexual function as the primary outcome. The authors found only two RCTs which showed some positive effects of PFMT on sexual function of women with POP [15]; however, the short-term improvement of sexual questionnaires described by Pauls et al. [10] was lost after 24 weeks [10]. One RCT [15] comparing 50 women with PFMT + lifestyle advice vs. 59 women lifestyle advice found that most of the women in the PFMT group reported unchanged sexual function on the standardized questionnaire following 6 months of training. However, based on the qualitative analysis of the semi-structured interview, the data revealed that 39% of women in the PFMT group experienced improvements in sexual function compared with 5% in the control group. Women reporting improvement in sexual function demonstrated the greatest increase in PFM strength and endurance. No significant change in the number of sexually active women was reported. The authors did not find any significant differences between groups regarding changes in frequency of sexual intercourse. The reported changes in sexual function included increased awareness, strength, and control of PFM; sensation of a "tighter" vagina; improved self-confidence, libido, and orgasms; resolution of pain experienced with intercourse; and partner reports of increased sexual gratification.

To date, there is low-quality evidence demonstrating that PFMT can improve sexuality in women with POP and virtually no evidence showing that PFMT can treat sexual dysfunction in this population [25].

6 The Impact of Pessaries for POP on Sexual Activity and Function

Vaginal pessaries are passive mechanical devices designed to support the pelvic organs while correcting their anatomical descent and improving the symptom of bulge. They are commonly used as the first-line management for symptomatic POP, especially in the elderly, prior to surgery or when the surgical repair is not chosen due to the patient's comorbidities or preferences. Different types and sizes of pessaries can be used, with the ring (as "support" type) and the Gellhorn or the cube (as "space-occupying" type) being the most used. It is recommended to remove the pessary during vaginal sexual activity; however, most of the female ring pessary users decide to maintain it to feel more comfortable during sexual intercourse as well as to improve genital image during sex. Some couples consider the pessary as a sexual toy.

According to a recent systematic review [30], there is sufficient evidence that, in sexually active women who successfully use a pessary for the treatment of their POP, there is no deterioration in sexual function and there is some evidence of an improvement. The improvement in sexual function is expected to be associated with the woman's self-perceived body image and the condition-specific bother from POP, which may improve after treatment [20, 21].

Unfortunately, there is insufficient evidence regarding the effect of pessary treatment on female sexuality among non-sexually active pessary users. In a subsequent multicenter prospective study of women with symptomatic POP with a 24-month follow-up period, 16.5% of women in the pessary group resumed their sexual activity, whereas 15.8% became sexually inactive [21].

These data should be considered with caution because the previously mentioned studies did not report the rate of women who were removing their pessary for sexual activity, neither did they report the type of sexual activity women engaged in, and most of the outcome measures only assess sexual function regarding vaginal activity [21, 30]. Despite this bias, women can probably be counseled that there are no available data on other forms of sexual activity, but it is reasonable to expect that they are even less likely to be negatively affected by pessary use, although more inclusive studies would be welcomed in this field [30].

7   The Impact of the Surgical Treatment for POP on Female Sexuality

Among women who present with POP throughout their lives, 12.6–19% will request a surgical treatment for the correction of their symptoms. Surgery has an important role in solving the symptoms experienced by women with an advanced stage of POP and restoring, as far as possible, the anatomy of the vagina. Data about the impact of surgical treatment for POP on female sexuality are controverted [31], due to a wide variety of surgical techniques (vaginal, abdominal, with native tissue or mesh, associated or not with an anti-incontinence technique), as well as for the diversity of the measuring instruments employed. Sexual activity and function seem to improve or remain the same after surgery for POP in most of the cases [2, 31]. Nevertheless, some women may complaint about sexual dysfunction, which can have a psychosocial or an organic origin. During a surgical process, psychological factors (stress, anxiety, fear, depression, apprehension) coexist and may affect the patient and their partner (if they have one) and cause a negative impact on the sexual life. Organic causes may include anatomical, physiological, vascular, neurological, or hormonal alterations. These variations may disrupt sensitivity and appropriate vaginal vasocongestion, thus affecting women's sexual response. Therefore, surgery in this region may affect innervation and alter sexual function [12]. A postoperative sexual dysfunction should be considered as a serious adverse event according to the impact of women's quality of life [32].

Currently, there is conflicting evidence, which does not allow for clear recommendations to be made to women regarding the modality of surgical treatment that may have a more positive effect on their sexuality.

7.1   Surgical Treatment and Sexual Activity

After POP surgery, a proportion of sexually inactive women will resume sexual activity, whereas some preoperative sexually active women will become sexually inactive.

The rate of women who become sexually active differs between different studies from 16.8% to 39.2% [16, 17, 21], regardless of surgery type [12]. Probably, women reporting a recovery of their sexual activity after surgery were mainly those who preoperatively described a higher negative effect of POP on their sexuality [17], as there was a significant decrease in the proportion of women who reported POP-related symptoms as a reason for sexual inactivity after surgery. It is of note that women having POP surgery had 2.62 times higher odds of changing from non-sexually active to sexually active than those who used a pessary [21].

The proportion of sexually active women in the preoperative period who postoperatively ceased their sexual activity was similar among the studies, ranging from 6.7% to 16.6% [16, 17, 21]. Many women who became sexually inactive reported reasons unrelated to surgery as the cause of their sexual inactivity (lack of interest, not having a partner, other health problems). However, in a subgroup of these women who discontinued their sexual activity after surgery (around 30%), bladder/intestinal/prolapse issues and pain were the cause of sexual inactivity [16, 17]. Therefore, it is crucial to continue assessing sexually inactive women in the postoperative period to detect potential complications of the surgical treatment in the sexual sphere.

Regarding sexually active women before POP surgery, positive effects on their sexual activity after surgical treatment have also been shown. Anglès-Acedo et al. [16, 17] observed a significant decrease in the proportion of sexually active women who avoided/restricted their sexual activity due to fear of bulging sensation. This finding could possibly justify an increase in the sexual frequency, which could explain why, analyzing sexual function of sexually active women, not only the condition-specific subscales but also global quality of life [16, 17] or arousal, orgasm, and partner relationship [17] significantly improved.

This difference regarding the impact of POP surgery on the different dimensions of sexuality between both articles reflects the reality of current literature, in which this point still remains controversial, with studies observing changes limited to POP-related dimensions [8, 22, 32], while others identify improvements in other dimensions [13, 23]. More research on the sexual impact of surgical treatment of POP is needed through studies with sufficient power, in which the main variable is the sexual sphere.

7.2   Surgical Treatment and Sexual Function

Dyspareunia seems to be a key factor for a worse postoperative sexual function [19]. A proportion of women will present this symptom before surgery, so the rate of preoperative dyspareunia should be mandatorily assessed. After surgical treatment, some of these patients will have their symptom solved, while it will persist in others, being the reason for postoperative sexual inactivity in a subgroup of patients. A group of patients without dyspareunia before surgery may present de novo postoperative dyspareunia (5.9–13.8%) [6, 16, 19, 21].

Postoperative dyspareunia may be due to a hypercorrection which causes vaginal introitus stenosis, scars in the vaginal walls, vaginal shortening, retraction and fibrosis, or exposure of the synthetic material (mesh). However, it seems that vaginal length after surgery does not influence sexual activity, nor sexual function [13, 17, 23]. Vaginal prolapse surgery negatively impacted the level of vaginal congestion and vaginal wall sensibility. However, the answer of "are these factors relevant for women sexual function?" remains unclear [12]. Therefore, it is necessary to know the positive and negative effects of the different surgical techniques based on biopsychosocial variables.

7.3   Surgical Treatment and Specific Considerations

Within the shared decision-making process to select different surgery options, female sexuality will be the main focus in some specific situations.

7.3.1   Mesh Surgery

Mesh surgery for POP is recommended only in selected patients after a comprehensive shared decision-making process focused on risks and benefits. Although retrospective studies have shown a lower rate of POP recurrence with these techniques, new complications have been described (mesh exposure, extrusion, or retraction) which may impact women's sexual health. Consequently, the used of mesh surgery is currently restricted worldwide.

According to the most recent systematic review on sexual function after POP surgery [12], comparisons are more robust between transvaginal synthetic mesh and native tissue repairs and show similar prevalence of de novo dyspareunia and sexual function scores. Total dyspareunia is higher after transvaginal synthetic mesh than sacrocolpopexy; however, difference regarding de novo dyspareunia and sexual function has not been found.

7.3.2   Obliterative Procedures

An obliterative procedure, such as colpocleisis, which involves the closure of the genital hiatus to avoid the POP descent, is a quick, safe, and durable alternative to traditional reconstructive repairs. However, it means the impossibility to maintain vaginal sexual activity in an irreversible way. So, it is key to inform our patient about that fact as well as to be sure that she understands and is aware of sexual consequences since it may affect inevitably all women who enjoy vaginal sexual activity or expect to do it in the future.

A recent review [33] found that most of the patients reported no regret after a colpocleisis, with bowel and bladder symptoms being the main reason of regret, whereas a few patients (0.6–12.8%) reported regret because of loss of vaginal sexual activity. In addition, the body image scores demonstrated a significant improvement after surgery. Finally, the authors found that women tended to remain sexually active, and some also regained sexual activities after surgery.

Therefore, as health care professionals, it is important to understand that within preoperative counseling on sexuality in the shared decision-making process, an obliterative procedure does not mean it is only an option to sexually inactive women, but it may be a valid option for those sexually active women not interested in vaginal sexual activity. Moreover, we should be aware that women's preference on sexual behavior (interest or not interest on vaginal sexual activity) is independent of the age, relationship status, or sexual orientation of our patient, and it is mandatory to avoid sexual assumptions based on these factors.

7.3.3   Uterine Preservation

There is increasing literature regarding uterine preservation. In a multicenter, cross-sectional study [34], patient preferences for uterine preservation vs. hysterectomy were evaluated in women with POP symptoms who were being subjected to an initial urogynecological evaluation. Patient treatment preference (uterine preservation vs. hysterectomy) was collected before meeting the physician. The rate of women who preferred uterine preservation was 46% if uterine preservation was superior to hysterectomy, 36% if both options had equal efficacy, and 20% despite uterine preservation being inferior to hysterectomy. It means, within the shared decision-making process, women considering surgery for apical POP may desire uterine preservation for multiple reasons that are different than those related to the surgical outcomes.

The main reasons to opt for a uterus-sparing surgery are directly linked with female sexuality as they may involve factors such as reproduction, female autonomy, identity, intimacy, and fear about consequences on sexual function.

Anglim et al. [35] found that uterine-sparing options exist and are desired by both pre- and postmenopausal women. From a biologic point of view, they are the only choice for women who wish to retain their fertility and whose families are not yet complete. Culture plays a large role in determining the importance of uterine preservation; for most women, the uterus is seen as an essential component of a woman's identity, being connected to her value, social status, and self-esteem, and, in certain communities, hysterectomy is associated with significant social stigma. In addition, sexual function is an important component of a woman with POP counseling. During surgical consultation for POP surgery, the patient's fears and preconceived ideas of the effect of hysterectomy on sexual function must be addressed.

---

8   Biopsychosocial Approach

POP and its treatment may affect female sexuality from the physical, psychological, and sociocultural perspective as it has been previously mentioned along this chapter (Figs. 1, 2). Benefits of female sexuality through the improvement of POP symptoms by different treatments have been previously discussed. However, conservative treatment, use of pessary, or surgical treatment may not be enough to provide a comprehensive assessment and treatment of the complex sexual issues presented by those women.

Sometimes, POP and its treatment directly affect the female's sexual response, altering sexual desire, as well as the arousal/lubrication ability, orgasm achievement, and sexual satisfaction; cause a decrease in the genital sensations or pain during sexual activity; and may produce difficulties in the mobility or communication during partnered sex which interfere or block pleasurable sexual behavior. Loss of control towards the own quality of life, both in the familiar and social sphere, frequently affects self-esteem, body image perception, and self-attraction perception, and even occasionally the own sexual identity. All these factors may have an impact on the relational field, both for people who are stable couple(s) and for those who are not couple who wish to initiate a new relationship (sporadic or stable), because it is difficult to communicate the need to jointly relearn a new sexuality which guarantees sexual pleasure to everyone involved.

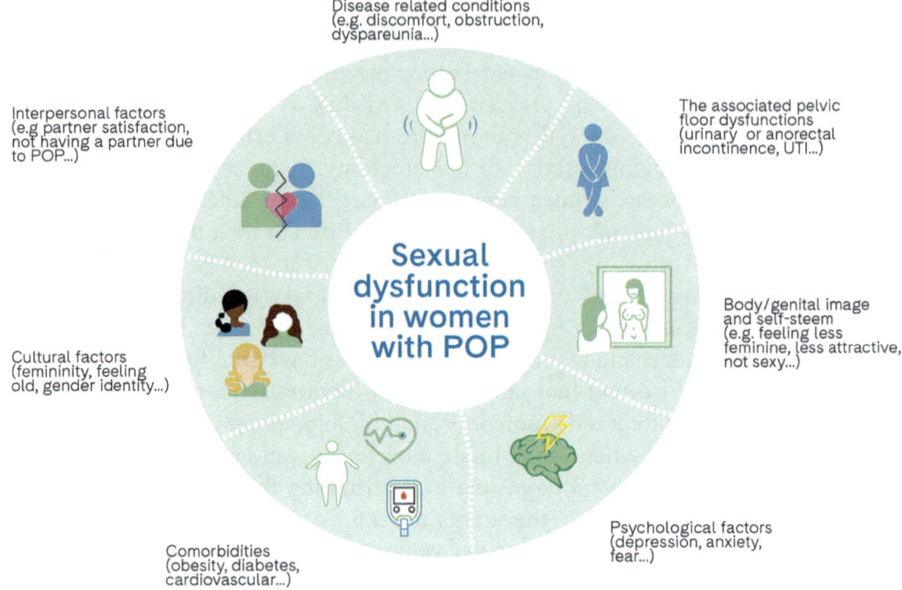

Fig 1 Sexual dysfunction in women with POP

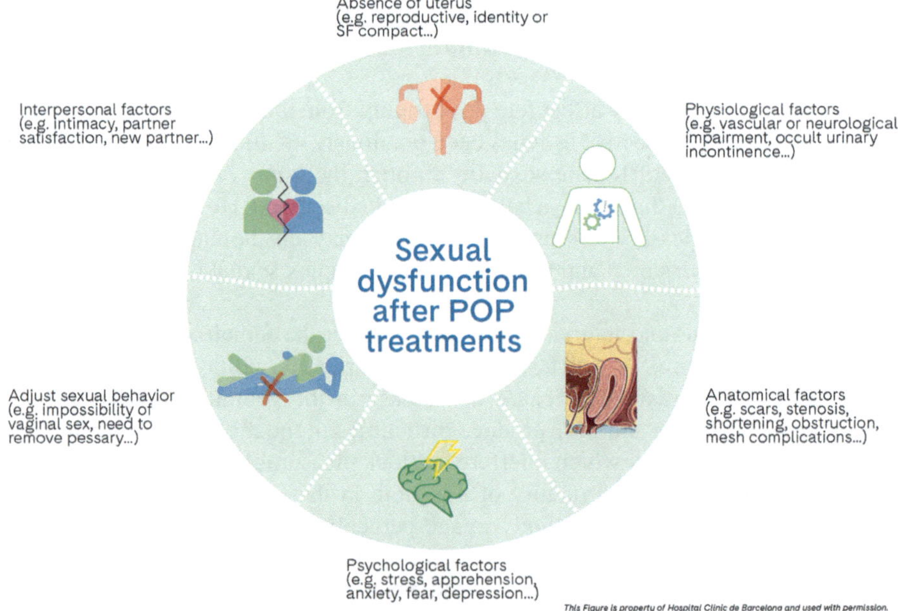

Fig 2 Sexual dysfunction after POP treatments

A multidisciplinary approach of sexual impairment is required to achieve significant and long-lasting improvement of sexual quality of life. We encourage to implement the extended PLISSIT model based on *permission* (which will always be the first step and may be followed by either of the next levels of intervention), *limited information*, *specific suggestion*, and *intensive therapy* [36]. It allows all the health care professionals (gynecologists, urologists, nurses, physiotherapists, sexologists, psychologists) to be involved in the sexual management of women with POP, according to their availability, knowledge, and skills in an easy, effective, and cost-effective way [37].

The *permission* step may solve some of the sexual concerns presented by patients with POP. It is known that sexual issues, as well as pelvic floor disorders like POP, are, still nowadays, tabu in most contexts (couple relationship, familiar, social), which can lead women with POP to loneliness, sadness, or frustration. Frequently, women's sexual distress can decrease only with the opportunity to talk about their sexual worries. For example, a homosexual woman may report concern about her partner's sexual experience (e.g., lower attraction, uncomfortable oral sex, lower sensation, or pain during vaginal activity), although partners (male or female) are frequently supportive and do not complain. It is not unusual for women to admit having this thought as a reason for sexual avoidance. It will be the health care professional's opportunity to reassure the woman, sharing with the patient that this is a common situation in her context (normalize the situation) and there probably are ways to get an improvement if she is interested, both actions contributing to a decrease in the woman's sexual distress.

Moreover, offering individualized *limited information* regarding their concerns may facilitate a significant change on thoughts or behavior related to a specific sexual issue. For example, a heterosexual woman with POP and pain during vaginal sexual activity (dyspareunia) may manifest sexual inactivity for this reason. Frequently, the avoidance of sexual intercourse becomes generalized to other intimate behaviors including mutual masturbation, kissing, and even hand-holding and hugging, resulting in an avoidance of any act of intimacy with the partner for the fear of an expectation for intercourse. In such case, limited information to address the concept of affectivity, as well as the concept of intimacy based on other pleasurable sexual behaviors, may help to improve the sexual health of that couple. Likewise, to provide *specific suggestions* about lubricants or local hormonal therapy, in addition to recommendations about sexual positions which can reduce the impact of POP during penetration (as lay down), may contribute to a further improvement in the couple's sexual health.

Finally, some patients may benefit from *intensive therapy* by a health care professional with specific skills on sexual therapy. Brief strategies, which can address women's sexual health from a biopsychosocial approach, may be easily implemented in comprehensive urogynecology units: for example, a communication-enhancing intervention to skillfully solicitate support or simply express own feelings and concerns (decreased self-esteem and feelings of embarrassment, shame, and guilt); sensate focus or pelvic floor muscle proprioception techniques that may provide a redirection of attention to avoid anticipatory fear/anxiety; coping-enhancing strategies; as well as renegotiation of sexual behaviors according to the current sexual needs and concerns.

In any case, it is important to center clinical treatment areas on the identified unmet needs, which frequently involve biological, psychological, and sociocultural aspects.

9   Conclusion

POP may affect sexual activity as well as sexual function of women affected. Physical, psychological, and sociocultural factors may have a role in sexual impairment on those women. Although POP treatment alternatives usually improve female sexuality, a subgroup of women can maintain, worsen, or develop a sexual dysfunction after those treatments. In this way, better awareness on the sexual impact of the different therapeutic options will permit us to provide better counseling to our patients at the time of treatment planning, considering their current sexual life and their expectations regarding their future sexuality. To comprehensively assess and treat women with POP considering their sexual health in the urogynecology units:

1. A systematic evaluation of sexual activity and function through condition-specific validated questionnaires before and after treatments is mandatory.
2. A multidisciplinary biopsychosocial approach based on extended PLISSIT model should be implemented in order to enhance the sexual quality of life of those women.

References

1. Developed by the Joint Writing Group of the American Urogynecologic Society and the International Urogynecological Association. Joint report on terminology for surgical procedures to treat pelvic organ prolapse. Int Urogynecol J. 2020;31(3):429–63;Erratum in: Int Urogynecol J. 2020 Jun;31(6):1283.
2. Maher C. Pelvic organ prolapse surgery. In: Abrams P, Cardozo L, Wagg A, Wein A, editors. International consultation on incontinence. 6th ed. London: Health Publications Ltd; 2017. p. 1855–991.
3. Manrique OJ, Adabi K, Martinez-Jorge J, Ciudad P, Nicoli F, Kiranantawat K. Complications and patient-reported outcomes in male-to-female Vaginoplasty - where we are today: a systematic review and meta-analysis. Ann Plast Surg. 2018;80(6):684–91.
4. Dreher PC, Edwards D, Hager S, Dennis M, Belkoff A, Mora J, et al. Complications of the neovagina in male-to-female transgender surgery: a systematic review and meta-analysis with discussion of management. Clin Anat. 2018;31(2):191–9.
5. Rogers RG, Pauls RN, Thakar R, Morin M, Kuhn A, Petri E, et al. An international Urogynecological Association (IUGA)/International Continence Society (ICS) joint report on the terminology for the assessment of sexual health of women with pelvic floor dysfunction. Neurourol Urodyn. 2018;37(4):1220–40.
6. Antosh DD, Kim-Fine S, Meriwether KV, Kanter G, Dieter AA, Mamik MM, et al. Changes in sexual activity and function after pelvic organ prolapse surgery: a systematic review. Obstet Gynecol. 2020;136(5):922–31.

7. Sobhgol SS, Alizadeli Charndabee SM. Rate and related factors of dyspareunia in reproductive age women: a cross-sectional study. Int J Impot Res. 2007;19(1):88–94.

8. Detollenaere RJ, den Boon J, Stekelenburg J, IntHout J, Vierhout ME, Kluivers KB, et al. Sacrospinous hysteropexy versus vaginal hysterectomy with suspension of the uterosacral ligaments in women with uterine prolapse stage 2 or higher: multicentre randomised non-inferiority trial. Br Med J. 2015;351:h3717.

9. Lukacz ES, Warren LK, Richter HE, Brubaker L, Barber MD, Norton P, et al. Quality of life and sexual function 2 years after vaginal surgery for prolapse. Obstet Gynecol. 2016;127(6):1071–9.

10. Pauls RN, Crisp CC, Novicki K, Fellner AN, Kleeman SD. Impact of physical therapy on quality of life and function after vaginal reconstructive surgery. Female Pelvic Med Reconstr Surg. 2013;19(5):271–7.

11. Pauls RN, Crisp CC, Novicki K, Fellner AN, Kleeman SD. Pelvic floor physical therapy: impact on quality of life 6 months after vaginal reconstructive surgery. Female Pelvic Med Reconstr Surg. 2014;20(6):334–41.

12. Lakeman MME, Laan E, Roovers JPWR. The effects of prolapse surgery on vaginal wall sensibility, vaginal vasocongestion, and sexual function: a prospective single centre study. Neurourol Urodyn. 2014;33(8):1217–24.

13. Gutman RE, Rardin CR, Sokol ER, Matthews C, Park AJ, Iglesia CB, et al. Vaginal and laparoscopic mesh hysteropexy for uterovaginal prolapse: a parallel cohort study. Am J Obstet Gynecol. 2017;216(1):38.e1–38.e11.

14. Barber MD, Visco AG, Wyman JF, Fantl JA, Bump RC, Continence Program for Women Research Group. Sexual function in women with urinary incontinence and pelvic organ prolapse. Obstet Gynecol. 2002;99(2):281–9.

15. Braekken IH, Majida M, Ellstrom Engh M, Bo K. Can pelvic floor muscle training improve sexual function in women with pelvic organ prolapse? A randomized controlled trial. J Sex Med. 2015;12(2):470–80.

16. Anglès-Acedo S, Ros-Cerro C, Espuña-Pons M, Valero-Fernandez EM. Sexual activity and function of women with severe pelvic organ prolapse subjected to a classical vaginal surgery. A multicentre study. Actas Urol Esp. 2019;43(7):389–95.

17. Anglès-Acedo S, Ros-Cerro C, Escura-Sancho S, Palau-Pascual MJ, Bataller-Sánchez E, Espuña-Pons M, et al. Sexual activity and function in women with advanced stages of pelvic organ prolapse, before and after laparoscopic or vaginal mesh surgery. Int Urogynecol J. 2021;32(5):1157–68.

18. Lowenstein L, Gamble T, Sanses TV, van Raalte H, Carberry C, Jakus S, et al. Sexual function is related to body image perception in women with pelvic organ prolapse. J Sex Med. 2009;6:2286–91.

19. Anglès-Acedo S, Ros-Cerro C, Escura-Sancho S, Palau-Pascual MJ, Bataller-Sánchez E, Espuña-Pons M, et al. Female sexuality before and after sacrocolpopexy or vaginal mesh: is vaginal length one of the key factors? Int Urogynecol J. 2022 Jan;33(1):143–52.

20. Lowenstein L, Gamble T, Sanses TV, van Raalte H, Carberry C, Jakus S, et al. Changes in sexual function after treatment for prolapse are related to the improvement in body image perception. J Sex Med. 2010;7(2 Pt 2):1023–8.

21. van der Vaart LR, Vollebregt A, Pruijssers B, Milani AL, Lagro-Janssen AL, Roovers JWR, et al. Female sexual functioning in women with a symptomatic pelvic organ prolapse; a multicenter prospective comparative study between pessary and surgery. J Sex Med. 2022;19(2):270–9.

22. van Zanten F, Brem C, Lenters E, Broeders IAMJ, Schraffordt Koops SE. Sexual function after robot-assisted prolapse surgery: a prospective study. Int Urogynecol J. 2018;29(6):905–12.

23. Ko YC, Yoo EH, Han GH, Kim YM. Comparison of sexual function between sacrocolpopexy and sacrocervicopexy. ObstetGynecol Sci. 2017;60(2):207–12.

24. Roos AM, Thakar R, Sultan AH, Burger CW, Paulus AT. Pelvic floor dysfunction: Women's sexual concerns unraveled. J Sex Med. 2014;11(3):743–52.

25. Bø K, Anglès-Acedo S, Batra A, Brækken IH, Chan YL, Jorge CH, et al. International urogynecology consultation chapter 3 committee 2; conservative treatment of patient with pelvic organ prolapse: pelvic floor muscle training. Int Urogynecol J. 2022;33(10):2633–67.
26. Mestre M. Validación de la versión española del PISQ-IR: The Pelvic Organ Prolapse/Incontinence Sexual Questionnaire, IUGA-Revised. Valoración de la salud sexual en mujeres con disfunciones del suelo pélvico. Universitat de Barcelona; 2022.
27. Hawton K, Catalan J. Prognostic factors in sex therapy. Behav Res Ther. 1986;24(4):377–85.
28. Robinson D, Prodigalidad LT, Chan S, Serati M, Lozo S, Lowder J, et al. International Urogynaecology Consultation chapter 1 committee 4: patients' perception of disease burden of pelvic organ prolapse. Int Urogynecol J. 2022;33(2):189–210.
29. Ferreira CH, Dwyer PL, Davidson M, De Souza A, Ugarte JA, Frawley HC. Does pelvic floor muscle training improve female sexual function? A systematic review Int Urogynecol J. 2015;26(12):1735–50.
30. Wharton L, Athey R, Jha S. Do vaginal pessaries used to treat pelvic organ prolapse impact on sexual function? A systematic review and meta-analysis. Int Urogynecol J. 2022;33(2):221–33.
31. Antosh DD, Dieter AA, Balk EM, Kanter G, Kim-Fine S, Meriwether KV, et al. Sexual function after pelvic organ prolapse surgery: a systematic review comparing different approaches to pelvic floor repair. Am J Obstet Gynecol. 2021;225(5):475.e1–475.e19.
32. Dunivan GC, Sussman AL, Jelovsek JE, Sung V, Andy UU, Ballard A, et al. Eunice Kennedy Shriver National Institute of Child Health and Human Development Pelvic Floor Disorders Network. Gaining the patient perspective on pelvic floor disorders' surgical adverse events. Am J Obstet Gynecol. 2019;220(2):185.e1–185.e10.
33. Felder L, Heinzelmann-Schwarz V, Kavvadias T. How does colpocleisis for pelvic organ prolapse in older women affect quality of life, body image, and sexuality? A critical review of the literature. Womens Health (Lond). 2022;18:17455057221111067.
34. Korbly NB, Kassis NC, Good MM, Richardson ML, Book NM, Yip S, et al. Patient preferences for uterine preservation and hysterectomy in women with pelvic organ prolapse. Am J Obstet Gynecol. 2013;209(5):470.e1–6.
35. Anglim B, O'Sullivan O, O'Reilly B. How do patients and surgeons decide on uterine preservation or hysterectomy in apical prolapse? Int Urogynecol J. 2018;29(8):1075–9.
36. Taylor B, Davis S. Using the extended PLISSIT model to address sexual healthcare needs. Nurs Stand. 2006;21(11):35–40.
37. Tuncer M, Oskay ÜY. Sexual counseling with the PLISSIT model: a systematic review. J Sex Marital Ther. 2022;48(3):309–18.

Male Sexuality and Prostate Cancer

Roger Matheu Riviere, Carmen Martinez Garcia,
and Juan Manuel Corral Molina

1   Introduction

About one man in eight will be diagnosed with prostate cancer (PCa) during his lifetime, being the second most common cancer in men worldwide. Modern treatments allow oncological healing or long survivals, even in metastatic disease, causing a great proportion of patients becoming a cancer survivor and dealing with treatment-associated side effects. All modalities of PCa treatment have a negative impact on sexual life, with erectile dysfunction (ED) being the most reported and studied. Nowadays, sexuality is understood more vastly than it was before, and practitioners should be aware that more domains will eventually change after the treatment. Some of them can be considered as more organic as orgasm, ejaculation, sexual continence, penile and body changes and other more psychologic as self-image, masculinity and sexual intimacy.

R. Matheu Riviere · C. Martinez Garcia
Urology Department, Clinical Institute of Nephrology and Urology, Hospital Clínic de Barcelona, Barcelona, Spain
e-mail: rmatheu@clinic.cat; cmartinez@clinic.cat

J. M. Corral Molina (✉)
Urology Department, Clinical Institute of Nephrology and Urology, Hospital Clínic de Barcelona, Barcelona, Spain

Clinical Sexology Working Group, Hospital Clinic de Barcelona, Barcelona, Spain
e-mail: jmcorral@clinic.cat

© The Author(s), under exclusive license to Springer Nature Switzerland AG 2024
C. Castelo-Branco, S. Anglès Acedo (eds.), *Medical Disorders and Sexual Health*, Trends in Andrology and Sexual Medicine,
https://doi.org/10.1007/978-3-031-55080-5_8

2 Part 1: Sexuality Assessment and Effects on Localised Treatments

2.1 Sexuality Assessment in Men with PCa

As PCa therapies have a direct impact on sexual function, an assessment should be performed before and after treatment as we suggest in Table 1. Indeed, before the treatment, 64% of patients consider their sexual activity at least "important" for their lives, even if at the moment of evaluation psychological reasons as stress, fear and frustration may alter from their basal status: 20% of the patients decreased their sexual activity, and 10% were unable to achieve an erection [1]. Feminine sexual dysfunction can be present at the same time of PCa diagnosis for half of the couples and should be assessed.

Nowadays, sexuality is understood more vastly, but most of the studies are focused on penetration capability in heterosexual couples. International Index of Erectile Function (IIEF), Sexual Health Inventory for Men (SHIM) and Expanded Prostate cancer Index Composite (EPIC) are the most used scales, but for some studies, just the penetrative capacity is considered.

However, more recent research is addressing changes in other aspects of sexuality as male identity, non-penetrative intercourses, body imaging and including non-heteronormative groups, but with lower level of evidence due to lack of big cohorts and reviews.

Table 1 Sexual assessment in PCa

- Comorbidities that can affect erectile function (HTA, diabetes, dyslipidaemia, vasculopathies, penile surgeries, etc.)
- Grade of PCa/potential need for adjuvant treatments
- Libido
- Sexual partner
  - Single/multiple
  - Collaborative/not interested
  - Gender
- Type of sexual activity
  - Solo sex
  - Partner masturbation
  - Oral sex
  - Vaginal penetrative sex
  - Anal penetrative sex
  - Anal receptive sex
- Orgasm relevance
- Ejaculation relevance
- Rigidity erection achieved (EHS) during
  - Sexual intercourse
  - Non-voluntary erections
  - Autoerotism
- Erection quality (SHIM or IIEF)
- Proportion of erections achieved when desired
- Use of PDE5i/ICI
- Use of vacuum device

2.2   Sexuality After Localised Treatments

For localised disease, radical prostatectomy (RP), radiotherapy and active surveillance are the three gold standards for patients suitable for treatment. All of them have negative effect on sexuality, even active surveillance [1]. RP and radiotherapy show similar oncological efficacy but with different side effects, and both are usually discussed with the patient. In this subchapter, we are going to review organic effects of PCa treatments.

2.2.1   Radical Prostatectomy

RP affects erectile function (EF) by damaging the neurovascular bundle (NVB). The most accepted pathophysiological theory is that even this damage can be definitive or temporary, and erection is considerably lowered or completely abolished for a period of time. Oxygen tension is 25–40 mmHg during flaccid state but 100 mmHg at erection, so penis usually oxygenates through voluntary and involuntary erections. During this variable period, penile hypoxia is developed which leads to definitive changes as decreased elasticity, smooth muscle apoptosis and fibrosis (Fig. 1). These will be the major factors responsible for ED, shortening of the penis and Peyronie's disease after RP.

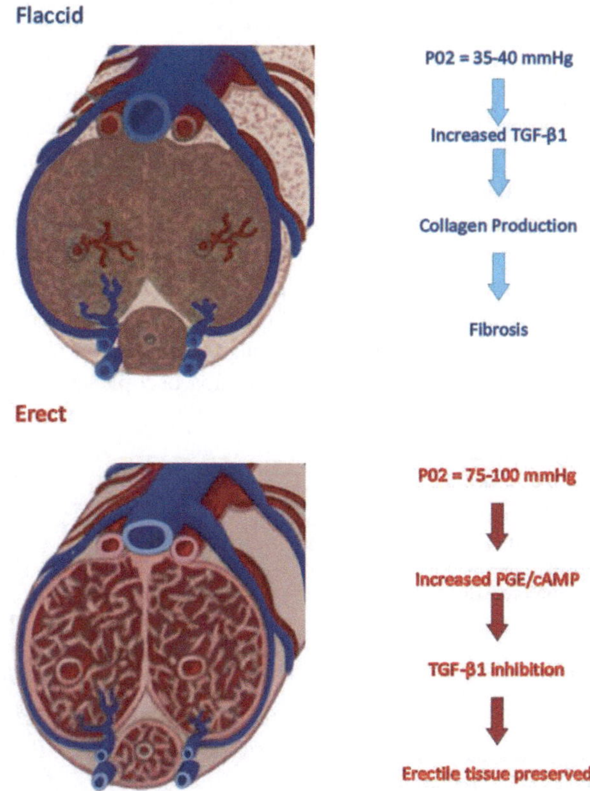

Fig. 1 In flaccid state, PO2 is the same as venous blood, which increases the amount of TGF-β1, a pro-fibrotic molecule. Voluntary and involuntary (nocturnal) erections contribute to oxygenating the penis by raising the PO2 to arterial levels and increasing prostaglandins and cyclic AMP, which will inhibit TGF-β1

Erectile Dysfunction

The effect of radical prostatectomy on sexuality has been studied since Walsh described in 1982 the NVB, and 1 year later, he modified the radical prostatectomy (RP) technique, preserving the NVB, which improved erectile function (EF) [2].

The incidence of post-RP ED is very variable in the published literature (20–90%), but this is explained because definitions, measurements and populations evaluated are also heterogeneous [3]. If we take a look at the studies which evaluated the rehabilitation effect of the PDE5i in a population of selected men with good prognostic factors (young, high proportion of bilateral intrafascial preservation, without pre-existing ED, interested in sexual function), less than 50% scored more than 22 points at the IIEF-5 (considered as "no ED") even when receiving PDE5i treatment [4–7].

Even if half of the patients will not develop a post-operative ED, in the counselling prior to the surgery, it should be taken into consideration that the quality of the erection will not be back to baseline for 75% of the patients [8]. In other words, just one in four men will preserve the erection they had before the surgery.

As explained before, NVB can receive a direct and irreversible damage, but it can also be temporary (neuropraxia) that recovers gradually. Neuropraxia is usually caused by indirect damage during PCa treatment as inflammation, thermal damage, grasping the NVB, etc. This is the reason why some patients will experience a complete lack of erections just before the surgery but will regain them later. It is usually accepted that EF will recover in the first 2 years post-operatively, but for some patients, it can take even longer [9].

The risk of ED can be assessed by nomograms. Preoperative factors include age, previous ED and comorbidity status [10]. Post-operatively, it is calculated by adding the grade of neurovascular preservation achieved, which can be estimated preoperatively by staging the tumour [11]. In clinical practice, these risk factors are easy to take into consideration for counselling.

Some factors during the RP procedure have demonstrated to be involved in EF. The grade of NVB preservation is an independent prognostic factor, as the more preservation is associated with lower ED rates [12]. For standardising the nomenclature, some planes of dissection have been proposed (Fig. 2). Preserving other structures as pudendal arteries or anterior NVB can also be important for maintaining EF [13]. With the introduction of new technologies, laparoscopic and robotic radical prostatectomies

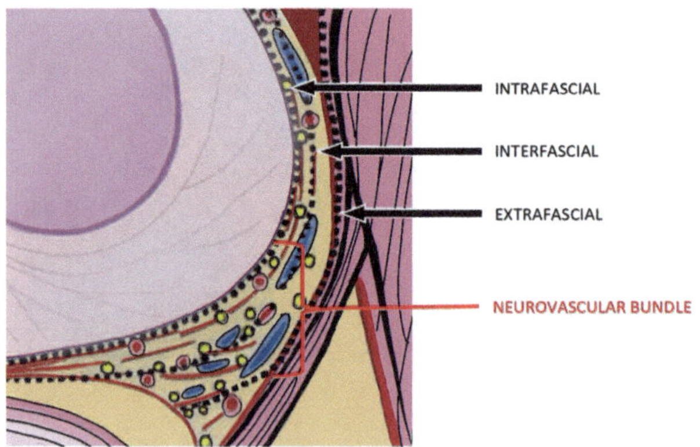

Fig. 2 Dissection planes in radical prostatectomy. Note that intrafascial plane is attached to prostate capsule, preserving the vast majority of neurovascular bundle, while extrafascial does not preserve it

are the new gold standards of PCa treatment. Compared with conventional open procedure, some studies show better results in EF [12], but this is still controversial. Regarding lymph node dissection, one study has found that extended lymphadenectomy is also associated with ED [14]. Discouragingly, despite all these efforts to mitigate the effects of RP on EF, in the last decade, there is no trend in improving it even with the new technologies and knowledge [15].

Penile rehabilitation is conceived as all the strategies to prevent hypoxia and secondary fibrosis and ultimately maintain erectile function. In this subject, a lot of studies regarding the effect of IPDE5, sildenafil, tadalafil and vardenafil, on different strategies (once a day, on demand) and doses were compared against placebo [4–7]. Tadalafil 5 mg once a day, sildenafil 100 mg once a day or on demand and vardenafil on demand presented better erectile function while they were given as treatment, but when the therapy was discontinued, there was no difference with placebo. These studies concluded that PDE5i could be given as post-RP ED treatment, but they did not have rehabilitation potential. However, those studies were designed for a treatment period less than 24 months (which is considered the regular time for recovering neuropraxia), and tadalafil 5 mg once a day demonstrated to reduce the penile length loss [7] and shortened the time to recover EF [16], which can be seen as an initial improvement of the fibrotic process.

Nevertheless, actual strategies should be more personalised and objective based in a multimodal strategy and should not rely on one-drug strategies. Current rehabilitation should encourage the patient to have quality erections more than once per week and should give them different tools to achieve it (PDE5i, intracavernosal injections (ICI), vacuum device, etc.) and include sexology support for the patient and the partner (if present). With this regard, the term sexual rehabilitation should be considered.

All the usual strategies for ED can be applied for post-RP ED. The election of the treatment should be discussed with the patient as multiple strategies are available. The most frequent strategy is based on PDE5i, and here two options are available. Once-a-day treatments do not need planification but require an adherence. On the other hand, on-demand strategies need more planification (taking a pill 30/60 min before) and do not provide this hypothetical stimulation of non-voluntary erections (preventing the penile hypoxia) [17]. In patients who do not respond satisfactorily to PDE5i, ICI or intraurethral prostaglandins on demand should be considered. Combination of these different treatments is also a valid option. For men who do not desire drug-based treatments, a vacuum device can be suggested or added to drug treatments. Finally, penile prosthesis is also a good option with high satisfaction among the patients and partners [18].

Low-intensity shock-wave therapy has a low level of evidence of improving EF post-RP and can be offered. Pelvic floor muscle training has currently not demonstrated clinical benefit. Platelet-rich plasma, neuromodulatory therapy, hyperbaric oxygenation and botulinum toxin currently have no enough evidence for being recommended outside from a clinical trial.

Urinary Incontinence

Urinary incontinence is also a major bothersome factor for patients after PCa treatments reducing quality of life. Stress urinary incontinence without climacturia after

RP or radiotherapy can cause sexual dysfunction on its own. Continual pad use and odour may be the causes of sexual avoidance, negative self-image, hygiene issues and depression.

Sexual incontinence includes climacturia, which is defined as the leak of urine during the orgasm, arousal leaks during foreplay and other leaks during sexual intercourse. It is not always associated with stress urinary incontinence, and it can be found after radiotherapy (5%), but it is more frequent after RP (28%). This rate increases if both treatments are applied. Frequently, sexual incontinence is inconstant and involves just some drops of urine. Even if this condition is not harmful for the patient nor the partner, it deeply affects own sexual perception: half of the patients are concerned about it, but partners are usually not bothered [19]. It can be the cause of sexual avoidance, which is more frequent in unpartnered men and men who have sex with men [20].

Multiple strategies can be applied to mitigate this condition. General hygienic recommendations as emptying the bladder before the intercourse limit fluid intake, and condoms can be applied. It is also demonstrated that the pelvic floor muscle training may have a role. An external compressive band or the "mini-jupette" (a urethral sling placed during the penile prosthesis insertion) can satisfactorily treat sexual incontinence [21].

Penile Changes

As we have previously explained, post-RP ED can lead to penile hypoxia, fibrosis and loss of elasticity, which may reduce its size. Half of the patients report a subjective penile shortening of at least 1 cm, which has been confirmed in some studies that measured the penis before and after RP with a variable mean loss [22].

Some treatments have demonstrated to prevent the shortening as the daily use of vacuum [23] or tadalafil 5 mg once a day [7] has shown a decrease in the mean shortening from 6 mm to 2 mm.

Incurvation of the penis can start before an RP but is commonly underdiagnosed especially in men who do not reach rigid erection. Peyronie's disease can be developed in 15% of the patients treated with RP with a mean curvature of 30°. Penile curvature can affect sexuality, especially penetrative sex, and should be treated specifically [24]. Specific populations as men who have sex with men experience significantly more psychosocial distress because of this [25].

Ejaculatory and Orgasmic Dysfunction

Anejaculation is expected after RP as the prostate and seminal vesicles are removed, but just 40% of the patients will be aware of this before the surgery. Healthcare providers should explain the difference between anejaculation and anorgasmia, and especially its consideration in fertility.

Anejaculation can be important in patients' sexuality: half of the patients regret its absence, and 8% will avoid sexual activity because of that [26]. No treatment is currently available to restore ejaculation after RP.

Altered feelings during orgasm are very frequent after PCa treatment (78%), but anorgasmia is rare (5–20%), with older age and no preservation of the NVB being the two main risk factors. Sixty per cent of the men also reported more prolonged sexual activity because it was more difficult to reach the orgasm. Usually, orgasmic sensation seems to decrease first and progressively improves [27]. There is no specific treatment for this condition.

Dysorgasmia is defined as pain during the orgasm. It is found in almost 10% of the men following RP and 12% after external beam radiotherapy (EBRT). One-third will report dysorgasmia at every orgasm, one-third occasionally and 19% rarely [28]. Symptoms tend to mitigate over time. It is believed to be caused by a reflex contraction of the bladder neck during orgasm, so giving tamsulosin has demonstrated an improvement in pain [29].

2.2.2 Radiotherapy

The pathophysiology of post-radiation ED is complex and mainly attributed to damage to arteries responsible for blood flow to the corpus cavernosum and endothelial cells in erectile tissues. Indeed, patients with post-radiotherapy ED present an arterial insufficiency in penile ultrasonography and an occlusive vascular disease in arteriography. Therefore, post-radiation ED can be considered mainly as a consequence of vascular damage, as neurogenic involvement is minimal and only observed in 3% of patients [30].

External Beam Radiotherapy

As mentioned, both RP and radiotherapy similarly affect erectile function, although the incidence in different series appears to be lower in radiotherapy. However, this tends to equal over time, as with RP the effects on EF are immediate but with radiotherapy the decay is progressive with rates close to 50% after 5 years of follow-up. Similarly to other PCa treatments, the probability of preserving sexual potency after radiotherapy depends on the patients' previous sexual function and comorbidities [30].

Another key factor is the dose received. A strong relationship between the dose/volume and the probability of maintaining potency after treatment is found. In fact, those patients who received 70 Grays or more have a very high risk of subsequently developing post-radiation therapy ED [31].

Particularly interesting is the effect of radiotherapy on ejaculation, because it significantly reduces the volume of semen in almost all the patients and can cause anejaculation [32]. Actually, there is no treatment for increasing seminal volume after radiotherapy. Radiotherapy is also associated with a decrease in orgasm in half of the patients, anorgasmia in a quarter of them and dysorgasmia in 12% [33]. Other effects of radiotherapy have been already explained or will be discussed.

Brachytherapy

Brachytherapy involves the placement of radioactive seeds in or near tumours for therapeutic purposes. Usually, it is indicated for low-risk disease or as a concomitant treatment with EBRT. The causes of ED secondary to brachytherapy are multifactorial, with underlying small-vessel disease, nerve injury, and dose in specific tissues as the bulb of the penis being the main factors. Similarly to external beam radiotherapy, the deterioration of EF is progressive, but initial sexual dysfunction is higher as it is related to post-treatment pain and ejaculatory discomfort. Indeed, initial dysorgasmia is very common (30%) after seed placement but then improves over the time [34].

Rates of EF preservation after brachytherapy vary from 50% to 86% according to different studies, which seems to be higher compared with RP or external radiotherapy. In addition, approximately 85% of patients would respond to treatment with PDE5i [35]. However, altered orgasm is referred by half of the patients, but anorgasmia is still rare (10%). Brachytherapy can cause also haematospermia in 15% of men that can be persistent in up to 6% [36].

2.2.3 Focal Therapy

Focal therapy has emerged as a potential treatment modality for localised prostate cancer, involving the selective treatment of cancerous foci and allowing preservation of healthy prostate tissue and adjacent structures such as urethral sphincter and NVB. The preservation of sexual function is one of the most important factors for patients when choosing between treatment options. Consequently, focal therapy, in contrast with radical treatments, was developed to achieve similar oncological outcomes while significantly reducing side effects, including the impact on sexual function.

Focal therapy encompasses various techniques, such as high-intensity focused ultrasound (HIFU), cryotherapy, electroporation and focal laser ablation, among others. However, there is insufficient present-day evidence regarding the detrimental effects of said therapies, as they are yet to gain widespread use. In current studies, just EF has been evaluated as a secondary outcome, and no information has been collected about other important aspects of sexuality that may alter as ejaculate volume or orgasm alterations. Although multiple therapies exist, we will proceed to expound on two of the most renowned.

Cryotherapy

Cryotherapy uses freezing techniques to induce cellular death through dehydration, which results in protein denaturation and subsequent direct rupture of cell membranes due to ice crystal formation, vascular stasis and microthrombi that impede microcirculation, leading to subsequent ischaemic apoptosis.

Prostate cryoablation is applicable from whole-gland treatment to targeted focal therapy. It is expected that when cryotherapy is used as a whole-gland therapy, the incidence of ED significantly rises up to 80% [37]. Nevertheless, when cryotherapy is employed as a focal therapy, it can effectively preserve sexual and urinary function in appropriately selected patients, attaining pre-treatment level of erectile function recovery approximately at 85% within the first 12 months, which increases slightly in the subsequent 18–24 months, with the only significant predictive factor being pre-treatment sexual function [38].

HIFU

This technique employs ultrasonic waves generated by a transducer, which accurately transfers thermal energy to the targeted area, resulting in tissue destruction.

The destruction of tissue occurs through thermal, mechanical and cavitation effects that create coagulative necrosis. Initially, thermal energy is generated by the absorption of mechanical energy. Furthermore, the mechanical effects are intricate and involve forces of diverse nature, such as shear, torque and streaming. Lastly, cavitation is produced by the formation of gas bubbles within cells due to the deposition of thermal and mechanical energy, which prompts oscillation of the bubbles.

When HIFU is employed as a treatment of the whole gland, ED can reach up to 40%. As a focal treatment, it shows similar results as cryotherapy, preserving EF in 69–80% at 6 months from the procedure, increasing up to 86% at 2 years [39].

3 Part 2: Hormonal Treatment, Biopsychosocial Assessment and Non-Heteronormative Groups

3.1 Sexuality After Hormonal Therapy

The growth and proliferation of prostate cells depend on androgens. Testosterone, although not oncogenic by itself, plays a fundamental role in the growth and perpetuation of tumour cells. Hormonal castration therapy deprives such stimulation, and prostate cancer cells undergo apoptosis [40]. Therefore, androgen deprivation therapy (ADT) is currently essential in the treatment of metastatic prostate cancer or is combined with radiotherapy in high-risk localised disease.

However, this treatment has a deleterious effect on sexual function and the general well-being. This is a consequence of the fundamental role that testosterone plays in male sexual sphere. The relative function of androgenic and estrogenic stimulation in male sexual behaviour is complex. Testosterone is deeply involved in regulating most aspects of sexual function, playing a role both centrally and peripherally. For example, in patients with hypogonadism, testosterone replacement therapy can improve sexual function, especially in increasing libido and, to a lesser extent, in regulating spinal and local erection. Nevertheless, erections are still possible in the absence of androgens [41].

Furthermore, many patients who receive androgen deprivation therapy (ADT) have already undergone treatments such as RP or radiotherapy, which could already have a significant impact on sexual function.

Some patients undergoing ADT have demonstrated maintaining sexual function. Current research suggests that the preservation of sexual behaviour post-treatment may not be associated with steroid receptor activation pathways. For instance, in one study, no correlation was found between sex steroid levels in areas of the brain related to sexual behaviour, such as the preoptic area, amygdala or hypothalamus. Moreover, the preservation of neuronal activity in the nucleus accumbens following sexual stimulation may be an important factor in maintaining sexual behaviour post-ADT treatment [42]. A neurobiological investigation on factors that differentiate patients with lower treatment-related impact on sexual function would be of great interest.

3.1.1 Effects on Sexual Functioning

Androgen deprivation therapy can lead to a significant decline in sexual function. Up to 82% of such patients presented with ED, and 64% experienced a significant decrease in sexual desire [43]. Although the proportion of patients who remain sexually active is low, it is challenging to estimate the exact percentage of cessation of sexual activity, given that most studies focus on erectile function and penetrative sex and may underestimate those men who, despite treatment, maintain non-penetrative sexual activity.

While these findings are not surprising, human sexual behaviour is complex and does not rely exclusively on biological factors but also involves psychological and social factors that cannot be ignored. When non-penetrative sexual activities are also evaluated, three in ten patients with prostate cancer undergoing androgen deprivation therapy recognised having some sort of sexual relationships with their partner [41].

3.1.2 Effect on Body Image

Physical appearance plays a vital role in the perception of masculinity, and therefore the body changes can affect sexual sphere. Nearly 60% of men receiving ADT experience negative changes in their body image. Testicles can become atrophic, penile size can decrease significantly (dropping of stretched penile length from a mean of 14.2 cm to 8.6 cm), body hair can be lost, some can develop fatigue or gain weight and hot flushes can also be bothersome and affect masculine self-perception as gynecomastia that will be developed by 20% of the patients. Some of these effects can be mitigated by treatments as tamoxifen for gynecomastia, gabapentin or medroxyprogesterone for hot flushes or exercises for both fatigue and overweight [44].

3.1.3 Effect on Libido

The correlation between ADT and sexual desire has been well established. The hypothalamus and limbic system are the main brain areas involved in regulating sexual desire. Androgen receptors are present in different areas of the brain, including the hypothalamic and limbic regions, indicating the role of testosterone in regulating sexual behaviour [41].

Even though the neurophysiological mechanisms underlying sexual desire are still not fully understood, several animal studies have suggested the pivotal role of testosterone. For instance, castrated rats exhibit compromised sexual behaviour, while the restoration of androgen levels in these rats seems to restore it [43].

However, even if libido in humans is multifactorial with other factors as hormones (prolactin), and psychosocial background, 90% of the patients on ADT will experience a decrease in sexual desire, fantasising and erotic dreams [41]. At the same time, the depressive or anxious state that often goes with diagnosis and treatment directly affects this loss of sexual desire.

3.1.4 Effect on Erectile Function

The relationship between erectile function and testosterone in humans remains controversial. Penile erection depends on the vasculature of the corpus cavernosum, its integrity and proper functioning, which is regulated by testosterone, through its effects on nitric oxide (NO), and the enzyme NO synthase, which is involved in the synthesis of NO in endothelial cells and non-adrenergic, non-cholinergic nerves. Animal studies suggest that testosterone upregulates the amount of endothelial and neuronal NO synthase [42].

Nocturnal erections are more related to androgen milieu than stimulated ones that depend also on psychological conditions. Chronic lack of involuntary and voluntary erections due to ADT can cause a penile hypoxia [45] and, by that, result in the same fibrous process as after RP. That would explain penile length loss and ED in ADT. Eighty-five per cent of the patients on ADT report having no erection at all, although 8% manifest having some erections while the rest report having few [46].

3.1.5 Effect on Ejaculation

The spinal nuclei responsible for regulation of ejaculation, such as the bulbocavernosus and ischiocavernosus nerve nucleus, are contingent upon androgens. Nevertheless, there is a scarcity of physiological evidence available concerning the association between testosterone and ejaculation in humans, with most of the evidence being deducted from animal models. However, it was found that perceived ejaculate volume was reduced in men undergoing ADT [47].

3.2 Biopsychosocial Assessment

Sexual functioning declines progressively with age, but the sense of sexual being remains important. As it has been showed, PCa treatment can alter sexuality significantly and abruptly. In most of the studies addressing sexuality in PCa patients, erectile function is defined by firmness and penetration, but when the patient gets asked, it is about satisfaction for them and their partner [48].

Psychological interventions have been assessed in sexual dysfunction after PCa, and it has been set that improving communication skills in a couple can improve early sexual satisfaction [49]. Also, sexual counselling in combination with ED treatments improves sexual function and adherence to treatments. Enhancing the idea of a multidisciplinary approach may be helpful [50, 51]. All of these interventions should have a different focus depending on male sexuality.

3.2.1 Sexual Intimacy

Men who experience ED after PCa usually refer to lacking confidence in sexual intercourses and fear of embarrassment. This is associated with emotions of sadness, anger, anxiety, intrusive thoughts of what was before, hopelessness and loss of self-esteem [46].

Some couples adapt to ED when reaching of orgasm cannot be fully restored with different stimulations, but usually the grief over the lost previous sexual life decreases relationship intimacy [52]. For mitigating the loss in intimacy, some included acts as kissing and hugging more often and others engaged in non-penetrative practices. Normally, female partners are less stressed by sexual changes than the patients [53] and usually undervalue penetrative sex [54], but 38% of them report not being sexually satisfied [55].

Sexual intercourse can be seen as unnatural due to ED treatments for the patient and the partner [54] and can be the cause of sexual discontinuation for some couples even when the ED is successfully recovered [56].

3.2.2 Relationship with Women

Heterosexual unpartnered men also experience an important change in the way they connect with women. Some of them relate to be more inattentive for sexual intimacy with the women they meet than previously did. Also, ED in unpartnered men makes them less likely to find new relationships and hide their diagnosis. In heterosexual couples, partners play a key role in emotional support, but most of the patients admit not discussing changes in sexuality with them or just blame them for the lack of interest in sex [57].

3.2.3 Sexual Imaging

Some men who are sexually inactive after PCa treatment experience a total lack of fantasising sexual intercourse with woman, making them feel nostalgic and missing masculine self-identity. This loss of libido is most notorious on ADT [57].

3.2.4 Masculinity

Masculinity is a social construct that can alter after PCa treatments. For localised treatment of prostate cancer, the lack of sex arousal and performance can be viewed as a gender disqualification. For some men, PCa diagnosis and treatment suppose a premature retirement from their job, and they perceive that also as loss of their masculine role and worthlessness [58].

Two well-defined psychological responses to this "loss of masculinity" have been addressed. One kind of patients consider it as a trade-off to preserve their health. They usually accept better the general changes in their life and feel less general discomfort with side effects. For them, regaining their previous sexuality is not a main objective, and they are more disposed to treatments. The others are men with firm "masculine" ideals. They tend to regret the loss of previous sexuality, feel more distress and are more reluctant to use erectile aids, which they consider "unmanly" [59]. Usually, younger patients are more affected by changes in masculinity [60].

As we have previously explained, hormonal treatments also add physical changes as loss in strength, hot flushes, gynecomastia and other body alterations (loss of body hair, increasing abdominal fat) and some emotional changes such as crying more often and becoming more emotional [57]. This is expressed as "feminising" by some patients and can cause distress [61].

3.3 Non-Heteronormative Groups

3.3.1 Men Who Have Sex with Men

Most of the data about ED is gathered from studies of heterosexual patients, but men who have sex with men (MSM) have specific demands regarding their sexuality, and many providers may lack of giving appropriate advice.

For anal penetration, a more rigid erection is needed than for vaginal. Only 40% of MSM who always engaged in anal insertive sex (always top) continued practicing it after treatment [62]. In that matter, there is a specific lack of data regarding heterosexual couples who have anal sex. Sexual conduit is diverse of sexual orientation, and usually this is not taken into consideration.

Receptive anal sex is also affected by PCa treatments as half of the patients report a loss of pleasure or for some of them even anorgasmia. Anodyspareunia is defined as pain during receptive anal sex and appears in one in six men. Anal dilatation is referred as a treatment by some patients without proper scientific evidence. Radiotherapy can cause ischaemia and fibrosis, which may result in long-term effects as anal bleeding and faecal incontinence affecting sexuality among these patients. Something worrying is that less than 10% of the patients received information from their practitioner regarding this subject [63].

Some MSM react to this by switching their predominant role. Switching the penetrative role is not as banal as it may seem because it can be an important part of the personality and in the couple functioning. But not just penetrative roles can alter. Some men may avoid sexual activity, and some may alter their sexual practice to non-penetrative sex such as oral sex, masturbation and role-play (bondage-discipline-sado-masochism). Psychologically, MSM can have more inferiority feelings because of the immediate visual comparison [62].

In addition, anejaculation is a major bothersome factor for MSM. Regardless of the preferred sexual activity, lack of ejaculation can cause fear of judgement by partners who might view it as a sign of failure, loss of male identity and self-worth [64].

3.3.2 Transgender Woman

PCa in transgender woman is severely not understood as just few case reports, retrospective studies and reviews are available with heterogeneity of the data collected and lack of large cohort or long-term follow-up. As we have seen, PCa is dependent on testosterone, and transgender women usually undergo androgen deprivation and/or hormonal replacement treatments. Data cannot always be extrapolated from cisgender man.

PCa incidence in transgender woman cohorts seems to be lower in retrospective studies compared to that reported in cisgender man, but this should be taken as a caution as the cohorts evaluated report a median age of 30 years. Some theorised that PCa was present before starting hormonal treatment and some influence of oestrogen in PCa cells [65].

A retrospective study found that 6 trans women out of 2281 had PCa. Among them, 5 had a Gleason grade $\geq$ 7 and the mean PSA was 18, highlighting the possibility that PCa diagnosed in transgender women can be more aggressive. As they are on hormonal treatment with castration levels of testosterone, another possibility is the selection of castration-resistant cells [66]. This is especially important for the systematic hormonal treatment in the era of androgen receptor-targeted treatment. However, more studies are needed to confirm this theory.

Diagnosis can be complicated in transgender women as hormonal treatment usually drops PSA levels, and no validation of MRI has been made for this subgroup of population. Specialists agree on an upper limit of PSA of 1 ng/mL. For patients that had vaginoplasty, digital examination of the prostate can be assessed vaginally, and prostate biopsy can also proceed with transvaginal probe [67].

Localised treatment should be considered as RP can be more challenging in patients with vaginoplasty with more risk of fistula, and radiotherapy could also lead to more risk of neovaginal stenosis. Also, having these treatments before the gender-affirming surgery increases the risks of rectal injury, fistula and incontinence and can even discourage it. However, labiaplasty can be performed without important risks. This should be discussed with the patient before PCa treatment.

Just one study addresses sexuality in transgender women with PCa. Some of them who did not receive vaginoplasty may experience ED after local treatments and may receive an approach similar to cisgender men. For patients with vaginoplasty, radiotherapy can cause neovaginal stenosis for which it is recommended increasing dilatation frequency [68].

In the biopsychosocial approach, we found just one recent study in all types of cancer in transgender population. This study included patients with different cancers and their perception of embodiment and identity of cancer diagnosis and healthcare and for some treatments with heterogeneous findings. They highlighted the fact that transgender women are usually reluctant to consult practitioners. In the case of PCa, one gay transgender woman felt more comfortable after the gynecomastia and the reduction of penis and testicles produced by the hormone therapy, which enhanced her embodiment. On the other hand, another transgender woman felt not adequately informed because gender affirmation surgery was formerly not recommended after RP complications [69].

4   Conclusion

Traditionally, ED has been central in the management of PCa survivors, but as we have reviewed, a lot of domains in sexuality may change. Even in non-sexually active patients, distress may occur due to changes in their sense of masculinity and self-image. Managing all these issues is technically impossible in a regular urology/ oncology office, so a multimodal approach with different professionals (specialised nurses, sexologists, psychologists, rehabilitators) may offer more resources for dealing with the secondary distress caused by sexual dysfunction.

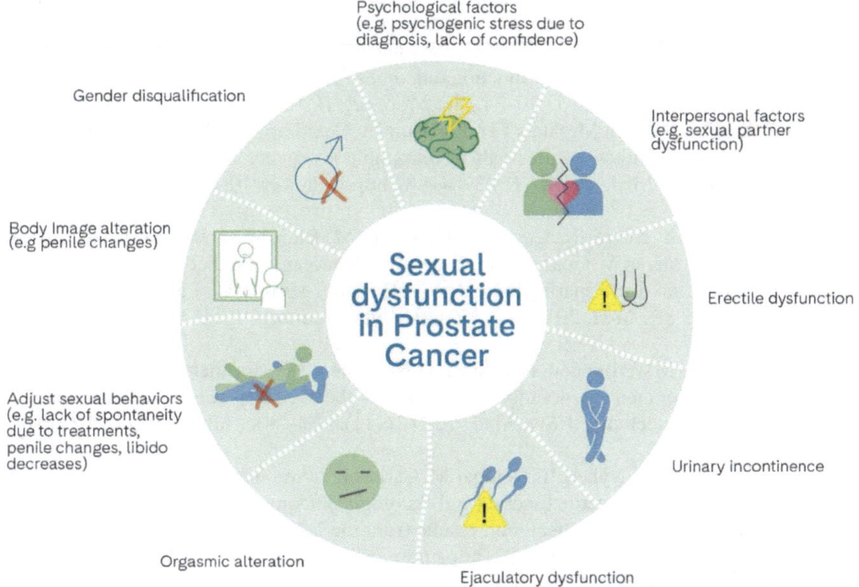

References

1. Incrocci L, Madalinska JB, Essink-Bot ML, Van Putten WL, Koper PC, Schröder FH. Sexual functioning in patients with localized prostate cancer awaiting treatment. J Sex Marital Ther. 2001;27:353–63.
2. Walsh PC, Lepor H, Eggleston JC. Radical prostatectomy with preservation of sexual function: anatomical and pathological considerations. Prostate. 1983;4(5):473–85. https://doi.org/10.1002/pros.2990040506.
3. Mulhall JP. Defining and reporting erectile function outcomes after radical prostatectomy: challenges and misconceptions. J Urol. 2009;181(2):462–71. https://doi.org/10.1016/j.juro.2008.10.047.
4. Padma-Nathan H, AR MC, Levine LA, Lipshultz LI, Siegel R, Montorsi F, Giuliano F, Brock G, Study Group. Randomized, double-blind, placebo-controlled study of postoperative nightly sildenafil citrate for the prevention of erectile dysfunction after bilateral nerve-sparing radical prostatectomy. Int J Impot Res. 2008;20(5):479–86. https://doi.org/10.1038/ijir.2008.33.
5. Pavlovich CP, Levinson AW, Su LM, Mettee LZ, Feng Z, Bivalacqua TJ, Trock BJ. Nightly vs. on-demand sildenafil for penile rehabilitation after minimally invasive nerve-sparing radical prostatectomy: results of a randomized double-blind trial with placebo. BJU Int. 2013;112(6):844–51. https://doi.org/10.1111/bju.12253.
6. Montorsi F, Brock G, Lee J, Shapiro J, Van Poppel H, Graefen M, Stief C. Effect of nightly versus on-demand vardenafil on recovery of erectile function in men following bilateral nerve-sparing radical prostatectomy. Eur Urol. 2008;54(4):924–31. https://doi.org/10.1016/j.eururo.2008.06.083.
7. Montorsi F, Brock G, Stolzenburg JU, Mulhall J, Moncada I, Patel HR, Chevallier D, Krajka K, Henneges C, Dickson R, Büttner H. Effects of tadalafil treatment on erectile function recovery

following bilateral nerve-sparing radical prostatectomy: a randomised placebo-controlled study (REACTT). Eur Urol. 2014;65(3):587–96. https://doi.org/10.1016/j.eururo.2013.09.051.

8. Levinson AW, Lavery HJ, Ward NT, Su LM, Pavlovich CP. Is a return to baseline sexual function possible? An analysis of sexual function outcomes following laparoscopic radical prostatectomy. World J Urol. 2011;29(1):29–34. https://doi.org/10.1007/s00345-010-0616-5.

9. Rabbani F, Schiff J, Piecuch M, Yunis LH, Eastham JA, Scardino PT, Mulhall JP. Time course of recovery of erectile function after radical retropubic prostatectomy: does anyone recover after 2 years? J Sex Med. 2010;7(12):3984–90. https://doi.org/10.1111/j.1743-6109.2010.01969.x.

10. Briganti A, Gallina A, Suardi N, Capitanio U, Tutolo M, Bianchi M, Passoni N, Salonia A, Colombo R, Di Girolamo V, Guazzoni G, Rigatti P, Montorsi F. Predicting erectile function recovery after bilateral nerve sparing radical prostatectomy: a proposal of a novel preoperative risk stratification. J Sex Med. 2010;7(7):2521–31. https://doi.org/10.1111/j.1743-6109.2010.01845.x.

11. Mulhall JP, Kattan MW, Bennett NE, Stasi J, Nascimento B, Eastham J, Guillonneau B, Scardino PT. Development of nomograms to predict the recovery of erectile function following radical prostatectomy. J Sex Med. 2019;16(11):1796–802. https://doi.org/10.1016/j.jsxm.2019.08.003.

12. Sooriakumaran P, Pini G, Nyberg T, Derogar M, Carlsson S, Stranne J, Bjartell A, Hugosson J, Steineck G, Wiklund PN. Erectile function and oncologic outcomes following open Retropubic and robot-assisted radical prostatectomy: results from the LAParoscopic prostatectomy robot open trial. Eur Urol. 2018;73(4):618–27. https://doi.org/10.1016/j.eururo.2017.08.015.

13. Walz J, Epstein JI, Ganzer R, Graefen M, Guazzoni G, Kaouk J, Menon M, Mottrie A, Myers RP, Patel V, Tewari A, Villers A, Artibani W. A critical analysis of the current knowledge of surgical anatomy of the prostate related to optimisation of cancer control and preservation of continence and erection in candidates for radical prostatectomy: an update. Eur Urol. 2016;70(2):301–11. https://doi.org/10.1016/j.eururo.2016.01.026.

14. van der Poel HG, Tillier C, de Blok W, van Muilekom E. Extended nodal dissection reduces sexual function recovery after robot-assisted laparoscopic prostatectomy. J Endourol. 2012;26(9):1192–8. https://doi.org/10.1089/end.2012.0011.

15. Capogrosso P, Vertosick EA, Benfante NE, Eastham JA, Scardino PJ, Vickers AJ, Mulhall JP. Are we improving erectile function recovery after radical prostatectomy? Analysis of patients treated over the last decade. Eur Urol. 2019;75(2):221–8. https://doi.org/10.1016/j.eururo.2018.08.039.

16. Moncada I, de Bethencourt FR, Lledó-García E, Romero-Otero J, Turbi C, Büttner H, Henneges C, Martinez Salamanca JI. Effects of tadalafil once daily or on demand versus placebo on time to recovery of erectile function in patients after bilateral nerve-sparing radical prostatectomy. World J Urol. 2015;33(7):1031–8. https://doi.org/10.1007/s00345-014-1377-3.

17. Montorsi F, Maga T, Strambi LF, Salonia A, Barbieri L, Scattoni V, Guazzoni G, Losa A, Rigatti P, Pizzini G. Sildenafil taken at bedtime significantly increases nocturnal erections: results of a placebo-controlled study. Urology. 2000;56(6):906–11. https://doi.org/10.1016/s0090-4295(00)00841-4.

18. Pillay B, Moon D, Love C, Meyer D, Ferguson E, Crowe H, Howard N, Mann S, Wootten A. Quality of life, psychological functioning, and treatment satisfaction of men who have undergone penile prosthesis surgery following robot-assisted radical prostatectomy. J Sex Med. 2017;14(12):1612–20. https://doi.org/10.1016/j.jsxm.2017.10.001.

19. Elliott S, Matthew A. Sexual recovery following prostate cancer: recommendations from 2 established Canadian sexual rehabilitation clinics. Sex Med Rev. 2018;6(2):279–94. https://doi.org/10.1016/j.sxmr.2017.09.001.

20. Salter CA, Bach PV, Miranda E, Jenkins LC, Benfante N, Schofield E, Nelson CJ, Mulhall JP. Bother associated with Climacturia after radical prostatectomy: prevalence and predictors. J Sex Med. 2020;17(4):731–6. https://doi.org/10.1016/j.jsxm.2019.12.016.

21. Mykoniatis I, van Renterghem K, Sokolakis I, Hatzichristodoulou G, Sempels M, Andrianne R. Climacturia: a comprehensive review assessing pathophysiology, prevalence, impact, and

treatment options regarding the "leak of pleasure". Int J Impot Res. 2021;33(3):259–70. https://doi.org/10.1038/s41443-020-0257-1.

22. Engel JD, Sutherland DE, Williams SB, Wagner KR. Changes in penile length after robot-assisted laparoscopic radical prostatectomy. J Endourol. 2011;25(1):65–9. https://doi.org/10.1089/end.2010.0382.

23. Raina R, Agarwal A, Ausmundson S, et al. Early use of vacuum constriction device following radical prostatectomy facilitates early sexual activity and potentially earlier return of erectile function. Int J Impot Res. 2006;18:77–81.

24. Tal R, Heck M, Teloken P, Siegrist T, Nelson CJ, Mulhall JP. Peyronie's disease following radical prostatectomy: incidence and predictors. J Sex Med. 2010;7(3):1254–61. https://doi.org/10.1111/j.1743-6109.2009.01655.x.

25. Salter CA, Nascimento B, Terrier JE, Taniguchi H, Bernie H, Miranda E, Jenkins L, Schofield E, Mulhall JP. Defining the impact of Peyronie's disease on the psychosocial status of gay men. Andrology. 2021;9(1):233–7. https://doi.org/10.1111/andr.12899.

26. Messaoudi R, Menard J, Ripert T, Parquet H, Staerman F. Erectile dysfunction and sexual health after radical prostatectomy: impact of sexual motivation. Int J Impot Res. 2011;23:81–6.

27. Frey A, Sønksen J, Jakobsen H, Fode M. Prevalence and predicting factors for commonly neglected sexual side effects to radical prostatectomies: results from a cross-sectional questionnaire-based study. J Sex Med. 2014;11(9):2318–26. https://doi.org/10.1111/jsm.12624.

28. Barnas JL, Pierpaoli S, Ladd P, Valenzuela R, Aviv N, Parker M, Waters WB, Flanigan RC, Mulhall JP. The prevalence and nature of orgasmic dysfunction after radical prostatectomy. BJU Int. 2004;94(4):603–5. https://doi.org/10.1111/j.1464-410X.2004.05009.x.

29. Barnas J, Parker M, Guhring P, Mulhall JP. The utility of tamsulosin in the management of orgasm-associated pain: a pilot analysis. Eur Urol. 2005;47:361–5.

30. Incrocci L. Sexual function after external-beam radiotherapy for prostate cancer: what do we know? Crit Rev Oncol Hematol. 2006;57(2):165–73. https://doi.org/10.1016/j.critrevonc.2005.06.006.

31. Fisch BM, Pickett B, Weinberg V, Roach M. Dose of radiation received by the bulb of the penis correlates with risk of impotence after three-dimensional conformal radiotherapy for prostate cancer. Urology. 2001;57(5):955–9. https://doi.org/10.1016/s0090-4295(01)00940-2.

32. Sullivan JF, Stember DS, Deveci S, Akin-Olugbade Y, Mulhall JP, Akin-Olugbade Y, et al. Ejaculation profiles of men following radiation therapy for prostate cancer. J Sex Med. 2013;10:1410–6.

33. Frey A, Pedersen C, Lindberg H, Bisbjerg R, Sønksen J, Fode M. Prevalence and predicting factors for commonly neglected sexual side effects to external-beam radiation therapy for prostate cancer. J Sex Med. 2017;14(4):558–65. https://doi.org/10.1016/j.jsxm.2017.01.015.

34. Merrick GS, Wallner K, Butler WM, Lief JH, Sutlief S. Short-term sexual function after prostate brachytherapy. Int J Cancer. 2001;96(5):313–9. https://doi.org/10.1002/ijc.1028.

35. Merrick GS, Butler WM, Dorsey AT, Lief JH, Donzella JG. A comparison of radiation dose to the neurovascular bundles in men with and without prostate brachytherapy-induced erectile dysfunction. Int J Radiat Oncol Biol Phys. 2000;48(4):1069–74. https://doi.org/10.1016/s0360-3016(00)00746-x.

36. Delaunay B, Delannes M, Salloum A, Delavierre D, Wagner F, Jonca F, Thoulouzan M, Plante P, Bachaud JM, Soulie M, Huyghe E. Orgasme après curiethérapie de prostate par implants permanents d'iode 125 pour cancer localisé de la prostate [orgasm after curietherapy with permanent iodine-125 radioimplants for localized prostate cancer]. Prog Urol. 2011;21(13):932–9. https://doi.org/10.1016/j.purol.2011.05.002.

37. Asterling S, Greene DR. Prospective evaluation of sexual function in patients receiving cryosurgery as a primary radical treatment for localized prostate cancer. BJU Int. 2009;103(6):788–92. https://doi.org/10.1111/j.1464-410X.2008.08042.x.

38. Shah TT, Peters M, Miah S, Eldred-Evans D, Yap T, Hosking-Jervis F, Dudderidge T, Hindley RG, McCracken S, Greene D, Nigam R, Valerio M, Winkler M, Virdi J, Arya M, Ahmed HU, Minhas S. Assessment of return to baseline urinary and sexual function following primary

focal cryotherapy for nonmetastatic prostate cancer. Eur Urol Focus. 2021;7(2):301–8. https://doi.org/10.1016/j.euf.2019.09.004.

39. Bakavicius A, Marra G, Macek P, Robertson C, Abreu AL, George AK, Malavaud B, Coloby P, Rischmann P, Moschini M, Rastinehad AR, Sidana A, Stabile A, Tourinho-Barbosa R, de la Rosette J, Ahmed H, Polascik T, Cathelineau X, Sanchez-Salas R. Available evidence on HIFU for focal treatment of prostate cancer: a systematic review. Int Braz J Urol. 2022;48(2):263–74. https://doi.org/10.1590/S1677-5538.IBJU.2021.0091.

40. Hull EM, Rodríguez-Manzo G. Male sexual behavior. In: Elsevier eBooks. Elsevier BV; 2009. p. 5–66. https://doi.org/10.1016/b978-008088783-8.00001-2.

41. Duthie CJ, Calich HJ, Rapsey CM, Wibowo E. Maintenance of sexual activity following androgen deprivation in males. Crit Rev Oncol Hematol. 2020;153:103064. https://doi.org/10.1016/j.critrevonc.2020.103064.

42. Morelli A, Filippi S, Zhang XH, Luconi M, Vignozzi L, Mancina R, Maggi M. Peripheral regulatory mechanisms in erection. Int J Androl. 2005;28(Suppl 2):23–7. https://doi.org/10.1111/j.1365-2605.2005.00550.x.

43. Mazzola CR, Mulhall JP. Impact of androgen deprivation therapy on sexual function. Asian J Androl. 2012;14(2):198–203. https://doi.org/10.1038/aja.2011.106.

44. Wibowo E, Wassersug RJ, Robinson JW, Matthew A, McLeod D, Walker LM. How are patients with prostate cancer managing androgen deprivation therapy side effects? Clin Genitourin Cancer. 2019;17(3):e408–19. https://doi.org/10.1016/j.clgc.2018.12.006.

45. Nguyen PL, Alibhai SM, Basaria S, D'Amico AV, Kantoff PW, Keating NL, Penson DF, Rosario DJ, Tombal B, Smith MR. Adverse effects of androgen deprivation therapy and strategies to mitigate them. Eur Urol. 2015;67(5):825–36. https://doi.org/10.1016/j.eururo.2014.07.010.

46. Hoffman RM, Hunt WC, Gilliland FD, Stephenson RA, Potosky AL. Patient satisfaction with treatment decisions for clinically localized prostate carcinoma. Results from the prostate cancer outcomes study. Cancer. 2003;97(7):1653–62. https://doi.org/10.1002/cncr.11233.

47. Corona G, Boddi V, Gacci M, Sforza A, Forti G, Mannucci E, Maggi M. Perceived ejaculate volume reduction in patients with erectile dysfunction: psychobiologic correlates. J Androl. 2011;32(3):333–9. https://doi.org/10.2164/jandrol.110.010397.

48. Bokhour BG, Clark JA, Inui TS, Silliman RA, Talcott JA. Sexuality after treatment for early prostate cancer: exploring the meanings of "erectile dysfunction". J Gen Intern Med. 2001;16(10):649–55. https://doi.org/10.1111/j.1525-1497.2001.00832.x.

49. Canada AL, Schover LR. Research promoting better patient education on reproductive health after cancer. J Natl Cancer Inst Monogr. 2005;2005:98–100.

50. Titta M, Tavolini IM, Dal Moro F, Cisternino A, Bassi P. Sexual counseling improved erectile rehabilitation after non-nerve-sparing radical retropubic prostatectomy or cystectomy—results of a randomized prospective study. J Sex Med. 2006;3:267–79.

51. Matthew A, Lutzky-Cohen N, Jamnicky L, Currie K, Gentile A, Mina DS, Fleshner N, Finelli A, Hamilton R, Kulkarni G, Jewett M, Zlotta A, Trachtenberg J, Yang Z, Elterman D. The prostate cancer rehabilitation clinic: a biopsychosocial clinic for sexual dysfunction after radical prostatectomy. Curr Oncol. 2018;25(6):393–402. https://doi.org/10.3747/co.25.4111.

52. Wittmann D. Emotional and sexual health in cancer: partner and relationship issues. Curr Opin Support Palliat Care. 2016;10(1):75–80. https://doi.org/10.1097/SPC.0000000000000187.

53. Garos S, Kluck A, Aronoff D. Prostate cancer patients and their partners: differences in satisfaction indices and psychological variables. J Sex Med. 2007;4(5):1394–403. https://doi.org/10.1111/j.1743-6109.2007.00545.x.

54. Wittmann D, Foley S, Balon R. A biopsychosocial approach to sexual recovery after prostate cancer surgery: the role of grief and mourning. J Sex Marital Ther. 2011;37(2):130–44. https://doi.org/10.1080/0092623X.2011.560538.

55. Wootten AC, Abbott JM, Farrell A, Austin DW, Klein B. Psychosocial interventions to support partners of men with prostate cancer: a systematic and critical review of the literature. J Cancer Surviv. 2014;8(3):472–84. https://doi.org/10.1007/s11764-014-0361-7.

56. Son H, Park K, Kim SW, Paick JS. Reasons for discontinuation of sildenafil citrate after successful restoration of erectile function. Asian J Androl. 2004;6(2):117–20.

57. Bowie J, Brunckhorst O, Stewart R, Dasgupta P, Ahmed K. Body image, self-esteem, and sense of masculinity in patients with prostate cancer: a qualitative meta-synthesis. J Cancer Surviv. 2022;16(1):95–110. https://doi.org/10.1007/s11764-021-01007-9.
58. Dieperink KB, Wagner L, Hansen S, Hansen O. Embracing life after prostate cancer. A male perspective on treatment and rehabilitation. Eur J Cancer Care (Engl). 2013;22(4):549–58.
59. Fergus KD, Gray RE, Fitch MI. Sexual dysfunction and the preservation of manhood: experiences of men with prostate cancer. J Health Psychol. 2002;7:303–16.
60. Chambers SK, Chung E, Wittert G, Hyde MK. Erectile dysfunction, masculinity, and psychosocial outcomes: a review of the experiences of men after prostate cancer treatment. Transl Androl Urol. 2017;6(1):60–8. https://doi.org/10.21037/tau.2016.08.12.
61. Muermann MM, Wassersug RJ. Prostate cancer from a sex and gender perspective: a review. Sex Med Rev. 2022;10(1):142–54. https://doi.org/10.1016/j.sxmr.2021.03.001.
62. Martin-Tuite PJ, Shindel AW. Prostate cancer and sexual consequences among men who have sex with men. Int J Impot Res. 2021;33(4):473–9. https://doi.org/10.1038/s41443-020-00392-6.
63. Wheldon CW, Polter EJ, Rosser BRS, Kapoor A, Talley KMC, Haggart R, Kohli N, Konety BR, Mitteldorf D, Ross MW, West W, Wright M. Pain and loss of pleasure in receptive anal sex for gay and bisexual men following prostate cancer treatment: results from the *Restore-1* study. J Sex Res. 2022;59(7):826–33. https://doi.org/10.1080/00224499.2021.1939846.
64. McInnis MK, Pukall CF. Sex after prostate cancer in gay and bisexual men: a review of the literature. Sex Med Rev. 2020;8(3):466–72. https://doi.org/10.1016/j.sxmr.2020.01.004.
65. Silverberg MJ, Nash R, Becerra-Culqui TA, et al. Cohort study of cancer risk among insured transgender people. Ann Epidemiol. 2017;27:499–501.
66. de Nie I, de Blok CJM, van der Sluis TM, Barbé E, Pigot GLS, Wiepjes CM, Nota NM, van Mello NM, Valkenburg NE, Huirne J, Gooren LJG, van Moorselaar RJA, Dreijerink KMA, den Heijer M. Prostate cancer incidence under androgen deprivation: Nationwide cohort study in trans women receiving hormone treatment. J Clin Endocrinol Metab. 2020;105(9):e3293–9. https://doi.org/10.1210/clinem/dgaa412.
67. Ingham MD, Lee RJ, MacDermed D, Olumi AF. Prostate cancer in transgender women. Urol Oncol. 2018;36(12):518–25. https://doi.org/10.1016/j.urolonc.2018.09.011.
68. Deebel NA, Morin JP, Autorino R, Vince R, Grob B, Hampton LJ. Prostate cancer in transgender women: incidence, Etiopathogenesis, and management challenges. Urology. 2017;110:166–71. https://doi.org/10.1016/j.urology.2017.08.032.
69. Ussher JM, Power R, Allison K, Sperring S, Parton C, Perz J, Davies C, Cook T, Hawkey AJ, Robinson KH, Hickey M, Anazodo A, Ellis C. Reinforcing or disrupting gender affirmation: the impact of cancer on transgender embodiment and identity. Arch Sex Behav. 2023;52(3):901–20. https://doi.org/10.1007/s10508-023-02530-9.

Male Sexual Dysfunctions in the Infertile Couple

Maurizio D'Anna and Josep Torremadé Barreda

1   Introduction

Infertility is a widespread condition that affects around 15% of couples [1, 2]. It is defined as the inability of a couple to conceive after 1 year of regular unprotected intercourse. According to the World Health Organization, male factors contribute to infertility in about 50% of cases [1].

Male sexual dysfunction is a broad term used to describe a range of problems that can affect sexual performance. Problems can occur at any stage of the sexual response cycle, which includes desire, arousal, orgasm and ejaculation. These sexual dysfunctions can be caused by various factors, including physical, psychological and social factors. Around 50% of the male population reports at least one sexual dysfunction during their lifetime, having a detrimental effect on their quality of life.

The association between male sexual dysfunctions and infertility is often bidirectional: infertility can be caused by male sexual dysfunctions, and these sexual dysfunctions can arise as a consequence of the infertility diagnosis and the psychopathological burden that it carries. Mainly, psychogenic erectile dysfunction (ED) and low sexual desire may be caused by the stress of having sexual intercourse with a procreative purpose [3].

Interestingly, according to some studies, infertile men have a higher Charlson Comorbidity Index than fertile controls, meaning that infertility may be a sign of poor general health [4], which in turn can cause male sexual dysfunctions.

M. D'Anna · J. Torremadé Barreda (✉)
Urology Department, Clinical Institute of Nephrology and Urology, Hospital Clínic de Barcelona, Barcelona, Spain

Clinical Sexology Working Group, Hospital Clinic de Barcelona, Barcelona, Spain
e-mail: danna@clinic.cat; torremade@clinic.cat

C. Castelo-Branco, S. Anglès Acedo (eds.), *Medical Disorders and Sexual Health*, Trends in Andrology and Sexual Medicine,
https://doi.org/10.1007/978-3-031-55080-5_9

Overall, male sexual dysfunctions are a not so common cause of infertility. Organic sexual dysfunctions cause between 2.3% and 5% of all infertility cases [2]. A study by the World Health Organization showed a prevalence of 2.3% in 7237 patients with infertility [5]. In another prevalence study from a cohort of 12,945 patients, male sexual dysfunctions caused 2.4% of all infertility cases [2]. Other studies report an even higher rate of 4.4% in 1737 patients, mainly because of ejaculatory disorders [6].

On the other hand, male infertility can have psychopathological consequences such as anxiety and depression disorders, which can be associated with male sexual dysfunctions [5]. If one person in the couple has a sexual dysfunction, the other person can develop feelings of guilt or lower self-esteem. Women whose partners have ED report decreased sexual satisfaction rates [7] and can also develop female sexual dysfunctions such as hypoactive sexual desire, arousal dysfunction and dyspareunia, and they can in turn worsen relational factors and male sexual dysfunctions. Thus, like infertility, sexual dysfunction in one individual in the relationship affects the couples' sexual function as a whole.

In this chapter, we will discuss different types of male sexual dysfunctions and its impact on the infertile couple.

2 Male Sexual Dysfunctions

2.1 Erectile Dysfunction

Erectile dysfunction (ED) is a common sexual dysfunction that affects millions of men worldwide. It is defined as the inability to get an erection or to maintain an erection long enough to have satisfactory sexual intercourse. ED's pathogenesis is complex and multifactorial. It can be caused by organic factors—which can be subdivided into vascular, metabolic, neurogenic and endocrine—relational factors and psychological factors—such as anxiety and depression. ED has a prevalence of 11–30% in patients with an infertility diagnosis [8].

A cause-effect relationship cannot be established because of the lack of prospective trials, but the association between depression, anxiety disorders and ED in men from infertile couples shows what the pathophysiology may be explained by the psychological distress caused by the infertility diagnosis. Also, as stated before, decreased general health can be associated with both ED and infertility [4].

ED can cause infertility when severe, such as in patients with insufficient erection for penetration. Less severe cases of ED can also lead to avoidance of sexual intercourse by the male partner with a negative effect on fertility.

Management of ED includes lifestyle modifications and control of the reversible causes of ED as the first measure. A stepwise approach is advised, based on the invasiveness of treatment. Oral phosphodiesterase-5 inhibitors (PDE5is) have shown a positive response in around 70% of patients. Currently, PDE5is in the market include sildenafil, tadalafil, vardenafil and avanafil, and the choice of the PDE5i depends on patient preference and tolerability.

Several studies confirm the safety of PDE5i in patients with infertility, with few studies suggesting even a positive effect on sperm mobility [9].

Other therapeutic alternatives are injectable vasodilator agents as prostaglandin E1 (PGE1), intraurethral or topical PGE1 and vacuum devices [2].

In young patients with sudden-onset ED after the infertility diagnosis, in which a psychological aetiology can be suspected, psychosexual therapy (individual or couple therapy) is advised.

2.2 Peyronie's Disease

Peyronie's disease is a highly prevalent disease, affecting 1.5–16.9% of men under 40 years old [2]. Aetiology is unknown, but the suggested pathophysiological mechanism is a repetitive microtrauma, which causes scar tissue with an abnormal healing that leads to a fibrotic plaque and a penile curvature. There is an acute phase, lasting up to 12–18 months, in which the most common symptoms are painful erections, a palpable nodule or plaque and a small curvature that might start to develop. Afterwards, a chronic phase follows, with disease stabilization. The penile curvature worsens in 21–48% of patients and stabilizes in 36–67% of patients in the chronic phase.

When severe, penile curvatures and deformity can make penetrative intercourse difficult and can lead to dyspareunia, with obvious negative effects on fertility.

In patients in the chronic phase with severe curvatures that affect the possibility to have penetrative intercourse, several surgical treatments are available. If the patient has no concomitant ED, the curvature is less than 60° and there are no other major deformities (hourglass deformity, indentation, etc.), a simple plication technique can be performed (tunica-shortening procedures). If curvature is higher than 60°, incision/excision techniques plus grafting are performed (tunica-lengthening procedures). Patients should be advised of a 20% risk of ED after grafting techniques.

In conclusion, Peyronie's disease can have negative effects on fertility due to dyspareunia, ED and sexual avoidance or aversion. Evaluation and management of these patients should be done as per the guideline recommendations [2]. Surgical treatment is the gold standard in patients with severe curvatures that have functional consequences.

2.3 Ejaculatory Disorders

The main ejaculatory disorders (EjDs) are the following:

- Anejaculation: absence of ejaculation, either in an antegrade or in a retrograde fashion. It is caused by failure of semen emission from the seminal vesicles, prostate and ejaculatory ducts into the urethra.
- Retrograde ejaculation: absence of antegrade ejaculation, and semen passes proximally through the bladder neck into the bladder. Patients may have a normal or decreased orgasmic sensation. Can be caused by neurogenic, pharmacological, urethral or bladder neck factors.

- Premature ejaculation: ejaculation that occurs almost always within 1 min of penetrative intercourse (lifelong premature ejaculation) or a significant reduction in latency time in about 3 min or less (acquired premature ejaculation), with inability to delay ejaculation and negative personal consequences, such as distress, frustration, bother and/or avoidance of sexual intimacy [10].
- Delayed ejaculation: marked delay, infrequency or absence of ejaculation on 75–100% of occasions that persists for at least 6 months and which causes personal distress [2].
- Painful ejaculation: mild to severe pain during or after ejaculation, which can involve the penis, scrotum and perineum.

Anejaculation is relatively rare, with a prevalence of 0.14% in the general population. It is frequently associated with neurological diseases or iatrogenic causes affecting peripheric nerves. The most common causes are retroperitoneal lymph node dissection (RPLND) and spinal cord injury (SCI), accounting for almost 90% of cases.

RPLND is most commonly performed in men with testicular cancer, which has a higher incidence in reproductive age. During this procedure, there may be injuries to the sympathetic chains, postganglionic sympathetic fibres and hypogastric plexus, thus damaging the ejaculatory reflex. Ejaculatory function is lost in up to 19% of men even after a nerve-sparing procedure [11].

Patients with SCI have a disruption of the autonomic nerves responsible for ejaculation. Only around 9% of patients with SCI can ejaculate during sexual intercourse or masturbation. Also, these patients have a higher rate of asthenozoospermia [11].

Treatment options include penile vibratory stimulation, electroejaculation and surgical sperm retrieval from the testes or epididymis.

Penile vibratory stimulation is a procedure that can be performed in office. It consists of applying a specific vibrator at the ventral side of the glans penis, set with a certain frequency and amplitude. Patients with a preserved ejaculatory reflex—depending on the level of the neurological injury—may be able to achieve a reflex ejaculation. Success of penile vibratory stimulation depends on the amplitude of the stimulating plate, achieving sperm retrieval rates of 54.4–98% [12].

Electroejaculation is a procedure performed under general anaesthesia with a transrectal probe, which delivers electric stimulation at a 60 Hz frequency with a current limited to usually 500 mA. The probe is activated in stimulus cycles, and ejaculation occurs in about 2–3 stimulation cycles. Sperm retrieval rate has been reported to be between 75% and 100%. In a study including both patients with SCI and RPLND as causes of anejaculation, ejaculation and sperm retrieval with a concentration of >10 M/mL were achieved in 75% of the patients with SCI and 87% of patients who had undergone RPLND [13].

Intracytoplasmic sperm injection (ICSI) is the most reliable assisted reproduction technique in patients with anejaculation. Surgical testicular sperm extraction (TESE) allows the retrieval of sperm from the testes to be used in ICSI.

Retrograde ejaculation occurs when semen is not expulsed in an antegrade fashion. This may be caused by incomplete closure of the bladder neck, leading to a retrograde ejaculation into the bladder. Diagnosis of true retrograde ejaculation is based on the finding of spermatozoa in urine after ejaculation.

Causes of retrograde ejaculation can be pharmacological, neurogenic, anatomic or iatrogenic. Alpha-blockers (e.g., tamsulosin, silodosin) can cause EjD with two proposed mechanisms: through relaxation of the bladder neck during ejaculation and through the absence of contractions of the seminal vesicles during orgasm, causing in some patients anejaculation and in others retrograde ejaculation [14].

Treatment of the ejaculatory dysfunction depends on the aetiology. In order to achieve antegrade ejaculation, different therapies have been tested in patients with retrograde ejaculation. Amoxapine, a tricyclic antidepressant, in a daily dose of 50 mg has been shown to be effective in 80% of patients compared to 16% of patients receiving vitamin B12 [15]. The effects of imipramine (another tricyclic antidepressant) 25 mg twice per day have also been studied, with a success rate of achieving antegrade ejaculation in around 38.5% of patients. Imipramine was compared in this study with pseudoephedrine 120 mg twice per day, which had a higher success rate, achieving antegrade ejaculation in around 50%. The combination of the two drugs achieved a success rate of 61.5%.

In patients with true retrograde ejaculation, sperm can also be retrieved from post-coital urine. In order to preserve sperm mobility, it is recommended to achieve urine alkalinization with sodium bicarbonate or potassium citrate. Sperm is then prepared using density gradient centrifugation, allowing to retrieve motile sperm.

Surgical treatments for benign prostatic enlargement (i.e. transurethral resection of the prostate, holmium-laser enucleation of the prostate, open simple prostatectomy) may cause retrograde ejaculation in up to 60–80% of patients. New minimally invasive surgical treatments as the water vapour therapy (Rezum), prostatic urethral lift (UroLift) and temporal implantable nitinol device (iTind) have been recently marketed to try to reduce ejaculatory dysfunction after prostatic treatment.

Premature ejaculation is the most common ejaculatory dysfunction in men, and it refers to the inability to control ejaculation during sexual activity. It can occur before or shortly after penetration and can be caused by psychological or physical factors. Premature ejaculation can affect fertility by reducing the time available for the sperm to be deposited in the female reproductive tract. This can reduce the chances of conception as the sperm may not be able to reach the egg.

There are mainly four subtypes of premature ejaculation: lifelong, acquired, variable and subjective premature ejaculation. It has been suggested that the aetiology of lifelong premature ejaculation is related to serotonin neurotransmission. Acquired premature ejaculation can be related to psychogenic causes or other organic dysfunctions.

Treatment of premature ejaculation may involve lifestyle modifications, psychosexual therapy and pharmacological therapy. Patients may benefit from the use of selective serotonin reuptake inhibitors (SSRIs) as dapoxetine, which is a short-acting SSRI and is the only currently approved drug for premature ejaculation in

Europe. Other SSRIs can be used off-label, such as sertraline, citalopram, escitalopram and fluoxetine. Off-label tramadol is another on-demand option. Topical lidocaine/prilocaine treatments have also been proved to be effective [2].

2.4 Low Sexual Desire

Male partners of infertile couples may suffer from low sexual desire. There are limited epidemiological studies correlating low sexual desire in infertile men, often performed with non-validated questionnaires. A case-control study [16] compared 448 men of infertile couples to 74 age-matched control men from fertile couples. In a subgroup analysis, men with azoospermia had significantly low sexual desire domain per the International Index of Erectile Function (IIEF) than men with normal semen parameters, 7.4 vs. 7.9 (p < 0.05). No differences in sexual desire were found between infertile men with oligospermia or with normal semen parameters compared to fertile men. In another case-control study, sexual desire was evaluated in three groups of patients: although without reaching statistical significance, men with non-obstructive azoospermia had an 8% low sexual desire prevalence, compared with 4% in men with oligospermia and 0% in men with normal semen parameters [17].

Another study showed that low sexual desire prevalence was higher in a group of 60 men of infertile couples compared with 52 male partners of routine gynaecologic patients, using the IIEF questionnaire [3].

A case-control study evaluated the association of hypogonadism in infertile men with oligospermia with fertile age-matched controls using the Sexual Complaints Screener for Men (SCS-M). Low sexual desire was more prevalent in infertile hypogonadal men in comparison to fertile controls, but not in infertile men with normal testosterone levels. Also, low sexual desire was significantly more reported by men who had completed infertility treatment compared to men at initial infertility assessment [OR (95% CI): 2.1 (1.2–3.8) vs. 1.1 (0.5–2.2); p < 0.05] [18].

Other studies described the prevalence of low sexual desire in male partners of infertile couples at 26.6%. In this study [19], the authors did not find an association between testosterone levels and low sexual desire. Therefore, they conclude that the high prevalence of low sexual desire in their group was caused by psychological factors related to the stress and anxiety of an infertility diagnosis and infertility treatments.

Based on the limited available publications, male partners of infertile couples have a higher risk of reporting low sexual desire, which can be reported in almost one-third of cases. Low sexual desire is more prevalent in azoospermic men than other groups of subfertile men and could be related to hormonal, psychological and interpersonal factors [8]. The lower sexual desire found in infertile couples is most probably related to the fact that sexual activity is focused on procreating rather than on recreation, having schedules for sexual intercourse and other intrusive medical interventions that may affect couple's intimacy.

2.5 Anorgasmia

Anorgasmia is the inability to achieve orgasm despite adequate sexual stimulation. It can occur in both men and women and can be caused by various factors, including physical and psychological factors. In men, anorgasmia can be caused by physical factors such as prostate surgery, SCI and hormonal imbalances. Psychological factors such as stress, anxiety and depression can also cause anorgasmia.

Orgasmic function in men in infertile couples has been rarely studied using validated questionnaires. Some studies report male orgasmic failures of 8–11% [20, 21]. In these studies, men reported severe anxiety and difficulties in retrieving a second sample for a semen analysis after diagnosis of abnormalities in one or more semen parameters in their first semen analysis. Compared to men having sexual intercourse for pleasure, men who have intercourse for reproductive reasons have lower orgasmic function total values using the IIEF-5 questionnaire [22]. In this study, the impact of subfertility diagnosis was measured evaluating 171 men aged 25–40 years old, who attended a fertility clinic. All the subjects responded to a modified IIEF questionnaire, made up of five questions: two regarding erectile function, one concerning orgasmic function, one question on sexual desire and one on satisfaction with intercourse. The intention was to evaluate questionnaire scores for spontaneous sex for pleasure and sex intended to procreate. Results showed sexual dysfunction in sexual intercourse for reproductive purposes in 23.7% of patients. Only 8.9% of these patients on the other hand had also sexual dysfunctions with sex for pleasure. This highlights the stressful situation that sexual relationships for reproductive purposes can become. Of note, in this study, there were no differences in semen parameters between patients with sexual dysfunctions and patients without sexual dysfunctions.

2.6 Psychological Disorders

Infertility can have a significant impact on the mental health and well-being of men. Men who experience infertility may feel a range of emotions, including sadness, anger, guilt and shame. They may also experience anxiety and depression, which can have a negative impact on their overall quality of life [21].

In addition to personal stress, infertility can also put great pressure on a relationship, as it can cause feelings of guilt and men can project these feelings to their partner.

One of the most significant psychological burdens of infertility in men is the feeling of inadequacy and emasculation. Men may feel that their masculinity is threatened by their inability to father a child, and they may worry about being seen as less of a man by their partner or society. This can lead to feelings of shame and embarrassment, which can further exacerbate the psychological burden of infertility and the development of sexual dysfunctions [22].

Another psychological burden of infertility in men is the feeling of isolation and loneliness. Men may feel like they are the only ones going through this experience, which can lead to a sense of isolation and detachment from others. This can make it difficult for men to seek support and can contribute to feelings of depression and anxiety.

ED and premature ejaculation are associated with psychological disorders, such as anxiety, depression and distress. The prevalence of ED has shown to be higher in patients with azoospermia than in other men with better semen analysis parameters or fertile controls [16]. Assessment of sexual function and psychological status of men in infertile couples is warranted.

3 Male Infertility, Male Sexual Dysfunctions and General Health Status

Male sexual dysfunctions and infertility are well-known index of worse general health status [23, 24]. Men in infertile couples have a higher rate of oncological and non-oncological diseases than age-matched men without an infertility diagnosis [25, 26]. Also, decreased general health status was found in patients with increased semen abnormalities. Fertility status may even predict later mortality. Among 43,277 men without azoospermia who consulted an infertility clinic, mortality decreased as the sperm concentration increased up to a threshold of 40 million/mL [27]. Also, better sperm motility and morphology parameters meant a decrease in mortality. The decrease in mortality in men with better semen quality was caused by a decrease in comorbidities and was found both among men with and without children. Therefore, it could not be attributed just to environmental and lifestyle factors; semen parameters may be a biomarker of overall health status (Fig. 1).

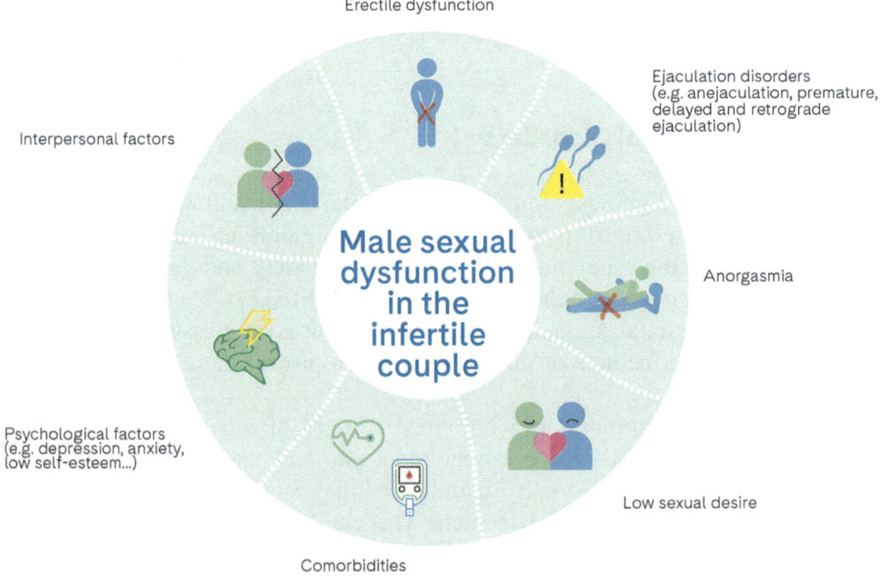

Fig 1 Male sexual dysfunction in the infertile couple

4   Fertility in Transgender and Non-Binary

The desire of transgender individuals to have children is similar to cisgender individuals. Between 37% and 76% of transgender individuals would consider fertility preservation before gender-affirming therapy. However, in a recent study of 189 transgender people, only 9.6% of trans women and 3.1% of trans men had undergone fertility preservation [28].

Hormonal treatment and surgical treatment for gender-affirming therapy are options to treat gender dysphoria, although with an obvious loss in reproductive function. Cryopreservation of sperm, oocytes and embryos should be discussed with transgender individuals before starting medical treatment [29].

In transgender women, hormonal therapy with antiandrogens and oestrogens is fundamental for the feminization. Long-term treatment with oestrogens caused maturation arrest of spermatogenesis in 80% of patients who underwent orchidectomy for gender-reaffirming surgery, and hypospermatogenesis with focal spermatid and mature spermatozoa in the other 20% [30]. In transgender men, testosterone exposure influences ovarian tissue, with stromal hyperplasia and luteinization, thickened ovarian cortex and accelerated follicular atresia. It can also produce an atrophic effect on the endometrium, potentially affecting implantation [29].

Taking all of this into account, the best option for transgender women who want to preserve fertility is cryopreservation before hormonal therapy or gender-reaffirming surgery. Sperm sample is usually obtained through masturbation, but it can be a burden to trans women. Hormonal treatment with antiandrogens and oestrogens can hinder erectile and ejaculatory function. Specimen retrieval can be aided with penile vibratory stimulation, electroejaculation or in some cases even TESE or microTESE. Surgical retrieval is more invasive and can also be performed at the time of gender-reaffirming surgery [29].

5   Conclusion

Male infertility and sexual dysfunctions have a bilateral cause-effect relationship. They can both affect quality of life and reproductive outcomes. Assessment of sexual function, general health and psychological status of infertile men is advisable to improve reproductive possibilities and sexual health.

When the diagnosis from a sexual dysfunction is independent from the infertility status, it should be treated as per guideline recommendations, trying to avoid treatments that decrease fertility rates.

Even though sexual dysfunctions are a rare cause of male infertility, every kind of sexual dysfunction has been seen in men from infertile couples. Low sexual desire and lack of satisfaction of sexual life are the most prevalent sexual dysfunctions in these patients. The psychological burden of an infertility diagnosis leaves patients often with feelings of inadequacy, stress and anxiety that worsen some of the sexual dysfunctions.

References

1. WHO. WHO manual for the standardized investigation and diagnosis of the infertile couple. Cambridge: Cambridge University Press; 2000.
2. Salonia A, Bettocchi C, Carvalho J, et al. EAU guidelines on sexual and reproductive health 2023.
3. Marci R, Graziano A, Piva I, Lo Monte G, Soave I, Giugliano E, Mazzoni S, Capucci R, Carbonara M, Caracciolo S, Patella A. Procreative sex in infertile couples: the decay of pleasure? Health Qual Life Outcomes. 2012;10:140. https://doi.org/10.1186/1477-7525-10-140.
4. Salonia A, Matloob R, Gallina A, Abdollah F, Saccà A, Briganti A, Suardi N, Colombo R, Rocchini L, Guazzoni G, Rigatti P, Montorsi F. Are infertile men less healthy than fertile men? Results of a prospective case-control survey. Eur Urol. 2009;56(6):1025–31. https://doi.org/10.1016/j.eururo.2009.03.001.
5. World Health Organization. Towards more objectivity in diagnosis and management of male fertility. Int J Androl. 1987;7:1–53.
6. Punab M, Poolamets O, Paju P, Vihljajev V, Pomm K, Ladva R, Korrovits P, Laan M. Causes of male infertility: a 9-year prospective monocentre study on 1737 patients with reduced total sperm counts. Hum Reprod. 2017 Jan;32(1):18–31. https://doi.org/10.1093/humrep/dew284.
7. Jiann BP, Su CC, Tsai JY. Is female sexual function related to the male partners' erectile function? J Sex Med. 2013;10(2):420–9. https://doi.org/10.1111/j.1743-6109.2012.03007.x.
8. Capogrosso P, Jensen CFS, Rastrelli G, Torremade J, Russo GI, Raheem AA, Frey A, Fode M, Maggi M, Reisman Y, Bettocchi C, Corona G. Male sexual dysfunctions in the infertile couple-recommendations from the European Society of Sexual Medicine (ESSM). Sex Med. 2021;9(3):100377. https://doi.org/10.1016/j.esxm.2021.100377.
9. Du Plessis SS, de Jongh PS, Franken DR. Effect of acute in vivo sildenafil citrate and in vitro 8-bromo-cGMP treatments on semen parameters and sperm function. Fertil Steril. 2004;81(4):1026–33. https://doi.org/10.1016/j.fertnstert.2003.09.054.
10. Serefoglu EC, McMahon CG, Waldinger MD, Althof SE, Shindel A, Adaikan G, Becher EF, Dean J, Giuliano F, Hellstrom WJ, Giraldi A, Glina S, Incrocci L, Jannini E, McCabe M, Parish S, Rowland D, Segraves RT, Sharlip I, Torres LO. An evidence-based unified definition of lifelong and acquired premature ejaculation: report of the second international society for sexual medicine ad hoc committee for the definition of premature ejaculation. Sex Med. 2014;2(2):41–59. https://doi.org/10.1002/sm2.27.
11. Fode M, Krogh-Jespersen S, Brackett NL, Ohl DA, Lynne CM, Sønksen J. Male sexual dysfunction and infertility associated with neurological disorders. Asian J Androl. 2012;14(1):61–8. https://doi.org/10.1038/aja.2011.70.
12. Sønksen J, Biering-Sørensen F, Kristensen JK. Ejaculation induced by penile vibratory stimulation in men with spinal cord injuries. The importance of the vibratory amplitude. Paraplegia. 1994;32(10):651–60. https://doi.org/10.1038/sc.1994.105.
13. Denil J, Ohl DA, McGuire EJ, Jonas U. Treatment of anejaculation with electroejaculation. Acta Urol Belg. 1992;60(3):15–25.
14. Pavone C, Abrate A, Li Muli P, Guzzardo C, Guarneri AG, Dioguardi S, Sanfilippo C, Vella M, Serretta V, Simonato A. Can we clinically distinguish Anejaculation from retrograde ejaculation in patients on α1A-blockers therapy for lower urinary tract symptoms? Urology. 2020;139:129–33. https://doi.org/10.1016/j.urology.2020.01.027.
15. Hu J, Nagao K, Tai T, Kobayashi H, Nakajima K. Randomized crossover trial of Amoxapine versus vitamin B12 for retrograde ejaculation. Int Braz J Urol. 2017;43(3):496–504. https://doi.org/10.1590/S1677-5538.
16. Lotti F, Corona G, Castellini G, Maseroli E, Fino MG, Cozzolino M, Maggi M. Semen quality impairment is associated with sexual dysfunction according to its severity. Hum Reprod. 2016;31(12):2668–80. https://doi.org/10.1093/humrep/dew246.
17. Giannouli C, Goulis DG, Lambropoulos A, Lissens W, Tarlatzis BC, Bontis JN, Papadimas J. Idiopathic non-obstructive azoospermia or severe oligozoospermia: a cross-sectional study

in 61 Greek men. Int J Androl. 2004;27(2):101–7. https://doi.org/10.1046/j.1365-2605.2003. 00456.x.

18. Kruljac M, Finnbogadóttir H, Bobjer J, Giraldi A, Fugl-Meyer K, Giwercman A. Symptoms of sexual dysfunction among men from infertile couples: prevalence and association with testosterone deficiency. Andrology. 2020;8(1):160–5. https://doi.org/10.1111/andr.12678.

19. Satkunasivam R, Ordon M, Hu B, Mullen B, Lo K, Grober E, Jarvi K. Hormone abnormalities are not related to the erectile dysfunction and decreased libido found in many men with infertility. Fertil Steril. 2014;101(6):1594–8. https://doi.org/10.1016/j.fertnstert.2014.02.044.

20. Saleh RA, Ranga GM, Raina R, Nelson DR, Agarwal A. Sexual dysfunction in men undergoing infertility evaluation: a cohort observational study. Fertil Steril. 2003;79(4):909–12. https://doi.org/10.1016/s0015-0282(02)04921-x.

21. Jain K, Radhakrishnan G, Agrawal P. Infertility and psychosexual disorders: relationship in infertile couples. Indian J Med Sci. 2000;54(1):1–7.

22. Elia J, Delfino M, Imbrogno N, Mazzilli F. The impact of a diagnosis of couple subfertility on male sexual function. J Endocrinol Investig. 2010;33(2):74–6. https://doi.org/10.1007/BF03346556.

23. Lotti F, Maggi M. Sexual dysfunction and male infertility. Nat Rev Urol. 2018;15(5):287–307. https://doi.org/10.1038/nrurol.2018.20.

24. Capogrosso P, Ventimiglia E, Boeri L, Capitanio U, Gandaglia G, Dehò F, Pederzoli F, Cazzaniga W, Scano R, Montorsi F, Salonia A. Sexual functioning mirrors overall men's health status, even irrespective of cardiovascular risk factors. Andrology. 2017;5(1):63–9. https://doi.org/10.1111/andr.12299.

25. Walsh TJ, Schembri M, Turek PJ, Chan JM, Carroll PR, Smith JF, Eisenberg ML, Van Den Eeden SK, Croughan MS. Increased risk of high-grade prostate cancer among infertile men. Cancer. 2010;116(9):2140–7. https://doi.org/10.1002/cncr.25075.

26. Eisenberg ML, Li S, Behr B, Pera RR, Cullen MR. Relationship between semen production and medical comorbidity. Fertil Steril. 2015 Jan;103(1):66–71. https://doi.org/10.1016/j.fertnstert.2014.10.017.

27. Jensen TK, Jacobsen R, Christensen K, Nielsen NC, Bostofte E. Good semen quality and life expectancy: a cohort study of 43,277 men. Am J Epidemiol. 2009;170(5):559–65. https://doi.org/10.1093/aje/kwp168;Erratum in: Am J Epidemiol. 2009 Dec 1;170(11):1453.

28. Auer MK, Fuss J, Nieder TO, et al. Desire to have children among transgender people in Germany: a cross-sectional multi-center study. J Sex Med. 2018;15(5):757–67. https://doi.org/10.1016/j.jsxm.2018.03.083.

29. Neblett MF 2nd, Hipp HS. Fertility considerations in transgender persons. Endocrinol Metab Clin N Am. 2019;48(2):391–402. https://doi.org/10.1016/j.ecl.2019.02.003.

30. Matoso A, Khandakar B, Yuan S, Wu T, Wang LJ, Lombardo KA, Mangray S, Mannan AASR, Yakirevich E. Spectrum of findings in orchiectomy specimens of persons undergoing gender confirmation surgery. Hum Pathol. 2018;76:91–9. https://doi.org/10.1016/j.humpath.2018.03.007.

Endocrine Disorders and Sexuality I: Hypothalamus-Pituitary Axes and Peripheral Thyroid and Adrenal Glands

Mireia Mora Porta, Felicia A. Hanzu, and Aida Orois Añón

1 Hypophysis Disorders and Sexual Dysfunction

Pituitary hormones are key to sexual development and function. Therefore, hypothalamic-pituitary (HP) disorders can cause sexual dysfunction in both men and women, due to the involvement of one or more of the different hormonal axes. Most of the literature refers to the gonadotropic axis, and especially how its involvement can cause erectile dysfunction (ED) in men or hypogonadotropic hypogonadism in women. Data on sexual and reproductive function in individuals with other pituitary conditions are still scarce. However, in addition to hypogonadism, other pituitary disorders have been associated with sexual dysfunction.

1.1 Gonadotropic Axis

The gonadotropic axis is the central axis involved in the development of sexual disorders. Central or secondary hypogonadism is defined as a clinical syndrome that results from failure of the testes or ovaries to produce physiological concentrations of sexual hormones (mainly testosterone and estrogens), due to HP suppression.

M. Mora Porta (✉) · F. A. Hanzu
Endocrinology and Nutrition Department, Clinical Institute of Digestive and Metabolic Diseases, Hospital Clínic de Barcelona, Barcelona, Spain

Institut d'Investigacions Biomèdiques August Pi i Sunyer, Barcelona, Spain
e-mail: mporta@clinic.cat; fhanzu@clinic.cat

A. Orois Añón
Endocrinology and Nutrition Department, Clinical Institute of Digestive and Metabolic Diseases, Hospital Clínic de Barcelona, Barcelona, Spain
e-mail: aorois@clinic.cat

© The Author(s), under exclusive license to Springer Nature Switzerland AG 2024
C. Castelo-Branco, S. Anglès Acedo (eds.), *Medical Disorders and Sexual Health*, Trends in Andrology and Sexual Medicine,
https://doi.org/10.1007/978-3-031-55080-5_10

Gonadotropin levels (luteinizing hormone (LH) and follicle-stimulating hormone (FSH)) are low or inappropriately normal. Most causes of central hypogonadism are functional, that is, caused by comorbid illness, medications, aging, etc., without structural HP disease [1]. Eating disorders, extreme sports, or severe physical or emotional stress and extreme obesity can lead to hypogonadotropic hypogonadism with sexual dysfunction and infertility. An example is the hypothalamic functional amenorrhea and anovulation suffered by some underweight female athletes, which can cause amenorrhea and osteoporosis ("the female athlete triad"). Also, the use and abuse of substances such as alcohol, opioids, glucocorticoids, or anabolic steroids can produce a functional deficit of sex steroids, mainly testosterone. This is of special interest in present-day society, where the abuse of opioids (such as fentanyl or methadone) constitutes a major public health problem in some countries such as the USA. As mentioned, eating disorders, and depletion or uncontrolled bulimic alterations of nutrient disposal, induce profound alterations in leptin, cortisol circadian rhythm, and LH secretion with long-term disturbance of the menstrual cycle and estrogen production in females and testosterone production in males.

Beyond functional hypogonadism, organic hypogonadotropic hypogonadism can result from many medical conditions, such as sellar or suprasellar tumors, head trauma, infiltrative or destructive diseases of the HP region, pituitary surgery, or hyperprolactinemia. Radiation must be taken into account, especially as a cause of late hypogonadism in childhood cancer survivors. Also, there are several syndromes causing congenital central hypogonadism, such as Kallmann syndrome or Prader-Willi syndrome.

In the case of pituitary neuroendocrine tumors (pituitary adenomas), hypogonadism is usually due to a mass effect that can cause hypopituitarism or stalk compression with subsequent hyperprolactinemia. Sexual dysfunction is more common in functioning pituitary adenomas than in nonfunctioning. Males with prolactinomas have the higher prevalence of sexual dysfunction (83%) [2]. Clinically functional gonadotroph pituitary tumors are extremely rare and are often confused with nonfunctioning tumors. It has been observed that transsphenoidal surgery for pituitary neuroendocrine tumors improves sexual function, and it is recommended to reassess a certain time after the surgery (about 6 months) whether or not gonadal replacement therapy is required [3].

Clinically, hypogonadotropic hypogonadism presents with delayed puberty or primary amenorrhea when it is congenital or very early. In adult life, it is associated with oligomenorrhea, infertility, decreased libido, ED, azoospermia, gynecomastia, or osteoporosis, among others. Although most of the literature refers to sexual dysfunction in men, in recent years, some tests have been proposed for the evaluation of sexual function in women with hypogonadotropic hypogonadism, such as the Female Sexual Function Index (FSFI) [4].

Gonadal replacement therapy improves different components of sexual function such as erectile function, sexual desire, orgasm, satisfaction with sexual intercourse, and sexual activity. It does not improve ejaculatory function. In the male, testosterone, administered parenterally or transdermally, is used. In women, treatment consists of estrogens together with progestogens (if intact uterus), either orally or transdermally. In some studies, it has been described that associating testosterone at low doses in women with hypogonadism can improve sexual function and body composition parameters, taking into account that serum androgen levels in these women are lower than in healthy women. However, given the scant evidence, it is not currently recommended.

For the discussion on clinical management of ovarian hypogonadisms with a pragmatic approach useful in the physician's daily clinical practice, the reader is referred to the chapter titled *Endocrine Disorders and Sexuality II: Ovary*.

1.2   Hypothalamus-Pituitary-Gonadal and Adrenal Axis in the Puberty and Sexual Health

The onset of puberty involves the reactivation of the HP-gonadal axis, induced by the effect of kisspeptin and the hypothalamic gonadotropin-releasing factor (GnRH) "pulse generator" neurons that activate LH and further gonadal steroid secretion. Puberty is typically earlier in females than in males. Pathological variations, namely, precocious and delayed puberty, are also possible. Gonadal puberty is typically preluded with 2–4 years by the adrenarche, the adrenal activation (discussed in the adrenal part).

Delayed puberty, due to the absence of physical signs of secondary sexual characteristics by age 12 in girls or 14 in boys, is mostly idiopathic and sometimes run in families. Other situations can be chromosomal abnormalities, chronic illnesses, tumors of the pituitary or hypothalamic region, hypopituitarism, abnormal development of the reproductive system, complete androgen insensitivity syndromes, other serious medical conditions, too much exercise, or severe eating disorders. Delayed puberty affects all sexual related functions and imprint quality of life and fertility. Pulsatile GnRH (in case of hypothalamic condition) or gonadotropins are used when fertility is desired or in order to stimulate puberty in both sexes.

Precocious puberty (PP) is considered the precocious sexual maturation/development of secondary sexual characteristics before age 8 in girls and before 9 in boys with an initial accelerated growth and stop before reaching the full genetic height potential. PP is becoming increasingly common due to a multitude of factors such as genetics, lifestyle changes, and exposure to endocrine-disrupting chemicals. PP can be central, due to an increased gonadotropin secretion, or peripheral, gonadotropin independent, due to an increased secretion in gonadal hormones. Causes can be tumors on the ovaries, testes (Sertoli and Leydig, dysgerminomas, teratomas, embryonal tumors), testotoxicosis, adrenal glands (congenital adrenal hyperplasia (CAH), other benign and malign adrenal tumors), pituitary, hypothalamus, and central nervous system (hamartoma, gliomas, astrocytoma, septo-optic dysplasia); other central nervous system injury; rare genetic syndromes (McCune-Albright, neurofibromatosis, kisspeptin gain-of-function mutation, Van Wyk and Grumbach syndrome); family history of idiopathic PP; and exogenous steroids. Removal of the tumor-secreting gonadal steroids is the treatment of choice. When not available, treatment with GnRH analogues in an expert multidisciplinary team must be considered in function of the evolution of the PP and the underlying etiology. Untreated PP can cause significant emotional and behavioral alterations such as substance abuse, social isolation, multiple sexual partners, and self-image concerns, mostly resolved if adequately treated in the early adulthood. Parents should be informed and receive education about how to manage and explain to their children and families the events [5].

1.3 Somatotropic Axis

1.3.1 Growth Hormone (GH) Excess

Gonadotropic and somatotropic are two pituitary axes very related to each other, especially for the development of puberty, producing the sex steroids and increase in GH levels. Besides, GH plays a positive role in the homeostasis of the vascular endothelium, regulating nitride oxide (NO) production and protecting the endothelium by a modulation of oxidative stress, so it could be directly involved in erectile function [6].

Although GH has a positive effect on gonadal function, when it is produced in excess, it has a deleterious effect. GH excess (and consequently insulin-like growth factor-1 (IGF-1)) is almost always due to a GH-producing pituitary neuroendocrine tumor, causing gigantism in childhood or acromegaly in adulthood. Acromegaly can induce problems in the sexual sphere in up to 50% of patients [7]. In fact, in the widely known AcroQoL (Acromegaly Quality of life test), one of the domains evaluated is sexual appetite and sexual relationships. This is due to multiple factors: On the one hand, we know that patients with acromegaly have a higher prevalence of cardiovascular disease and metabolic comorbidities, such as hypertension, diabetes, or obstructive sleep apnea syndrome, directly related to sexual dysfunction. On the other hand, the aforementioned participation of GH in the homeostasis of the vascular endothelium could also interfere with sexual function, although the pathophysiological bases are poorly understood to date. In addition, patients with acromegaly often have associated symptoms such as anxiety, depression, and body image distortion that can worsen the sexual dysfunction [8].

It is still unknown if control of acromegaly reverses sexual dysfunction. Currently, a hypothetical beneficial effect of drugs used in acromegaly on sexual health, such as somatostatin analogues or pegvisomant, has not been demonstrated. The efficacy of classic treatment for ED (phosphodiesterase 5 inhibitors) in patients with acromegaly has not been studied. It has to be noted, however, that elevated GH levels directly correlate with the severity of ED in men with acromegaly.

Regarding fertility in men with acromegaly, recent data do not support reduced semen quality in acromegaly [9].

1.3.2 GH Deficiency

GH deficiency usually appears in the context of other pituitary deficits. In addition, replacement therapy is usually only offered when several hormonal axes are altered, making it difficult to discern the direct effect of GH on sexual function. Likewise, GH deficiency is associated with cardiovascular complications, which can also influence sexual involvement. For all, it is not possible to directly link GH deficiency with the appearance of sexual complications, although an extremely high prevalence of sexual dysfunctions (71.2%) in patients with GH deficiency of both sexes has been described [10].

1.4 Adrenal Axis

1.4.1 Corticotropin (ACTH) Overproduction and Glucocorticoid Excess

Impact of increased glucocorticoid levels on gonadal function and sexuality is complex due to the alteration at both metabolic and cardiovascular levels. Although endogenous Cushing is a rare disease, exogenous Cushing affects 1% of general population in Western countries, which incidence is expected to increase due to the rise of inflammatory, autoimmune, and neoplastic disorders that need glucocorticoid therapy. Endogenous hypercortisolism can be due to tumors producing ACTH of pituitary or ectopic origin or due to tumors of the adrenal secreting directly cortisol and other androgens. Pituitary ACTH-producing adenomas, called Cushing disease, present with metabolic and cardiovascular comorbidities such as central obesity, hypertension, thromboembolism, insulin resistance, diabetes, and osteoporosis, which usually affect sexual function due to endothelial dysfunction and altered coagulability pathways among others. Even more, hypercortisolism induces central hypogonadism and hypothyroidism and can be associated with an overproduction of androgens. All these conditions are associated with a higher prevalence of psychiatric disturbances like depression [11]. Thus, the clinical, physical, and psychological manifestations of Cushing severely impact the gonadal function and sexuality of the subjects, and evaluation of the quality of life of this patients should be routinely performed employing specific questionnaires like the CushingQoL and Tuebingen CD-25 [12]. Even in patients with functional hypercortisolism, the so-called pseudo-Cushing (increased cortisol levels in the context of other chronic pathologies such as alcoholism, depression, or obesity, in subjects without pituitary or adrenal disorders), a higher prevalence of ED has been described. In fact, it has been suggested that the negative effect of stress on libido could be mediated by serum cortisol levels, also in patients without pituitary or adrenal pathology. As with other diseases, women report a greater influence of the aesthetic and psycho-emotional impact of the disease on sexuality, and women with Cushing have lower scores on the FSFI test in all domains of sexuality [13]. Among men, ED is one of the most frequent manifestations. In addition, common symptoms such as fatigue and decreased sexual desire can seriously affect the sexual life of these people and their partners.

As mentioned, chronic treatment with exogenous glucocorticoids at supraphysiological doses can also have, depending on the dose and time, the same consequences as the endogenous Cushing disease.

1.4.2 ACTH Deficiency and Glucocorticoid Deficiency

Central glucocorticoid deficiency has been studied mostly together with other anterior pituitary hormonal deficiencies. There are some studies on the affectation of sexuality in primary adrenal insufficiency (Addison's disease) extended in the adrenal pathology part.

However, we do not have studies on sexual dysfunction in patients with isolated central adrenal insufficiency, for example due to head trauma, transsphenoidal surgery, or radiotherapy.

1.5 Lactotroph Axis

Hyperprolactinemia is known to cause central hypogonadism, due to disruption of GnRH pulsatility and gonadotropin secretion.

One of the main causes of hyperprolactinemia are prolactin-producing pituitary tumors (micro- or macroprolactinomas), which are in fact the most common pituitary tumors. In these cases, prolactin levels are quite high, usually above 50 ng/mL. Manifestations include oligomenorrhea/amenorrhea and galactorrhea in women, while in men, decreased libido or ED is more common. The symptoms in men are frequently less noticeable, so the diagnosis is typically later, when the tumor is already larger than 1 cm. Other types of tumors in the HP area can also increase prolactin levels due to a mass effect. They can produce compression of the HP stalk, preventing the inhibitory effect of hypothalamic dopamine on pituitary lactotroph cells, producing secondary hyperprolactinemia. In these cases, serum prolactin levels are usually lower than prolactinomas, and the symptoms are generally milder: Serum prolactin levels are directly related to the severity of symptoms of gonadal dysfunction.

Most of the studies on sexual dysfunction and hyperprolactinemia are done in patients with hyperprolactinemia of pharmacological cause, due to drugs that act on the dopaminergic pathway. Antipsychotics or antidepressants deserve special attention. Treatment with drugs to reduce prolactin levels (mainly dopamine agonists) has been shown to restore or at least improve sexual function in these patients.

1.6 Thyrotrophic Axis

Overt hypothyroidism or hyperthyroidism can affect fertility and the sexual sphere. However, the involvement of thyrotropin-releasing hormone (TRH) or thyroid-stimulating hormone (TSH) and its relationship with sexual dysfunction have been only scarcely studied. As mentioned before, any tumor at the base of the skull (such as TSHoma) can induce sexual problems due to hypopituitarism or hyperprolactinemia. In addition, TRH is a stimulating factor for prolactin too, so a prolonged primary hypothyroidism (typically Hashimoto disease) may result in hyperprolactinemia. In any case, we will expand the information in the section on thyroid pathology and sexual dysfunction.

1.7   Other HP Hormones

Vasopressin and oxytocin are neuropeptides synthesized in the hypothalamus and secreted by the neurohypophysis. Vasopressin is involved in water metabolism, and its involvement in sexual function is difficult to investigate because most patients with vasopressin deficiency (diabetes insipidus) also have panhypopituitarism. Oxytocin, colloquially known as the "love hormone," is especially important during childbirth. Its levels also increase during sexual intercourse, reaching its peak during orgasm, so it is thought that it may be involved in mental and sexual emotions. Although oxytocin is important in causing sexual arousal, the use of this peptide or its analogues to stimulate sexual arousal is still being investigated [14].

2   Thyroid Disorders and Sexual Dysfunction

Sexual function requires normal libido, an intact hypothalamic-pituitary-gonadal axis, neurovascular integrity to genitalia, as well as physiological levels of sexual hormones. The association between thyroid disorders and sexual dysfunction has recently been studied. Twenty years ago, no studies were performed and no information was available. In the last 15 years, an increasing number of studies have been done suggesting a correlation between thyroid disorders and sexual dysfunction.

Hypothyroidism and hyperthyroidism are common medical disorders and are more frequent in women compared to men (5–8 times). Prevalence of hypothyroidism is about 4.6% (including overt and subclinical), while prevalence of hyperthyroidism is about 1.3% (including overt and subclinical) [12]. Hypothalamic release of TRH stimulates production of pituitary TSH, which finally promotes the production of thyroxine (T4) and tri-iodothyronine (T3) in the thyroid gland, which are involved in essential metabolic activities, such as regulation of temperature; fat, protein, and carbohydrate metabolism; as well as bone and neural development. Moreover, positive and negative feedback regulates the production and release of TRH and TSH. Overt hypothyroidism can be diagnosed by decreased levels of free T4 with low levels of TSH (central or secondary hypothyroidism) or high levels of TSH (primary hypothyroidism), while overt hyperthyroidism is detected by increased levels of free T4 with high levels of TSH (central or secondary hyperthyroidism) or low levels of TSH (primary hyperthyroidism). It is important to consider that thyroid dysfunction can be subclinical, characterized by elevated (subclinical hypothyroidism) or decreased (subclinical hyperthyroidism) levels of TSH with normal free T4 and T3 levels. Treatment of hypothyroidism includes replacement therapy with synthetic T4 until the patient is euthyroid; on the other hand, treatment of hyperthyroidism can include antithyroid medication, radioactive iodine, and thyroidectomy [15].

2.1   Proposed Mechanisms and Basic Research

The mechanisms by which thyroid disorders drive sexual dysfunction are not well understood. However, recent studies have shown that thyroid alterations exert effects on circulating sex hormone levels through peripheral and central pathways and provoke indirect psychiatric and autonomic dysregulation that can impair sexual function. For a long time, the gonads were thought to be unresponsive to thyroid hormones and receptors. However, recent studies have demonstrated the presence of thyroid receptors in epididymis and penis in men, and in all ovary cell types, endometrium, vaginal epithelium, and striated and smooth musculatures of the vagina in women [16]. In this sense, a direct T3 effect on erectile tissues and smooth muscle cells of the genital tract can be hypothesized; nevertheless, the molecular mechanism remains unclear.

Patients with hypothyroidism present decreased levels of total and free testosterone, sex hormone-binding globulin (SHBG), dehydroepiandrosterone (DHEA) and its sulfate (DHEAS), and estrogenic metabolites of DHEAS compared to healthy controls, as well as elevated levels of prolactin, leading to a hypogonadotropic hypogonadism. Hypothyroidism-mediated elevation of TRH increases the production of prolactin, and hyperprolactinemia inhibits the pulsatile release of GnRH, leading to reduced levels of testosterone, DHEA, and estrogen production. Moreover, hypothyroidism is clinically associated with fatigue, somnolence, and mood disorders (refractory depression and anxiety), and even an increase of weight that can contribute to a lower interest in sexual activity. Metabolic syndrome potentiates the development of cardiovascular disease and type 2 diabetes, which can independently drive the development of sexual dysfunction [15].

On the contrary, hyperthyroidism enhances sensitivity to catecholamines upregulating B-adrenergic receptor density, alters serotonin turnover, exerts effects on thyroid hormone receptors found in human cavernosal tissues, and impairs NO-dependent relaxation of corpora cavernosa suggesting an effect of thyroid hormones on penile NO formation [15]. Moreover, hyperthyroidism increases SHBG, leading to a relative hyperestrogenism and reduced bioavailable testosterone, which has an important role in both male and female sexual desire and libido. Moreover, NO synthase activity in the clitoris has been hypothesized to be under testosterone regulation [14]. On the other hand, hyperthyroidism is associated with fatigue, myalgias, and mood disturbances such as irritability and depression, which can contribute to sexual dysfunction.

2.2   Thyroid Disorders and Male Sexual Dysfunction

The prevalence of sexual dysfunction in men with hypothyroidism is about 59–63% [14]. There are several reports demonstrating an association between sexual dysfunction and hypothyroidism in men, especially in relation to ED, ejaculatory dysfunction, hypoactive sexual desire disorder (HSDD), and alterations in sperm characteristics and fertility. ED is probably the most studied. A study with 44 hypothyroid men and 71 healthy controls observed significant differences between the reported ED (63% vs. 34%, hypothyroid vs. control men) with a positive correlation between free T4 levels and negative correlation with TSH and Sexual Health Inventory for Men (SHIM) [15], with no association with thyroid antibodies. Moreover, they found a significant decrease in the prevalence of ED after thyroid treatment. Veronelli et al. [17] analyzed 55 hypothyroid men and 109 healthy controls, reporting that 55% of hypothyroid men had some form of ED. Krysiak et al. [18] compared 12 men with overt hypothyroidism (TSH >20 mUI/L and low T4 and T3), with subclinical hypothyroidism and 12 controls. Men with overt hypothyroidism had lower scores in all International Index of Erectile Function (IIEF) domains compared with controls, and 83% met the criteria for ED vs. 8% in controls. After treatment with T4, incidence of ED decreased to 25%, similar to controls. Men with subclinical hypothyroidism only had lower score in erectile function IIEF domain, which normalized after treatment. A large cross-sectional study of 5471 patients (2269 men from general population that participated in the European Male Aging Study (EMAS) and 3202 from a sexual medicine clinic (UNIFI cohort)) reported a prevalence of hypothyroidism of 1.1% in general population and 2.5% in sexual clinic population. In the EMAS population, no differences in erection were observed between hypothyroid and euthyroid men; however, in UNIFI cohort, a significant inverse correlation between TSH levels and the ability to have erections sufficient for intercourse was detected [19]. Several reports have suggested a relationship between hypothyroidism and ejaculatory dysfunction, wherein both delayed ejaculation and premature ejaculation (PE) [15].

In men, the prevalence of hyperthyroidism in patients presenting for sexual disorders has been estimated between 3.4% and 57.1%. On the other hand, the prevalence of sexual dysfunction in patients presenting hyperthyroidism ranges from 48 to 77% [14]. A Taiwanese study conducted by Keller et al. [20] with 6310 patients newly diagnosed of ED and 18,930 matched controls found that men with ED were 1.64 times more likely to have prior diagnosis of hyperthyroidism. In the study of Corona et al. [19] with EMAS and UNIFI cohort including 3369 unselected men and 3203 presenting with sexual dysfunction, similar rates of overt primary hyperthyroidism were observed in men with sexual dysfunction and general population (0.2% vs. 0.3%), but overt hyperthyroidism was strongly associated with ED (subjects reporting never having erections had higher free T4 levels). The relationship between premature ejaculation (PE) and hyperthyroidism is an area of special interest. In another study of Corona et al. [21] with 755 men with sexual dysfunction, those with PE had a higher prevalence of hyperthyroidism (TSH <0.2 mU/L). A recent meta-analysis has observed a correlation between TSH levels and mean intravaginal ejaculation latency time (IELT), with an improvement of the mean IELT measures with the treatment of thyroid disorders [22]. There have been reports of decreases in libido associated with hyperthyroidism; however, no studies have established a significant association.

2.3 Thyroid Disorders and Female Sexual Dysfunction

Although hypo- and hyperthyroidism are frequent in females, the association with sexual dysfunction is still unknown. Thyroid disorders have been associated with alterations in reproductive physiology such as menstrual irregularities and infertility; however, sexual function has not been studied.

The prevalence of sexual dysfunction in women with hypothyroidism is about 22–46%, while the prevalence of sexual dysfunction in women with hyperthyroidism is estimated to be ranging from 44% to 60% [15].

Several studies have shown that hypothyroidism was associated with decreased scores in every FSFI domain (including desire, arousal/lubrication, orgasm, pain) and overall scores [23–25] with a normalization of the desire, satisfaction, and pain domains after reaching an euthyroid state but still decreased in comparison to controls in arousal/lubrication and orgasm domains. Veronelli et al. [26] found an inverse correlation between antithyroid antibodies and FSFI score.

On the other hand, studies regarding the impact of subclinical hypothyroidism or euthyroid Hashimoto thyroiditis on female sexual function are conflicting and incomplete, but it seems that the presence of antibodies is implicated in the pathogenesis of sexual dysfunction in women [25, 27]. In a study with 168 subclinical hypothyroid women and 951 controls, no increased risk of female sexual dysfunction (FSD) or differences in FSFI were observed [27]. A recent meta-analysis, including 7 studies with 88 women with hypothyroidism, 337 with subclinical hypothyroidism, and 2056 controls, observed that patients with hypothyroidism scored lower in all FSFI dimensions, especially lubrication, while only arousal and orgasm were decreased in subclinical hypothyroidism.

Regarding hyperthyroidism, two studies have found a higher prevalence of FSD in hyperthyroid women compared to control, with significant worse total FSFI. Also, an inverse correlation has been described with free T3 and T4, and direct correlation with TSH, with normalization after 3 months of treatment with methimazole. However, another study failed to find a relationship, and no differences in the rate of FSD, total FSFI score, or its domains were found, except for desire, which was lower than that in controls [27].

3 Adrenal Disorders and Sexual Dysfunction

The cortical adrenal gland is crucial for life, maturation, immune response, and metabolism. Adrenal cortex secretes glucocorticoids, mineralocorticoids, and androgens. A complex enzymatic chain covers this intricate synthesis. Both hypersecretions as insufficient function due to genetic or acquired diseases affect sexual development and maturation and fertility due to the disbalance between androgens and glucocorticoids [28].

3.1   Congenital Adrenal Hyperplasia (CAH)

Among inherited adrenal enzymatic diseases, CAH is the most common genetic disorder, caused by a partial or total deficiency of the 21-hydroxylase enzyme (codified by the CYP21A2 gene) in majority of cases. This led to an excessive production of androgens and to relative or absolute cortisol and aldosterone deficiency. Neonatal screening of 17-OH-progesterone should be incorporated in all newborn screening. Severe forms of the rare classic CAH, with sexual development disorders (SDSs, condition associated with atypical development of the urogenital tract and external genital structures), and adrenal insufficiency are diagnosed at birth and in the early infancy. Milder forms are diagnosed during adolescence or in the adulthood due to accelerated skeletal maturation with short stature, premature puberty/adrenarche, hirsutism, and a higher risk for metabolic syndrome. The non-classic CAH, a partial common form of CAH (prevalence of 1/500 cases), is the main differential diagnosis of polycystic ovary syndrome (PCOS) and should be ruled out in all studies of hyperandrogenism.

Treatment of CAH is focused on the control of adrenal androgen overproduction, hormonal supplementation without excessive glucocorticoid exposure, and in severe cases surgical correction of the SDS-affected structures. Multidisciplinary pediatric and adults' expert management of fertility and genetic and psychological counseling are key points in the care of CAH.

Overall, congenital disorders affecting adrenal function may be associated with SDS in both 46,XX and 46,XY people. In 46,XX women, the adrenal overproduction of androgens is responsible for the genital anomalies, while in 46,XY patients, SDS results from the testicular dysfunction and lack of androgens.

In CAH besides SDS, fertility is affected in women by the suppression of the HP-gonadal axis through the inhibition of ovulation by high levels of progesterone and the disbalanced rise in estrogens due to peripheral aromatization of adrenal androgens. In males, the reproductive function can be affected through the presence of testicular steroid cell masses, which can have a mechanical and paracrine effect on spermatogenesis [29].

3.2   Other Congenital SDSs of Adrenal Origin

As mentioned, 21-hydroxylase deficiency is by far the most prevalent followed by the 11β-hydroxylase deficiency. Lipoid congenital adrenal hyperplasia due to STAR defects and cytochrome P450scc and P450c17 deficiencies induce SDS in 46,XY newborns. Mutations in *SF1* may also result in combined adrenal and testicular failure leading to SDS in 46,XY individuals. Finally, impaired activities of 3βHSD2 or POR may lead to SDS in both 46,XX and 46,XY individuals [30].

3.3 Adrenal Androgens, Adrenarche, and Sexuality

Sexual physiological maturation related to puberty comprises adrenal secretion of androgens (the adrenarche) followed by the HP-gonadal axis maturation and function. Adrenarche activation mechanisms are still under research and seem to be related to intra-adrenal weight-dependent mechanisms and early-life programming. Secretion of adrenal androgens, like DHEA and 11-oxygenated androgens (11-OHA), emerged from the development of the reticular zone of the adrenal cortex and is clinically manifested by pubarche and other low androgenic changes and an increased libido. Adrenarche is the messenger for the preparation of puberty [31].

Androgen receptors are expressed in various female tissues and are essential for many physiological processes including sexual, cardiovascular, bone, muscle, and brain health. They are also involved in adipose tissue and liver function. Low libido and an altered female sexual function index have been associated with decreased androgen levels. Adrenal androgen prohormone DHEA increases early in puberty and decreases after the third decade of life independently of menopausal status. Potential beneficial effect of the treatment with DHEA has been very recently summarized in a systematic meta-analysis. Hereby, data show some benefits in quality of life and mood but not on sexual function in women with primary or secondary adrenal insufficiency or anorexia, but no consistent beneficial effects for menopausal symptoms, sexual function, cognition, or overall well-being in normal women. Local administration of DHEA shows benefit in vulvovaginal atrophy, while the use of DHEAS in the induction of ovary response is not recommended [32]. 11-OHA is a very recently discovered adrenal androgen through mass spectrometry techniques. 11-Ketotestosterone (11-KT) has been established as the most important adrenal androgen in women. As reported by recent studies, 11-KT is involved in precocious adrenarche and in PCOS and, contrary to DHEAS, increases in menopause and is the main androgen observed in aging women [33].

Fetal brain development under the presence or absence of adrenal androgens could have a role in sexual orientation. Therefore, although subject to over- and underestimation, interestingly, a recent published analysis showed that assigned females at birth (46,XX) with CAH had a greater likelihood to not have an exclusively heterosexual orientation than females from the general population, whereas no assigned males at birth (46,XY or 46,XX) with CAH identified themselves as nonheterosexual [34]. However, more research is necessary in sexual diversity population.

3.4 Adrenal Hormonal Secretory Tumors and Sexuality

Adrenal benign and malign tumors can profoundly alter the sexual function due to the secretion of glucocorticoids or androgens.

Glucocorticoid oversecretion, as depicted in the *Cushing syndrome* (CS) paragraph previously, alters ovulation and fertility, decreases sexual desire, causes depression, induces central hypogonadism with erectile and ejaculatory dysfunction in men and anovulation and amenorrhea in women, and decreases libido with an altered quality of life in 90% of CS patients [35, 36].

As mentioned before, hypercortisolism does not only affect sexual function but also leads to several comorbidities, which themselves might deteriorate sexual well-being. Diabetes, hypertension, cardiovascular diseases, coagulopathy, and hypothyroidism are frequent in CS.

Oversecretion of androgens and precursors can be observed also in CS, being higher in ectopic forms. In rare forms of *adrenal cancer*, very increased secretion of androgens can lead to clinical virilization and a temporary increase in sexual drive. Secretion of estrogen, even more rare, can be associated in males with feminization and ED and loss of sexual drive [37].

Medullary tumors secreting increased amount of catecholamines, named *pheochromocytomas and paragangliomas*, can induce sexual dysfunction and loss of libido affecting sexuality and fertility in both females and males [38].

Primary hyperaldosteronism induces ED in men, through direct aldosterone action and due to the severe vascular hypertension, as in other vascular affecting diseases. In women, Conn's syndrome also leads to sexual dysfunction as decreased libido, but there are no mechanistic studies [39].

Early diagnosis and treatment of the secretory syndrome, if possible, through surgical removal of the tumor, are therefore the main objective in these diseases.

After cure, in CS, possible chronic adrenal insufficiency and metabolic acquired alteration, as well as glucocorticoid fingerprint at tissue level, can perpetuate the alteration of the fertility and affect the quality of life.

3.5   Adrenal Insufficiency

Adrenal insufficiency (AI) can be due to primary or secondary, genetic, and acquired disease. Primary AI is usually autoimmune (Addison's disease) or of infiltrative origin (sarcoidosis, metastasis, etc.), and it is frequently associated with other systemic pathologies.

Adrenarche is missing in young patients with Addison's disease that will present a minimal pubarche as gonadal puberty progresses. During adult life, probably due to the adrenal androgen depletion, women with Addison's disease present a reduced fertility scale, while sexual dysfunction presents contradictory results in the published studies to date. In an early study, they did not report any sexual dysfunction showing equal pleasure and discomfort than controls [40]. A recent study revealed significantly different scores for desire, arousal, lubrication, and overall sexual satisfaction in women with AI compared to matched controls, using the adapted FSFI-6 and Sexual Distress Scale. The presence of sexual distress was moreover related to cortisol levels [41]. In males, onset of autoimmune AI is associated with sexual dysfunctions that reverse after initiating replacement hormone therapy. Glucocorticoid and aldosterone deficiency seems to play an important role in the genesis of ED although the mechanism of their activity is not clear [42].

ED and fertility will be furthermore affected during the lifetime treatment with glucocorticoids in both males and females due to the overtreatment or deficient adaptation to stress, acute disease, exercise, and circadian rhythm. This has direct deleterious effects on metabolism, gonadal function, and vasculature increasing cardiometabolic and vascular burden and therefore affecting fertility and sexual function. Adequate treatment and new hormonal formulation that permit a more physiologic adaptation of the hormonal replacement treatment are therefore the focus in all adrenal chronic pathologies that need prolonged hormonal replacement treatment like CAH and primary adrenal insufficiency [43].

3.6 Endocrine Disruptors and the Pituitary, Thyroid, and Adrenal Sexual Function

Accumulating evidence indicates that several persistent organic pollutants (as pesticides or flame retardants, for example) are endocrine-disrupting chemicals (EDCs) and may impact on multiple levels the sexual function affecting pituitary, adrenal, and gonadal sexual maturation and thyroid function [44, 45]. Humans are exposed daily to EDCs through food or polluted air, among others. Prenatal and perinatal period, infancy, childhood, and puberty are critical moments particularly sensitive to hormonal disruptions. Exposure to environmental chemicals with estrogenic or antiandrogenic action may disrupt reproductive and sexual differentiation and function, leading to infertility or sexual dysfunction [46].There is also growing evidence that EDCs modify behavioral sexual dimorphism in children, presumably by interacting with the hypothalamic-pituitary-gonadal axis [47].

4 Conclusion

Endocrine disorders of the HP axis and peripheral thyroid and adrenal disturbances can induce a great variety of sexual alterations, decrease of fertility, and altered quality of life. Clinical evaluation, anamnesis, and management of the patient with dysfunction in these axes should include the sexual sphere.

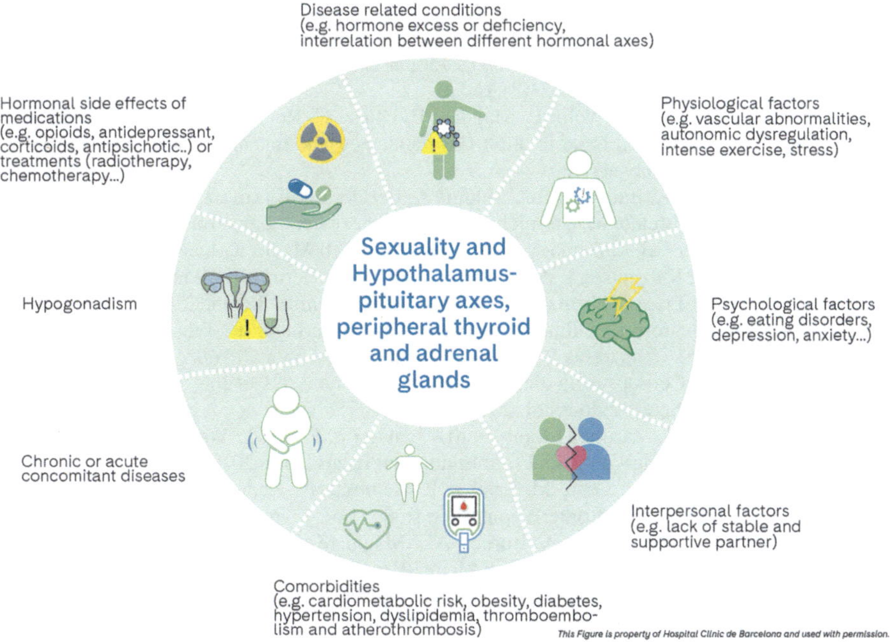

References

1. Grossmann M, Matsumoto AM. A perspective on middle-aged and older men with functional hypogonadism: focus on holistic management. J Clin Endocrinol Metab. 2017;102(3):1067–75.
2. Zhou WJ, Ma SC, Zhao M, Liu C, Guan XD, Bao ZS, Jia GJ, Jia W. Risk factors and the prognosis of sexual dysfunction in male patients with pituitary adenomas: a multivariate analysis. Asian J Androl. 2018;20(1):43–9.
3. Baydar AT, Ozercan AY, Divanlioglu D, Daglar Z, Balci M, Tuncel A. The impact of minimally invasive pituitary surgery on male and female sexual dysfunction in patients with pituitary adenoma. Urol Int. 2021;105(11-12):956–62.
4. Barut MU, Çoksüer H, Sak S, Bozkurt M, Ağaçayak E, Hamurcu U, Kurban D, Eserdağ S. Evaluation of sexual function in women with hypogonadotropic hypogonadism using the female sexual function index (FSFI) and the Beck depression inventory (BDI). Med Sci Monit. 2018;24:5610–8.
5. Cheuiche AV, da Silveira LG, de Paula LCP, Lucena IRS, Silveiro SP. Diagnosis and management of precocious sexual maturation: an updated review. Eur J Pediatr. 2021;180(10):3073–87.
6. Caicedo D, Devesa P, Alvarez CV, Devesa J. Why should growth hormone (GH) be considered a promising therapeutic agent for arteriogenesis? Insights from the GHAS TrialCells. 2020;9:886.
7. Salvio G, Martino M, Balercia G, et al. Acromegaly and male sexual health. Rev Endocr Metab Disord. 2022;23:671–8.
8. Pivonello R, Auriemma RS, Delli Veneri A, Dassie F, Lorusso R, Ragonese M, Liotta M, Sala E, Zarino B, Lai E, Urbani C, Bogazzi F, Mantovani G, Cannavò S, Maffei P, Chiodini P, Colao A. Global psychological assessment with the evaluation of life and sleep quality and sexual

and cognitive function in a large number of patients with acromegaly: a cross-sectional study. Eur J Endocrinol. 2022;187(6):823–45.

9. Andreassen M, Juul A, Feldt-Rasmussen U, Jørgensen N. Semen quality in hypogonadal acromegalic patients. Pituitary. 2020;23(2):160–6.

10. Monzani ML, Pederzoli S, Volpi L, Magnani E, Diazzi C, Rochira V. Sexual dysfunction: a neglected and overlooked issue in adult GH deficiency: the management of AGHD study. J Endocr Soc. 2021;5(3):bvab002.

11. Fleseriu M, Auchus R, Bancos I, Ben-Shlomo A, Bertherat J, Biermasz NR, Boguszewski CL, Bronstein MD, Buchfelder M, Carmichael JD, Casanueva FF, Castinetti F, Chanson P, Findling J, Gadelha M, Geer EB, Giustina A, Grossman A, Gurnell M, Ho K, Ioachimescu AG, Kaiser UB, Karavitaki N, Katznelson L, Kelly DF, Lacroix A, McCormack A, Melmed S, Molitch M, Mortini P, Newell-Price J, Nieman L, Pereira AM, Petersenn S, Pivonello R, Raff H, Reincke M, Salvatori R, Scaroni C, Shimon I, Stratakis CA, Swearingen B, Tabarin A, Takahashi Y, Theodoropoulou M, Tsagarakis S, Valassi E, Varlamov EV, Vila G, Wass J, Webb SM, Zatelli MC, Biller BMK. Consensus on diagnosis and management of Cushing's disease: a guideline update. Lancet Diabetes Endocrinol. 2021;9(12):847–75.

12. Santos A, Resmini E, Martínez Momblán MA, Valassi E, Martel L, Webb SM. Quality of life in patients with Cushing's disease. Front Endocrinol (Lausanne). 2019;10:862.

13. Keskin FE, Özkaya HM, Ortaç M, Salabaş E, Kadıoğlu A, Kadıoğlu P. Sexual function in women with Cushing's syndrome: a controlled study. Turk J Urol. 2018;44(4):287–93.

14. Corona G, Isidori AM, Aversa A, Burnett AL, Maggi M. Endocrinologic control of Men's sexual desire and arousal/erection. J Sex Med. 2016;13(3):317–37.

15. Gabrielson AT, Sartor RA, Hellstrom WJG. The impact of thyroid disease on sexual dysfunction in men and women. Sex Med Rev. 2019;7(1):57–70.

16. Carosa E, Lenzi A, Jannini EA. Thyroid hormone receptors and ligands, tissue distribution and sexual behavior. Mol Cell Endocrinol. 2018;467:49–59.

17. Veronelli A, Masu A, Ranieri R, Rognoni C, Laneri M, Pontiroli AE. Prevalence of erectile dysfunction in thyroid disorders: comparison with control subjects and with obese and diabetic patients. Int J Impot Res. 2006;18(1):111–4.

18. Krysiak R, Szkróbka W, Okopień. The effect of L-thyroxine treatment on sexual function and depressive symptoms in men with autoimmune hypothyroidism. Pharmacol Rep. 2017;69:432–7.

19. Corona G, Wu FC, Forti G, Lee DM, O'Connor DB, O'Neill TW, Pendleton N, Bartfai G, Boonen S, Casanueva FF, Finn JD, Giwercman A, Han TS, Huhtaniemi IT, Kula K, Lean ME, Punab M, Vanderschueren D, Jannini EA, Mannucci E, Maggi M, EMAS Study Group. Thyroid hormones and male sexual function. Int J Androl. 2012;35(5):668–79.

20. Keller J, Chen YK, Lin HC. Hyperthyroidism and erectile dysfunction: a population-based casecontrol study. Int J Impot Res. 2012;24:242–6.

21. Corona G, Petrone L, Mannucci E, Jannini EA, Mansani R, Magini A, Giommi R, Forti G, Maggi M. Psycho-biological correlates of rapid ejaculation in patients attending an andrologic unit for sexual dysfunctions. Eur Urol. 2004;46(5):615–22.

22. Cihan A, Esen AA. Systematic review and meta-analysis for the value of thyroid disorder screening in men with ejaculatory dysfunction. Int J Clin Pract. 2021 May;28:e14419.

23. Bates JN, Kohn TP, Pastuszak AW. Effect of thyroid hormone derangements on sexual function in men and women. Sex Med Rev. 2020;8(2):217–30.

24. Krysiak R, Drosdzol-Cop A, Skrzypulec-Plinta V, Okopien B. Sexual function and depressive symptoms in young women with thyroid autoimmunity and subclinical hypothyroidism. Clin Endocrinol. 2016;84(6):925–31.

25. Luo H, Zhao W, Yang H, Han Q, Zeng L, Tang H, Zhu J. Subclinical hypothyroidism would not lead to female sexual dysfunction in Chinese women. BMC Womens Health. 2018;18(1):26.

26. Veronelli A, Mauri C, Zecchini B, Peca MG, Turri O, Valitutti MT, Dall'Asta C, Pontiroli AE. Sexual dysfunction is frequent in premenopausal women with diabetes, obesity, and

hypothyroidism, and correlates with markers of increased cardiovascular risk. A preliminary report J Sex Med. 2009;6(6):1561–8.

27. Pasquali D, Maiorino MI, Renzullo A, Bellastella G, Accardo G, Esposito D, Barbato F, Esposito K. Female sexual dysfunction in women with thyroid disorders. J Endocrinol Investig. 2013;36(9):729–33.

28. Claahsen-van der Grinten HL, Speiser PW, Ahmed SF, Arlt W, Auchus RJ, Falhammar H, Flück CE, Guasti L, Huebner A, Kortmann BBM, Krone N, Merke DP, Miller WL, Nordenström A, Reisch N, Sandberg DE, Stikkelbroeck NMML, Touraine P, Utari A, Wudy SA, White PC. Congenital adrenal hyperplasia - current insights in pathophysiology, diagnostics, and management. Endocr Rev. 2022;43(1):91–159.

29. Uslar T, Olmos R, Martínez-Aguayo A, Baudrand R. Clinical update on congenital adrenal hyperplasia: recommendations from a multidisciplinary adrenal program. J Clin Med. 2023;12(9):3128.

30. Finkielstain GP, Vieites A, Bergadá I, Rey RA. Disorders of sex development of adrenal origin. Front Endocrinol (Lausanne). 2021;12:770782.

31. Witchel SF, Azziz R, Oberfield SE. History of polycystic ovary syndrome, premature Adrenarche, and Hyperandrogenism in pediatric endocrinology. Horm Res Paediatr. 2022;95(6):557–67.

32. Wierman ME, Kiseljak-Vassiliades K. Should dehydroepiandrosterone be administered to women? J Clin Endocrinol Metab. 2022;107(6):1679–85.

33. Storbeck KH, O'Reilly MW. The clinical and biochemical significance of 11-oxygenated androgens in human health and disease. Eur J Endocrinol. 2023;188(4):R98–R109.

34. Daae E, Feragen KB, Waehre A, Nermoen I, Falhammar H. Sexual orientation in individuals with congenital adrenal hyperplasia: a systematic review. Front Behav Neurosci. 2020;14(38):5.

35. Keskin FE, Özkaya HM, Ortaç M, Salabaş E, Kadıoğlu A, Kadıoğlu P. Sexual function in women with Cushing's syndrome: a controlled study. Turk. J Urol. 2018;44(4):287–93.

36. Pivonello R, Isidori AM, De Martino MC, Newell-Price J, Biller BM, Colao A. Complications of Cushing's syndrome: state of the art. Lancet Diabetes Endocrinol. 2016;4(7):611–29.

37. Fassnacht M, Dekkers OM, Else T, Baudin E, Berruti A, de Krijger R, Haak HR, Mihai R, Assie G, Terzolo M. European Society of Endocrinology Clinical Practice Guidelines on the management of adrenocortical carcinoma in adults, in collaboration with the European Network for the Study of Adrenal Tumors. Eur J Endocrinol. 2018;179(4):G1–G46.

38. Kantorovich V, Eisenhofer G, Pacak K. Pheochromocytoma: an endocrine stress mimicking disorder. Ann N Y Acad Sci. 2008;1148:462–8.

39. Chang CH, Chueh SJ, Wu VC, Chen L, Lin YH, Hu YH, Wu KD, Tsai YC. Risk of severe ED in primary hyperaldosteronism: a population-based propensity score matching cohort study. Surgery. 2019;165(3):622–8.

40. Erichsen MM, Husebye ES, Michelsen TM, Dahl AA, Løvås K. Sexuality and fertility in women with Addison's disease. J Clin Endocrinol Metab. 2010;95(9):4354–60.

41. Zamponi V, Lardo P, Maggio R, Simonini C, Mazzilli R, Faggiano A, Pugliese G, Stigliano A. Female sexual dysfunction in primary adrenal insufficiency. J Clin Med. 2021;10(13):2767.

42. Granata A, Tirabassi G, Pugni V, Arnaldi G, Boscaro M, Carani C, Balercia G. Sexual dysfunctions in men affected by autoimmune Addison's disease before and after short-term gluco- and mineralocorticoid replacement therapy. J Sex Med. 2013;10(8):2036–43.

43. Giordano R, Guaraldi F, Marinazzo E, Fumarola F, Rampino A, Berardelli R, Karamouzis I, Lucchiari M, Manetta T, Mengozzi G, Arvat E, Ghigo E. Improvement of anthropometric and metabolic parameters, and quality of life following treatment with dual-release hydrocortisone in patients with Addison's disease. Endocrine. 2016;51(2):360–8.

44. Dickerson SM, Gore AC. Estrogenic environmental endocrine-disrupting chemical effects on reproductive neuroendocrine function and dysfunction across the life cycle. Rev Endocr Metab Disord. 2007;8(2):143–59.

45. Castiello F, Suárez B, Gómez-Vida J, Torrent M, Fernández MF, Olea N, Freire C. Exposure to non-persistent pesticides and sexual maturation of Spanish adolescent males. Chemosphere. 2023;324:138350.
46. Beszterda M, Frański R. Endocrine disruptor compounds in environment: as a danger for children health. Pediatr Endocrinol Diabetes Metab. 2018;24(2):88–95.
47. Winneke G, Ranft U, Wittsiepe J, Kasper-Sonnenberg M, Fürst P, Krämer U, Seitner G, Wilhelm M. Behavioral sexual dimorphism in school-age children and early developmental exposure to dioxins and PCBs: a follow-up study of the Duisburg cohort. Environ Health Perspect. 2014;122(3):292–8.

Endocrine Disorders and Sexuality II: Ovary

Camil Castelo-Branco and Iuliia Naumova

1 Introduction

1.1 Evidence of the Role of Estrogens in Sexual Function

With the onset of perimenopause, which begins 4–6 years before cessation of menses, women often experience hot flushes, sweats, cognitive complaints, mood changes, and disrupted sleep [1]. Genitourinary syndrome of menopause (GUSM) may give rise to dyspareunia, which negatively impacts sexual function. While vasomotor symptoms usually improve over the time, vulvovaginal atrophy, if untreated, may worsen with time [2]. Menopause, however, is not a perfect model to assess the effect of estrogens on sexual function, since changes in testosterone are also observed. Spontaneous menopause has gradual changes in testosterone levels with aging [3], while surgical menopause implies a sharp and acute decrease in circulating levels at the time of bilateral oophorectomy [4]. Moreover, using surgical menopause as a model for studying the effects of estrogen on sexuality also presents additional inconveniences such as the fact that women undergoing surgery regularly have underlying pathology, e.g., myomas and endometriosis, which may

C. Castelo-Branco (✉)
Gynecological Department, Clinical Institute of Gynecology, Obstetrics and Neonatology, Hospital Clinic de Barcelona, Barcelona, Spain

Clinical Sexology Working Group, Hospital Clinic de Barcelona, Barcelona, Spain

Surgery and Medical-Surgical Specialties, Faculty of Medicine and Health Sciences, Universitat de Barcelona (UB), Barcelona, Spain

Institut d'Investigacions Biomèdiques August Pi i Sunyer, Barcelona, Spain
e-mail: castelobranco@ub.edu; ccastelo@clinic.cat

I. Naumova
Department of Obstetrics and Gynecology, Faculty of Medicine, Saratov State Medical University n.a. V. I. Razumovsky of the Ministry of Health of Russia, Saratov, Russia

cause pelvic pain or abnormal uterine bleeding; consequently, sexual function may improve in these cases due to the treatment of the underlying gynecologic complaint independent of the hormonal status [5, 6]. Alternatively, bilateral oophorectomy in premenopausal women originates premature ovarian failure and negatively affects sexual self-image and function [7].

Lack of estrogens may develop sexual dysfunction in different ways: primarily due to vaginal atrophy and dyspareunia [8], but often also accompanied secondarily by decreased sexual interest, arousal, and response [7, 9]. Skin sensitivity of sexual areas is also related to estrogen status. Vasomotor complaints often presented with sleep disturbances, fatigue, and impaired quality of life will also have a negative impact on sexual function [10]. Therefore, estrogen therapy may improve sexual function by treating GUSM and vasomotor symptoms [11].

1.2 Evidence of the Role of Androgens in Sexual Function

Androgens deserve an important role in female sexual function. This statement is supported by numerous studies showing that clinical conditions associated with low androgen levels are related to sexual complaints including hypoactive desire, arousal difficulties, and orgasmic disorder. Physiological low androgen states include aging and menopause. Whether these low levels are associated with natural or surgical menopause, it is clinically manifested by decreased sexual function, increased levels of personal distress, and anxiety [12]. Other conditions that are related to androgen deficiency are early menopause, premature ovarian insufficiency, adrenal insufficiency, and hypopituitarism [13].

Although sexual complaints of any nature increased with age, sexual dysfunction as distressing problems peaked in women younger than 65 and, in fact, lowdown in elder women. In addition, an increased prevalence of low sexual desire has been observed with age and among surgically and naturally menopausal women compared to premenopausal women [14]. Several population-based studies have attempted to find a relationship between androgen levels and sexual function, but in many of them, those levels were not associated with any aspects of female sexual functioning [15]. However, a recent meta-analysis suggested that there appears to be a moderate association between total testosterone and sexual desire/global sexual function and that similar results on desire were obtained for free testosterone and free androgen index, while DHEAS only showed a positive association with global sexual function [16].

1.3 Evidence of the Role of Progestins in Sexual Function

In multiple animal and human studies, the effects of progesterone and other sexual steroids were observed through classical signaling pathways of estrogen, androgen, and P4 receptors. However, nonclassical signaling via transmembrane receptors also appears to play a significant role in the action of sexual steroids [17]. Data from

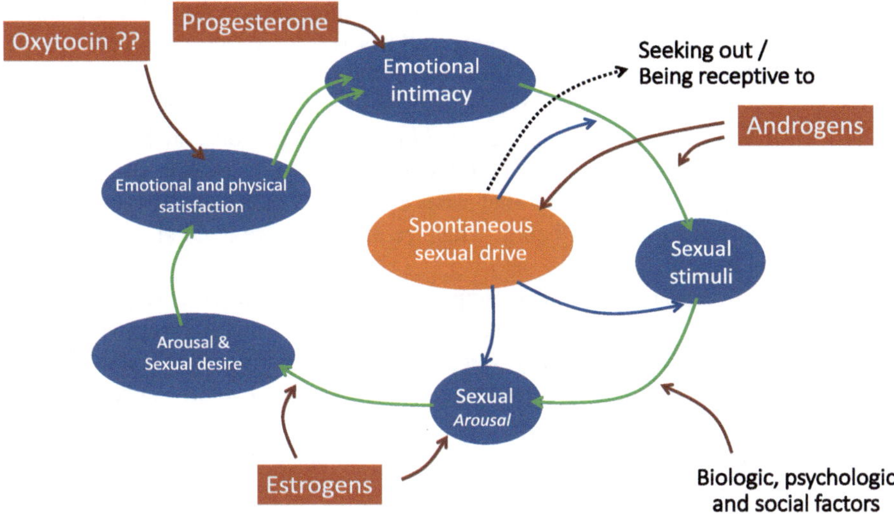

Fig. 1 Female sexual response: biopsychosocial model and the role of sexual hormones

animal studies, including nonhuman primates, suggest that sexual attractiveness, proceptivity, and receptivity are highest in situations of high estrogen and declined when a progestin is added [18]. This fact was observed both in the natural cycle and in experimental conditions.

Notwithstanding some discrepancies on the effect of sexual steroids in female sexual function, data suggest that estrogen has a facilitatory action while progestin has a certain inhibitory role. However, it is to note that hormonal actions may also be modified by previous conditioning influences. In this sense, it is important to consider other biopsychosocial factors, such as the risk of unwanted conception, that will also influence female sexual functioning across the cycle (Fig. 1).

2   Part I: Sexual Dysfunction in Hypogonadisms

2.1   Menopause

Sexual dysfunction may appear at any time in women's lifespan but is most common around menopause. Aging process and menopause are two conditions that may concurrently affect female sexuality. Sexual complaints can be a prominent feature of the transition to menopause and can be a source for concern if the cause is the concurrent hormone deficiency. The low estrogen levels associated with menopause cause epithelial thinning and reduced lubrication and vasocongestion during sexual arousal that progresses to GUSM and dyspareunia. Other bothersome sexual complaints of the menopause, particularly decreased libido and sexual activity, can be attributed to the decline in testosterone levels. It is to note that at the age of 45, testosterone levels in most women are halved compared to those at the beginning of adulthood in their 20 s.

Sexual dysfunction associated with menopause may not reverse unless therapy is started as its cause, hormone deficiency, will not resolve on its own. Menopause-related sexual dysfunction is a complex condition; therefore, therapeutic measures must be engaged in a comprehensive manner embracing the multifactorial etiology of this disorder. This is important, because in certain situations, such as hormonal deficiency typical of menopause, where the etiology seems obvious, the complaint may have been present for so long that it has additionally affected the patient's psychological and relational well-being, which requires a more general or biopsychosocial approach.

Sexual dysfunction related to menopause is more severe and frequent among women who suffer surgical menopause. Nearly three out of four women who had undergone bilateral oophorectomy were at risk of suffering sexual dysfunction, mainly arousal and desire disorders; this risk was increased when less than 5 years since surgical menopause had elapsed [7].

There are multiple options for the therapeutic approach to menopause-related sexual dysfunction. Following a biopsychosocial model, they can be classified into actions focused on the psychosocial area (mindfulness, *sex corporel*, psychotherapy, couple therapy, and social interventions), mechanical-physical (lubricants, physiotherapy, vaginal dilators, vibrators, and vacuum therapy), and pharmacological (menopausal hormone therapy with estrogens and progestins or estrogens alone, testosterone therapy alone or with menopausal hormone therapy, tibolone, pain medications, antidepressants, vasodilators) therapies [19].

2.2 Premature Ovarian Insufficiency

Premature ovarian insufficiency (POI) is a common cause of infertility affecting about 1% of young women. This disorder has significant psychological sequelae and major health implications [20]. The main features are absence of ovulation, amenorrhea, and elevated serum levels of gonadotropins. While in most cases the etiology remains undefined, several infrequent conditions have been related. Possible causes of POI include iatrogenic factors (bilateral oophorectomy, radiation therapy, or chemotherapy), environmental factors, viral infections, metabolic and autoimmune diseases, and genetic variations. The traditional indicators to evaluate ovarian aging are age, serum hormonal levels, anti-Mullerian hormone, and antral follicle count.

Many factors, including biomedical (low sexual steroid levels, age, infertility, other physical health problems, etc.), psychological (depression, anxiety, self-esteem, distress, etc.), and social (intimacy, couple relationship, interpersonal relationships, etc.), contribute to sexual dysfunction in women with POI. In general, women with POI had reduced general and sexual well-being and were less satisfied with their sexual lives, and additionally, they had fewer sexual fantasies and masturbated less frequently [21].

Women with POI refer to less sexual arousal, reduced lubrication, and increased genital pain during sexual intercourse, and suffering from these sexual symptoms has been associated with significant distress. However, the frequency of actual sexual contact with the partner, as well as the frequency of desire to have sexual contact, did not differ between healthy women and those with POI. In general, women with ovarian insufficiency, both POI and gonadal dysgenesis, presented worse quality of life and poor sexual functioning than age-matched healthy women [22]. Therefore, sexuality in women with POI mandatorily requests consideration because of the young age and the distressing impact of such a life-changing diagnosis. Interestingly when comparing women affected with spontaneous POI with gonadal dysgenesis and healthy females, the most important differences were encountered between POI and healthy controls in most of the domains and in total score of FSFI [22]. These results could be interpreted as an important complaint of these patients regarding their sexual life, and although hormone replacement therapy with estrogens and progestins (HRT) is the standard management for women with premature ovarian failure, these pharmacological regimens do not completely mimic natural steroid production and testosterone supplementation would probably also be recommended for these women.

After corroborating the diagnosis of POI and excluding major genetic causes, it is accepted that the gold standard treatment for POI is hormone replacement therapy, at least until the usual age of natural menopause. These women have an increased risk of premature death, mainly from cardiovascular disease, and POI has a potentially devastating influence on bone, with an increased risk of fracture, and on many other body targets severely affecting the quality of life and well-being of these women. An extensive variety of treatment modalities are reported, but there is no clear evidence of best practice. Physiological sexual steroid replacement appears to recover many aspects of life functioning; however, both age at POI and underlying etiology seem to play a role in the success of the therapeutic approach.

2.3   Gonadal Dysgenesis

Sexuality in women with gonadal dysgenesis (GD) has been found to be an important determinant of self-esteem and social adjustment [23]. The different studies agree that sexual function is impaired in women with GD. Data suggest a low rate of sexual activity compared to similar age women; only half of the patients diagnosed with Turner syndrome declare sexual activity [22].

One of the factors that have consistently shown to affect sexual function of patients with Turner syndrome is the height. Patients without sexual activity are significantly shorter than those with sexual activity, while the tallest women have shown higher scores in sexual functioning [22, 23].

The existence of a sexual partner is a factor that influences sexual activity. Among women with Turner syndrome who had couple relationship, sexual functioning was overall within normal range, and their general evaluation of the sexual activity could be considered satisfying [22]. However, this group represents a minority as less than one-third of women with gonadal dysgenesis included in studies on this topic were married or in a relationship [23]. Interestingly, hearing status, degree of dysmorphology, and noncardiac comorbidities such as renal malformations, high blood pressure, hypothyroidism, dyslipidemia, diabetes mellitus, hypertransaminasemia, or osteoporosis have not been recognized as factors influencing the sexual functioning in women with gonadal dysgenesis [22, 23].

2.4   Hypogonadotropic Ovarian Dysfunction

Women with hypothalamic amenorrhea present sexual steroid deficiency due to the disruption of hypothalamic-pituitary-ovarian axis. Due to the lack of estrogens, they may complaint about urogenital atrophy and other symptoms of hypoestrogenism, but vasomotor symptoms are often not present. Among hypogonadotropic hypogonadisms, those of central origin, the congenital ones must be differentiated from those that appear in the reproductive years. Non-congenital hypothalamic amenorrhea is typically caused by excess stress, intensive exercise (athlete triad), eating disorders (anorexia, bulimia), or other physiologic or psychologic factors. There are scant data on sexual function in these conditions. Since hormone therapy (both physiological and hormonal contraceptives) is usually prescribed to young women with hypothalamic amenorrhea to preserve bone mineral density, maintenance of vaginal health would be an expected benefit.

Women with congenital hypogonadotropic hypogonadism are more prone to start and maintain sexual intercourse and activity than women with congenital gonadal dysgenesis and POI [22]. However, large differences have been detected in arousal, lubrication, orgasm, and pain when compared to healthy women in their age range [22]. These complaints could be related to the lack of hormones, as although many of these women receive a standard hormone replacement therapy, it may not fully mimic the ovaries' natural production of steroids. In addition, their delayed sexual development compared to their peers may make them feel uncomfortable or ashamed (Fig. 2).

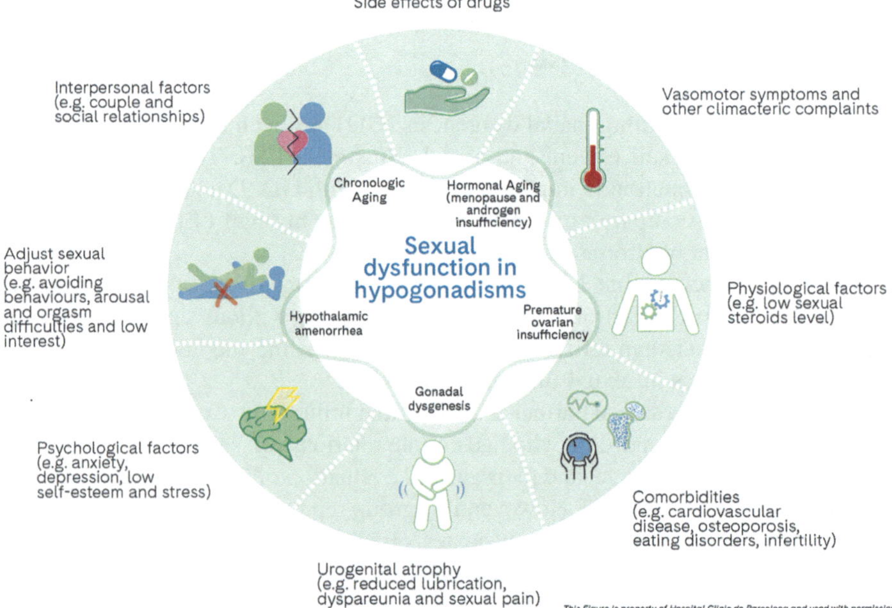

Fig. 2 Factors related to sexual dysfunction among hypogonadal women

3 Management of Sexuality in Young Women with Hypogonadism

The management of sexuality problems in women with hypogonadism of any age, but specifically in those of younger ages, must be multidisciplinary and consider all the biopsychosocial aspects that may be involved. Medical treatments should be part of such a management considering that this is an atypical cohort of women who have lack of ovarian hormones from naissance in some cases or beyond the average age of natural menopause in others. For those women, hormone therapy is a real replacement. Except in cases where there is an absolute contraindication for the use of estrogens, all guidelines agree on the need to prescribe them to reduce the risk of deleterious consequences of the lack of sexual steroids such as osteoporosis, cardiovascular disease, cognitive decline, and urogenital atrophy and therefore to maintain sexual health and quality of life. The addition of progestogens is mandatory in women with an intact uterus, while in the hypothetical case that spontaneous ovarian activity may occur, combined estrogen and progestogen contraception should also be considered to avoid the risk of pregnancy.

There is an imparity in the management of sexual symptoms with hormones specifically in young women since most studies have focused on postmenopausal women. Common sense and knowledge on the different treatments should help us to make the correct choice of drugs.

For hormone replacement, natural estradiol is preferred. 17-β-Estradiol, especially in non-oral routes, has less effect on sex hormone binding globulin and therefore in the bioavailable testosterone levels. Similarly, the use of birth control pills containing estradiol or estetrol should be preferred over those containing ethinylestradiol. Other options for hormone therapy include tibolone and androgens. Tibolone is mainly used in the treatment of menopausal symptoms like hot flashes and vaginal atrophy, and postmenopausal osteoporosis. It has similar effectiveness compared to other hormone replacement medications and shares a similar safety profile. It has also been investigated as a possible treatment for female sexual dysfunction in postmenopausal women [24] but again no valuable data on its use for sexual complaints in young women. Local therapies including estrogens and prasterone are effective in moving back urogenital atrophy symptoms, as well as dyspareunia and other associated sexual disorders, but again most of the studies are based on women in their postmenopausal years. Despite being the most logical option, in some cases, the standard hormone replacement does not completely solve sexual problems since as commented, it does not entirely mirror the actual complete steroid distribution in women. For this reason, some authors proposed to include androgens as a part of the management.

Hormone therapy is the gold standard in the management of ovarian insufficiency in young women; however, some of them may present contraindications to estrogens, and then, alternative nonhormonal strategies to manage short-term and long-term consequences of these maintained low estrogen levels over the years should be considered. Healthy lifestyle promotion, mindfulness, vitamin-mineral-oligonutrient supplementation, and other medication and therapeutic approaches can be used.

Selective serotonin-norepinephrine reuptake inhibitors have demonstrated to be useful in the management of vasomotor symptoms; however, these symptoms are infrequent in gonadal dysgenesis and in hypogonadotropic amenorrhea, and additionally, these drugs may present sexual dysfunction as an adverse event in a large amount of patients.

The first-line therapy, in all guidelines, for the management of GUSM symptoms is lubricants and moisturizers. Other strategies include the use of vibrators, psychosexual therapy, and pelvic floor reeducation, with the use of laser for this purpose being controversial.

4　Conclusion

Women with hypogonadisms at any age but especially those at younger ages merit specific attention as the premature lack of sexual steroids leads to a large quantity of complaints, including sexual dysfunction that may also severely affect the quality of life.

The adequate management of sexual dysfunction should be done from a biopsychosocial perspective that includes early and precise diagnosis of the hypogonadism, facilitating the patient's openness and communication, giving understandable information, offering sensitive advice, and personalized treatment that must include hormone therapy and in many occasions psychosexual counseling.

5　Part II: Sexual Dysfunction in Polycystic Ovary Syndrome

5.1　Introduction

Polycystic ovary syndrome (PCOS) is the most common endocrine disorder in women of reproductive age; according to various data, its prevalence in the population reaches 6–15% and 21% in high-risk groups [25, 26].

To date, PCOS is one of the most studied conditions; nevertheless, the pathogenesis of PCOS is not well understood and is considered multifactorial, although it is reliably known that among the main causes of this pathology are the patient's genetic predisposition and lifestyle [27].

Polycystic ovary syndrome is a clinically heterogeneous disorder characterized by three key features: anovulation, hyperandrogenism, and polycystic ovarian morphology [28]. However, the diagnosis of PCOS is based on certain criteria, which differ according to the scientific data of the association that issued them [29].

Women suffering from PCOS face many challenges including reproductive issues (irregular menstrual cycles, infertility, and pregnancy complications) [30], metabolic disorders (insulin resistance, abdominal and visceral obesity, prediabetes, type 2 diabetes), and cardiovascular risk factors [31]. In addition, many recent studies have clearly shown that PCOS is associated with anxiety and depressive symptoms [32] and with a poorer quality of life [33]. A high prevalence of eating disorders, such as anorexia nervosa, bulimia nervosa, and binge eating disorder, has also been observed in PCOS, particularly in the presence of anxiety and depression [34].

The issue of impaired sexuality in patients with PCOS currently remains debatable.

The published results of most studies show a decrease in the level of sexual well-being in women with PCOS. Thus, problems in the sexual sphere are identified in more than 30% of women with PCOS, with obesity being largely predominant among complainers [35].

The etiology of sexual dysfunction in women with PCOS has not been definitively established. However, endocrine disorders and discomfort in emotional and social spheres associated with the syndrome could have the major role.

5.2   Complaints Related to Sexual Functioning

Overweight, infertility, and features of hyperandrogenic dermopathy are the most bothersome symptoms commonly reported by PCOS women. Poor body image, dissatisfaction with one's appearance, low self-esteem, perception of oneself as not feminine, and unattractive for a partner can markedly affect women's emotional and sexual well-being [36].

Some studies have demonstrated a high prevalence of difficulties with arousal, poor lubrication, orgasm, and pain during intercourse and high degree of sexual dissatisfaction [37, 38].

Obesity has been documented to have a negative effect on sexuality, but in women with PCOS, the results remain mixed [39].

Thus, a recent meta-analysis demonstrated that sexual attractiveness and satisfaction with sex life were impaired in women with PCOS, and body image had an impact on sexuality in patients with syndrome [40]. Conversely, some studies report that PCOS women are more susceptible to impaired stimulation, reduced lubrication, satisfaction, and pain vs. controls. However, weight excess did not correlate with sexual function [41].

Hirsutism, together with obesity, has been described to have aversive effects on sexuality by causing body dissatisfaction and affecting feminine identity [42].

Data suggest that excessive body hair concern and acne-related concern are markedly associated with low sexual satisfaction in both PCOS women and their partners [43].

Menstrual cycle disorders: The majority of PCOS women experience menstrual cycle disorders; approximately two-thirds of them present with anovulation and face the problem of subfertility or infertility [33]. Some hormonal changes specific for the syndrome and anovulation might affect sexual function. There is evidence of the impact of progesterone and LH on reduced sexual satisfaction, and association between the level of testosterone and pain during sexual intercourse in PCOS patients.

Contradictory data is presented regarding the association between sexual dysfunction and androgen circulating levels, with some studies demonstrating a positive correlation, others showing negative, whereas others showing no significant association [39, 42, 44].

Infertility is the third most troubling symptom of PCOS after weight concerns and menstrual problem [45]. In a large community-based cohort study, infertility was reported in 72% of women with PCOS compared with 16% in those without; its incidence was 15-fold higher in women reporting PCOS, independent of BMI [46].

Infertility of any cause is associated with complex biological, psychological, social, and ethical issues [47]. Of note, more than half of women suffering from subfertility and infertility face the risk of depression, anxiety disorders, and social dysfunction. Infertility is a two-person problem, and being a burden, infertility affects the marriage and sex life of any couple. Sexual problems are common among infertile couples and are reported to affect between 5% and 55% of women in infertile couples [48].

The impact of this aspect of PCOS on sexual well-being is mediated by high level of emotional distress among patients with infertility.

Self-esteem: PCOS-related concerns including (but not limited to) obesity, acne, androgenic alopecia, and hirsutism play the greatest role in self-perception as they largely interfere with outer appearance and social norms and lead to the loss of self-esteem in most of the patients.

Literature on self-esteem and sexuality supports a positive relationship between these two variables. Low self-esteem can also adversely affect a person's body image and in this way negatively influence sexuality [49].

Psychological issues: According to the literature, the frequency of anxiety and depressive symptoms in patients with PCOS can reach 14–67% [50], while in the general population, its prevalence does not exceed 6–10% [51].

Some studies showed that respondents with depressive and anxiety symptoms were much more likely to have difficulty in achieving an orgasm than those without mood disorders [52]. Anxiety and depression along with poor body image in PCOS patients are psychosocial risk factors for impaired sexual functioning and sexual dissatisfaction [53]. In turn, women with PCOS with the lowest sexual satisfaction are more prone to anxiety and depression than other women [54].

Since sexual dysfunction in women with PCOS is not an independent nosology, but is the result of a complex effects of the clinical manifestations of the syndrome on female identity and emotional well-being, the management of patients with sexual dysfunction associated with PCOS should be aimed at relieving symptoms and overcoming the consequences of the disease (Fig. 3).

5.2.1 Treatment

For patients not actively attempting to conceive, first-line treatment of PCOS is lifestyle interventions for weight loss and hormonal oral contraceptive pills (OCPs).

Lifestyle modification includes caloric restriction, increased physical activity, and behavioral interventions aimed at weight loss, improving endocrine profile and insulin resistance, and decreasing androgen levels. Since obesity aggravates the

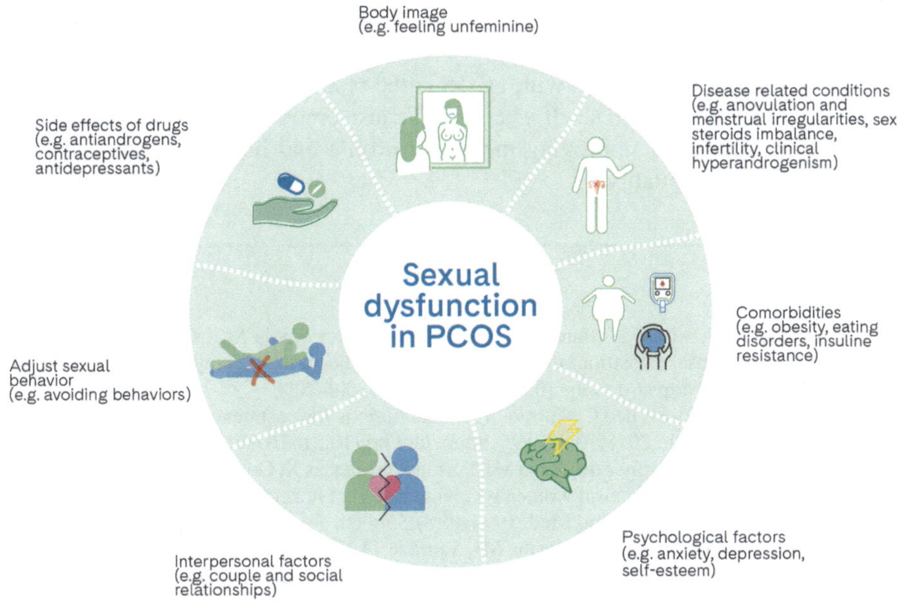

Fig. 3 Factors related to sexual dysfunction in women complaining with PCOS

symptoms of PCOS, weight management has been proposed as an initial treatment strategy. A meta-analysis of lifestyle interventions demonstrates improvements in body weight, free androgen index, and BMI with weight loss from lifestyle interventions [55].

However, it is not clear how these interventions affect sexual function.

Numerous studies in the general population have shown that weight loss is associated with improvement in sexual function. Specifically, significant improvements in sexual function are observed in those who experience the greatest weight loss. However, there are no data on the impact of weight loss on sexual function in PCOS patients [56].

OCPs, suppressing ovarian hyperandrogenism, are effective in treating irregular cycles and superior for the treatment of hirsutism and acne compared to progestin-only preparations in women with PCOS; however, its effect on sexuality is controversial [57].

However, data on the effect of taking OCPs on the sexual function of women with PCOS are limited. Some surveys reported the improvement of female sexuality and social self-esteem—increasing frequency of sexual intercourse and of orgasm during the sixth and the ninth cycle of OCPs' use in normal-weight PCOS patients [58].

Some studies demonstrate that the combination of OCPs and intensive lifestyle interventions resulted in significant improvement in sexual function and reduced sexual distress [59].

6   Conclusion

Sexual dysfunction in women with PCOS is the result of a complex of factors that someway reduce a woman's self-esteem and cause emotional distress. Therapeutic interventions aimed at improving metabolic profile and body image may have a positive effect on sexuality.

References

1. Gava G, Orsili I, Alvisi S, Mancini I, Seracchioli R, Meriggiola MC. Cognition, mood and sleep in menopausal transition: the role of menopause hormone therapy. Medicina (Kaunas). 2019;55(10):668. https://doi.org/10.3390/medicina55100668.
2. Naumova I, Castelo-Branco C. Current treatment options for postmenopausal vaginal atrophy. Int J Women's Health. 2018;10:387–95. https://doi.org/10.2147/IJWH.S158913.
3. Castelo-Branco C, Martínez de Osaba MJ, Fortuny A, Iglesias X, González-Merlo J. Circulating hormone levels in menopausal women receiving different hormone replacement therapy regimens. A comparison. J Reprod Med. 1995;40(8):556–60.
4. Castelo-Branco C, Martínez de Osaba MJ, Vanrezc JA, Fortuny A, González-Merlo J. Effects of oophorectomy and hormone replacement therapy on pituitary-gonadal function. Maturitas. 1993;17(2):101–11. https://doi.org/10.1016/0378-5122(93)90005-3.
5. Gracia M, Martínez-Zamora MA, Castelo-Branco C, Carmona F. The influence of laparoscopic benign hysterectomy in sexual function. Clin Exp Obstet Gynecol. 2023;50(2):38. https://doi.org/10.31083/j.ceog5002038.
6. Dedden SJ, Werner MA, Steinweg J, Lissenberg-Witte BI, Huirne JAF, Geomini PMAJ, Maas JWM. Hysterectomy and sexual function: a systematic review and meta-analysis. J Sex Med. 2023;20(4):qdac051. https://doi.org/10.1093/jsxmed/qdac051.
7. Castelo-Branco C, Palacios S, Combalia J, Ferrer M, Traveria G. Risk of hypoactive sexual desire disorder and associated factors in a cohort of oophorectomized women. Climacteric. 2009;12(6):525–32. https://doi.org/10.3109/13697130903075345.
8. Palacios S, Castelo-Branco C, Currie H, Mijatovic V, Nappi RE, Simon J, Rees M. Update on management of genitourinary syndrome of menopause: a practical guide. Maturitas. 2015;82(3):308–13. https://doi.org/10.1016/j.maturitas.2015.07.020.
9. Nappi RE, Kokot-Kierepa. Vaginal health: insights, views & attitudes (VIVA)—results from an international survey. Climacteric. 2012;15(1):36–44. https://doi.org/10.3109/1369713 7.2011.647840.
10. El Khoudary SR, Greendale G, Crawford SL, Avis NE, Brooks MM, Thurston RC, Karvonen-Gutierrez C, Waetjen LE, Matthews K. The menopause transition and women's health at midlife: a progress report from the study of Women's health across the nation (SWAN). Menopause. 2019;26(10):1213–27. https://doi.org/10.1097/GME.0000000000001424.
11. Mendoza N, Ramírez I, de la Viuda E, Coronado P, Baquedano L, Llaneza P, Nieto V, Otero B, Sánchez-Méndez S, de Frutos VÁ, Andraca L, Barriga P, Benítez Z, Bombas T, Cancelo MJ, Cano A, Branco CC, Correa M, Doval JL, Fasero M, Fiol G, Garello NC, Genazzani AR, Gómez AI, Gómez MÁ, González S, Goulis DG, Guinot M, Hernández LR, Herrero S, Iglesias E, Jurado AR, Lete I, Lubián D, Martínez M, Nieto A, Nieto L, Palacios S, Pedreira M, Pérez-Campos E, Plá MJ, Presa J, Quereda F, Ribes M, Romero P, Roca B, Sánchez-Capilla A, Sánchez-Borrego R, Santaballa A, Santamaría A, Simoncini T, Tinahones F, Calaf J. Eligibility criteria for menopausal hormone therapy (MHT): a position statement from a consortium of scientific societies for the use of MHT in women with medical conditions. MHT Eligibility Criteria Group Maturitas. 2022;166:65–85. https://doi.org/10.1016/j.maturitas.2022.08.008.

12. West SL, D'Aloisio AA, Agans RP, Kalsbeek WD, Borisov NN, Thorp JM. Prevalence of low sexual desire and hypoactive sexual desire disorder in a nationally representative sample of US women. Arch Intern Med. 2008;168:1441–9.

13. Naamneh Elzenaty R, du Toit T, Flück CE. Basics of androgen synthesis and action. Best Pract Res Clin Endocrinol Metab. 2022;36(4):101665. https://doi.org/10.1016/j.beem.2022.101665.

14. Clayton AH, Goldstein I, Kim NN, Althof SE, Faubion SS, Faught BM, Parish SJ, Simon JA, Vignozzi L, Christiansen K, Davis SR, Freedman MA, Kingsberg SA, Kirana PS, Larkin L, McCabe M, Sadovsky R. The International Society for the Study of Women's sexual health process of Care for Management of hypoactive sexual desire disorder in women. Mayo Clin Proc. 2018;93(4):467–87. https://doi.org/10.1016/j.mayocp.2017.11.002.

15. Rosato E, Sciarra F, Anastasiadou E, Lenzi A, Venneri MA. Revisiting the physiological role of androgens in women. Expert Rev Endocrinol Metab. 2022;17(6):547–61. https://doi.org/1 0.1080/17446651.2022.2144834.

16. Maseroli E, Vignozzi L. Are endogenous androgens linked to female sexual function? A systemic review and meta-analysis. J Sex Med. 2022;19(4):553–68. https://doi.org/10.1016/j. jsxm.2022.01.515.

17. Pillerová M, Pastorek M, Borbélyová V, Riljak V, Frick KM, Hodosy J, Tóthová L. Sex steroid hormones in depressive disorders as a basis for new potential treatment strategies. Physiol Res. 2022;71(S2):S187–202. https://doi.org/10.33549/physiolres.935001.

18. Beach FA. Sexual attractivity, proceptivity, and receptivity in female mammals. Horm Behav. 1976;7:105–38.

19. Al-Azzawi F, Bitzer J, Brandenburg U, Castelo-Branco C, Graziottin A, Kenemans P, Lachowsky M, Mimoun S, Nappi RE, Palacios S, Schwenkhagen A, Studd J, Wylie K, Zahradnik HP. Therapeutic options for postmenopausal female sexual dysfunction. Climacteric. 2010;13(2):103–20. https://doi.org/10.3109/13697130903437615.

20. Hernández-Angeles C, Castelo-Branco C. Early menopause: a hazard to a woman's health. Indian J Med Res. 2016;143(4):420–7. https://doi.org/10.4103/0971-5916.184283.

21. van der Stege JG, Groen H, van Zadelhoff SJ, Lambalk CB, Braat DD, van Kasteren YM, van Santbrink EJ, Apperloo MJ, Weijmar Schultz WC, Hoek A. Decreased androgen concentrations and diminished general and sexual Well-being in women with premature ovarian failure. Menopause. 2008;15(1):23–31. https://doi.org/10.1097/gme.0b013e3180f6108c.

22. Ros C, Alobid I, Balasch J, Mullol J, Castelo-Branco C. Turner's syndrome and other forms of congenital hypogonadism impair quality of life and sexual function. Am J Obstet Gynecol. 2013;208(6):484.e1–6. https://doi.org/10.1016/j.ajog.2013.01.011.

23. Garrido Oyarzún MF, Castelo-Branco C. Sexuality and quality of life in congenital hypogonadisms. Gynecol Endocrinol. 2016;32(12):947–50. https://doi.org/10.1080/09513590.201 6.1241229.

24. Ziaei S, Moghasemi M, Faghihzadeh S. Comparative effects of conventional hormone replacement therapy and tibolone on climacteric symptoms and sexual dysfunction in postmenopausal women. Climacteric. 2010;13(2):147–56. https://doi.org/10.1080/13697130903009195.

25. Yu HF, Chen HS, Rao DP, Gong J. Association between polycystic ovary syndrome and the risk of pregnancy complications: a PRISMA-compliant systematic review and meta-analysis. Medicine (Baltimore). 2016;95(51):e4863. https://doi.org/10.1097/MD.0000000000004863.

26. Bozdag G, Mumusoglu S, Zengin D, Karabulut E, Yildiz BO. The prevalence and phenotypic features of polycystic ovary syndrome: a systematic review and meta-analysis. Hum Reprod. 2016;31(12):2841–55. https://doi.org/10.1093/humrep/dew218.

27. Bednarska S, Siejka A. The pathogenesis and treatment of polycystic ovary syndrome: What's new? Adv. Clin Exp Med. 2017;26(2):359–67. https://doi.org/10.17219/acem/59380.

28. Rotterdam ESHRE/ASRM-Sponsored PCOS Consensus Working Group. Revised 2003 consensus on diagnostic criteria and long-term health risks related to polycystic ovary syndrome (PCOS). Hum Reprod. 2004;19:41–7.

29. National Institute of Health. Evidence-based Methodology Workshop on Polycystic Ovary Syndrome. Final report. 2012. https://prevention.nih.gov/docs/programs/pcos/FinalReport. pdf. Accessed 1 Nov 2015.

30. Boomsma CM, Eijkemans MJ, Hughes EG, Visser GH, Fauser BC, Macklon NS. A meta-analysis of pregnancy outcomes in women with polycystic ovary syndrome. Hum Reprod Update. 2006;12(6):673–83. https://doi.org/10.1093/humupd/dml036.
31. Apridonidze T, Essah PA, Iuorno MJ, Nestler JE. Prevalence and characteristics of the metabolic syndrome in women with polycystic ovary syndrome. J Clin Endocrinol Metab. 2005;90(4):1929–35. https://doi.org/10.1210/jc.2004-1045.
32. Naumova I, Castelo-Branco C, Casals G. Psychological issues and sexual function in women with different infertility causes: focus on polycystic ovary syndrome. Reprod Sci. 2021;28(10):2830–8. https://doi.org/10.1007/s43032-021-00546-x.
33. Castelo-Branco C, Naumova I. Quality of life and sexual function in women with polycystic ovary syndrome: a comprehensive review. Gynecol Endocrinol. 2020;36(2):96–103. https://doi.org/10.1080/09513590.2019.1670788.
34. Borghi L, Leone D, Vegni E, Galiano V, Lepadatu C, Sulpizio P, Garzia E. Psychological distress, anger and quality of life in polycystic ovary syndrome: associations with biochemical, phenotypical and socio-demographic factors. J Psychosom Obstet Gynaecol. 2018;39(2):128–37. https://doi.org/10.1080/0167482X.2017.1311319.
35. Stapinska-Syniec A, Grabowska K, Szpotanska-Sikorska M, Pietrzak B. Depression, sexual satisfaction, and other psychological issues in women with polycystic ovary syndrome. Gynecol Endocrinol. 2018;34(7):597–600. https://doi.org/10.1080/09513590.201 8.1427713.
36. Lee I, Cooney LG, Saini S, Smith ME, Sammel MD, Allison KC, Dokras A. Increased risk of disordered eating in polycystic ovary syndrome. Fertil Steril. 2017;107(3):796–802. https://doi.org/10.1016/j.fertnstert.2016.12.014.
37. Kogure GS, Ribeiro VB, Lopes IP, Furtado CLM, Kodato S, Silva de Sá MF, Ferriani RA, Lara LADS, Maria Dos Reis R. Body image and its relationships with sexual functioning, anxiety, and depression in women with polycystic ovary syndrome. J Affect Disord. 2019;253:385–93. https://doi.org/10.1016/j.jad.2019.05.006.
38. Asik M, Altinbas K, Eroglu M, Karaahmet E, Erbag G, Ertekin H, Sen H. Evaluation of affective temperament and anxiety-depression levels of patients with polycystic ovary syndrome. J Affect Disord. 2015 Oct;1(185):214–8. https://doi.org/10.1016/j.jad.2015.06.043.
39. Ferraresi SR, Lara LA, Reis RM, Rosa e Silva AC. Changes in sexual function among women with polycystic ovary syndrome: a pilot study. J Sex Med. 2013;10(2):467–73. https://doi.org/10.1111/jsm.12011.
40. Jedel E, Waern M, Gustafson D, Landén M, Eriksson E, Holm G, Nilsson L, Lind AK, Janson PO, Stener-Victorin E. Anxiety and depression symptoms in women with polycystic ovary syndrome compared with controls matched for body mass index. Hum Reprod. 2010;25(2):450–6. https://doi.org/10.1093/humrep/dep384.
41. Benetti-Pinto CL, Ferreira SR, Antunes A Jr, Yela DA. The influence of body weight on sexual function and quality of life in women with polycystic ovary syndrome. Arch Gynecol Obstet. 2015;291(2):451–5. https://doi.org/10.1007/s00404-014-3423-1.
42. Rellini AH, Stratton N, Tonani S, Santamaria V, Brambilla E, Nappi RE. Differences in sexual desire between women with clinical versus biochemical signs of hyperandrogenism in polycystic ovarian syndrome. Horm Behav. 2013;63(1):65–71. https://doi.org/10.1016/j.yhbeh.2012.10.013.
43. De Frène V, Verhofstadt L, Loeys T, Stuyver I, Buysse A, De Sutter P. Sexual and relational satisfaction in couples where the woman has polycystic ovary syndrome: a dyadic analysis. Hum Reprod. 2015;30(3):625–31. https://doi.org/10.1093/humrep/deu342.
44. Ercan CM, Coksuer H, Aydogan U, Alanbay I, Keskin U, Karasahin KE, Baser I. Sexual dysfunction assessment and hormonal correlations in patients with polycystic ovary syndrome. Int J Impot Res. 2013;25(4):127–32. https://doi.org/10.1038/ijir.2013.2.
45. Jungheim ES, Lanzendorf SE, Odem RR, Moley KH, Chang AS, Ratts VS. Morbid obesity is associated with lower clinical pregnancy rates after in vitro fertilization in women with polycystic ovary syndrome. Fertil Steril. 2009;92(1):256–61. https://doi.org/10.1016/j.fertnstert.2008.04.063.

46. Joham AE, Teede HJ, Ranasinha S, Zoungas S, Boyle J. Prevalence of infertility and use of fertility treatment in women with polycystic ovary syndrome: data from a large community-based cohort study. J Womens Health (Larchmt). 2015;24(4):299–307. https://doi.org/10.1089/jwh.2014.5000.

47. Massarotti C, Gentile G, Ferreccio C, Scaruffi P, Remorgida V, Anserini P. Impact of infertility and infertility treatments on quality of life and levels of anxiety and depression in women undergoing in vitro fertilization. Gynecol Endocrinol. 2019;35(6):485–9. https://doi.org/10.1080/09513590.2018.1540575.

48. Bakhtiari A, Basirat Z, Nasiri-Amiri F. Sexual dysfunction in women undergoing fertility treatment in Iran: prevalence and associated risk factors. J Reprod Infertil. 2016;17(1):26–33.

49. Larson JH, Anderson SM, Holman TB, Niemann BK. A longitudinal study of the effects of premarital communication, relationship stability, and self-esteem on sexual satisfaction in the first year of marriage. J Sex Marital Ther. 1998;24(3):193–206. https://doi.org/10.1080/00926239808404933.

50. Dokras A, Clifton S, Futterweit W, Wild R. Increased risk for abnormal depression scores in women with polycystic ovary syndrome: a systematic review and meta-analysis. Obstet Gynecol. 2011;117(1):145–52. https://doi.org/10.1097/AOG.0b013e318202b0a4.

51. Kiejna A, Piotrowski P, Adamowski T, Moskalewicz J, Wciórka J, Stokwiszewski J, Rabczenko D, Kessler R. The prevalence of common mental disorders in the population of adult Poles by sex and age structure - an EZOP Poland study. Psychiatr Pol. 2015;49(1):15–27. https://doi.org/10.12740/PP/30811.

52. Dashti S, Latiff LA, Hamid HA, Sani SM, Akhtari-Zavare M, Abu Bakar AS, Binti Sabri NA, Ismail M, Esfehani AJ. Sexual dysfunction in patients with polycystic ovary syndrome in Malaysia. Asian Pac J Cancer Prev. 2016;17(8):3747–51.

53. Pastoor H, Timman R, de Klerk C, Bramer M, W, Laan ET, Laven JS. Sexual function in women with polycystic ovary syndrome: a systematic review and meta-analysis. Reprod Biomed Online. 2018;37(6):750–60. https://doi.org/10.1016/j.rbmo.2018.09.010.

54. Fliegner M, Richter-Appelt H, Krupp K, Brunner F. Sexual function and socio-sexual difficulties in women with polycystic ovary syndrome (PCOS). Geburtshilfe Frauenheilkd. 2019;79(5):498–509. https://doi.org/10.1055/a-0828-7901.

55. Lim SS, Hutchison SK, Van Ryswyk E, Norman RJ, Teede HJ, Moran LJ. Lifestyle changes in women with polycystic ovary syndrome. Cochrane Database Syst Rev. 2019;3(3):CD007506. https://doi.org/10.1002/14651858.CD007506.pub4.

56. Sarwer DB, Wadden TA, Spitzer JC, Mitchell JE, Lancaster K, Courcoulas A, Gourash W, Rosen RC, Christian NJ. 4-year changes in sex hormones, sexual functioning, and psychosocial status in women who underwent bariatric surgery. Obes Surg. 2018;28(4):892–9. https://doi.org/10.1007/s11695-017-3025-7.

57. Caruso S, Palermo G, Caruso G, Rapisarda AMC. How does contraceptive use affect Women's sexuality? A novel look at sexual acceptability. J Clin Med. 2022;11(3):810. https://doi.org/10.3390/jcm11030810.

58. Caruso S, Rugolo S, Agnello C, Romano M, Cianci A. Quality of sexual life in hyperandrogenic women treated with an oral contraceptive containing chlormadinone acetate. J Sex Med. 2009;6(12):3376–84. https://doi.org/10.1111/j.1743-6109.2009.01529.x.

59. Steinberg Weiss M, Roe AH, Allison KC, Dodson WC, Kris-Etherton PM, Kunselman AR, Stetter CM, Williams NI, Gnatuk CL, Estes SJ, Sarwer DB, Coutifaris C, Legro RS, Dokras A. Lifestyle modifications alone or combined with hormonal contraceptives improve sexual dysfunction in women with polycystic ovary syndrome. Fertil Steril. 2021;115(2):474–82. https://doi.org/10.1016/j.fertnstert.2020.08.1396.

Endocrine Disorders and Sexuality III: Diabetes and Sexual Disorders

Irene Vinagre and Aida Orois

1   Introduction

Diabetes can be related to the appearance of long-term chronic complications, including sexual dysfunction, both in men and women. The number of publications and citations regarding sexual function and diabetes has steadily increased over the few past decades [1]. In a recent study, one-third of adults with type 1 (T1D) or type 2 diabetes (T2D), men or women, reported a sexual dysfunction, associated with distress, low emotional well-being, and anxiety symptoms [2]. Also, it has been described that sexual orientation can influence diabetes, reporting higher levels of noncompliance with diabetes management guidelines among sexual minorities [3]. This information can be used to develop appropriate interventions to improve diabetes management for this population.

Erectile dysfunction, retrograde ejaculation, and low sexual desire may appear in men with diabetes, especially when there is a chronic poor metabolic control. In the case of women with diabetes, sexual dysfunction is characterized by low sexual desire, vaginal lubrication disorders, anorgasmia, or dyspareunia, among others. Next, we will describe the aforementioned alterations in men and women in greater detail.

I. Vinagre (✉) · A. Orois
Endocrinology and Nutrition Department, Clinical Institute of Digestive and Metabolic Diseases, Hospital Clínic de Barcelona, Barcelona, Spain
e-mail: ivinagre@clinic.cat; aorois@clinic.cat

2　Sexual Dysfunction in Men with Diabetes

2.1　Erectile Dysfunction

Erectile dysfunction is characterized by a persistent inability to achieve and maintain an erection sufficient to allow satisfactory sexual activity. It is the most common sexual complication in men with advanced diabetes: Its prevalence is 35–75%, being three times higher than in the general population of the same age, worsening the quality of life of men and their partners. The pathophysiology is multifactorial, as a result of metabolic, vascular, and neurological abnormalities. Thus, there is impaired relaxation of the smooth muscle of the corpus cavernosum in subjects with diabetes in response to reduced production of nitric oxide of neural and endothelial origin, due, in part, to the accumulation of advanced glycosylation products. Likewise, there is an increase in the expression of certain vasoconstrictor products produced by the endothelium, such as endothelin-1 and its receptor, and an increase in the release of norepinephrine from the adrenergic endings, which maintains the state of vasoconstriction and flaccidity.

Obviously, the presence of other pathologies and concomitant treatments also have an influence: hypertension, smoking, or dyslipidemia can affect the endothelium, and drugs such as antihypertensive and antidepressants could affect sexual function. Regarding the effect of antidiabetic treatments in sexual function, there is still small evidence and mainly in nonhuman models [4]. Treatment with metformin in patients with erectile dysfunction and poor response to sildenafil reduced the insulin resistance and improved erectile function, but diabetes was an exclusion criterion [5]. The novel classes of antihyperglycemic drugs, that are associated with loss of weight (GLP1 analogs and SGLT2 inhibitors), could indirectly improve the gonadal axis. In fact, some studies have begun to link the use of GLP1 analogs with the improvement of serum testosterone levels [6].

Also, there is a progressive reduction of testosterone levels associated with age, but more intense in patients with T2D and obesity compared with healthy subjects [7]. The relationship between diabetes and testosterone is thought to be bidirectional: On the one hand, subjects with diabetes often have hypogonadism, which worsens sexual dysfunction, and on the other hand, patients with hypogonadism have greater insulin resistance and risk of developing diabetes.

In T1D, C-peptide deficiency may be involved, at least partially, in the development of sexual/reproductive dysfunction [8]. When exposed to C-peptide, cavernosal smooth muscle cells increase the production of nitric oxide. C-peptide in rats with diabetes improves sperm count, sperm motility, testosterone levels, and nerve conduction compared to non-treated diabetic rats [9]. However, further studies in humans are needed.

2.1.1　Diagnosis

The evaluation of the subject with diabetes and impotence should be based on taking a detailed clinical history to characterize the symptoms (defining whether the erectile dysfunction is primary or secondary, the time of evolution, the form of onset, etc.). It is important that health care professionals proactively ask the patient about this problem, which, although it does not compromise life, can be very relevant for both the patient and his environment, as it may be sometimes a taboo subject due to psychosocial barriers. Moreover, evidence suggests that erectile dysfunction can represent an early marker of cardiovascular disease in people with diabetes, so early diagnosis is very important [9].

In order to quantify the degree of erectile dysfunction, the use of certain brief questionnaires may be useful. If there are normal erections under certain circumstances, the erectile mechanism will be preserved. A normal maximum erection followed by intravaginal detumescence before orgasm will suggest a psychogenic etiology. On the contrary, organic alterations will always be accompanied by incomplete erections, with a tendency to improve slightly at the moment of climax.

Diagnostic tests to arrive at the etiology of erectile dysfunction are not very specific. Erectile response can be verified by administering vasodilator drugs (prostaglandin E1) with application of a tourniquet at the base of the penis for 2 min and evaluation of tumescence, angle, and rigidity at 15 and 30 min. A complete erection of 1 h or more will be considered positive and will report vascular normality. Penile echo-Doppler ultrasonography analyzes the vascular component in more detail. The functional study of the venous component can be completed by dynamic cavernometry and cavernography. To detect nocturnal penile tumescence, characterized by the appearance of spontaneous erections in certain phases of sleep, generated from the central nervous system without the effect of the cerebral cortex, the recording of nocturnal erections is used. The most informative method is the RigiScan®, provided with two rings that simultaneously record changes in girth and rigidity at the base and tip of the penis. This record must be made during three nights to obtain representative information.

2.1.2 Treatment

Treatment includes lifestyle changes, such as quitting tobacco and alcohol, reducing body weight, and including physical activity in the daily routine. Within the specific treatments, first-line treatments of erectile dysfunction are specific inhibitors of the enzyme phosphodiesterase type 5 (PDE5i). When oral treatment is not possible or effective, intracavernous injections, intraurethral suppositories, vacuum erection systems, and penile prostheses are other therapeutic alternatives, which are described below [10].

Phosphodiesterase Type 5 Inhibitors

PDE5is are considered the first-line therapy for erectile dysfunction of any etiology. They prevent the degradation of cGMP in the muscle cell, amplifying the myocyte's response to normal erection stimuli. Thus, they improve and prolong erections mediated by sexual stimuli and nocturnal erections. They do not act if there is no sexual arousal, they are administered on demand, and their effect is appreciated after 1 h of oral administration. They do not cause priapism. The effect of the drug increases after the first doses. The first marketed drug was sildenafil, and later vardenafil, tadalafil, and avanafil were developed. Udenafil and mirodenafil are

Table 1 Characteristics of the main Phosphodiesterase type 5-inhibitors (PDE5i)

	SILDENAFIL	VARDENAFIL	TADALAFIL	AVANAFIL
Dose (mg)	25-50-100	5-10-20	5-10-20	50-100-200
Tmax (hours)	0.7–0.9	1	2	0.5–0.75
Half life (hours)	3–5	3–5	18	3–5
Effective interval (hours after intake)	1–6	1–6	1–36	0.5–6
Absolute contraindications	Treatment with nitrates Blood pressure <90/50 mmHg Active or unstable ischemic heart disease NYHA class III-IV heart failure Recent episodes (3–6 months) of heart attack, stroke, or congestive heart failure Anterior ischemic optic neuropathy			
Relative contraindications	Risk factors for priapism Active digestive ulcer Hepatic or renal failure -adjust dose- Retinitis pigmentosa			
Caution	Hypertension treated with multiple drugs, Orthostatic hypotension Treatment with α-blockers Treatment with CYP3 inhibitors (indinavir, ritonavir, erythromycin, ketoconazole…)			

T_{max} maximal concentration in plasma

approved in very few countries. Nowadays, superiority of one PDE5i over the others cannot be clearly determined [11], with the duration of the effect being the main difference between them. Also, different doses and regimens of treatment have been proposed [12]. Table 1 describes the most important characteristics of the main PDE5i and their contraindications. They are effective in 50–65% of subjects with diabetes and erectile dysfunction, compared with 20–25% of placebo responders. Its benefit is lower in subjects with diabetes compared to the general population. Up to 50% of patients drop out from treatment despite being effective, which reveals that isolated symptomatic treatment is not effective and psychological support must be associated with psychosexual and couple's education.

Intracavernous Injection of Drugs

The most commonly used intracavernous erection-inducing drugs are papaverine hydrochloride (smooth muscle relaxant), prostaglandin E1 (PGE1) (acts on vascular prostanoid receptors), and phentolamine (α-receptor blocker). The indications for intracavernous treatment include the entire spectrum of etiologies, with erectile dysfunction of neurological origin being the one that responds best. It is not a treatment for libido or anorgasmia problems. Small doses of papaverine (5–15 mg) or PGE1 (5–10 μg) are usually enough, although when the cause is vascular, it may be necessary to increase the dose up to 40 mg papaverine or 20–30 μg PGE1 or use combinations of both drugs in compound preparation (papaverine 30 mg and PGE1 20 μg). Good instruction and counseling for self-injection by patients are essential. Intracavernous injection can be applied to subjects undergoing anticoagulant treatment, but it is not recommended in states of blood hyperviscosity or risk of priapism (sustained erection for more than 4 h without sexual stimulation), such as multiple myeloma, polycythemia, or anemia of sickle cells. The most common side effects of intracavernous treatment are pain in the injection area, bruising, appearance of fibrotic nodules that can sometimes cause curvature, urethral injuries due to failed injection, and priapism. This last complication can cause tissue hypoxia and irreversible damage to erectile tissue if it lasts for more than 6 h. For this reason, patients must be informed that if the erection persists after 4 h of self-injection, without sexual stimulation, it is advisable to perform physical exercise first and, if it does not subside, seek urgent medical help.

Intraurethral Suppositories

An alternative to the treatment of erectile dysfunction is prostaglandin suppositories (alprostadil), which are administered intraurethrally. It is administered using a disposable applicator that inserts a small alprostadil suppository about the size of half a grain of rice into the tip of the penis. The suppository, placed about 5 cm into the urethra, is absorbed by the erectile tissue in the penis, increasing the blood flow that will produce an erection. The advantage over the other two previous methods is that it can be used during sexual activity and it works in the short term. It can be useful for patients that dislike injectable therapies, although its efficacy is lower compared to intracavernous injection. Patients with diabetes, especially those using insulin therapy, have higher compliance with self-injections compared to those without diabetes [13]. Contraindications are the same as for intracavernous injection of prostaglandins. As adverse effects, there may be burning at the urethral level, pain, small bleeding in the urethra, fibrous tissue formation, dizziness, and also irritation of the partner's mucosa, if a condom is not used.

Topical Treatments

Alprostadil cream administered into the external urethral meatus promoted adequate erection in 74–83% of patients with similarly good results in populations with diabetes and those unresponsive to PDE5i according to several studies [14].

Vacuum Erection Systems (Vacuum)

Systems that induce erection by negative pressure or vacuum represent another viable alternative, being effective in 85% of patients regardless of the etiology. It consists of a rigid and transparent cylinder that fits at the base of the penis, sealed with lubricant. With a manual or electric suction pump, a vacuum is produced so that blood flows into the penis and engorgement occurs. Once sufficient rigidity has been achieved, an elastic constriction ring is applied to the base of the penis (to retain blood in the corpora cavernosa) and the cylinder is removed. It can be kept for a maximum of 30 min. Some studies suggest that the combination of a vacuum erectile device with electromagnetic low-intensity extracorporeal shock has better results in the treatment of patients with diabetes and erectile dysfunction who were unresponsive to PDE5i [15]. The main contraindications for the use of vacuum systems would be treatment with anticoagulants, penile deformities, or urinary incontinence.

Surgical Treatment

When other treatments are not effective or satisfactory, the implantation of a penile prosthesis is the best therapeutic option in men with diabetes and erectile dysfunction. In this case, the satisfaction is more than 95% of the subjects. However, it is an irreversible treatment since the prostheses replace the cavernous erectile tissue, occupying its entire volume. There is also an incidence of more than 10% of infections or intolerance to the prosthesis in subjects with diabetes, especially in those with other advanced chronic complications [16]. There are malleable, inexpensive prostheses that are practically free of mechanical problems, which are implanted with a simple surgery that requires only locoregional anesthesia, although they have the drawback of having an unphysiological appearance at rest. Thus, the most commonly used prostheses today are hydraulic or inflatable, which consist of the presence of internally empty cylinders that can be filled with liquid from a reservoir that is pumped at will. However, the connections can fail with some frequency and experience fluid leaks from the system. These prostheses are more expensive and require a long and aggressive surgical intervention under general or epidural anesthesia. Its main advantage is that during penis deflation, it looks quite similar to the physiological one.

On the other hand, arterial reconstructive surgery is limited to entities such as atheromatous occlusions of the aortic bifurcation or the proximal portion of the iliac arteries (Leriche syndrome), as long as the distal arterial territory is preserved.

2.2   Retrograde Ejaculation

Anterograde ejaculation is a complex reflex controlled by the medullary vegetative centers and depends on the coordination of three neurological processes: emission of secretions from the prostate, the deferential ampullae, and the seminal vesicles into the posterior urethra; the closure of the internal and external urethral sphincter, which is accompanied by the sensation of imminent orgasm; and the expulsion phase, which depends on the parasympathetic, during which the external sphincter opens and the semen is expelled to the exterior by the clonic contractions of the perineal muscles.

In subjects with diabetes and neuropathy, proximal sphincter muscle tone may decrease, and the ejaculate travels upward toward the bladder during the ejection phase, known as retrograde ejaculation. Its prevalence is 10–30% of patients with T1D of more than 10 years of evolution [17]. This process has also been described in patients being treated with tamsulosin for prostatic hyperplasia. It is clinically manifested by a reduction in the volume of the ejaculate, with the consequent sterility, although the sensation of orgasm is usually preserved. Flowmetry and dynamic and postvoid bladder ultrasound can be performed to study the contractile capacity of the neck and bladder residue. Mechanical treatment can be useful in cases of incomplete or intermittent retrograde ejaculation and consists of increasing pressure on the bladder neck to keep the proximal sphincter closed. This can be achieved by keeping the bladder full and assuming the standing position at the time of ejaculation. Alternative pharmacological strategies to restore antegrade ejaculation temporarily in order to help close the bladder neck are anticholinergics, antihistamines, and alpha-adrenergics. With regard to fertility, spermatozoa can be recovered in post-orgasm urine for being used in assisted reproductive techniques.

2.3 Low Sexual Desire

Type 2 diabetes, especially if associated with obesity or metabolic syndrome, has been related to low levels of total testosterone and free testosterone, with a prevalence of hypogonadism of 25–50% depending on the series. This hypoandrogenism causes a decrease in libido with a reduction in the frequency of erotic thoughts and sexual activity and decreases the quality of orgasm and the volume of semen. The quantity and quality of voluntary and reflex erections also depend on the serum testosterone concentration. Although the results are controversial, some studies support that testosterone treatment in hypogonadal men with diabetes decreases weight and improves glycemic control by reducing insulin resistance [18], with the effect on sexual function being less evident. On the other hand, in the corpus cavernosum, the nitric oxide pathway is partly regulated by testosterone levels. Thus, the administration of testosterone in hypogonadal men potentiates the effects of sildenafil (PDE5i) and achieves an effect in those individuals who initially do not respond to this drug [19].

2.4 Psychological Interventions

It is known that the prevalence of depression and distress is high in patients with diabetes. Nevertheless, no evidence currently exists on the effectiveness of psychological therapies for men with diabetes. In fact, the psychological approach is not even mentioned in the therapeutic algorithms, which are focused on biological factors.

3 Sexual Dysfunction in Women with Diabetes

Several studies have shown a significantly higher prevalence of sexual dysfunction among women with T1D compared with healthy controls, but the causes, types, and risk factors are still unclear. There are many causes for the increased incidence of sexual dysfunction in women with T1D, including organic and psychosocial factors. The involvement of psychological and social factors in the expression of female sexuality is complex, and they are strongly associated with biological factors. Female sexual dysfunction is characterized by low sexual desire, vaginal lubrication disorders, anorgasmia, and dyspareunia. Although both physicians and patients tend to ignore female sexual dysfunction and it is probably underdiagnosed, the known prevalence is 25–70% in women with T1D and 40–50% in women with T2D, remaining double the rate for women of the same age without diabetes [20, 21]. Some studies show a higher frequency of sexual dysfunction in women with chronic complications of diabetes, although other authors do not confirm this affirmation. However, a recent meta-analysis of 26 observational studies showed a higher prevalence of sexual dysfunction in women with any type of diabetes and any duration (OR 2.02) compared with controls [22].

3.1 Factors Affecting Sexual Dysfunction in Women with Diabetes

There are some organic factors, such as autonomic neuropathy, decreased blood supply due to vascular damage, hormonal changes, and a greater risk of genitourinary tract infections, that can favor sexual dysfunction in women with diabetes (Fig. 1). Moreover, high or low blood glucose levels can also lead to vaginal dryness, pain during sex, and a lack of ability to have an orgasm, which may affect sexual function in women. In addition, people with diabetes may also present depression more frequently, and this is associated with reduced sexual desire. Specific problems related to diabetes can affect body image such as wearing medical devices or lipohypertrophy from injection sites. The need to test glucose prior to

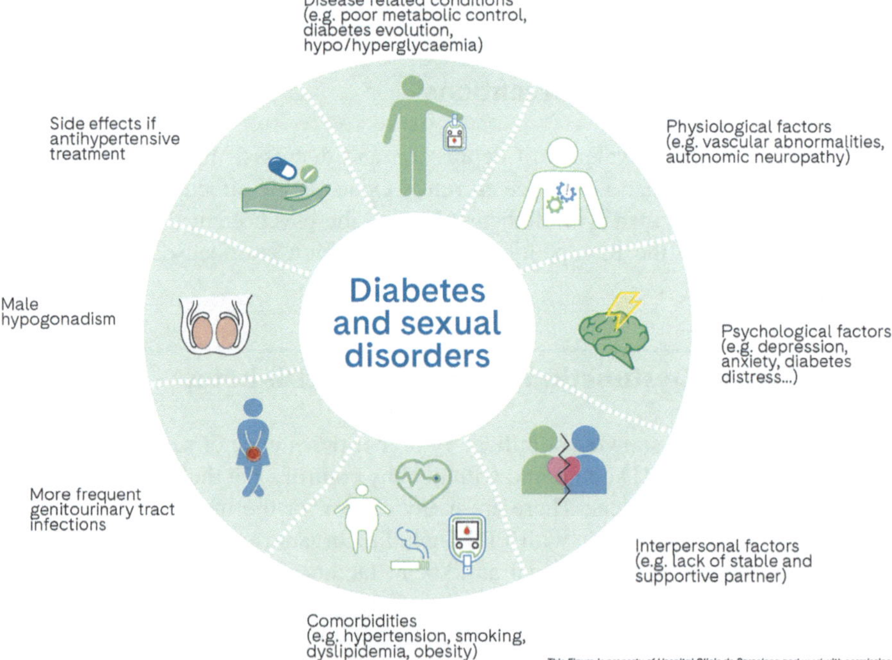

Fig. 1 Factor influencing the development of sexual dysfunction among patients complaining with diabetes

sexual act to avoid hypoglycemia, or the fear of having a hypoglycemia during sex, can affect its quality too. And finally, there is also an association between decreased sexual desire and diabetes distress, as it is highlighted in the study of Van Cauwenberghe et al. [2]. This study also reported a significant correlation between sexual dysfunction and impaired psychological well-being in women with T1D. Accordingly, a study from a Norwegian cohort also indicated that having a stable and supportive partner seemed to be important in dealing with the sexual challenges [23]. Likewise, two previous systematic reviews of the literature emphasized that social support and greater marital satisfaction were associated with better diabetes outcomes [24, 25].

3.2   Identification and Assessment of Sexual Dysfunction in Women with Diabetes

Identification of sexual dysfunction in women with diabetes may be difficult. On the one hand, up to 50% of women are unaware that sexual dysfunction might be diabetes related. On the other hand, health care professionals are not sufficiently aware of sexual problems in women. As an example, structured education programs do not discuss sexual dysfunction in women with diabetes, perhaps because this is not recognized as a problem in diabetes guidelines. Moreover, diabetes specialists are probably more concerned about preventing unplanned pregnancy in women with diabetes, rather than sexual problems. And finally, although sexual dysfunction is considered important to the well-being of men with diabetes, the impact of sexual dysfunction for women may remain unnoticed.

All the domains of sexual cycle in women including desire, arousal, lubrication, orgasm, and satisfaction have been reported to be affected in both T1D and T2D patients. However, diabetes seems to have a greater impact on desire than on the other sexual domains, maybe both by a disorder of primary interest due to the hormonal effects, but also secondary to alterations in arousal, lubrication, and pain, which make sexual activity non-pleasurable, and therefore, interest is lost secondarily. Genital arousal and lubrication are neurovascular events that represent an interplay between smooth muscle relaxation and contraction, similar to the process involved in male. Accordingly, similar to what is observed in erectile dysfunction, genital arousal disorder in women with diabetes might be related to neurovascular alterations due to chronic hyperglycemia and vascular impairment in genital areas with altered genital response to sexual stimuli. As reported for men, hormonal medium can affect sexuality in women with diabetes too. Available data are mainly derived from animal models. Insulin and insulin-like growth factors (IGFs) can regulate the activities of aromatase and 3β-hydroxysteroid dehydrogenase, which are involved in steroid synthesis. Some experimental data also suggest that insulin can contribute to maintaining estrogen receptor expression at the hypothalamus level, having a role in sexual behavior in female rats. In addition, peripherally, both insulin and other growth factors stimulate the proliferation of mouse vaginal epithelial cells and, in the vagina, estrogens seem to stimulate the production of IGF and

IGF-binding proteins. Sexual pain is another important issue related to women sexuality. Unexplained vulvodynia has been proposed as an unrecognized sign of diabetic neuropathic syndrome, although recent consensus did not support diabetes as a potential pathogenic mechanism [26]. Instead, dyspareunia could be explained by neuropathy and vascular impairment, as well as due to vaginal candidiasis.

On the other hand, sexual dysfunction is known to be associated with cardiovascular complications in men, and there is evidence that women with diabetes and sexual dysfunction can also have cardiovascular and neurological complications. In the Diabetes Control and Complications Trial/Epidemiology of Diabetes Interventions and Complications (DCCT/EDIC), women with T1D and sexual dysfunction had more risk of developing cardiovascular autonomic neuropathy (OR 1.52) [27]. Moreover, in a study comparing 30 women with diabetes and 20 normal sexually active women, the first group had reduced sensation around genital sites, although it was not associated with sexual dysfunction score on the Female Sexual Function Index (FSFI) [28]. Then, the presence of sexual dysfunction in women could be a sign of advanced diabetes complications and would require further investigation of other diabetes complications.

3.3 Treatment

There are some pharmacological options and non-pharmacological interventions, as we will explain above.

3.3.1 Phosphodiesterase 5 Inhibitors

It is thought that PDE5i may also improve blood flow to the clitoris and restore some sexual function for women. Although some improvements in sexual function could be established from the results of the studies, such as improvements in arousal and orgasm, no effect on desire, the main sexual disorder, was found. In addition, these drugs do not work improving the psychological sexual response, which is an important issue in women's sexual dysfunction. Therefore, they are not accepted for the treatment of women with sexual dysfunction and T1D as the evidence for their use is inconclusive. On the other hand, for women with T2D, PDE5i has been tested to improve heart failure rather than to treat sexual dysfunction [26].

3.3.2 Menopausal Hormone Therapy

Menopausal hormone therapy (MHT) includes estrogen with or without progesterone, and it is known that it can improve sexual functioning in postmenopausal women. However, MHT increases the risk of breast cancer and thromboembolism; therefore, it is now only prescribed as the treatment for menopausal symptoms at lowest effective doses and during the time required. In women, higher plasma levels of estrogen and testosterone are associated with insulin resistance and incidence of T2D. Testosterone treatment is thought to boost sexual function in postmenopausal women when it is added to conventional hormonal therapy, but specific studies for women with diabetes are lacking [26].

3.3.3   Antidepressant Therapy

There is some evidence to suggest that treating depression in diabetes can lead to improved sexual function. However, selective serotonin reuptake inhibitors (SSRIs) such as paroxetine and venlafaxine are associated with reduction in sexual functioning, while mirtazapine would be the one that least affects. Instead, bupropion, an atypical antidepressant (a norepinephrine-dopamine reuptake inhibitor) commonly used in smoking cessation and to treat major depressive disorder (MDD), has demonstrated improvements in sexual energy scores in women with T2D and MDD, but in the analysis of secondary data [26].

3.3.4   Weight Loss

Reducing weight and thereby improving perceived body image may be a useful strategy for the treatment of sexual dysfunction in women with diabetes. The Look AHEAD trial demonstrated that women with T2D and obesity who participated in the intensive lifestyle intervention arm had a significant improvement in sexual function, based on the FSFI, compared with controls [29]. Improvements in sexual function have also been demonstrated in women with diabetes who have undergone bariatric surgery. While the use of metformin is known to have a beneficial effect on male and female reproductive function, the novel classes of antihyperglycemic drugs (GLP1 analogs and SGLT2 inhibitors) have shown effect on weight loss and could be an interesting, although indirect, way to improve the gonadal and sexual function in women complaining of sexual dysfunction [4].

3.3.5   Psychological Interventions

Psychological interventions to improve sexual dysfunction in women have been made. As an example, the Permission, Limited Information, Specific Suggestions, and Intensive Therapy (PLISSIT) framework has been developed to assist the treatment of sexual problems. Results showed a significant improvement in satisfaction, orgasm, lubrication, arousal, and sexual desire in women with gynecologic and breast cancer and sexual dysfunction [30]. Nevertheless, limited evidence currently exists on the effectiveness of the PLISSIT framework for women with diabetes.

4   Conclusion

Sexual dysfunction is frequently observed in men and women with diabetes, especially when there is poor metabolic chronic control or long evolution. Among individuals with diabetes, it can correlate with depression, anxiety, and difficulties in living with diabetes, including body image issues and hyper- or hypoglycemia. In addition, it can severely impair the quality of life, eventually leading to relationship difficulties and breakdown, resulting in worse metabolic control and poor therapeutic compliance. Moreover, sexual dysfunction can be an early marker of cardiovascular disease in both men and women, and it should be routinely investigated. A timely identification of the problem and an adequate approach can allow lifestyle modifications and better metabolic control. Including sexual health as part of diabetes follow-up could give a more comprehensive health service for people with diabetes, and holistic treatments need to be available in diabetes services.

References

1. Meng F, Liao X, Chen H, Sheng Deng S, Wang L, Zhao M, et al. Bibliometric and visualization analysis of literature relating to diabetic erectile dysfunction. Front Endocrinol (Lausanne). 2022;13:1091999. https://doi.org/10.3389/fendo.2022.1091999.
2. Van Cauwenberghe J, Enzlin P, Nefs G, Ruige J, Hendrieckx C, De Block C, et al. Prevalence of and risk factors for sexual dysfunctions in adults with type 1 or type 2 diabetes: results from diabetes MILES - Flanders. Diabet Med. 2022;39(1):e14676. https://doi.org/10.1111/dme.14676.
3. Tran P, Tran L, Tran L. Influence of sexual orientation on diabetes management in US adults with diabetes. Diabetes Metab. 2021;47(1):101177. https://doi.org/10.1016/j.diabet.2020.07.004.
4. Corona G, Isidori AM, Aversa A, Bonomi M, Ferlin A, Foresta C, et al. Male and female sexual dysfunction in diabetic subjects: focus on new antihyperglycemic drugs. Rev Endocr Metab Disord. 2020;21(1):57–65. https://doi.org/10.1007/s11154-019-09535-7.
5. Rey-Valzacchi GJ, Costanzo PR, Finger LA, Layus AO, Gueglio GM, Litwak LE, et al. Addition of metformin to sildenafil treatment for erectile dysfunction in eugonadal nondiabetic men with insulin resistance. A prospective, randomized, double-blind pilot study. J Androl. 2012;33(4):608–14. https://doi.org/10.2164/jandrol.111.013714.
6. Shao N, Yu XY, Yu YM, Li BW, Pan J, Wu WH, et al. Short-term combined treatment with exenatide and metformin is superior to glimepiride combined metformin in improvement of serum testosterone levels in type 2 diabetic patients with obesity. Andrologia. 2018;50(7):e13039. https://doi.org/10.1111/and.13039.
7. Corona G, Monami M, Rastrelli G, Aversa A, Sforza A, Lenzi A, et al. Type 2 diabetes mellitus and testosterone: a meta-analysis study. Int J Androl. 2011;34(6 Pt 1):528–40. https://doi.org/10.1111/j.1365-2605.2010.01117.x.
8. Pujia R, Maurotti S, Coppola A, Romeo S, Pujia A, Montalcini T. The potential role of C-peptide in sexual and reproductive functions in type 1 diabetes mellitus: an update. Curr Diabetes Rev. 2022;18(1):e051021196983. https://doi.org/10.2174/1573399817666211005093434.
9. Yamada T, Hara K, Umematsu H, Suzuki R, Kadowaki T. Erectile dysfunction and cardiovascular events in diabetic men: a meta-analysis of observational studies. PLoS One. 2012;7(9):e43673. https://doi.org/10.1371/journal.pone.0043673.
10. Redrow GP, Thompson CM, Wang R. Treatment strategies for diabetic patients suffering from erectile dysfunction: an update. Expert Opin Pharmacother. 2014;15(13):1827–36. https://doi.org/10.1517/14656566.2014.934809.
11. Liao X, Qiu S, Bao Y, Wang W, Yang L, Wei Q. Comparative efficacy and safety of phosphodiesterase type 5 inhibitors for erectile dysfunction in diabetic men: a Bayesian network meta-analysis of randomized controlled trials. World J Urol. 2019;37(6):1061–74. https://doi.org/10.1007/s00345-018-2583-1.
12. Yıldırım Ç, Salman MY, Yavuz A, Bayar G. Comparison of three different tadalafil regimens for erectile dysfunction treatment in patients with diabetes mellitus microvascular complications. Andrologia. 2022;54(10):e14536. https://doi.org/10.1111/and.14536.
13. Perimenis P, Gyftopoulos K, Athanasopoulos A, Barbalias G. Diabetic impotence treated by intracavernosal injections: high treatment compliance and increasing dosage of vaso-active drugs. Eur Urol. 2001;40(4):398–402.; discussion 403. https://doi.org/10.1159/000049806.
14. Rooney M, Pfister W, Mahoney M, Nelson M, Yeager J, Steidle C. Long-term, multicenter study of the safety and efficacy of topical alprostadil cream in male patients with erectile dysfunction. J Sex Med. 2009;6(2):520–34. https://doi.org/10.1111/j.1743-6109.2008.01118.x.

15. Tao R, Chen J, Wang D, Li Y, Xiang J, Xiong L, et al. The efficacy of Li-ESWT combined with VED in diabetic ED patients unresponsive to PDE5is: a single-center, randomized clinical trial. Front Endocrinol (Lausanne). 2022;13:937958. https://doi.org/10.3389/fendo.2022.937958.

16. Lipsky MJ, Onyeji I, Golan R, Munarriz R, Kashanian JA, Stember DS, et al. Diabetes is a risk factor for inflatable penile prosthesis infection: analysis of a large statewide database. Sex Med. 2019;7(1):35–40. https://doi.org/10.1016/j.esxm.2018.11.007.

17. Fedder J, Kaspersen MD, Brandslund I, Højgaard A. Retrograde ejaculation and sexual dysfunction in men with diabetes mellitus: a prospective, controlled study. Andrology. 2013;1(4):602–6. https://doi.org/10.1111/j.2047-2927.2013.00083.x.

18. Andlib N, Sajad M, Kumar R, Thakur SC. Abnormalities in sex hormones and sexual dysfunction in males with diabetes mellitus: a mechanistic insight. Acta Histochem. 2023;125(1):151974. https://doi.org/10.1016/j.acthis.2022.151974.

19. Grant P, Jackson G, Baig I, Quin J. Erectile dysfunction in general medicine. Clin Med. 2013;13(2):136–40. https://doi.org/10.7861/clinmedicine.13-2-136.

20. Ahmed MR, Shaaban MM, Sedik WF, Mohamed TY. Prevalence and differences between type 1 and type 2 diabetes mellitus regarding female sexual dysfunction: a cross-sectional Egyptian study. J Psychosom Obstet Gynaecol. 2018;39(3):176–81. https://doi.org/10.108 0/0167482X.2017.1318123.

21. Enzlin P, Mathieu C, van den Bruel A, Vanderschueren D, Demyttenaere K. Prevalence and predictors of sexual dysfunction in patients with type 1 diabetes. Diabetes Care. 2003;26(2):409–14. https://doi.org/10.2337/diacare.26.2.409.

22. Pontiroli AE, Cortelazzi D, Morabito A. Female sexual dysfunction and diabetes: a systematic review and meta- analysis. J Sex Med. 2013;10(4):1044–51. https://doi.org/10.1111/jsm.12065.

23. Buskoven M, Kjørholt E, Strandberg R, Søfteland E, Haugstvedt A. Sexual dysfunction in women with type 1 diabetes in Norway: a qualitative study of women's experiences. Diabet Med. 2022;39(7):e14856. https://doi.org/10.1111/dme.14856.

24. Strom JL, Egede LE. The impact of social support on outcomes in adult patients with type 2 diabetes: a systematic review. Curr Diab Rep. 2012;12:769–81. https://doi.org/10.1007/s11892-012-0317-0.

25. Rintala TM, Jaatinen P, Paavilainen E, Astedt-Kurki P. Interrelation between adult persons with diabetes and their family: a systematic review of the literature. J Fam Nurs. 2013;19:3–28. https://doi.org/10.1177/1074840712471899.

26. Winkley K, Kristensen C, Fosbury J. Sexual health and function in women with diabetes. Diabet Med. 2021;38(11):e14644. https://doi.org/10.1111/dme.14644.

27. Hotaling JM, Sarma AV, Patel DP, Braffett BH, Cleary PA, Feldman E, et al. Cardiovascular autonomic neuropathy, sexual dysfunction, and urinary incontinence in women with type 1 diabetes. Diabetes Care. 2016;39(9):1587–93. https://doi.org/10.2337/dc16-0059.

28. Erol B, Tefekli A, Sanli O, Ziylan O, Armagan A, Kendirci M, et al. Does sexual dysfunction correlate with deterioration of somatic sensory system in diabetic women? Int J Impot Res. 2003;15(3):198–202. https://doi.org/10.1038/sj.ijir.3900998.

29. Wing RR, Bond DS, Gendrano IN, Wadden T, Bahnson J, Lewis CE, et al. Effect of intensive lifestyle intervention on sexual dysfunction in women with type 2 diabetes: results from an ancillary look AHEAD study. Diabetes Care. 2013;36(10):2937–44. https://doi.org/10.2337/dc13-0315.

30. Chun N. Effectiveness of PLISSIT model sexual program on female sexual function for women with gynecologic cancer. J Korean Acad Nurs. 2011;41(4):471. https://doi.org/10.4040/jkan.2011.41.4.471.

Sexuality in People with Obesity

José M. Balibrea, Albert Caballero, Pau Moreno, and Jordi Tarascó

1 Introduction: Obesity as a Global Health Problem

Obesity is currently recognized as a disease in itself responsible for one of the main health problems and is considered a worldwide epidemic. According to the World Health Organization (WHO) and the European Association for the Study of Obesity (EASO), overweight and obesity are defined as an abnormal or excessive accumulation of fat that can damage health. It is a chronic and recurrent disease that is also associated with other comorbidities that result in a decrease in life expectancy and quality of life. For its typification, WHO, EASO, or the Centers for Disease Control and Prevention (CDC) still use the body mass index (BMI) to better define these terms, considering a BMI of 25–29.9 kg/m^2 as overweight and $\geq$30 kg/m^2 as obese. However, this "numerical" definition is increasingly being questioned since ultimately the degree of adiposity and especially the amount of metabolically active fat tissue are what determine the occurrence of the pathophysiological phenomena associated with obesity. That is, the essence of obesity is excess adipose tissue in the body (not a ratio of height and weight), so BMI can only serve as an indirect estimate of obesity. Excess fat is usually conceived as an indicator of poor health and, in turn, constitutes a risk factor for a number of diseases such as diabetes, ischemic heart disease, hyperlipidemia, sleep apnea, among others. A more correct definition of obesity states that it is the result of a long-term positive energy balance in which energy intake exceeds energy expenditure. It is important to remember that body weight is a physiologically regulated parameter, and thus, obesity is considered a

J. M. Balibrea (✉) · A. Caballero · P. Moreno · J. Tarascó
Endocrine-Metabolic and Bariatric Surgery Unit, Germans Trias I Pujol University Hospital (Badalona), Barcelona, Spain

Department of Surgery, Autonomous University of Barcelona, Barcelona, Spain

© The Author(s), under exclusive license to Springer Nature Switzerland AG 2024
C. Castelo-Branco, S. Anglès Acedo (eds.), *Medical Disorders and Sexual Health*, Trends in Andrology and Sexual Medicine,
https://doi.org/10.1007/978-3-031-55080-5_13

disease of body weight regulation. Thus, there are many factors that can contribute to the development of obesity, such as genetics, age, lifestyle, medications, and hormonal problems.

Currently, although obesity is considered a disease, it is accepted that there is a high degree of individual variability and even specific types with particular functional properties (phenotypes). This phenotyping beyond BMI should not be limited to physiological or anatomical variables. Biochemical and molecular profiles will also be helpful in individualizing the potential for obesity mortality. In addition, BMI can be subdivided using psychometric instruments to try to identify phenotypes based on traits such as disinhibition and tendency to pathological eating behaviors.

The prevalence of obesity has been increasing exponentially since the early 1980s, having doubled in more than 70 countries. In the United States, it currently stands at about 42.4%. If we look at class III obesity (body mass index [BMI] $\geq$40 kg/m^2), the figure is close to 9%. Globally, more than 620 million adults suffer from obesity worldwide. This prevalence has been increasing similarly in both men and women. In a particularly relevant way, we can say that the prevalence of obesity in low- to middle-income countries has increased in the last 10 years to around 38%.

People with obesity present profound endocrine alterations as well as alterations in sexual function and satisfaction. If we transfer this to the psycho-social sphere, it should not be forgotten that as in other forms of stigmatization based on race, class, ability, gender or sexual orientation, the stigma of obesity can have devastating social and health consequences. Prejudice about people's weight or appearance has significant physiological and psychological consequences, leading to increased depression and anxiety, eating disorders and low self-esteem. They can even affect the quality of care for patients with obesity [1].

2   Obesity and Sexual Function

Obesity and associated comorbidities have a detrimental impact on sexual function as well as quality of sexual life. This relationship between obesity and sexual dysfunction appears to be especially prevalent in individuals with greater adiposity. The origin of sexual dysfunction in people with obesity is manifold, but in general terms it can be said to be the combination of the direct effects of adipose tissue on sexual response, the impact of obesity-related comorbidities on sexual desire and functioning, and the influence of psycho-affective factors (Fig. 1).

Nearly 70% of women and more than half of men who are treated in multidisciplinary teams for obesity report some form of sexual dysfunction. In cohort studies conducted among candidates for bariatric surgery (i.e., highly selected individuals predisposed to seek a solution to their problem), 26% of women and 12% of men reported having no sexual desire and 33% of women and 25% of men reported having no sexual activity at all. Half of the women and men reported being dissatisfied with their sex life.

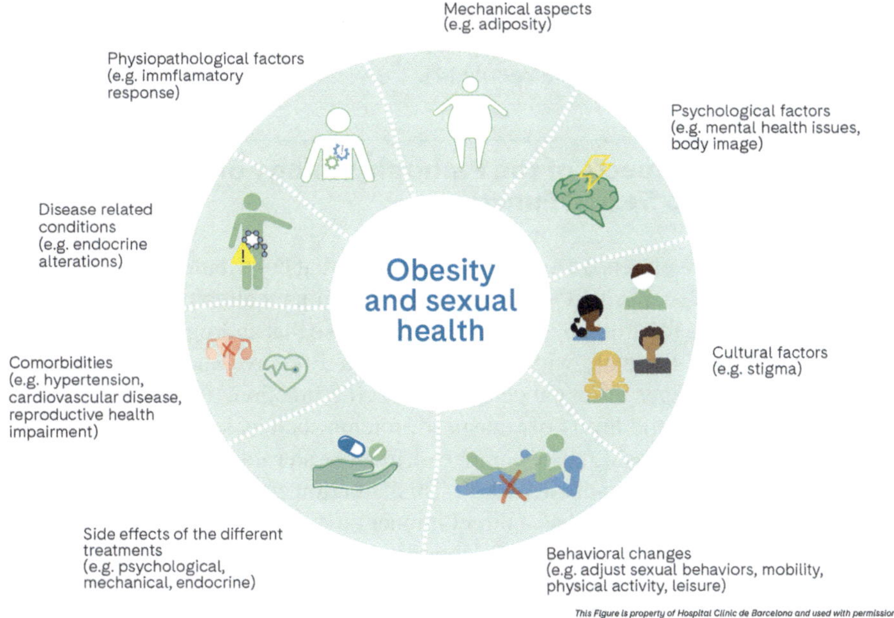

Fig. 1 Factors influencing the impairment of sexual health and the development of sexual dysfunction among obese patients

In most cases, it is declining physical health that limits sexual activity. While in women, age, urinary incontinence, depressive symptoms, and antidepressant use are clearly related to worse sexual function, in men, in addition to age, depressive symptoms, and antidepressant use are also associated with worse sexual function [2].

The relationship between BMI and sexual dysfunction is unclear. While for some people, preoccupation with physical appearance and body image may negatively influence sexual desire and activity, for others (minority) it is not only an impediment but may also be the source of increased attractiveness to others or to the obese person him/herself. In general, dissatisfaction with body image makes people with obesity reluctant to engage in sexual practices. Similarly, the physical limitations associated with extreme obesity can make sexual activity unpleasant, difficult, painful, or outright impossible. On the other hand, it is important to note that in most cases this happens in the context of an interpersonal relationship. That is, other problems or issues in a romantic relationship may contribute to the onset of sexual dysfunction [3].

People with obesity not only have a greater amount of adipose tissue in their body, but it may also have an altered distribution. Firstly, depending on the location of the adipose deposits, body image can be seriously distorted and even lead to serious problems of self-esteem or sexual identity. On the other hand, both mobility and access to body areas involved in sexual relations (especially genitalia) may be severely limited. Also, the impossibility of maintaining sexual relations in certain postures or simply to maintain some type of sexual activity can generate an important degree of frustration in these people [4].

3 General Aspects of the Pathophysiology of Obesity Related to Sexual Function

Obesity has negative effects on a series of hormones that contribute to sexual behavior and reproductive capacity. One of the most determinant alterations is the potential of adipose tissue for aromatization of sex steroids so that androgens are converted to estrogens. While the male with obesity presents a relative androgen deficiency that is related to changes in sexual desire and erectile function, women with obesity present alterations in the levels of transport proteins such as sex hormone binding globulin (SHBG), increasing the clearance of free sex steroids such as testosterone, dihydrotestosterone, and androstenediol. This situation results in a compensatory hyperandrogenemic state that has a direct impact on ovarian cycles.

On the other hand, metabolically dominant adipose tissue (especially intra-abdominal) is responsible for the release of various mediators that perpetuate a state of meta-inflammation responsible for both the persistence of adiposity and the appearance of many of the associated comorbidities. Some of these mediators have a direct influence on the corticotroph-adrenal axis, peripheral steroid aromatization, or the generation of oxidative stress, negatively impacting sperm function and fertility in general, both in men and women [5, 6].

Moreover, comorbidities associated with obesity (especially hypertension, diabetes, and joint dysfunction) and even their treatment can have a clear negative impact on sexual functioning. In men, hypertension and type 2 diabetes are clear risk factors for erectile dysfunction both because of peripheral neuropathic involvement and associated vascularization alterations. In fact, the increased cardiovascular risk associated with the presence of both conditions is also a predisposing factor for sexual dysfunction. Those patients with poorer control of their hypertension or diabetes are at greater risk for either form of sexual dysfunction. In addition, the relationship between comorbidities and sexual function are often influenced by age-related physiological changes. Erection quality and lubrication decrease with age; time to orgasm increases in both women and men. In women, sexual function decreases with menopause due to lower estrogen production, which causes atrophy of the vaginal epithelium, dryness, and less elasticity of the vaginal tissue, which can lead to dyspareunia [7].

Pharmacological treatment of obesity-related diseases can also adversely affect sexual function. For example, antihypertensives have been associated with sexual dysfunction as some of them have sympatholytic, beta-blocking, and diuretic effects. A significant proportion of people with obesity (40%) take psychotropic drugs. Drugs such as selective serotonin reuptake inhibitors and serotonin-norepinephrine reuptake inhibitors are associated with some degree of sexual dysfunction in most patients.

Finally, it should be taken into consideration that in most people with obesity there are permanent alterations in the brain circuits of satiety and reward. While the former tend to show less activity, the mechanisms associated with reward tend to prevail in those promoted by immediate stimuli related especially to the ingestion of high-energy foods. In the same way that obesity is associated (before and after treatment) with eating disorders as well as with other types of substance abuse, it has not been studied in depth whether this phenomenon also occurs in the brain circuits usually involved in sexual function at a cognitive level. Probably, the influence of a multitude of psychological factors related to obesity itself makes this a difficult aspect to clarify [8].

4 Sexual Dysfunction as a Comorbidity Associated with Obesity

4.1 Obesity, Sexual Orientation, and Identity

Although both sexual identity and sexual orientation or preferences are complex aspects that could be influenced by a large number of factors, obesity could influence at least the determination of the phenotype and, secondarily, condition other aspects. On the other hand, obesity may also be a more prevalent disease in certain groups of people depending on their sexual orientation or identity. Some studies have found that lesbian and bisexual women may have a higher risk of obesity. For men the disparities have not been studied as deeply. Some work suggests that bisexual men have a higher risk of obesity and type 2 diabetes than heterosexual and gay men.

There is epidemiological work indicating that black and Latina bisexual women as well as black and white lesbians had higher body mass indexes (BMIs) than white heterosexual women and, on the other hand, that gay men of all races/ethnicities tend to have lower BMIs than white heterosexual men. Other studies have noted that black lesbian and bisexual women had the highest prevalence of food insecurity, while white heterosexual women had the highest prevalence of food insecurity. In reality, it is very likely that this food insecurity is indeed associated with obesity but is actually more of a marker of social status.

As for the possible relationship between sexual orientation and the presence of comorbidities typically associated with obesity, type 2 diabetes and cardiovascular disease are the best studied. Although it is difficult to establish causality, some studies have reported HbA1c glycosylated hemoglobin levels in the diagnostic range of diabetes and increased risk of associated obesity in bisexual men and lesbian and bisexual women. In fact, some observational studies indicate that individuals (especially women) belonging to sexual minorities during adolescence and young adulthood are more likely to have type 2 diabetes in adulthood than heterosexual women [9, 10].

4.2   Effects on Female Sexual and Reproductive Function

Obesity has been correlated in women with the so-called hyperandrogenic syndrome: anovulation, menstrual irregularity, and reduced fertility [9–17]. These phenomena are much more frequent in women with a BMI >40 kg/m^2. The origin of these alterations is, as already mentioned, the excess of aromatized sex steroids produced as a consequence of adiposity. As it occurs in males, obesity is associated with important alterations in sex hormones such as reproductive sex hormone binding globulin (SHBG), follicle stimulating hormone (FSH), or testosterone. However, other phenomena, such as the elevation of leptin levels typical of obesity, can disrupt the hormonal balance of women, causing alterations in the menstrual cycle and fertility. One of the most prevalent comorbidities in women with obesity is polycystic ovary syndrome (PCOS), which serves as an example of the typical alterations in women with obesity, since it is also associated with insulin resistance, cardiovascular diseases, and endometrial cancer, as well as psychological well-being [11]. It is often associated with female sexual dysfunction (prevalence is close to 25%) among premenopausal women. The origin is in the excess of androgens and psychosocial changes often generated by low self-esteem in relation to lack of acceptance of body image can severely affect their sexual function [12]. The reader is referred to chapter titled "Endocrine Disorders and Sexuality II: Ovary (Part II)", for a comprehensive discussion on PCOS and sexuality.

4.3   Effects on Male Sexual and Reproductive Function

The effects of obesity on male fertility have not been studied as much as on female fertility. We can state that the vast majority of obese males live in a state of hypogonadism which, in turn, is associated with a tendency towards progressive and sustained weight gain. Generally speaking, obese males have lower testosterone levels along with lower sexual satisfaction and fertility compared to normal weight males. It can be stated that for every 9 kg of overweight, the chances of male infertility increase by 10%. This fact is reflected at the epidemiological level if we take into account that since the end of the 1970s of the last century the number of obese people has doubled and, at the same time, the quality of semen has been decreasing. Obese men have a lower overall production of androgens than non-obese individuals and, in addition, excess adiposity leads to a greater peripheral aromatization of androgens, which are transformed into estrogens. Thus, we can find lower plasma concentrations of sex hormone binding globulin (SHBG) and testosterone. Consequently, we will have a blockage of the gonadotropic axis at the hypothalamic level together with a characteristic hypofunction of the Sertoli cells. On the other hand, the redistribution of body fat can lead to an increase in scrotal adiposity and thus to an increase in local temperature, which is deleterious for spermiogenesis [13–15].

5   Obesity During Sexual Development, Social Exclusion, Risky Behaviors

Obesity can have important implications in sexual development, especially in adolescents. In the West, the rate of childhood and adolescent obesity continues to grow, especially in large urban centers. Its estimated prevalence is 20% in individuals between 12 and 19 years of age. Among adolescents as a whole, obesity is more prevalent in sexual minorities (people who identify themselves as gay/lesbian or bisexual, or who are unsure of their sexual identity), regardless of the origin or ethnicity of their parents. The origin of this phenomenon is not clear since, on the one hand, they have less physical activity and also a higher prevalence of eating disorders, or at least disordered eating behaviors. Other factors such as individual and family socioeconomic status, educational level, place of residence, and work performed may play a role. Obesity during adolescence is also associated with victimization and psychological violence in schools. In this context, the social, emotional, and even physical environment also play a fundamental role. Also, people with obesity have a higher prevalence of history of sexual abuse during childhood-adolescence than other people [16].

In addition, obesity may be related to sexual behaviors considered risky, mainly by increasing the likelihood of contracting sexually transmitted diseases as well as unwanted pregnancies. Both overweight and obesity may influence the sexual behavior of adolescents since BMI is associated with psychological determinants related to physical attractiveness. This association has been explained in two ways: (1) the psychosocial determinants of obesity decrease the ability to have healthy affective relationships and secondarily, to negotiate safe sexual practices; (2) the increased risk is related to early sexual initiation due to early sexual maturation related to the presence of obesity in childhood and excessive production of sex steroids. Many women of childbearing age with obesity have highly irregular ovarian cycles and menstrual disturbances. This may lead them to consider themselves as "people with a very low risk of pregnancy" and so they sometimes opt for risky sexual practices [17].

Obesity is a source of stigma and discrimination. If the so-called normative sexual behaviors can already be the object or motive of discrimination against people with obesity (both in terms of quantity and quality), in the case of sexual minorities this phenomenon is even greater. On the other hand, fear of rejection and exclusion is often related to a higher prevalence of obesity. For example, there is a higher risk of overweight and obesity among men of heterosexual identity who reported having same-sex sexual relations. These contextual and structural factors may be determinants in perpetuating phenomena of sexual dis-orientation. The existence of "safe" environments in which inclusive policies are promoted for LGBTQ groups has been correlated with a lower prevalence of obesity, especially in the university setting [18].

6 Obesity, Relationships, and Sexual Practices

When dealing with the issue of sexual relationships in people with obesity, we must never lose the perspective of these people. In many occasions, the stigma is maintained and quickly transformed into judgment, reaching morbid terms by the media and general opinion. The disregard for the sexuality of people with obesity has sometimes been defined as a reflection of a voyeuristic fixation of the media that ends up presenting it as a sordid entertainment spectacle.

People with obesity have trouble forming emotional relationships for a variety of reasons. For many, the stigma persists even after they have lost weight, achieved healthy lifestyle habits or emotional stability. This is due in many cases to the fear of a relapse of the disease (which is extremely frequent). There is also the fetishization of fat bodies and there are exclusive dating sites for fat people. The tendency to experience sexual attraction to people with obesity is called anastimaphilia. It is classified as a type of paraphilia that refers to the behavior of people who are sexually attracted to people with obesity. It is grouped, like acrophilia, with the set of sexual preferences towards larger people.

Obese people can also be part of complex sexual practices, often included as part of BDSM (bondage/discipline domination/submission and sadism/masochism) such as "feederism." In feederism, food is used as a means of control, as the feeder decides what the other person eats and thus controls the changes in his or her body. It is important to note that some people with obesity enjoy this practice and find satisfaction in it. However, others have felt that fetishism was imposed on them without their consent in a surreptitious way over the course of a long-term romantic relationship. Likewise, obesity as an object of desire is part of the subject matter of pornography as well as sex work, and the demand for this type of services and content is very high, surpassing that generated through terms such as "skinny" or "thin" [18, 19].

7 Changes in Sexuality After Obesity Treatment, Bariatric Surgery, and Sexual Function

Currently, the treatment of obesity is multidisciplinary and is beginning to target some mechanisms of the pathophysiology of the disease. Although the achievement of healthy habits is desirable and one of the main objectives, it is not always feasible to do so in a lasting way due to the complexity of the disease. Overall, weight loss induced by lifestyle changes has a beneficial effect, for example, on testosterone levels and may improve semen quality. However, as already discussed, it is very difficult to maintain weight loss in the long term with this strategy alone.

Current treatment of obesity includes measures aimed at improving lifestyle, drugs, endoscopic treatments, psychological-psychiatric interventions, and surgery. It is essential to design a personalized strategy adapting the type of treatment to the characteristics of each patient as well as his or her objectives and expectations. The appearance of drugs such as glucagon-like peptide-1 receptor agonists (GLP-1ra), capable of achieving weight loss of around 15% of total body weight, has been a great advance in the treatment of obesity. Although long-term results are not yet available, it is very likely that they will become a key element in the management of this type of patient. However, as with endoscopic treatments, we do not know if they have any effect on sexual function in people with obesity. Bariatric surgery is the most effective treatment for durable weight loss in patients with obesity as well as for the resolution of associated comorbidities. Although obesity-associated sexual dysfunction is not an indication for surgery per se, polycystic ovarian syndrome, the desire to improve fertility or the prevention of hormone-dependent cancers may be. Almost half of the patients who undergo bariatric surgery present some type of sexual dysfunction. While in women the vast majority of studies claim that bariatric surgery can improve fertility and reduce pregnancy complications, the true effects of bariatric surgery on semen quality and male sex hormones are unclear [20].

7.1   Changes in Male and Female Sexuality

Bariatric surgery is generally associated with improved female sexual health when using scores such as the Female Sexual Functioning Index (FSFI) or commonly used questionnaires such as the Pelvic Organ Prolapse/Urinary Incontinence Sexual Questionnaire (PISQ-12). In general, improvements are seen in sexual desire, arousal, lubrication, orgasm, overall sexual satisfaction, and a reduction in dyspareunia. However, many of the women with obesity have pelvic floor disorders; when these are present, PISQ-12 and FSFI scores do not usually improve after surgery. The underlying mechanisms responsible for this increase in women's sexual function are several. Among them, the increase in estrogen, FSH, LH, and SHGB along with the decrease in testosterone and DHEA-S. On the other hand, modifications of psychological and mental conditions after weight loss could benefit sexual function. Likewise, partial resolution or complete remission of some comorbidities (especially type 2 diabetes) may play a crucial role in the improvement of sexual health in these patients, as significant improvements in peripheral nerve involvement have been observed. In men, after bariatric surgery, an increase in total and free testosterone levels has been observed. In terms of activity, if we take the International Index of Erectile Function (IIEF) score as a reference, after bariatric surgery a significant increase in erectile function is usually observed. Likewise, LH, FSH, and SHBG levels also increase while estradiol (free and total) and prolactin levels decrease. However, and very strikingly, these hormonal changes do not correlate with improved sperm quality nor with alterations in DHEA, androstenedione, or inhibin B levels. The worsening of sperm quality despite the hormonal changes described above could have its origin in nutritional deficiencies associated with surgery. Nutritional imbalances sometimes observed in hypoabsorptive surgeries can alter GnRH secretion in the same way that iron, calcium, and vitamin deficiencies negatively affect spermatogenesis. On the other hand, massive loss of adipose mass can be associated with the initial accumulation and subsequent release of fat-soluble toxic substances, contributing to spermatogenesis deficit [21, 22].

7.2   Other Phenomena Observed After Treatment of Obesity

As previously mentioned, people with obesity usually present dissatisfaction with their physical appearance and body image, which has a negative influence on sexual behavior. A priori, weight loss after surgery should positively affect these patients. In principle, the massive loss of adipose tissue improves self-esteem, reduces anxiety and depressive symptoms. However, some patients develop dysmorphophobic disorders or are simply dissatisfied with the aesthetic result after weight loss. Large weight losses can generate significant skin flaps that some patients do not accept aesthetically and may even affect their mobility or hygiene. For this reason, perhaps the best time to evaluate the improvement or not of sexual health is after body contouring surgery (abdominoplasty, reduction mammoplasty, brachy or cruroplasty…) if performed at all; that is, about 2 years after bariatric surgery [23, 24].

Operated patients who achieve a satisfactory weight loss and who also manage to maintain an anthropomorphic pattern that satisfies them usually experience a very notable increase that correlates with an increase in their self-esteem and affective relationships. In some cases, bariatric surgery implies an important biographical rupture that is associated with changes in romantic relationships, separations, or the search for new options or multiple partners. Many times these people begin to feel socially accepted and even desired so that their social interactions tend to increase exponentially. In addition, the increase in fertility parallel to the increase and regularization of ovarian cycles has been related, especially in adolescents, with an increase in unwanted pregnancies as risky behaviors prevail along with a parallel increase in the number of sexual relationships and partners [18, 25].

8   Conclusions

Obesity is a systemic disease of enormous prevalence that affects sexual health in many aspects. Both the pathophysiology of the disease itself and its comorbidities have a clear effect on it. In addition, obesity has an impact on sexual behaviors and can influence behavioral aspects but also others related to identity or orientation. The treatment of obesity is clearly multidisciplinary and should consider sexual dysfunction as one of the problems to be treated. Likewise, although there are effective treatments with excellent results on other comorbidities, due to the complexity and the large number of factors involved, the overall effect on sexual health must be analyzed individually.

References

1. Quinn N, Zeglin RJ, Boggs C, Glusenkamp H, Rule M, Hicks-Roof K, Terrell KR. Sex at every size: a content analysis of weight inclusivity in sexual functioning research. Body Image. 2022;43:420–8. https://doi.org/10.1016/j.bodyim.2022.10.010.
2. Al Qurashi AA, Qadri SH, Lund S, Ansari US, Arif A, Durdana AR, Maryam R, Saadi M, Zohaib M, Khan MK, Waseem A, Dar S, Almas T. The effects of bariatric surgery on

male and female fertility: a systematic review and meta-analysis. Ann Med Surg (Lond). 2022;80:103881. https://doi.org/10.1016/j.amsu.2022.103881.

3. Loh HH, Shahar MA, Loh HS, Yee A. Female sexual dysfunction after bariatric surgery in women with obesity: a systematic review and meta-analysis. Scand J Surg. 2022;111(1):14574969211072395. https://doi.org/10.1177/14574969211072395.

4. Smith SJ, Teo SYM, Lopresti AL, Heritage B, Fairchild TJ. Examining the effects of calorie restriction on testosterone concentrations in men: a systematic review and meta-analysis. Nutr Rev. 2022;80(5):1222–36. https://doi.org/10.1093/nutrit/nuab072.

5. Emami MR, Safabakhsh M, Khorshidi M, Moradi Moghaddam O, Mohammed SH, Zarezadeh M, Alizadeh S. Effect of bariatric surgery on endogenous sex hormones and sex hormone-binding globulin levels: a systematic review and meta-analysis. Surg Obes Relat Dis. 2021;17(9):1621–36. https://doi.org/10.1016/j.soard.2021.05.003.

6. Subramanian A, Idkowiak J, Toulis KA, Thangaratinam S, Arlt W, Nirantharakumar K. Pubertal timing in boys and girls born to mothers with gestational diabetes mellitus: a systematic review. Eur J Endocrinol. 2021;184(1):51–64. https://doi.org/10.1530/EJE-20-0296.

7. Liu S, Cao D, Ren Z, Li J, Peng L, Zhang Q, Cheng B, Cheng Z, Ai J, Zheng X, Liu L, Wei Q. The relationships between bariatric surgery and sexual function: current evidence based medicine. BMC Urol. 2020;20(1):150. https://doi.org/10.1186/s12894-020-00707-1.

8. Nguyen NTK, Fan HY, Tsai MC, Tung TH, Huynh QTV, Huang SY, Chen YC. Nutrient intake through childhood and early menarche onset in girls: systematic review and meta-analysis. Nutrients. 2020;12(9):2544. https://doi.org/10.3390/nu12092544.

9. Loh HH, Yee A, Loh HS, Kanagasundram S, Francis B, Lim LL. Sexual dysfunction in polycystic ovary syndrome: a systematic review and meta-analysis. Hormones (Athens). 2020;19(3):413–23. https://doi.org/10.1007/s42000-020-00210-0.

10. Moxthe LC, Sauls R, Ruiz M, Stern M, Gonzalvo J, Gray HL. Effects of bariatric surgeries on male and female fertility: a systematic review. J Reprod Infertil. 2020;21(2):71–86.

11. Castelo-Branco C, Naumova I. Quality of life and sexual function in women with polycystic ovary syndrome: a comprehensive review. Gynecol Endocrinol. 2020;36(2):96–103. https://doi.org/10.1080/09513590.2019.1670788. Epub 2019 Sep 27. PMID: 31559883.

12. Naumova I, Castelo-Branco C, Casals G. Psychological issues and sexual function in women with different infertility causes: focus on polycystic ovary syndrome. Reprod Sci. 2021;28(10):2830–8.

13. Jäger P, Wolicki A, Spohnholz J, Senkal M. Review: sex-specific aspects in the bariatric treatment of severely obese women. Int J Environ Res Public Health. 2020;17(8):2734. https://doi.org/10.3390/ijerph17082734.

14. Gao Z, Liang Y, Deng W, Qiu P, Li M, Zhou Z. Impact of bariatric surgery on female sexual function in obese patients: a meta-analysis. Obes Surg. 2020;30(1):352–64. https://doi.org/10.1007/s11695-019-04240-5.

15. Xu J, Wu Q, Zhang Y, Pei C. Effect of bariatric surgery on male sexual function: a meta-analysis and systematic review. Sex Med. 2019;7(3):270–81. https://doi.org/10.1016/j.esxm.2019.06.003.

16. Montenegro M, Slongo H, Juliato CRT, Minassian VA, Tavakkoli A, Brito LGO. The impact of bariatric surgery on pelvic floor dysfunction: a systematic review. J Minim Invasive Gynecol. 2019;26(5):816–25. https://doi.org/10.1016/j.jmig.2019.01.013.

17. Lee Y, Dang JT, Switzer N, Yu J, Tian C, Birch DW, Karmali S. Impact of bariatric surgery on male sex hormones and sperm quality: a systematic review and meta-analysis. Obes Surg. 2019;29(1):334–46. https://doi.org/10.1007/s11695-018-3557-5.

18. VanKim NA, Laska MN. Sexual orientation and obesity: what do we know? Curr Obes Rep. 2021;10(4):453–7. https://doi.org/10.1007/s13679-021-00454-w.

19. Glina FPA, de Freitas Barboza JW, Nunes VM, Glina S, Bernardo WM. What is the impact of bariatric surgery on erectile function? A systematic review and meta-analysis. Sex Med Rev. 2017;5(3):393–402. https://doi.org/10.1016/j.sxmr.2017.03.008.

20. Escobar-Morreale HF, Santacruz E, Luque-Ramírez M, Botella Carretero JI. Prevalence of 'obesity-associated gonadal dysfunction' in severely obese men and women and its

resolution after bariatric surgery: a systematic review and meta-analysis. Hum Reprod Update. 2017;23(4):390–408. https://doi.org/10.1093/humupd/dmx012.

21. Corona G, Rastrelli G, Monami M, Saad F, Luconi M, Lucchese M, Facchiano E, Sforza A, Forti G, Mannucci E, Maggi M. Body weight loss reverts obesity-associated hypogonadotropic hypogonadism: a systematic review and meta-analysis. Eur J Endocrinol. 2013;168(6):829–43. https://doi.org/10.1530/EJE-12-0955.

22. Pizzol D, Smith L, Fontana L, Caruso MG, Bertoldo A, Demurtas J, McDermott D, Garolla A, Grabovac I, Veronese N. Associations between body mass index, waist circumference and erectile dysfunction: a systematic review and meta-analysis. Rev Endocr Metab Disord. 2020;21(4):657–66. https://doi.org/10.1007/s11154-020-09541-0.

23. Iafrate M, Ermacora C, Morlacco A, Dal Moro F, Di Vincenzo A, Rossato M. Metabolic syndrome and andrological diseases. Panminerva Med. 2022;64(3):324–8. https://doi.org/10.23736/S0031-0808.22.04628-6.

24. Louters M, Pearlman M, Solsrud E, Pearlman A. Functional hypogonadism among patients with obesity, diabetes, and metabolic syndrome. Int J Impot Res. 2022;34(7):714–20. https://doi.org/10.1038/s41443-021-00496-7. Epub 2021 Nov 13.

25. Wiss DA, Brewerton TD, Tomiyama AJ. Limitations of the protective measure theory in explaining the role of childhood sexual abuse in eating disorders, addictions, and obesity: an updated model with emphasis on biological embedding. Eat Weight Disord. 2022;27(4):1249–67. https://doi.org/10.1007/s40519-021-01293-3.

Sexual Health in Inflammatory Bowel Disease

Agnès Fernández-Clotet, Berta Caballol,
and Marta Gallego

1   Introduction

Inflammatory bowel disease (IBD) is a chronic inflammatory disorder of the gastro-intestinal tract that is characterized by periods of clinical activity and remission. The main representative forms are Ulcerative Colitis (UC) and Crohn's Disease (CD) both of which have been shown to significant impact health-related quality of life. IBD is associated with distressing and embarrassing symptoms such as fecal urgency, anal incontinence, bloody diarrhea, abdominal pain, malnutrition, and fatigue. Extra-intestinal presentations can affect the joints, liver, skin, and the eyes. The disease can cause a psychological burden from attempting to live a normal life while living in fear of symptoms [1]. IBD has a high incidence and prevalence in young individuals (more than 50% of patients are diagnosed before 35 years) when sexual and interpersonal identities are developing and affecting people in their reproductive years [2].

Sexual dysfunction (SD) is defined as a sexual problem that is persistent or recurring and causes personal distress or interpersonal difficulty. SD in women includes a lack of sexual desire, inability to orgasm, impaired arousal, or pain with sexual activity. The most recognized disorders in men are erectile dysfunction, abnormal ejaculation, and decreased libido [3]. SD is a common and little-known problem in IBD: the unpredictable nature of IBD symptoms, pelvic-floor disorders, fatigue, and psychological factors can influence body image perception, sexual desire, and intimacy. Moreover, relationship status, education, misconceptions about the disease, fertility concerns in both men and women, and erectile function also affect sexual

A. Fernández-Clotet (✉) · B. Caballol · M. Gallego
Inflammatory Bowel Disease Unit, Department of Gastroenterology,
Clinical Institute of Digestive and Metabolic Diseases, Hospital Clínic de Barcelona,
Barcelona, Spain
e-mail: AGFERNANDEZ@clinic.cat; CABALLOL@clinic.cat; MGALLEGO@clinic.cat

    229
C. Castelo-Branco, S. Anglès Acedo (eds.), *Medical Disorders and Sexual Health*, Trends in Andrology and Sexual Medicine,
https://doi.org/10.1007/978-3-031-55080-5_14

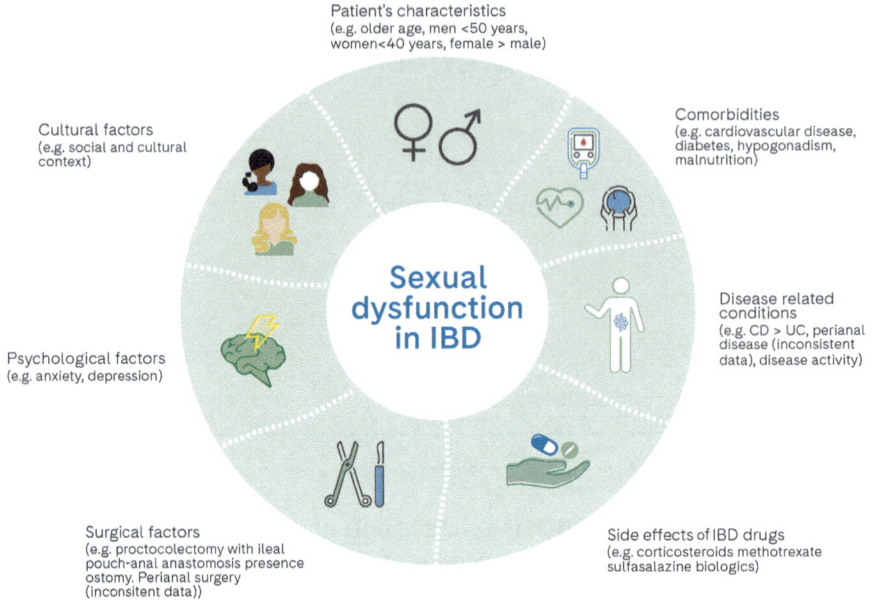

Fig. 1 Factors involved in the development of sexual dysfunction in inflammatory bowel disease

satisfaction and patient wellbeing. The etiology of SD in IBD remains unclear but is likely to be multifactorial, including disease flares, psychosocial factors, surgical interventions, perianal complications, and side effects of drugs (Fig. 1) [4]. Although the impact of IBD on sexual function is a frequent concern in patients, physicians rarely consider this issue when discussing therapeutic goals with them [5]. Improved clinician awareness and understanding of the etiology, risk factors, and impact of SD in IBD may result in an early diagnosis, and ultimately better health and wellbeing for this population.

2 Sexual Dysfunction Assessment Tools

Most SD assessment tools are non-specific for IBD patients. The scale that evaluated the quality of life in the IBD (IBD-Q) contains a few items referring to general sexual function. For this reason, most of the studies related to SD in IBD have used the Female Sexual Function Index [6] and the International Index of Erectile Function [7] as a reference tools, despite they are non-IBD-specific. The Female Sexual Function Index consists of 19 items with 5-point Likert scale to assess six primary domains of female sexual function including desire, arousal, lubrication, orgasm, satisfaction, and pain. This scale has been validated in numerous clinical and research settings [6]. The International Index of Erectile Function evaluates 15 items with five categories: erectile function, orgasm, sexual desire, sexual satisfaction, and general satisfaction. Higher scores reflect better sexual functioning [7].

Recently, new IBD-specific scales have been developed: a specific scale to assess sexual function in men (IBD-Male Sexual Dysfunction Scale or IDB-MSDS) [8] and a specific scale for women (IBD-specific Female Sexual Dysfunction Scale or IBD-FSDS) [9]. The IBD-FSDS correlates positively with the Female Sexual Function scale and includes questions which address the impact of IBD-specific medications, symptoms, and surgical procedures on sexual functioning. These scales assess how IBD symptoms interfere with sexual function; however, their use is not yet widespread (Table 1).

Table 1 Summary of scales and questionnaires for assessing sexual dysfunction

Questionnaire	Target population	IBD specific	Items	Domains	Cutoff for SD
Female Sexual Function Index	Women heterosexual and homosexual	NO	19 (original)	1. Desire 2. Arousal 3. Lubrication 4. Orgasm 5. Satisfatction 6. Pain	Total score ≤ 26: SD Lower score indicates higher severity of sexual dysfunction
International Index of Erectile Function	Men from community and medical populations	NO	15 (original)	1. Erectile function 2. Orgasmic function 3. Sexual desire 4. Intercourse satisfaction 5. Overall satisfaction	Erectile function range 0–30 (6–10: severe; 11–15: moderate; 17–25: mild; 26–30: non) Orgasmic function, sexual desire, and overall satisfaction ranges from 0 to 10 Intercourse satisfaction range 0–15

(continued)

Table 1 (continued)

Questionnaire	Target population	IBD specific	Items	Domains	Cutoff for SD
IBD-Specific Female Sexual Dysfunction Scale (IBD-FSDS)	Women with IBD	YES	15	1. Sexual distress 2. Preventing sexual activity or relationship 3. Delayed sexual activity 4. Causing problems during sex 5. Awareness of disease during intercourse 6. Worried about symptoms during intercourse (abdominal or pelvic or rectal pain) 7. Desire or arousal 8. Fatigue 9. Negative feelings towards sexual activity 10. Sexual satisfaction	Maximal score: 92 Each item was scored individually from 0 to 4 points on a Likert-type scale Higher scores indicate greater severity of SD
IBD-Male Sexual Dysfunction Scale (IBD-MSDS)	Men with IBD	YES	10	1. Desire 2. Participating in sexual activity 3. Preventing having sex 4. Causing problems during sex 5. Feeling guilty about sex 6. Fatigue or lack of energy 7. Other symptoms (abdominal or pelvic pain, bowel movements, anal bleeding or discharge, anal pain, discomfort, or irritation)	Maximal score: 40 Each item was scored individually from 0 to 4 points on a Likert-type scale Higher scores indicate greater severity of SD

3   Inflammatory Bowel Disease and Its Impact on Sexual Health

Some factors related to IBD are likely to negatively affect sexual function. There is a complex, multidimensional, and not fully known or recognized network of different IBD aspects affecting physical appearance, self-confidence, fair, psychosocial emotions, disturbances, and changes in hormone pathways among others. These factors interact and ultimately lead to a reduction in sexual satisfaction and, consequently, a reduction in global quality of life in IBD patients.

Patients with active disease report more frequently sexual problems. Anemia has been associated with a higher risk of SD (OR 7.34, [95% CI 1.14–40.51]) [10]. In men, active disease patients report higher rates of SD (36.1%) compared to patients in remission (18.8%). Active patients referred more orgasm and erectile problems (58.3% vs 40%), and less sexual desire and satisfaction have been described in active patients compared to patients in remission. Additionally, female patients with active disease seems to have higher rates of SD (63.1% vs 44%) experiencing more frequent lubrication problems and dyspareunia compared to patients in remission [11].

Surprisingly, perianal Crohn's disease (active or passed) has not been significantly linked to higher SD even in women and in male. However, in most studies, the results for this factor are inconsistent, with confidence intervals too wide to provide conclusive evidence for the effects of these infrequent situations [10, 12–14].

In the IMPACT study, a wide European study including almost 5000 IBD patients recruited by patients' associations, 40% reported that IBD-related symptoms prevented them from pursuing intimate relationships [15]. Despite the evidence of the decreased frequency of sexual activity in patients with IBD, some authors have reported that the rate of sexual activity in IBD patients would be similar to healthy individuals, but with a lower satisfaction rate [10].

Physical consequences of malnutrition, cosmetic side effects of drug therapies, Crohn's-related fistulas, surgical scars, ostomies and IBD-related symptoms like fatigue, diarrhea, urgency and incontinence, and abdominal pain prevent 40% patients of intimate relationships [16].

Indeed, SD rates are higher in patients with IBD than in the general population, and they may also be present even before the IBD diagnosis: it affects up to 60% of women and 15% of men with IBD compared with 30% in women and 5% in men in general population [10]. Around 40% of IBD men suffer from erectile dysfunction versus 15% of men of the same age in the general population. A study based on the Danish medical register that included more than 31,000 IBD and non-IBD men reflected that erectile dysfunction treatments were more often used by IBD patients [12% vs 10%, HR 1.22 (1.18–1.27)] [17].

It seems not to be differences in SD according to IBD diagnosis (UC or CD), but interestingly its prevalence is inversely associated with longer disease duration [10, 12, 13]. Consistently, in different studies, despite most patients remain sexually active after IBD diagnose a significant proportion (30–45%) of patients report a worsening in their sexual life after IBD diagnosis. Fatigue is reported by patients as the main complaint for the worsening of sexual life in both men and women in a Spanish cohort.

Body image and intimacy are some of the major concerns of IBD patients: significantly, a higher proportion of IBD patients (35% of the women and 13% of the men) compared to healthy population (16% and 3%, respectively) refers frequent problems with their body image [14].

In addition to impacting the overall sexual health, IBD may contribute to impairment in specific domains of SD. For example, a study conducted by Marin et al. [14] demonstrated a reduced sexual functioning scores in all measured domains among a cohort of 202 women, while a separate case-control study found that among 222 women with IBD, decreased frequency of intercourse was the only commonality in comparison to controls. The same study also showed that one third of men considered that sexual desire and satisfaction worsened after the diagnosis of IBD. Despite the finding of lower SD scores in all the International Index of Erectile Function domains, only erectile dysfunction, and sexual desire domains were significantly affected ($p = 0.044$ and $p = 0.031$, respectively) [14].

The etiology of SD in IBD is multifactorial, including biological factors, psychological factors, surgical interventions, and side effects of drugs, which are discussed below:

1. Biological Factors

    Similar to the general population, older age and the coexistence of depression and anxiety could play a role in SD, showing lower levels of sexual interest and satisfaction, and lower quality of life in IBD patients [18]. However, related to age, a recent meta-analysis that included 8 studies found that younger IBD patients (men <50 years and women <40 years) had a higher risk of SD compared to those of older age. The authors attributed this finding to the age of IBD diagnosis, which occurs regularly between 15 and 35 years of age, impacting early and negatively the sexual development of individuals in the context of chronic disease [19].

    Related to other medical conditions, hypogonadism may be present in IBD patients related to chronic inflammation and the use of some drugs. It is known that hypogonadism is associated with SD; therefore, it is recommended to rule out this condition in IBD patients who report alterations in sexual functioning [20]. Nonetheless, there are no evidence related to the use of testosterone replacement in men with IBD with SD and hypogonadism, so its indication must be individualized. Malnutrition is highly prevalent in patients with IBD, and poor nutritional status can cause SD, especially in men with zinc deficiency (that has been related to infertility). Additionally, comorbidities such as cardiovascular disease, diabetes [14], and lifestyle habits (smoking and alcohol consumption) may also contribute to SD.

2. Inflammatory Bowel Disease Drugs

    It is important to differentiate the effect of the drugs on sexual and reproductive health. Despite that some of IBD drugs can reduce fertility; the literature recognizes a limited influence on SD. Evidence shows no effect on sexual function of mesalamine and azathioprine. Corticosteroids have been associated with impaired sexual function due to their impact on body image in women and due to hypogonadism and decreased levels of testosterone in men which cause erectile dysfunction and low libido, the major cause of SD in men, with a high prevalence in IBD patients and a higher need of erectile dysfunction drugs usage than general population [17]. Also, corticosteroid therapy has been linked with low pleasure and orgasm score [13]. Methotrexate has been associated with erectile dysfunction and reduced libido in a few case reports mainly in rheumatoid arthritis and dermatological disorders, but the quality of evidence is low and has not clearly stablished this association [21, 22]. Other studies have not shown association between methotrexate or azathioprine an erectile dysfunction [17]. Biologic agents are generally not associated with SD, although there is some contradictory data Marin et al. in a cohort of 355 IBD patients reported the need for biological agents to be an independent risk factor for SD only in males, but this probably reflects a more severe disease instead of a concrete effect of these drugs [14]. Date from other immune-mediated diseases showed that anti-TNFα prescription was associated with an improve in SD in male patients with ankylosing spondylitis in addition to reducing disease activity, and only one case of a possible association between adalimumab and priapism in rheumatoid arthritis is reported [23, 24] so they are generally not considered to have a bad effect on sexual function.

Non-specific IBD drugs but often prescribed in IBD patients like psychotropic drugs and opioids are recognized as important SD inducers. For example, selective serotonin reuptake inhibitors widely used for the treatment of depression and opioids can produce erectile and ejaculatory problems until 80% of patients and increase the risk of premature ejaculation by three-fold [21, 25].

3. Surgical Factors

Medical treatment for patients with IBD has evolved over the years, in particular with the emergence of biologic therapy; however, surgery continues to play a significant role in treating IBD patients, a meta-analysis found that nearly half of CD patients and 16% of UC patients required surgery within 10 years of diagnosis [26].

Patients often develop concerns or worries related to their disease, and having surgery and carrying an ostomy bag were rated among the first five in importance in six countries of the overall level of concern assessing with the scale Rating Form of Inflammatory Bowel Disease Patient Concerns [27]. In addition, sexual function after surgery is a concern of many patients. Surgical procedures can include colectomy, perianal fistula, limited resection with intestinal continuity, ileal pouch-anal anastomosis, restorative proctocolectomy, proctectomy, and stoma construction.

There is an increased prevalence of SD after surgery in patients with IBD that affects patient's quality of life and can differ significantly in women and men. Surgery can impact sexual function by dyspareunia, erectile problems, retrograde ejaculation or no ejaculation, satisfaction or orgasms lower [20]. There have been numerous studies investigating the effect of sexual function in patients who underwent surgery, and most of the studies assessing SD are related to restorative proctocolectomy with ileal pouch-anal anastomosis. Some studies have shown that the majority of patients with UC after an ileal pouch-anal anastomosis considered that the overall general satisfaction with their sexual life had normalized considerably after surgeries [28], but other studies, have revealed that there is a higher incidence of dyspareunia after restorative proctocolectomy in female patients with UC, although, this does not have a negative effect on sexual function overall [29].

Female gender and surgery for IBD are risk factors for a negative view of body image, libido, and frequency of sexual activity. A greater proportion of women reported decreased frequency of sexual activity, as did operated subjects (female 66.3% versus male 40.5%, $P < 0.0001$; operated 68.5% versus non-operated 50.4%, $P = 0.0113$). Women and operated subjects also more often reported decreased libido (female 67.1% versus male 41.9%, $P = 0.0005$; operated 67.4% versus non-operated 52.6%, $P = 0.035$) [30].

The introduction of laparoscopic approach has minimized surgical scars and stoma formation. A total laparoscopic approach, including rectal dissection, should be preferred an ileal pouch-anal anastomosis to preserve erectile function in men.

Enterostomy therapy nurses are vital resources for patients because they offer specialized care and counseling regarding concerns before and after surgery, the impact of the ostomy on activities of daily life and sexual counseling.

For all of the above reasons, it is important to discuss the impact of surgery on sexual function with the patient in the consultation room because sexual well-being is an important outcome in patients undergoing surgery.

4. Psychological and Social Factors

Mood disturbances are higher in patients with IBD than in overall population, and one of the most important psychological factors related to sexuality disorders. The comorbidity of depression and anxiety in patients with IBD is between 29% and 35% during remission, and as high as 80% for anxiety and 60% for depression during active disease. Women with IBD had a higher probability of experiencing anxiety symptoms than men with IBD, particularly women with CD [31].

Psychological disorders and body image perceptions and changes may influence the sexual health of patients with IBD. Male and female individuals with IBD might have an increased prevalence of SD by more than 41% and 76%, respectively [19].

When addressing body image many patients were concerned about physical disturbances because IBD and treatment can impact on change appearance of the body. Negative body image can be as a result of weight loss secondary to malnutrition, hair loss, muscle loss, swollen face, acne, presence of setons and perianal fistulas, effects of scars and stoma by surgical management, dermatologic manifestations or symptom burden, and all of this can lead to withdrawing into the comfort zone and reducing social and leisure activities. For this reason, body image is a psychosocial factor that critically impacts patients' quality of life and can be involved in the development of SD. In a study of 330 patients with IBD, body image dissatisfaction was greater in females and was associated with greater depression, anxiety, and poor quality of life with feelings of shame and low self-worth and linked to decreased sexual satisfaction although not with sexual activity [32].

Depression is reported as frequent psychological comorbidity in IBD and the major factor for SD. It has significant impact on erectile function and satisfaction for male and has impact on most sub-domains of sexual function (pain, desire, arousal, lubrication, orgasm, satisfaction, and quality) for female individuals [33]. However, multivariate analysis in different published studies untie the disease activity of SD and mainly associate it to depression (OR for SD 6.23, [95% CI 1.96–20.05]), and also to anxiety and fatigue secondary to the disease [10–13, 16]. Although patients with active disease report higher levels of depressive mood, higher levels of fatigue, lower disease-related quality of life, and a more negative body image, these variables were all associated with worse sexual functioning; the effect of active disease on sexual functioning has been mainly mediated by depression indicating that active IBD impacts sexual functioning mainly through the impact of active disease on mood [11].

Gastroenterologists should address in clinics the impact of living with IBD that could lead to identify comorbidities for psychological disease that might be contributing SD and consider necessary treatment of current psychiatric disease that may improve overall quality of life.

4   Sexual Dysfunction Management and Challenges in Sexual Assessment Among IBD Patients

Unfortunately, there are no recommendations or clinical guidelines about how to assess and manage SD in IBD patients. Mostly, IBD patients are attended by gastroenterologists and gastrointestinal surgeons, who do not have specific training about sexual disorders. Moreover, there continues to be a taboo surrounding sexuality and the lack of consensus on how to specifically and correctly evaluate sexual function in IBD patients, as previously described in this chapter. This results in sexual function in IBD patients being clearly not well evaluated and consequently not well managed in clinical practice. This situation has been documented: a questionnaire proposed to IBD French gastroenterologists revealed that more than 80% of physicians acknowledge no addressing the topic of sexuality with their IBD patients mainly because they think they do not have strategies or solutions to offer in case of detecting troubles. This contrasts with the patient's point of view where more than 50% of them expect to discuss sexuality with their specialists [10]. This situation likely requires multidisciplinary management involving gastroenterologists and surgeons to control the intestinal burden of the disease and optimize treatments, IBD nurses and psychologists to address patients' feelings, fears, and IBD-associated anxiety, and specialists in SD to treat and manage patients with these issues. Consensus and clinical guidelines established by major scientific societies would help disseminate this knowledge widely and facilitate the creation of these teams.

5 Conclusions and Key Messages

- Sexual disorders are a common problem among inflammatory bowel disease patients, affecting more women and during the first years of the disease.
- The etiology of sexual dysfunction in inflammatory bowel disease is multifactorial, including biological factors, psychosocial factors, surgical interventions, and side effects of drugs.
- Fatigue, anxiety, and changes in self-body image related to inflammatory bowel disease have been related to sexual dysfunction.
- Intrinsic disease factors like inflammatory bowel disease activity and anemia could have an impact on sexual function.
- Most specific inflammatory bowel disease medical treatments have not been associated to sexual dysfunction with the exception of corticosteroids and methotrexate.
- Defining specific tools for evaluating, detecting, and managing sexual disorders in inflammatory bowel disease patients and create clinical guidelines is crucial to improve their detection, management, and consequently patients' quality of life.

References

1. Kemp K, Griffiths J, Lovell K. Understanding the health and social care needs of people living with IBD: a meta-synthesis of the evidence. World J Gastroenterol [Internet]. 2012 [cited 2023 Mar 7];18(43):6240–9. https://pubmed.ncbi.nlm.nih.gov/23180944/.
2. Torres J, Mehandru S, Colombel JF, Peyrin-Biroulet L. Crohn's disease. Lancet (London, England) [Internet]. 2017 [cited 2022 May 5];389(10080):1741–55. https://pubmed.ncbi.nlm.nih.gov/27914655/.
3. McCabe MP, Sharlip ID, Atalla E, Balon R, Fisher AD, Laumann E, et al. Definitions of sexual dysfunctions in women and men: a consensus statement from the fourth international consultation on sexual medicine 2015. J Sex Med [Internet]. 2016 [cited 2023 Mar 7];13(2):135–43. https://pubmed.ncbi.nlm.nih.gov/26953828/.
4. de Arce EP, Quera R, Barros JR, Sassaki LY. Sexual dysfunction in inflammatory bowel disease: what the specialist should know and ask. Int J Gen Med [Internet]. 2021 [cited 2023 Mar 7];14:2003–15. https://pubmed.ncbi.nlm.nih.gov/34079340/.
5. Maunder R, Toner B, De Rooy E, Moskovitz D. Influence of sex and disease on illness-related concerns in inflammatory bowel disease. Can J Gastroenterol [Internet]. 1999 [cited 2023 Mar 7];13(9):728–32. https://pubmed.ncbi.nlm.nih.gov/10633825/.
6. Rosen R, Brown C, Heiman J, Leiblum S, Meston C, Shabsigh R, et al. The Female Sexual Function Index (FSFI): a multidimensional self-report instrument for the assessment of female sexual function. J Sex Marital Ther [Internet]. 2000 [cited 2023 Mar 7];26(2):191–205. https://pubmed.ncbi.nlm.nih.gov/10782451/.
7. Rosen RC, Riley A, Wagner G, Osterloh IH, Kirkpatrick J, Mishra A. The international index of erectile function (IIEF): a multidimensional scale for assessment of erectile dysfunction.

Urology [Internet]. 1997 Jun [cited 2023 Mar 7];49(6):822–30. https://pubmed.ncbi.nlm.nih.gov/9187685/.

8. O'Toole A, De Silva PS, Marc LG, Ulysse CA, Testa MA, Ting A, et al. Sexual dysfunction in men with inflammatory bowel disease: a new IBD-specific scale. Inflamm Bowel Dis [Internet]. 2018 [cited 2023 Mar 7];24(2):310–6. https://pubmed.ncbi.nlm.nih.gov/29361102/.

9. de Silva PS, O'Toole A, Marc LG, Ulysse CA, Testa MA, Julsgaard M, et al. Development of a sexual dysfunction scale for women with inflammatory bowel disease. Inflamm Bowel Dis [Internet]. 2018 [cited 2023 Mar 7];24(11):2350–9. https://pubmed.ncbi.nlm.nih.gov/30165525/.

10. Rivière P, Zallot C, Desobry P, Sabaté JM, Vergniol J, Zerbib F, et al. Frequency of and factors associated with sexual dysfunction in patients with inflammatory bowel disease. J Crohns Colitis [Internet]. 2017 [cited 2023 Mar 7];11(11):1347–52. https://pubmed.ncbi.nlm.nih.gov/28981625/.

11. Bel LGJ, Vollebregt AM, Van der Meulen-de Jong AE, Fidder HH, Ten Hove WR, Vliet-Vlieland CW, et al. Sexual dysfunctions in men and women with inflammatory bowel disease: the influence of IBD-related clinical factors and depression on sexual function. J Sex Med [Internet]. 2015 [cited 2023 Mar 22];12(7):1557–67. https://pubmed.ncbi.nlm.nih.gov/26054013/.

12. Timmer A, Bauer A, Kemptner D, Fürst A, Rogler G. Determinants of male sexual function in inflammatory bowel disease: a survey-based cross-sectional analysis in 280 men. Inflamm Bowel Dis [Internet]. 2007 [cited 2023 Mar 22];13(10):1236–43. https://pubmed.ncbi.nlm.nih.gov/17508419/.

13. Timmer A, Kemptner D, Bauer A, Takses A, Ott C, Fürst A. Determinants of female sexual function in inflammatory bowel disease: a survey based cross-sectional analysis. BMC Gastroenterol. 2008;8:45.

14. Marín L, Mañosa M, Garcia-Planella E, Gordillo J, Zabana Y, Cabré E, et al. Sexual function and patients' perceptions in inflammatory bowel disease: a case-control survey. J Gastroenterol [Internet]. 2013 [cited 2023 Mar 7];48(6):713–20. https://pubmed.ncbi.nlm.nih.gov/23124604/.

15. Ghosh S, Mitchell R. Impact of inflammatory bowel disease on quality of life: results of the European Federation of Crohn's and Ulcerative Colitis Associations (EFCCA) patient survey. J Crohns Colitis [Internet]. 2007 [cited 2023 Mar 7];1(1):10–20. https://pubmed.ncbi.nlm.nih.gov/21172179/.

16. Leenhardt R, Rivière P, Papazian P, Nion-Larmurier I, Girard G, Laharie D, et al. Sexual health and fertility for individuals with inflammatory bowel disease. World J Gastroenterol. 2019;25(36):5423–33.

17. Friedman S, Magnussen B, O'Toole A, Fedder J, Larsen M, Nørgård B. Increased use of medications for erectile dysfunction in men with ulcerative colitis and Crohn's disease compared to men without inflammatory bowel disease: a nationwide cohort study. Am J Gastroenterol [Internet]. 2018 [cited 2023 Mar 7];113(9):1355–62. https://pubmed.ncbi.nlm.nih.gov/29988041/.

18. Eluri S, Cross RK, Martin C, Weinfurt KP, Flynn KE, Long MD, et al. Inflammatory bowel diseases can adversely impact domains of sexual function such as satisfaction with sex life. Dig Dis Sci [Internet]. 2018 [cited 2023 Mar 7];63(6):1572–82. https://pubmed.ncbi.nlm.nih.gov/29564672/.

19. Zhao S, Wang J, Liu Y, Luo L, Zhu Z, Li E, et al. Inflammatory bowel diseases were associated with risk of sexual dysfunction in both sexes: a meta-analysis. Inflamm Bowel Dis [Internet]. 2019 [cited 2023 Mar 7];25(4):699–707. https://pubmed.ncbi.nlm.nih.gov/30476074/.

20. Ghazi LJ, Patil SA, Cross RK. Sexual dysfunction in inflammatory bowel disease. Inflamm Bowel Dis [Internet]. 2015 [cited 2023 Mar 7];21(4):939–47. https://pubmed.ncbi.nlm.nih.gov/25504236/.

21. Hammami MB, Mahadevan U. Men with inflammatory bowel disease: sexual function, fertility, medication safety, and prostate cancer. Am J Gastroenterol [Internet]. 2020 [cited 2023 Mar 22];115(4):526–34. https://pubmed.ncbi.nlm.nih.gov/32022719/.

22. Aguirre MA, Vélez A, Romero M, Collantes E. Gynecomastia and sexual impotence associated with methotrexate treatment. J Rheumatol. 2002;29(8):1793.

23. Kreitenberg AJ, Ortiz EC, Arkfeld DG. Priapism after tumor necrosis factor alpha inhibitor use. Clin Rheumatol [Internet]. 2015 [cited 2023 Mar 22];34(4):801–2. https://pubmed.ncbi.nlm.nih.gov/25579651/.

24. Oh JS, Heo HM, Kim YG, Lee SG, Lee CK, Yoo B. The effect of anti-tumor necrosis factor agents on sexual dysfunction in male patients with ankylosing spondylitis: a pilot study. Int J Impot Res [Internet]. 2009 [cited 2023 Mar 22];21(6):372–375. https://pubmed.ncbi.nlm.nih.gov/19759542/.

25. Semet M, Paci M, Saïas-Magnan J, Metzler-Guillemain C, Boissier R, Lejeune H, et al. The impact of drugs on male fertility: a review. Andrology [Internet]. 2017 [cited 2023 Mar 22];5(4):640–63. https://pubmed.ncbi.nlm.nih.gov/28622464/.

26. Frolkis AD, Dykeman J, Negrón ME, deBruyn J, Jette N, Fiest KM, et al. Risk of surgery for inflammatory bowel diseases has decreased over time: a systematic review and meta-analysis of population-based studies. Gastroenterology [Internet]. 2013 [cited 2018 Jul 25];145(5):996–1006. http://www.ncbi.nlm.nih.gov/pubmed/23896172.

27. Levenstein S, Li Z, Almer S, Levenstein S, Marquis P, Moser G, et al. Cross-cultural variation in disease-related concerns among patients with inflammatory bowel disease. Am J Gastroenterol [Internet]. 2001 [cited 2023 Apr 17];96(6):1822–1830. https://pubmed.ncbi.nlm.nih.gov/11419836/.

28. Berndtsson I, Öresland T, Hultén L. Sexuality in patients with ulcerative colitis before and after restorative proctocolectomy: a prospective study. Scand J Gastroenterol [Internet]. 2004 [cited 2023 Apr 17];39(4):374–9. https://pubmed.ncbi.nlm.nih.gov/15125470/.

29. Cornish JA, Tan E, Teare J, Teoh TG, Rai R, Darzi AW, et al. The effect of restorative proctocolectomy on sexual function, urinary function, fertility, pregnancy and delivery: a systematic review. Dis Colon Rectum [Internet]. 2007 [cited 2023 Apr 17];50(8):1128–38. https://pubmed.ncbi.nlm.nih.gov/17588223/.

30. Muller KR, Prosser R, Bampton P, Mountifield R, Andrews JM. Female gender and surgery impair relationships, body image, and sexuality in inflammatory bowel disease: patient perceptions. Inflamm Bowel Dis [Internet]. 2010 [cited 2023 Apr 17];16(4):657–63. https://pubmed.ncbi.nlm.nih.gov/19714755/.

31. Barberio B, Zamani M, Black CJ, Savarino EV, Ford AC. Prevalence of symptoms of anxiety and depression in patients with inflammatory bowel disease: a systematic review and meta-analysis. Lancet Gastroenterol Hepatol [Internet]. 2021 [cited 2023 Apr 17];6(5):359–70. https://pubmed.ncbi.nlm.nih.gov/33721557/.

32. McDermott E, Mullen G, Moloney J, Keegan D, Byrne K, Doherty GA, et al. Body image dissatisfaction: clinical features, and psychosocial disability in inflammatory bowel disease. Inflamm Bowel Dis [Internet]. 2015 [cited 2023 Apr 17];21(2):353–60. https://pubmed.ncbi.nlm.nih.gov/25569732/.

33. Chen B, Zhou B, Song G, Li H, Li R, Liu Z, et al. Inflammatory bowel disease is associated with worse sexual function: a systematic review and meta-analysis. Transl Androl Urol [Internet]. 2022 [cited 2023 Apr 17];11(7):959–73. https://pubmed.ncbi.nlm.nih.gov/35958893/.

Lower Gastrointestinal Cancer and Sexual Function

Sara Tavares Nogueira and Isis Araujo

1 Introduction

Lower gastrointestinal cancer is defined as cancer arising between the colon and the anal canal, with the most frequent and studied entity being adenocarcinoma of the colon and rectum or colorectal cancer (CRC). Approximately one third of those cases are localized in the rectum [1, 2].

The incidence of CRC has increased in most European countries over the last decade, also among younger subjects aged 20–49 years [2] although this is not associated to a similar rise in mortality. The overall prevalence is hoped to decrease due to screening strategies [3]. Squamous cell carcinoma of the anus is not a frequent cause of cancer, counting for 2% of all gastrointestinal malignancies. It has a trend to be diagnosed at a younger age and has a relatively long-term survival rate [4, 5]. In the last decades, there have been advances in the treatment of CRC resulting in an improvement in survival rates that is estimated to be of 56% at 5 years [6].

Management of the disease focuses on the oncological outcomes and traditionally involves interventions such as radical surgery, chemotherapy, and/or radiotherapy with the associated morbidity and mortality. As survival has shifted in the last years, so did the importance of improving the quality of life (QoL) of survivors with long-term sequelae.

Frequent changes associated with surgery are fecal incontinence, urgency, variation in frequency of stools, or LARS (low anterior resection syndrome). It is estimated that about 50–90% of rectal cancer patients will present with those symptoms [7].

S. Tavares Nogueira (✉)
General and Digestive Surgery, Clinical Institute of Digestive and Metabolic Diseases, Hospital Clínic de Barcelona, Barcelona, Spain

I. Araujo
Endoscopy and Gastrointestinal Motility Unit, Clinical Institute of Digestive and Metabolic Diseases, Hospital Clínic de Barcelona, Barcelona, Spain

Data on sexual dysfunction (SD) is variable due to different terminology used and time of evaluation after surgery, but it can be present in 68% of men and 93% of women after rectal cancer treatment [8]. Causes are complex and involve functioning and psychosocial features. Local anatomical factors like pelvic nerve damage, vaginal strictures, loss of continence or the presence of a stoma can intervene and can also affect the patient's way to relate to others and their self-perception [7–9].

In previous publications [10, 11], the importance of defining quality of sexual life and sexual dysfunction was pointed out in a way to standardize the terminology used, as sometimes the absence of sexual activity is used as a surrogate of SD, without taking into consideration the individual's desire and opportunity. Quality of sexual life involves the patient's evaluation of their sexual function, whereas SD refers to the organic aspects. In male, this is reflected in erectile or ejaculation dysfunction and in women as lack of lubrication, dyspareunia, or the inability to achieve orgasm [12].

Although this seems to be a prevalent concern after treatment for rectal or anal cancer, physicians rarely address sexual function, and there seems to be a need to improve the communication on SD with their patients [13, 14]. Educational strategies to aid patients and their partners to adjust to changes during and after treatment need to be addressed and there is previous data that reports an improvement in self-reported sexual response [15].

Overall, as survival rate has improved constantly, QoL measures should be continued to be addressed, trying to enhance communication with patients to establish realistic expectations after treatment and still focusing on a curative procedure.

In this chapter, we overview the problem of sexual dysfunction in patients with CRC, its epidemiology, pathophysiology, risk factors, clinical presentation, diagnosis, and management.

2 Pathophysiology of Sexual Dysfunction

Data evaluating CRC outcomes usually focuses on morbidity, mortality, disease-free survival, and overall survival. Recent studies have also described quality of life (QoL) in which sexual function plays an important role [16].

Although sexual dysfunction lacks a standardized definition and comparison of results is difficult, there is some evidence available regarding its pathophysiology and risk factors among this population. A growing number of studies have been reporting the rate of sexual dysfunction following CRC treatment, especially in patients with rectal cancer.

The multimodal treatment consisting of radiotherapy, chemotherapy, and surgery for CRC patients may cause and contribute to different physiologic changes, all implicated in sexual dysfunction. This is summarized in Table 1 [17].

Table 1 Physiologic changes associated with sexual dysfunction in multimodal treatment for CRC

Physiologic changes	Radiotherapy	Chemotherapy	Surgery
Vascular, sensory, and continence	Vascular scarring—decreased genital blood flow (erection dysfunction; decreased vaginal lubrication)	Change in senses—taste bud changes; increased sensitivity to smells; peripheral neuropathy changes sensation of touch	Urinary/fecal incontinence—type of surgery affects risk
Skin changes	Skin changes—texture/color changes can affect body image; can remind partner of patient's diagnosis. Although tattoos are small, they can be a reminder to the patient or partner of diagnosis	Skin sensitivity changes—some chemo causes extreme reaction to cold which affects food that can be eaten on dates; neuropathy affects enjoyment of skin touch; hand/foot (palmar/plantar) syndrome can affect enjoyment of activity with partner/affect ease of touching partner if skin peeling off hands; skin rash can occur; affect color of nails	Surgical scars—body image changes; affect partner's ease in being with patient
Fatigue	Affects social interaction, libido	Affects social interaction, libido	Affects social interaction, libido
Vaginal vault changes	Shortening of vagina; decreased lubrication; risk of dyspareunia; vaginal stenosis	Decreased lubrication; risk of dyspareunia; increased risk of vaginal infection from tiny tears; Mucositis—can affect oral or vaginal cavity	Postoperative adhesions if they occur do not usually affect the vaginal vault unless surgery was done in that specific location

(continued)

Table 1 (continued)

Physiologic changes	Radiotherapy	Chemotherapy	Surgery
Sexual pattern alterations	If fatigue, may need to change usual positions or time of day for activity; affect spontaneity; if decreased lubrication will need to use artificial lubricant to avoid tears and possible infection; if radiotherapy causes diarrhea, will affect usual pattern if apprehensive; if fecal incontinence will affect spontaneity, change in positions	If nausea/vomiting, will decrease desire; affects dating pattern; if taste bud changes, may avoid French kissing/oral stimulation; if fatigue, may need to change usual positions or time of day for activity; affect spontaneity; if decreased lubrication will need to use artificial lubricant to avoid tears and possible infection	If stoma will need to remember to empty appliance prior to sexual activity; perhaps wear cover on appliance to prevent it "sticking" to body; if patient irrigates, may decide to do prior to activity so can wear smaller "security pouch"; change in usual position so appliance can lie to the side; if waterplay activity part of sexual pattern may want to irrigate, prior so do not have to wear appliance; avoid "gassy" food on date or use "gas filters"; loss of rectal sexual pleasuring if rectum removed
Nerve damage	Skin sensitivity decreased; decreased vaginal lubrication/erection dysfunction	Skin sensitivity decreased; decreased vaginal lubrication/erection dysfunction	Skin sensitivity decreased; decreased vaginal lubrication/erection dysfunction
Hair pattern	Alopecia—(only in the site of radiation treatment) affects body image; daily reminder of treatment/diagnosis; if loss of pubic hair may be pleasurable or may be emotionally upsetting to the patient or partner if they feel "childlike"	Alopecia/hair thinning—affects body image; if single, may affect desire to date; daily reminder of treatment/diagnosis; if loss of pubic hair may be pleasurable or may be emotionally upsetting to patient or partner if they feel "childlike"	No effects
Fertility impact	Location/dose affect risk; premature ovarian failure	Type/dose affect risk	Usually not for CRC. Abdominal adhesions can increase risk of female infertility post-treatment; pelvic exenteration (hysterectomy); A/P resection = retrograde ejaculation
Fear of recurrence	Impacts libido of patient and/or partner	Impacts libido of patient and/or partner	Impacts libido of patient and/or partner

(continued)

Table 1 (continued)

Physiologic changes	Radiotherapy	Chemotherapy	Surgery
Delayed complications	Risk of fecal or urinary incontinence due to fibrosis (risk factors for postoperative incontinence included preoperative incontinence, female gender, perioperative blood loss, preoperative bladder emptying difficulties, autonomic nerve damage, and presence of a permanent stoma)	Peripheral neuropathy may be permanent, and it can affect sensations/enjoyment; taste bud changes may be permanent and will affect sexuality	Adhesions can cause pelvic pain during coitus; nerve damage may be permanent and affect sensations

Adapted from Averyt et al. [17]

3 Risk Factors for Sexual Dysfunction

Sexual dysfunction in CRC patients is complex and tend to result from an interaction of factors (Table 2) that include patient, tumor, and treatment-related issues:

3.1 Patient-Related Factors

3.1.1 Age

Age has been evaluated as a potential risk factor for sexual dysfunction with evidence suggesting a clear correlation. *Lindau* and colleagues evaluated sexual function in a national reference group of adults and revealed that 73% of participants aged 57–64, 53% aged 65–74, and 26% of patients aged 75–85 years were sexually active, with women presenting lower rates than men in every age group [18]. Although there has been an increase in CRC diagnosis in the young population, most patients suffering from this condition tend to be over 50 years old.

Data published has used different age cutoffs to evaluate sexual dysfunction after treatment but one common aspect to all is that the rate of sexual dysfunction increases with age [19].

3.1.2 Gender

Both men and women suffer a decline in sexual function after CRC treatment, but the evidence suggests that sexual dysfunction in men is higher (23–69% versus 19–62%) [20].

There are three main aspects that must be addressed regarding these findings. First, male sexual dysfunction is often described as ejaculatory and erectile dysfunction. Those definitions are easier and more objective to evaluate than the

Table 2 Risk factors associated to sexual dysfunction

Patient-related	Tumor-related	Treatment-related
Age	Location	Radiation therapy
Gender		Surgical procedure
Psychological and social issues	Clinical stage	Ostomy creation
Preoperative function		

multifactorial, complex, and variable definition for female sexual dysfunction that include loss of libido, vaginal dryness, dyspareunia, and the ability to reach orgasm [21].

Second, male sexual dysfunction has been the focus of many studies of QoL after CRC treatment and only recently female sexual function has been analyzed.

Third, studies on sexual function are often limited to small cohorts and are characterized by low response rates, especially in female patients.

3.1.3 Psychological and Social Issues

Adaptation and coping with a recent cancer diagnosis and treatment challenges can have an important impact on QoL and sexual function in patients with colorectal cancer. Adding to that, relationship status and dynamics, body image and acceptance, depressive symptoms and fatigue can all play a role in causing or aggravating sexual dysfunction in CRC survivors [16].

3.1.4 Preoperative Sexual Function

The available literature lacks information on the assessment of pretreatment sexual function, with most patients being evaluated after diagnosis. As expected, pretreatment function is a strong predictor of results, and patients with previous sexual dysfunction will persist after treatment [20].

3.2 Tumor-Related Factors

3.2.1 Location

Comparison studies between colon cancer patients and rectal cancer patients show the latter experience worst sexual function, meaning that rectal and anal cancer patients are at higher risk of sexual dysfunction than colon cancer patients [16, 21].

3.2.2 Clinical Stage

There is previous data that suggests that TNM staging score for colorectal cancer is strongly associated with patient's prognosis [22]. T stage is also associated with sexual dysfunction. Patients with highly invasive tumors may have greater dysfunction because of distorted anatomy and pelvic organ invasion (vagina, uterus, prostate). The dysfunction can be related to symptoms, or the more complex and extensive surgery required [20, 23].

3.3 Treatment-Related Factors

3.3.1 Radiation Therapy

Neoadjuvant treatment is a crucial part of the multimodal treatment of rectal cancer. Either radiotherapy or combined chemo-radiotherapy have been shown to improve local control and reduce the risk of local recurrence in patients with locally advanced disease [24]. More recently, the possibility of achieving complete response has also positioned radiotherapy and chemo-radiotherapy as definitive treatments for rectal cancer patients [25].

Radiation acts by promoting oxidative stress damage targeting nuclear DNA transcription in both direct and indirect pathways. This effect is first seen in cells with high turnover, fulfilling the main goals of the therapy to eradicate or debulk the tumor, improving the chances for an R0 resection. Despite the clear oncologic benefits, radiotherapy also adds morbidity to surgery. Patients who received radiation-reported SD in spite of increased QoL [24]. Previous randomized trials have identified no difference between short- or long-course radiotherapy treatments [26, 27].

3.3.2 Surgical Treatment

Surgery is the cornerstone of CRC treatment. For colon cancer, the procedure has little to no impact on sexual function, unless it involves the creation of a stoma, something to be discussed further down.

For rectal cancer, surgical technique, and surgical procedure, both play an important role. Surgical treatment for rectal cancer has evolved greatly from the first procedure described in 1826 by Lisfranc to total mesorectal excision (TME) presented by Heald in 1982 [28]. Currently, TME is the gold standard for rectal cancer treatment, and it implies a meticulous dissection through embryologic planes to remove the rectum, mesorectum, and its fascial envelope as one. This dissection is done in close contact to nerve plexuses responsible for an adequate urogenital function: *nervi erigentes*, inferior hypogastric plexus, superior hypogastric plexus. Damage to those nerves may result in sexual and urinary dysfunction after rectal cancer surgery [23].

Tumor location in the rectum (upper, middle, or inferior third) (Fig. 1), sphincter invasion, anorectal function, and patient characteristics (age, comorbidities, performance status) are important aspects in the selection of the surgical procedure to perform: anterior resection (AR) or abdominoperineal resection (APR). At first, the rectum is removed following the TME principles and an anastomosis is performed for bowel reconstruction. In the latter, the rectum and anal canal are removed also following the TME principles but with no reconstruction, leaving the patient with a terminal colostomy. Available evidence suggests that patients submitted to APR may have worst sexual function than patients submitted to AR. In the study from Tekkis and colleagues with 295 women, patients who underwent APR were significantly less likely to be sexually active, had lower frequency of intercourse, were less likely to achieve arousal and had worst dyspareunia [23].

Fig. 1 Segmentation of
the rectum by thirds:
inferior, medium, superior

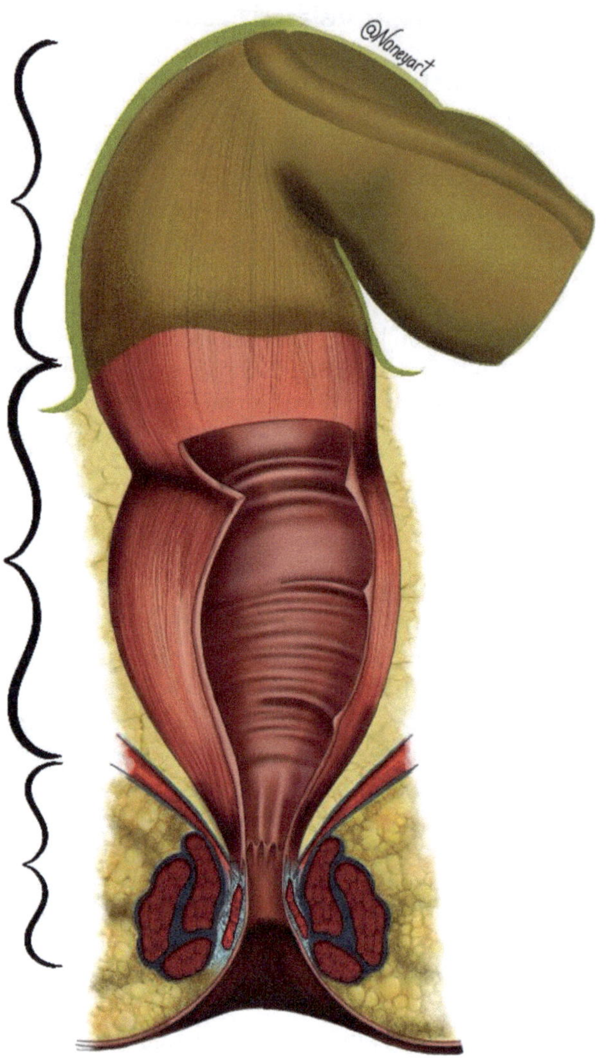

3.3.3 Ostomy Creation

Ostomy creation, either temporary or definitive, may be a consequence or necessity in CRC patients' treatment. Historically, the presence of a stoma has been associated with the worst quality of life (QoL), but this notion was challenged by a Cochrane review that found no significant differences between patients with stomas and patients without stomas [29].

When focusing on sexual function, data is inconclusive and insufficient. In a recent study from Thyø and colleagues, female patients with a permanent stoma had an increase odds ratio for loss of desire, dyspareunia, bleeding during intercourse and reduced vaginal dimension [21]. Engel et al. reported that having a stoma was significantly associated with worse sexual function and male sexual problems [30].

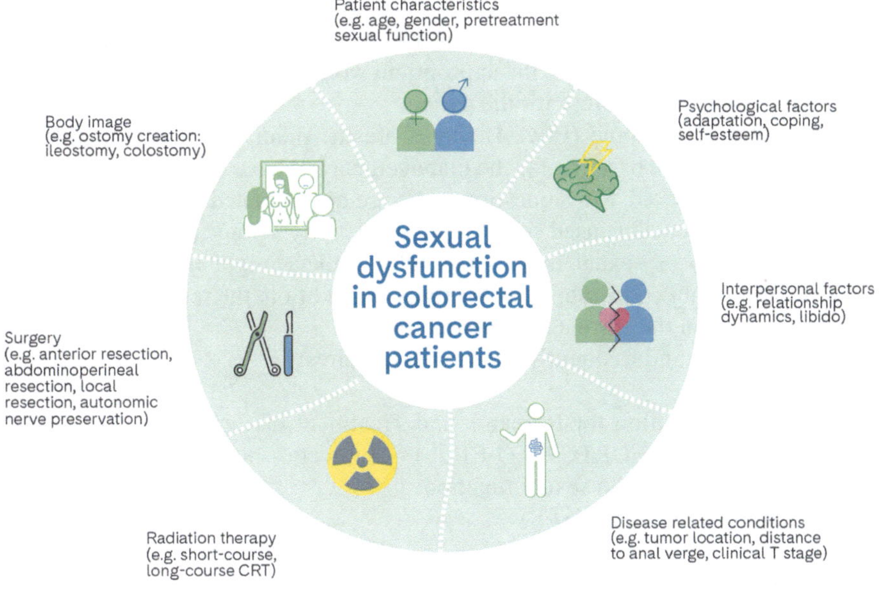

Fig. 2 Factor influencing the development of sexual dysfunction among colorectal cancer survivors

In conclusion, more studies with higher cohort numbers and higher response rates are needed to determine the relationship between stoma creation and sexual function (Fig. 2).

4   Clinical Presentation of Sexual Dysfunction

Sexual dysfunction in CRC survivors can present itself as erectile dysfunction and ejaculation problems in men, dyspareunia and vaginal dryness in women, and decrease in sexual desire, decrease in the frequency of intercourse, and difficulty in reaching orgasm in both sexes [6].

5   Diagnosis of Sexual Dysfunction

As discussed in previous sections, sexual dysfunction does not have a standard definition and varies between genders. One of the main challenges in obtaining objective and reproducible data on sexual function after CRC treatment is the difficulty in reaching a diagnosis.

History and physical examination play an important role, as with any other condition, but here we must highlight the importance of the physician's role in engaging the patient on the subject. Many patients, especially after going through the fear of malignant disease, have difficulties mentioning sexual difficulties and may even dismiss them. The physician needs to be aware of the possibility of sexual dysfunction after CRC treatment, to seek the appropriate wording and questions, in order to create an environment of safety for the patient.

Patient-reported outcome (PROM) scores are the main tool used to reach the diagnosis and to have a baseline for the management but have important limitations that need to be addressed. Most questionnaires are not validated and do not provide definitions for the concepts used such as "sexual activity." Some patients will interpret sexual activity as sexual intercourse, while others might feel that intimacy, touching, and kissing constitute sexual activity. In addition, the results obtained are highly dependent on the correct completion of data.

These are useful and frequently used questionnaires:

- European Organization for Research and Treatment of Cancer Quality of Life Questionnaire C38 (EORTC QLQ-CR38)—colorectal-specific supplement with three subscales related to sexual function:
  - Sexual Function Score (SFS)
  - Sexual Enjoyment Score (SES)
  - Gender-specific sexual problem score
- Female Sexual Function Index (FSFI)—scores between 2 and 36, being considered abnormal a score below 26.5.
- International Index of Erectile Function Questionnaire (IIEF)—scores between 5 and 75, being considered abnormal a score below 42.9.

6 Management of Sexual Dysfunction

As there is no consensus in the definition and diagnosis of sexual dysfunction in CRC patients, there is no structured and defined management. Patients should be treated individually, according to their symptoms and expectations.

The key message on management should focus on addressing the possibility of sexual dysfunction at the time of diagnosis and most importantly after the treatment, so that patients can have a space to discuss these difficulties when they are present.

When sexual dysfunction is identified, patients should be managed with a multidisciplinary team including a psycho-oncologist and referred to the appropriate specialist according to findings.

7 Conclusion

In the last decades, there have been many advances in the treatment of lower gastrointestinal cancer, leading to an increase in survival rates. As this happens, studies have focused on evaluating the QoL of survivors and the many features that can be influenced by the disease and its treatment, one being sexual function. Many factors can influence sexual function in patients that have survived a lower gastrointestinal cancer: patient-related, tumor-related and treatment-related. Overall, SD is a prevalent concern among this group of patients that needs to be more visible in order to be addressed by treating physicians so that an appropriate management can be sought.

Another aspect that needs further development is the management of sexual dysfunction in sexually diverse populations. Most of the information currently available focuses on SD in heterosexual cis-gender individuals and does not take into account, for example, the impact of rectal cancer and anal cancer surgical treatment in the population of men who have sex with men. There is a growing need to acknowledge the differences in the treated population and to learn how to address them.

References

1. Canty J, Stabile C, Milli L, Seidel B, Goldfrank D, Carter J. Sexual function in women with colorectal/anal cancer. Sex Med Rev. 2019;7:202.
2. Vuik FE, Nieuwenburg SA, Bardou M. Increasing incidence of colorectal cancer in young adults in Europe over the last 25 years. Gut. 2019;68:1820.
3. Miller KD, Siegel RL, Lin CC. Cancer treatment and survivorship statistics. CA Cancer J Clin. 2016;66:271.
4. Corrigan KL, Rooney MK, De B, Ludmir ED, Das P, Smith GL, Taniguchi C, Minsky BD, Koay EJ, Koong A, Morris VK, Messick CA, Nogueras-Gonzalez G, Holliday EB. Patient-reported sexual function in long-term survivors of anal cancer treated with definitive intensity modulated radiation therapy and concurrent chemotherapy. Pract Radiat Oncol. 2022;12(5):e397–405.
5. Gondal TA, Chaudhary N, Bajwa H, Rauf A, Le D, Ahmed S. Anal cancer: the past, present and future. Curr Oncol. 2023;30(3):3232–50.
6. Almont T, Bouhnik AD, Charif AB, Bendiane MK, Huyghe E. Sexual health problems and discussion in colorectal cancer patients two years after diagnosis: a national cross-sectional study. J Sex Med. 2018;16:96–110.
7. Pang JH, Jones Z, Myers OB, Popek S. Long term sexual function following rectal cancer treatment. Am J Surg. 2020;220(5):1258–63.
8. Attaallah W, Ertekin C, Tinay I, Yegen C. High rate of sexual dysfunction following surgery for rectal cancer. Ann Coloproctol. 2014;30(5):210–5.
9. Benedict C, Philip EJ, Baser RE, Carter J, Schuler TA, Jandorf L, Duhamel K, Nelson C. Body image and sexual function in women after treatment for anal and rectal cancer. Psychooncology. 2016;25(3):316–23.
10. Traa MJ, Orsini RG, den Oudsten BL, de Vries J, Roukema JA, Bosman SJ, Dudink RL, Rutten HJT. Measuring the health-related quality of life and sexual functioning of patients with rectal cancer: does type of treatment matter? Int J Cancer. 2014;134(4):979–87.
11. Perry WRG, Abd El Aziz MA, Duchalais E, Grass F, Behm KT, Mathis KL, Kelley SR. Sexual dysfunction following surgery for rectal cancer: a single-institution experience. Updates Surg. 2021;73(6):2155–9.
12. Celentano V, Cohen R, Warusavitarne J, Faiz O, Chand M. Sexual dysfunction following rectal cancer surgery. Int J Colorectal Dis. 2017;32(11):1523–30.
13. Flynn KE, Reese JB, Jeffery DD, Abernethy AP, Lin L, Shelby RA, Porter LS, Dombeck CB, Weinfurt KP. Patient experiences with communication about sex during and after treatment for cancer. Psychooncology. 2012;21(6):594–601.
14. Park ER, Norris RL, Bober SL. Sexual health communication during cancer care: barriers and recommendations. Cancer J. 2009;15:74.

15. Brotto LA, Erskine Y, Carey M, Ehlen T, Finlayson S, Heywood M, Kwon J, McAlpine J, Stuart G, Thomson S, Miller D. A brief mindfulness-based cognitive behavioral intervention improves sexual functioning versus wait-list control in women treated for gynecologic cancer. Gynecol Oncol. 2012;125(2):320–5.
16. Den Oudsten BL, Traa MJ, Thong MSY, Martijn H, van de Poll-Franse LV. Higher prevalence of sexual dysfunction in colon and rectal cancer survivors compared with the normative population: a population-based study. Eur J Cancer. 2012;48:3161.
17. Averyt JC, Nishimoto PW. Addressing sexual dysfunction in colorectal cancer survivorship care. J Gastrointest Oncol. 2014;5:388.
18. Lindau ST, Schumm LP, Laumann EO, Levinson W, Waite LJ. A study of sexuality and health among older adults in the United States. N Engl J Med. 2007;357:762.
19. Li K, He X, Tong S, Zheng Y. Risk factors for sexual dysfunction after rectal cancer surgery in 948 consecutive patients: a prospective cohort study. Eur J Surg Oncol. 2021;47:2087.
20. Ho VP, Lee Y, Stein SL, Temple LKF. Sexual function after treatment for rectal cancer: a review. Dis Colon Rectum. 2011;54:113.
21. Thyo A, Elfeki H, Laurberg S, Emmersten KJ. Female sexual problems after treatment for colorectal cancer—a population-based study. Colorectal Dis. 2019;21:1130.
22. Gao P, Song YX, Wang ZN, Xu YY, Xu HM. Is the prediction of prognosis not improved by the seventh edition of the TNM classification for colorectal cancer? Analysis of the surveillance, epidemiology, and end results (SEER) database. BMC Cancer. 2013;13:123.
23. Tekkis PP, Cornish JA, Remzi FH, Tilney HS, Fazio VW. Measuring sexual and urinary outcomes in women after rectal cancer excision. Dis Colon Rectum. 2009;52:46.
24. Zwart WH, Hotca A, Hospers GAP, Goodman KA, Garcia-Aguilar J. The multimodal management of locally advanced rectal cancer: making sense of the new data. ASCO Educational Book. 2022. p. 264.
25. Habr-Gama A, Perez RO, Proscurshim I, Gama-Rodrigues J. Complete clinical response after neoadjuvant chemoradiation for distal rectal cancer. Surg Oncol Clin N Am. 2010;19:829.
26. Pietrzak L, Bucko K, Nowacki MP. Quality of life, anorectal and sexual functions after preoperative radiotherapy for rectal cancer: report of a randomised trial. Radiother Oncol. 2007;84:217.
27. McLachlan SA, Fisher RG, Zalcberg J. The impact on health-related quality of life in the first 12 months: a randomised comparison of preoperative short-course radiation versus long-course chemoradiation for T3 rectal cancer (Trans-Tasman Radiation Oncology Group Trial 01.04). Eur J Cancer. 2016;55:15.
28. Heald RJ, Husband EM, Ryall RD. The mesorectum in rectal cancer surgery—the clue to pelvic recurrence? Br J Surg. 1982;69:613.
29. Pachler J, Wille-Jorgensen P. Quality of life after rectal resection for cancer, with or without permanent colostomy. Cochrane Database Syst Rev. 2005.
30. Engel J, Kerr J, Schlesinger-Raab A, Eckel R, Holzel D. Quality of life in rectal cancer patients: a four-year prospective study. Ann Surg. 2003;238:203.

Sexuality in Adult Patients with Cancer in the Era of Precision Oncology

Carme Font, Lydia Gaba, and Esther Gomez-Gil

1 Introduction

The general development of medicine and in particular the novel anticancer therapies achieved in recent years has led to a progressive lengthening in the survival of patients with cancer [1, 2]. Survivorship begins at the time a cancer is detected and addresses healthcare issues beyond diagnosis and acute treatment. Thus, the population of cancer survivors includes: (1) patients receiving active radical anticancer therapies with curative intent; (2) patients already treated with cancer in remission; and (3) patients with advanced uncurable cancer receiving mid- or long-term anticancer therapies along with supportive and palliative care approaches to relieve symptoms. In this context, new clinical scenarios continuously emerge, and there is a trend towards the development of new models of care and the expansion of subspecialties overlapping oncology, such as cardio-oncology or oncogeriatrics and the integration of early palliative care aimed at optimizing the growing needs of patients with cancer [3].

In line with the above, issues related to sexual health have also gained increasing attention as an area of knowledge and concern in recent years and have been included in the agenda of international scientific societies involved in the care of oncological patients [4, 5]. Sexual function may be profoundly altered in patients with cancer due to multiple and complex variety of insults to the physical and psychosocial dimensions of sexuality [6]. Sexual impairment may occur in cancer survivors due to the disease itself or anticancer treatments including surgery, chemotherapy, hormonal treatments, targeted therapies, and/or immunotherapy. The above potential aetiologic factors and their clinical consequences leading to sexual dysfunction (SD) in women and men are summarized in Fig. 1 and Table 1. Notably,

C. Font (✉) · L. Gaba · E. Gomez-Gil
Clinical Sexology Working Group, Hospital Clinic de Barcelona, Barcelona, Spain
e-mail: cfont@clinic.cat; lgaba@clinic.cat; esgomez@clinic.cat

C. Castelo-Branco, S. Anglès Acedo (eds.), *Medical Disorders and Sexual Health*, Trends in Andrology and Sexual Medicine,
https://doi.org/10.1007/978-3-031-55080-5_16

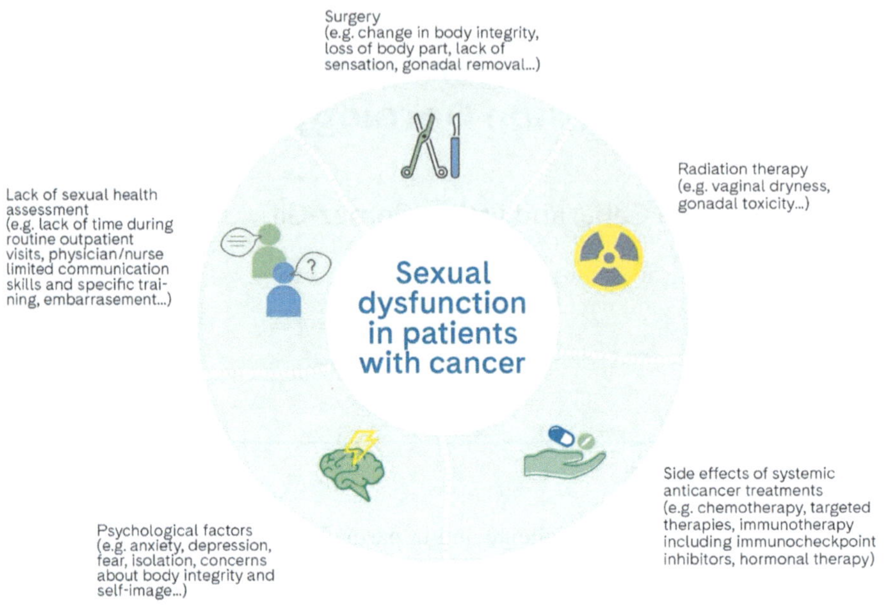

Fig. 1 Risk factors for sexual dysfunction in patients with cancer

the potential causes of SD frequently overlap, and the outcomes may vary depending on the type of cancer, the type of treatment(s), the age of the patient at the time of treatment, the amount of time that has passed since treatment, the reversibility of the physical and psychological sequelae, and other personal health factors (comorbidities, psychosocial factors) [7].

Despite the potential negative impact of SD on the quality of life (QoL) of both cancer survivors and their sexual partners, sexual health has largely remained unexplored in prospectively designed studies specifically addressing sexual health in this setting. Thus, most of the limited data available on this topic are from a great heterogeneity of studies including trials evaluating the safety/efficacy of anticancer treatments [4, 5], observational studies focused on fertility preservation after cancer therapy [8], and management of anxiety and depression in oncology [9]. Overall, although SD is considered common and frequently long lasting in cancer survivors [4, 5, 10], a wide range of rates (0–97%) of SD have been reported depending on the tumour type, study design, and the outcome measures used for SD assessment [7].

In this chapter, we provide a general concise overview of the most common sexual problems experienced by cancer survivors. There are specificities related to the sequelae of anticancer treatments due to female/male cancers involving the sexual organs, as well as commonalities related to other types of cancers involving both sexes. We review the current barriers for the SD assessment in daily practice and the potential interventions for the management of SD in the setting of

Table 1 Potential etiologic factors (general and cancer-associated) and their clinical consequences leading to sexual dysfunction (SD) in women and men

General factors influencing sexual health	Cancer-associated factors potentially influencing sexual health	Symptoms of sexual dysfunction in cancer survivors
Biological factors Age Gender Physical illness Genetic vulnerability Immune function Endocrine function Cardiovascular function Neurochemistry Stress reactivity Medication effects	**Cancer therapies:** • **Sexual organ surgery:** orchiectomy, penectomy, vulvectomy, hysterectomy • **Pelvic radiation** inducing vaginal fibrosis and stenosis • **Chemotherapy side effects:** hair loss, fatigue, gastrointestinal symptoms, lower oestrogen/testosterone levels (gonadal toxicity), haematologic toxicity (anaemia) • **Hormonal treatments:** androgen or testosterone deprivation therapy • **Immunotherapy:** endocrine side effects, hypogonadism • **Targeted therapies:** vascular, dermatological, respiratory and/or digestive side effects **Pain and fatigue** induced by cancer itself and their treatments **Change in body integrity or morphology affecting self-image** **Changes in body sensation** **Change in body physiology**	**Female** • Loss or low sexual desire • Decreased arousal • Orgasm absent delayed, infrequent, or lacks intensity (anorgasmia) • Pain/dyspareunia **Male** • Loss or low sexual desire • Decreased arousal • Ejaculation problems such as premature ejaculation; Failure to ejaculate • Erectile dysfunction • Orgasm problems such as anorgasm, delayed orgasm, or painful orgasm
Psychology factors Learning—Memory Personality—Temperament Attitudes—Behaviours—Beliefs Motivation—Self-efficacy Intelligence—Coping skills Self-esteem—Emotions Past trauma	**Increased emotional distress:** anxiety, depression **Cognitive shifts towards negative thinking:** fear of intimacy, impair of body image, negative thinking, diminished feelings of attractiveness **Increased barriers to effective communication:** embarrassment, prejudice, stigma	
Social and interpersonal context Family background and circumstances Social support Peer relationships Cultural values—Social norms Religious traditions Social and economic status Education/Sex education Spirituality	Diminished or discordant social relationship Isolation from peers and partners during anticancer treatment Decreased feelings of being attractive Increased barriers to effective communication (with partners and healthcare providers) Limited availability of specific resources Difficulties in the marital relationship	

patients with cancer, including the subgroup of adolescents and young adults (AYAs) [11]. We also identify areas that warrant further research in order to integrate sexual health as part of the best supportive and palliative care for cancer survivors.

2   Cancer Involving Sexual Organs in Females

The five main types of gynaecologic cancer are: cervical, ovarian, uterine, vaginal, and vulvar. A sixth type of gynaecologic cancer is the very rare fallopian tube cancer [1, 12]. Women diagnosed with primary gynaecological cancers frequently present SD during and after anticancer treatment, with prevalence ranging from 65 to 90%, being the higher rates reported in African and American women compared to women from Asia and Europe [12].

Most studies emphasize the physical aspects of sexuality, while psychosocial concerns involved in sexual health remain under-assessed [12]. For instance, patients with cervical cancer report persistent changes in vaginal anatomy (insufficient vaginal lubrication for sexual intercourse, short vagina, insufficiently elastic vagina and moderate or much distress due to vaginal changes and dyspareunia) compromising sexual activity [13]. Additionally, other common treatments in this setting such as oophorectomy and pelvic radiation can cause premature ovarian insufficiency and therefore a climacteric syndrome. This syndrome includes local (urinary tract disturbances, vaginal dryness, and dyspareunia) and systemic symptoms (hot flashes, joint pain), sleep disturbances and mood changes, which, in turn, may affect the libido and the sexual well-being [12, 14].

Regarding the clinical assessment of sexual problems in patients with cancer, it has to be taken into account that the physical changes due to gynaecological cancer treatment may have an impact in pelvic examinations that can be extremely painful, impossible, or traumatic [4, 5, 7]. Moreover, gynaecological cancer survivors and clinicians report communication barriers to address sexual health-related symptoms derived from inadequate training of clinicians in how to hold discussions related to sexual health, perceived lack of time, prioritization of other concerns, lack of provider comfort with the topic, embarrassment, and limited awareness about treatment. International guidelines recommend discussing the potential sexual impact of a planned anticancer treatment and inquiring about sexual health at regular intervals during follow-up [4, 5, 7].

There is no gold standard tool for the assessment of SD in women [15, 16]. Most authors recommend the use of the *Brief Sexual Symptom Checklist for Women (BSSC-W)* as a primary screening tool to assess the presence of SD and allow health providers to distinguish between a lack of sexual desire (i.e., libido, depression, anxiety, drugs, etc.) and/or physical inability to engage in sexual activity (i.e., due to pain or lack of physiological arousal, oestrogen deprivation, problems with orgasm, etc.). After this initial evaluation, the *Female Sexual Function Index (FSFI)* is commonly used for more in-depth evaluation of SD in women. Other more specific tools aimed at evaluating the six domains of sexuality (desire, arousal, lubrication, orgasm, satisfaction, and pain), body image, and aspects related to QoL include the *Sexual Adjustment and Body Image Scale (SABIS),* the *Sexual Adjustment and Body Image Scale-Gynaecologic Cancer (SABIS-G),* the *European Organization for Research and Treatment of Cancer Quality of Life Questionnaire (QLQ-C30),* the *Sexual function-Vaginal changes Questionnaire (SVQ),* the *Gynaecologic Leiden Questionnaire (GLQ),* the *Information on Sexual Health Questionnaire (SHQ),* the *Sexual Satisfaction Questionnaire (SSQ),* and the *Sexual Activity Questionnaire (SAQ),* among others [4, 5, 15, 16]. Moreover, *Patient-Reported Experience Measures (PREMs) and Patient-Reported Outcomes Measures (PROMs)* are valuable tools for evaluating clinical health-related QoL outcomes and can also be used in daily practice and/or for clinical research depending on the target and particularities of specific populations such as for those with minority sexual orientation [17].

For further sexual health evaluation, a holistic, patient-centred, and multidisciplinary approach, that may include primary care, gynaecology, urology, oncology, psychology, and rehabilitation medicine, is suggested to prevent and reduce the impact of cancer treatment in these patients. A broader integrative approach should be integrated as part of their optimal supportive care and survivorship rehabilitation programme during and after cancer treatment [4, 5, 7]. When appropriate, the comprehensive evaluation of GC survivors should include the patient's partner participation and should address concerns related to fertility, contraceptive methods, prescribed medications can negatively impact libido such as antidepressants and/or other psychological issues. The evaluation of menopausal status may include endocrine biomarkers such as oestradiol levels, follicle-stimulating hormone (FSH), anti-Mullerian hormone and inhibin, which may provide additional information on ovarian function.

Treatments and interventions aimed at relieving symptoms of SD in women with cancer are summarized in Table 2 [4, 5, 7]. Notably, for the management of climacteric syndrome and low libido, the use of systemic hormonal treatments such as oestrogen or testosterone are particularly controversial because of safety concerns in survivors of hormone-mediated cancers [18]. The creation of a specialized clinic dedicated to education and counselling on sexual health issues have been reported useful with high levels of patient satisfaction [19, 20].

Table 2 Suggested treatment options for sexual symptoms in women with cancer

Sexual symptoms	Treatment options

Vaginal atrophy and dryness	**Vaginal moisturizers**: without parabens, with acid pH and low osmolarity for regular use. Better containing hyaluronic acid
	Lubricants: Water-based: can use with silicone sex toys
	  Silicone-based: longer lasting, not for use with silicone sex toys
	  Oil-based: degrades condoms
	Low dose of vaginal oestrogen products: only in refractory cases following a risk/benefit discussion. Rings and suppositories are preferred over creams due to minimal systemic absorption

Low or lack of sexual desire or intimacy (Hypoactive sexual desire disorder)	**Psychosexual counselling**: address contributing psychosocial problems **Sensate focus techniques,** mindfulness **Exercise**
Orgasm absent delayed, infrequent, or lacks intensity (anorgasmia)	**Use of vibrator or clitoral stimulatory devices** **Pelvic physical therapy**
Pain with sexual activity/dyspareunia	**Topical vaginal therapies** for vaginal dryness **Progressive vaginal dilators**: help prevent or reverse correct scarring for patients with fibrosis/stenosis **Pelvic physical therapy**: pelvic floor physical therapy to lower pain, improve bladder retention, improve bowel function, and increase the flow of blood to the area **Topical anaesthetic such as aqueous lidocaine**: applied around the vestibule or opening the vagina before penetrative sexual activity
Global symptoms of distress, anxiety, depression, or other psychological concerns	**Psychotherapy** and multidisciplinary clinics led by nurses, psychologists, and/or other trained professionals – Communication and education interventions aimed to increase awareness about sexual health during anticancer therapies – Address concerns about potential side effects of anticancer treatments – Questions or concerns about fertility, infection, or bleeding – Optimize the management of common side effects of anticancer treatments: pain, fatigue, hair loss – Optimize the management of common psychological symptoms: sadness, loss of interest in activities, or trouble sleeping – Information to prevent pregnancy while receiving anticancer treatment for childbearing age patients – Education about the use of condoms to avoid the contact of the partner with some chemotherapies in vaginal secretions **Support groups for patients** **Online resources**: https://www.cancer.gov/about-cancer/treatment/side-effects/sexuality-women

3   Cancer Involving Sexual Organs in Males

Sexual impairment is common in male patients treated for cancers involving the sexual organs due to mutilating surgery and pelvic radiation which can potentially damage blood vessels and the autonomic nervous system leading to erectile dysfunction. Moreover, hormonal therapies, chemotherapy, and other anticancer treatments may all contribute to SD [21, 22].

In patients with prostate cancer, the most common cancer in men [1], the incidence of erectile dysfunction has been reported in 20–90% of patients [7, 21]. Radical prostatectomy surgery is associated with SD, with a majority of men never regaining preoperative levels of function. Bilateral nerve-sparing has been associated with better sexual outcomes whereas extended (versus limited) pelvic lymph node dissection has not been found to increase the risk of erectile dysfunction. In addition, for qualified candidates, robotic prostatectomy offers additional potential benefits over traditional open prostatectomy regarding bladder control and erectile function [21]. Other factors associated to erectile dysfunction after radical prostatectomy include the preoperative erectile function, the patient age, postoperative erectile haemodynamics, surgeon experience, surgeon volume, vascular comorbidities, and serum testosterone levels [22]. Regarding radiation therapy for prostate cancer, both external beam radiation therapy and brachytherapy can also lead to erectile dysfunction, with the highest rates resulting from external beam radiation therapy and brachytherapy used in combination [21]. Moreover, the androgen deprivation therapy is associated to hypogonadism and may produce additional adverse effects such as hot flashes, fatigue, gynaecomastia, emotional lability, and self-image impairment [23].

Penile cancer is a rare and aggressive neoplasm with great geographical disparities in the incidence of disease ranging from 2.8 to 6.8 per 100,000 in the developing world vs. 0.3 per 100,000 in western countries [1]. Squamous cell carcinoma of the penis has traditionally been treated with partial penectomy with a 2-cm margin. There is very limited data from small retrospective cohorts regarding the incidence and clinical manifestations of SD in patients with penile cancer. Notably, erection is possible after partial penectomy, and orgasms and ejaculation continue to be possible, but the body image is affected [21].

Testicular cancer ranks as the 20th leading type of cancer worldwide, being the most common cancer in young men in Europe [1]. Retroperitoneal lymph node dissection, orchiectomy and chemotherapy can all have major short- and long-term physical and psychological effects leading to SD. The rates of erectile dysfunction are reported as being between 12 and 84% [21]. Long-term (beyond 12 months) erectile dysfunction has been associated with dose-dependent chemotherapy and radiotherapy in this group of patients.

The rate and degree of erectile dysfunction in males with cancers involving the sexual organs, depends on several factors including the age, pre-cancer potency level, comorbidities, type of cancer, type of treatment (surgery, radiotherapy, chemotherapy, and hormonal therapy), and psychosocial factors. Evaluation of sexual function should be carried out at the baseline prior to starting anticancer therapy and at regular intervals. Moreover, prevalence of major sexual problems, the chronology of recovery, strategies to minimize long-term effects, and approaches to treat adverse effects should be routinely discussed, with referral to a sexual medicine clinician pre-therapy, if appropriate. However, as stated for women above, several barriers frequently prevent physicians and patients from discussing sexual concerns, including time constraints, unfamiliarity with treatment options, prioritizing other physical symptoms, ageism, as well as clinician lack of training, discomfort or embarrassment, physician bias and physician projection [21].

There is no gold standard for screening of SD in cancer survivors [16]. However, several valid psychometric screening tools have been developed for broad use including *the Expanded Prostate Cancer Index Composite* (EPIC), and the *International Index of Erectile Function (IIEF-5)* [24]. In addition, the *Sexual Health Inventory for Men (SHIM)* [25] is a quantitative questionnaire widely used for the screening, diagnosis, and to assess the severity of erectile dysfunction and can be considered for monitoring the outcomes and response of specific therapies. Moreover, a comprehensive evaluation of the male patients with SD requires to rule out cardiovascular, psychosocial problems, relationship issues, drug or alcohol, and other medications use such as hormone therapy or opioids. In addition, a targeted physical exam of the chest (for gynaecomastia), abdomen, phallus, scrotum/testicles, and cord structures should be performed [4, 5, 7, 21]. Complementary tests such as penile duplex Doppler ultrasonography may be used to assess blood flow and erectile haemodynamics to differentiate vasculogenic versus psychogenic erectile dysfunction. In addition, male hypogonadism should be evaluated based on sub-physiological concentrations of androgen hormones [26]. Androgen deficiency might be an important cause of muscle wasting in both cancer cachexia and sarcopenia.

The treatment options available for SD in men including the management of erectile dysfunction are summarized in Table 3. The management should be individualized using a tailored shared decision-making patient-centred approach and include couple counselling, if appropriate, as an integral part of the anticancer treatment. Oral PDE5i drugs are currently used as the standard first-line treatment, with several studies supporting their efficacy and tolerability in patients with cancer and survivors. The patient should be periodically monitored to evaluate side effects, and any significant change in health status. Invasive interventions such as intraurethral alprostadil suppositories, penile self-injection with intracavernous vasodilators, vacuum constriction, or penile prosthesis implantation can be considered after balancing the pros and cons of each treatment [21]. Some patients with advanced cancer and androgen deficiencies may benefit from receiving testosterone-replacement therapy for alleviating cancer cachexia symptoms and improving QoL.

Table 3 Potential interventions for the management and prevention of sexual dysfunction in male patients with cancer. (Adapted from Vodnezensky [21])

Intervention	Description
Modification of risk factors	**Smoking** cessation Avoiding excess **alcohol consumption** Increasing **physical activity** **Weight loss** if obesity or overweight
Psychosocial interventions: – Learning communication skills by healthcare providers – Psychotherapy – Individual or couple counselling	– Shared decision-making considering the benefits and risk/burdens associated to each treatment modalities choice – Manage the spiral downwards: loss of sexual confidence, reduced sexual satisfaction, loss of self-esteem, sexual avoidance, changes in relationship satisfaction, female sexual dysfunction – Dealing with impaired body image, fertility problems, social disruptions, disclosure of cancer, and dating new partners during and following cancer treatment
Phosphodiesterase type 5 inhibitors (PDE5i) (sildenafil, tadalafil, vardenafil) for the treatment of ED	**Advantages**: easy to use in pill form and fast onset of action **Relative contraindications:** concomitant administration of alpha-blockers; with use of nitrites for chest pain, history of heart failure, unstable angina, life-threatening arrhythmia in the past 6 months **Adverse effects**: facial flushing, stuffy nose, upset stomach, priapism, headache **Disadvantages:** less effective in men with diabetes or after some treatments for prostate cancer; cost if not covered by insurance
Vacuum erection device for ED	**Advantages**: can be combined with PDE5i. One-time expense **Adverse effects**: penile bruising, discomfort, numbness, or coldness **Potential disadvantages:** mechanical difficulties, blocked erection, insufficient erections
Intraurethral suppository (alprostadil) that creates a vasodilatory effect on the blood vessels of the penis for the management of ED	**Advantages**: easy to use. Alternative in patients failing PDE5i and/or vacuum erection device **Adverse effects:** penile and/or urethral pain or burning, priapism **Disadvantages:** efficacy is poor (about 30%); cost if not covered by public healthcare systems or insurance
Self-injection therapy directly into the base or side of the penis (alprostadil, papaverine, phentolamine, or combination) for the management of ED and penile rehabilitation	**Advantages**: easy to use. Can be used on demand **Adverse effects:** penile pain or fibrosis, priapism **Disadvantages:** some patients uncomfortable with injection to penis

(continued)

Table 3 (continued)

Intervention	Description
Inflatable penile prosthesis for medically refractory ED	**Advantages:** effective in majority of men; inflatable types are not visible; erection looks and feels natural; usually covered by insurance **Adverse effects:** destruction of natural erectile tissue **Potential disadvantages:** device repairs require surgery; hand dexterity needed to operate, not a reversible treatment, risk of infection

Depending on the treatment you are receiving, condom use may be advised

https://www.cancer.gov/about-cancer/treatment/side-effects/sexuality-men

ED erectile dysfunction, *SD* sexual dysfunction

4   Malignancies Other than Those Affecting Sexual Organs

Cancer in the pelvis, such as colorectal cancer and bladder cancer, may lead to erectile dysfunction due to local infiltration, sequelae of surgery affecting the neurovascular pathways responsible for erection, and the pelvic radiation therapy that may also cause toxicity to the pelvic blood supply and nerves [21]. In patients undergoing surgery for colorectal cancer, the nerve damage can result in erectile and ejaculatory disorders for men and lead to dyspareunia, decreased libido, and changes in orgasm for women. Moreover, the challenges following these treatments are not only physical; patients with ostomy may affect self-image. Overall, the prevalence of postoperative sexual dysfunction in survivors of colorectal cancer has been reported to range from 23 to 69% in men vs. 19–62% in women depending on the assessments used [21, 27]. Bladder cancer may also have a significant impact on sexual function in both male and female patients. Standard radical cystectomy (involving removal of prostate and seminal vesicles) results in high rates of erectile dysfunction for men, and SD for women and men. The rate of erectile dysfunction in patients undergoing radical cystectomy has been found to be up to 86%, being lower if patients undergo a nerve-sparing procedure [21]. In addition, ostomies for urinary diversion may also contribute to impair sexual function [4, 5, 7].

Head and neck cancer survivors may also have a great impact on sexual health as they frequently struggle with disfigurement, poor body image, and increased isolation. Additional adverse effects of treatment in this group of patients, such as loss of natural saliva, can make acts of intimacy difficult. Moreover, the changing demographics of this type of cancers observed in recent years (early age at onset, increased number of female patients) [1] in relation to sexually transmitted oncogenic human papillomavirus infection [1, 4, 5, 7], feelings of guilt, and responsibility may impact the sexuality and intimacy [21].

5 Adolescent and Young Adult Cancer Survivors

The trends in the number of adolescent and young adults (AYA) cancer survivor (between 15 and 39 years of age) continue to grow. About 7% of all the new cancer diagnoses in the USA occur in the AYA group, including either survivors of previous cancer treated during childhood or in young adulthood [1]. The AYA group can be diagnosed with any type of cancer. The diagnosis, treatment, and late medical effects related to cancer itself and anticancer therapies may directly or indirectly affect their sexual health. The improvements in survival rates and QoL outcomes in current oncology may leave adolescent and young patients behind due to poor participation in clinical trials and the age-related particularities. Life stage differences experiencing distinct unmet psychosocial age-specific needs [28] as summarized in Table 4.

AYA cancer survivors represent a challenging subgroup of patients in whom aspects related to sexual well-being are frequently unaddressed or only marginally assessed in contrast to issues related to contraceptive methods and fertility. While there is a lack of appropriate assessment tools and intervention by healthcare providers, AYA survivors themselves neglect their sexuality. However, a relevant proportion are sexually active with fewer than half reporting condom use [28].

The Children's Oncology Group, and within this group, the AYA Oncology Discipline Committee was formed to address the compelling medical and psychosocial needs of this group of patients with cancer and is primarily focused on the hormonal and physiological aspects of sexual function and fertility. This committee has recently created the interdisciplinary AYA Sexual Health Task Force to develop specific research and provide recommendations regarding concerns overlapping sexual well-being, affective relationships, and body image [11].

Table 4 Framework of symptoms and concerns influencing sexual health in adolescent and young adult with cancer, and unmet needs in communications regarding sexual health. (*Adapted from Frederick NN, 2019 Multinational Association of Supportive Care in Cancer (MASCC meeting)*)

Physical and psychosocial concerns affecting sexual health in adolescent and young adult with cancer	Unmet needs in communications regarding sexual health in adolescent and young adult with cancer and recommendations
Coping with physical symptoms and concerns • Physical effects of anticancer treatment • Structural damage, disfigurement and changes in body image • Pain • Fatigue • Fertility problems **Psychosocial issues** • Negative thinking • Worsening self-efficacy • Concerns about feeling desirable • Uncertainty with their own body • Difficulties in forming relationships particularly among younger who are isolated from peers and partners during cancer treatment • Risky health behaviours (including risky sexual health behaviours) by young survivors of cancer at rates equivalent to age-matched peers • Use of contraception less often than their healthy peers • The sexual health usually is focused primarily on sexual function (hormonal and physiological aspects) vs. psychosocial aspects (formation of romantic relationships, attainment of sexual milestones) and therefore, usually do not receive comparable attention	**Unmet needs in communication:** **Professionals: oncology providers** • Sexual health is **not routinely included** as part of assessments through disease treatment and survivorship • Oncology providers often **underestimate the relevance** of psychosexual issues • There is often a lack of **knowledge/training** by the medical team, and therefore, excessive assumptions, and a lack of anticipatory guidance • Often scarce **information details** about potential side effects of treatments on sexual health **Adolescents and young adults with cancer** • Young adults with cancer are generally uncomfortable initiating conversations about sexual health. Therefore, they need privacy/time alone with providers to address sexual well-being and discuss sensitive matters such as repercussions in sexual functions, fertility, or masturbation, in a more empathetic and open environment **Environment** • **Individualize the approach:** consider culture, modesty, use appropriate nomenclature • **Initiate the conversation at routine examinations** most women are relieved and respond positively • **Ensure a quiet and safe place to talk with patients**: avoid interruptions and lack of intimacy • **Reassure** patients that the symptoms usually are reversible • **Emphasize the option of non-systemic treatment** **Unmet needs and recommendations for appropriate interventions: (age-specific, skilled, and timely)** • No one size fits all solutions. Better to offer tailored approaches to individual needs and preferences • Multidisciplinary teams: include nurse practitioners, sexologists, and other clinicians. Refer to specialists (if indicated) • Innovation in resources: in-person and online tools • Clinical research specifically designed to assess how to screen for and address sexual dysfunction in young cancer survivors

6   Identification of Areas that Warrant Further Research and Development

Sexual function is often unaddressed in both the daily practice and clinical research of patients with cancer even though SD is common and represents a distressing reality for a high proportion of patients affected by different types of cancers.

There is very limited evidence about how each anticancer treatment impacts the sexual health, the optimal approaches for the assessment, and the efficacy and safety of therapeutic interventions. Thus, several aspects warrant further research with prospectively designed studies addressing sexual-related biological, physical, and psychosocial outcomes in oncology considering the multidimensional nature of sexuality.

6.1   Biological Aspects

It would be crucial to integrate sexual health outcome measures in the evaluation of anticancer treatment with specific subpopulation analysis. Routine measurement of LH, FSH, and oestradiol or testosterone at baseline and during follow-up should be included in prospective clinical trials. Expanding the overall knowledge about the sexual-related impact of anticancer therapies such as surgery [29], chemotherapy [30], novel targeted therapies, and immunotherapy including immune checkpoint inhibitor (ICI) agents [31, 32], is of particular interest in the setting of adjuvant treatments in order to improve the counselling regarding fertility and sexual health.

ICI have emerged as a first-line anticancer treatment of a growing number of cancers alone or in combination with chemotherapy with subpopulation of patients achieving durable cancer response or long-term complete remission. The ICI-related endocrine toxicities are common and tend to be irreversible and require life-long hormonal substitution. The most frequent endocrine complications are thyroid dysfunction (30%) and hypophysitis (5.6–11%) with potential panhypopituitarism and secondary hypogonadism albeit limited data about the levels of the pituitary gonadotropins have been rarely assessed [31, 32]. However, little is known about the direct impact of ICIs on gonadal function as ICI-related primary hypogonadism has not been properly assessed in the pivotal trials. Real-world data registries aimed to collect information about fertility, menopause status, sex hormone levels, and sexual health-related QoL would be helpful to assess the gonadal function in reproductive-age men and women undergoing ICIs and other anticancer therapies.

6.2   Psychosocial Aspects and Models of Care

The development of models of care of issues related to sexual health should be integrated as part of the global movement of supportive care of patients with cancer [33]. The 5As rule (Ask, Advise, Assess, Assist, and Arrange follow-up)

Table 5 The 5As rule framework for promoting communication about sexual health. (*Adapted from Frederick NN, 2019 Multinational Association of Supportive Care in Cancer (MASCC meeting)*)

Ask	Advise	Assess	Assist	Arrange Follow-up
Create a safe and **appropriate environment** Respect **confidentiality** **Individualize** conversations **Don't make assumptions** Introduce the topic of sexual health and **ask the patient for permission** to proceed with the conversation	Provide a **brief overview** on a specific topic Depending on patient needs, **consider discussing** the following: • Puberty/development • Contraception/fertility • Safe sex practices • Sexual function • Infection • Bleeding	Ask additional questions to **understand patient education and support needs**	Provide **brief counselling** based on conversation/assessment Give **appropriate handouts,** pamphlets, website links, etc. Make **referrals as necessary:** • Urology • Reproductive endocrinology • Adolescent medicine • Psychology	**Schedule a follow-up visit** to renew problems or concerns identified

summarized in Table 5 may be useful as a framework to promote communication and interventions in sexual health.

The implementation of specific interventions in the field of sexual health should cover several areas:

- Educational interventions: Health education in this field should be accessible, cost-effective, sustainable, and aimed to facilitate open discussion about sexual health. In this regard, digital healthcare approaches may potentially overcome barriers of inadequate staff time and training [34].
- Development of clinical assessment tools to explore sexual health including different languages and cross-cultural validation.
- Psychosocial interventions such as couples therapy, supportive group counselling, psychiatry consult, individual counselling, cognitive-behavioural therapy, and sex therapy technique.
- The permission (P), limited information (LI), specific suggestions (SS), and intensive therapy (IT) or PLISSIT model of sex therapy, commonly used to individualize the level of intervention in sexology, should be assessed in cancer survivors of different types of cancer [35].

6.3 Research and Development to Integrate Diversity

It is important to integrate diversity in a broad sense of the term, to prevent disparities in the care of selected groups. First, in the era of globalization, languages, cultures, religious beliefs, geographic differences, and ethnic differences must be considered. Similarly, particularities associated to socioeconomic status and academic level need to be considered. Moreover, the adaptation of sexual health-related resources should be sensitive with age including the AYA group and older cancer survivors [11, 36]. Additional tailored interventions should consider diversity related to relationship vulnerabilities when survivors are single, widowed, or divorced. In the same line, biological sex, gender identities, and sexual orientation including binary, nonbinary, or transgender patients [37, 38].

6.4   Sexuality and Palliative Care

There is a growing number of patients with advanced incurable cancer treated in the setting of palliative care [3, 33]. Sexual health of patients is also frequently neglected in this setting. In a recent systematic literature review [9, 39], numerous barriers had been identified from addressing patient sexuality, being lack of knowledge and poor confidence levels being among the most common. In a recent pilot study [40], 69% of palliative care providers with an anonymous survey, responded that rarely or never discussed sexuality with their patients. The majority acknowledged the need of more training.

6.5   Implementation of Models of Care

The development and implementation of different models of care should be adapted to each reality. For instance:

- Sexual-health multidisciplinary (physicians, nurses, psychotherapists, physiotherapists) dedicated clinic in referee academic cancer centres versus the training of a specific member of the clinical team.
- The integration of sexual health issues management in a separate dedicated clinic versus integrated with other services such as fertility, mental health services, and/or survivorship programmes.
- The development of sexual health rehabilitation programmes as standard of survivorship care linked to medical oncology and other specialities in hospitals or tertiary care hospitals versus connected to primary care and/or other community services, and how to build bridges between the different levels of care.

7   Conclusions

Sexual health usually remains unexplored in patients with cancer due to several barriers in daily care albeit the potential impact of sexual well-being in QoL. Future studies are needed to develop and validate specific tools for the assessment of sexual issues in patients with different types of cancer. Moreover, further research is needed to explore the feasibility of the implementation of specific interventions in this field in the era of precision oncology.

References

1. Miller KD, Nogueira L, Devasia T, et al. Cancer treatment and survivorship statistics, 2022. CA Cancer J Clin. 2022;72(5):409–36.
2. Shapiro CL. Cancer survivorship. N Engl J Med. 2018;379(25):2438–50.
3. Hui D, Bruera E. Integrating palliative care into the trajectory of cancer care. Nat Rev Clin Oncol. 2016;13(3):159–71.
4. Carter J, Lacchetti C, Andersen BL, et al. Interventions to address sexual problems in people with cancer: American Society of Clinical Oncology clinical practice guideline adaptation of cancer care Ontario guideline. J Clin Oncol. 2018;36(5):492–511.
5. NCCN Guidelines Version 1.2020 Survivorship: sexual function (female and male). https://acrobat.adobe.com/link/review?uri=urn:aaid:scds:US:f21b249c-09ed-3256-8cf4-4760e5447e6a.
6. World Health Organization (SUI) Definition of sexuality and sexual health. Geneva: The World Health Organization. http://www.who.int/health-topics/sexual-health#tab=tab_1
7. Bober SL, Varela VS. Sexuality in adult cancer survivors: challenges and intervention. J Clin Oncol. 2012;30(30):3712–9.
8. Pereira N, Schattman GL. Fertility preservation and sexual health after cancer therapy. J Oncol Pract. 2017;13(10):643–51.
9. Andersen BL, Lacchetti C, Ashing K, et al. Management of anxiety and depression in adult survivors of cancer: ASCO guideline update. J Clin Oncol. 2023;41:JCO2300293.
10. Heyne S, Taubenheim S, Dietz A, et al. Physical and psychosocial factors associated with sexual satisfaction in long-term cancer survivors 5 and 10 years after diagnosis. Sci Rep. 2023;13(1):2011.
11. Lehmann V, Laan ETM, den Oudsten BL. Sexual health-related care needs among young adult cancer patients and survivors: a systematic literature review. J Cancer Surviv. 2022;16(4):913–24.
12. Chang CP, Wilson CM, Rowe K, et al. Sexual dysfunction among gynecologic cancer survivors in a population-based cohort study. Support Care Cancer. 2022;31(1):51.
13. Tramacere F, Lancellotta V, Casà C, et al. Assessment of sexual dysfunction in cervical cancer patients after different treatment modality: a systematic review. Medicina (Kaunas). 2022;58(9):1223.
14. Mension E, Alonso I, Tortajada M, Matas I, Gómez S, Ribera L, et al. Genitourinary syndrome of menopause assessment tools. J Midlife Health. 2021;12:99–102.
15. Tounkel I, Nalubola S, Schulz A, Lakhi N. Sexual health screening for gynecologic and breast cancer survivors: a review and critical analysis of validated screening tools. Sex Med. 2022;10(2):100498.
16. Hatzichristou D, Rosen RC, Derogatis LR, et al. Recommendations for the clinical evaluation of men and women with sexual dysfunction. J Sex Med. 2010;7:337–48.
17. Ruseckaite R, Bavor C, Marsh L, Dean J, Daly O, Vasiliadis D, Ahern S. Evaluation of the acceptability of patient-reported outcome measures in women following pelvic floor procedures. Qual Life Res. 2022;31(7):2213–21.
18. Portman DJ, Gass MLS, Vulvovaginal Atrophy Terminology Consensus Conference Panel. Genitourinary syndrome of menopause: new terminology for vulvovaginal atrophy from the International Society for the Study of Women's Sexual Health and the North American Menopause Society. J Sex Med. 2014;11(12):2865–72.
19. Bober SL, Reese JB, Barbera L, et al. How to ask and what to do: a guide for clinical inquiry and intervention regarding female sexual health after cancer. Curr Opin Support Palliat Care. 2016;10(1):44–54.
20. Barbera L, Fitch M, Adams L, Doyle C, Dasgupta T, Blake J. Improving care for women after gynecological cancer: the development of a sexuality clinic. Menopause. 2011;18(12):1327–33.
21. Voznesensky M, Annam K, Kreder KJ. Understanding and managing erectile dysfunction in patients treated for cancer. J Oncol Pract. 2016;12(4):297–304. Erratum in: J Oncol Pract 2016; 12(6): 596.

22. Madan R, Dracham CB, Khosla D, et al. Erectile dysfunction and cancer: current perspective. Radiat Oncol J. 2020;38(4):217–25.
23. Elliott S, Latini DM, Walker LM, et al. Androgen deprivation therapy for prostate cancer: recommendations to improve patient and partner quality of life. J Sex Med. 2010;7:2996–3010.
24. Neijenhuijs KI, Holtmaat K, Aaronson NK, et al. The international index of erectile function (IIEF)—a systematic review of measurement properties. J Sex Med. 2019;16(7):1078–91.
25. Cappelleri JC, Rosen RC. The sexual health inventory for men (SHIM): a 5-year review of research and clinical experience. Int J Impot Res. 2005;17(4):307–19.
26. Vigano A, Piccioni M, Trutschnigg B, et al. Male hypogonadism associated with advanced cancer: a systematic review. Lancet Oncol. 2010;11(7):679–84.
27. Traa MJ, De Vries J, Roukema JA, et al. The sexual health care needs after colorectal cancer: the view of patients, partners, and health care professionals. Support Care Cancer. 2014;22:763–72.
28. Rosenberg AR, Bona K, Ketterl T, et al. Intimacy, substance use, and communication needs during cancer therapy: a report from the "resilience in adolescents and young adults" study. J Adolesc Health. 2017;60(1):93–9.
29. Opławski M, Grabarek BO, Średnicka A, et al. The impact of surgical treatment with adjuvant chemotherapy for ovarian cancer on disorders in the urinary system and quality of life in women. J Clin Med. 2022;11(5):1300.
30. Kuderer NM, Desai A, Lustberg MB, Lyman GH. Mitigating acute chemotherapy-associated adverse events in patients with cancer. Nat Rev Clin Oncol. 2022;19(11):681–97.
31. Özdemir BC. Immune checkpoint inhibitor-related hypogonadism and infertility: a neglected issue in immuno-oncology. J Immunother Cancer. 2021;9(2):e002220.
32. Martins F, Sofiya L, Sykiotis GP, et al. Adverse effects of immune checkpoint inhibitors: epidemiology, management and surveillance. Nat Rev Clin Oncol. 2019;16:563–80.
33. Scotté F, Taylor A, Davies A. Supportive care: the "keystone" of modern oncology practice. Cancers (Basel). 2023;15:3860. https://doi.org/10.3390/cancers15153860.
34. Matthew AG, Yang ZG. Online interventions for sexual health in cancer. Curr Opin Support Palliat Care. 2020;14(1):80–6.
35. Almeida NG, Britto DF, Figueiredo JV, Moreira TMM, Carvalho REFL, Fialho AVM. PLISSIT model: sexual counseling for breast cancer survivors. Rev Bras Enferm. 2019;72(4):1109–13.
36. Kagan SH, Holland N, Chalian AA. Sexual issues in special populations: geriatric oncology—sexuality and older adults. Semin Oncol Nurs. 2008;24(2):120–6.
37. Griggs J, Maingi S, Blinder V, et al. American Society of Clinical Oncology position statement: strategies for reducing cancer health disparities among sexual and gender minority populations. J Clin Oncol. 2017;35:2203–8.
38. Coleman E, Radix AE, Bouman WP, et al. Standards of Care for the Health of transgender and gender diverse people, version 8. Int J Transgend Health. 2022;23(Suppl 1):S1–S259.
39. Williams M, Addis G. Addressing patient sexuality issues in cancer and palliative care. Br J Nurs. 2021;30(10):S24–8.
40. Bramati P, Dai J, Urbauer DL, Bruera E. Attitudes of palliative care specialists toward assessing sexual dysfunction in patients with cancer. J Pain Symptom Manag. 2023;66(2):e185–8.

Allogeneic Stem Cell Transplantation and Sexual Disorders

Carmen Martínez 🔟

1   Allogeneic Hematopoietic Stem Cell Transplantation

Allogeneic hematopoietic stem cell transplantation (alloHSCT) has become a well-established curative therapy for a variety of malignant and non-malignant hematological disorders. It is currently integrated as an essential part in many treatment concepts and protocols [1]. AlloHSCT consists in the administration of healthy hematopoietic stem cells from a donor to replace the patient own stem cells that have been destroyed by treatment with high doses of chemotherapy with or without radiotherapy named conditioning regimen (Fig. 1). Healthy stem cells may come from the blood or bone marrow of a related donor or from an unrelated donor who are genetically similar to the patient.

The main complications of alloHSCT are relapse of hematologic disease, complications arising from post-transplant immunosuppression, and graft-versus-host disease (GVHD) (Fig. 1). Relapse of hematologic disease usually occurs in the first 2–3 years after transplantation and is generally associated with a very poor prognosis. Medical advances in recent decades have significantly reduced the incidence and severity of infectious complications and GVHD, with a consequent decrease in mortality and an increase in the number of long-term surviving patients. Thus, the probability of long-term survival reaches 80% in those patients who survive the first 2 years after transplantation [2].

AlloHSCT is a medically very complex procedure, with frequent post-transplant complications and hospital readmissions, which may have a negative impact on

C. Martínez (✉)
Hematopoietic Stem Cell Transplantation Unit, Hematology Department, Clinical Institute of Hematology and Oncology, Hospital Clínic de Barcelona, Barcelona, Spain

Clinical Sexology Working Group, Hospital Clinic de Barcelona, Barcelona, Spain

Institut d'Investigacions Biomèdiques August Pi i Sunyer, Barcelona, Spain
e-mail: cmarti@clinic.cat

C. Castelo-Branco, S. Anglès Acedo (eds.), *Medical Disorders and Sexual Health*, Trends in Andrology and Sexual Medicine,
https://doi.org/10.1007/978-3-031-55080-5_17

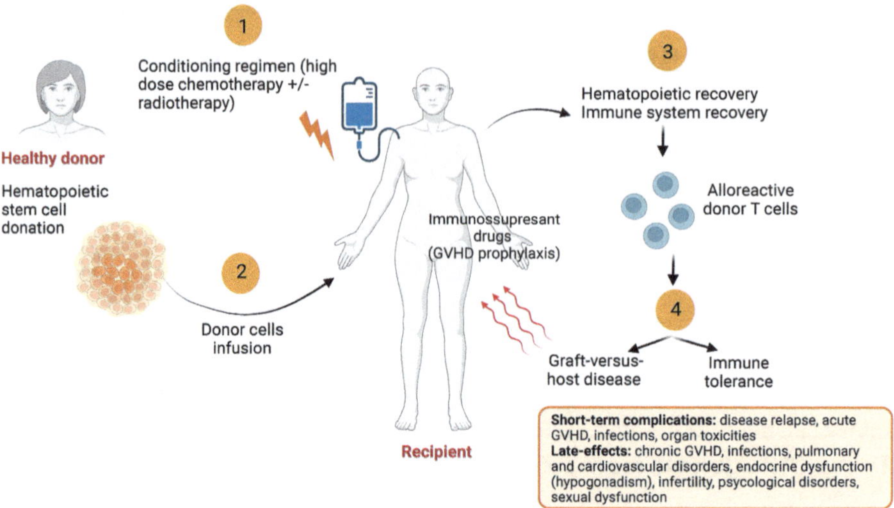

Fig. 1 Allogeneic hematopoietic stem cell transplantation: description of the procedure and complications (Figures are property of Hospital Clínic of Barcelona and used with permission)

patients' and their relatives' health-related quality of life concerning physical, emotional, cognitive, and social constraints. These patients also face a broad range of significant late effects including GVHD, hypogonadism, infertility, and sexual and emotional health problems.

2 Chronic Graft-Versus-Host Disease and Its Impact on Sexual Health

GVHD is one of the most serious complications after transplant [3]. GVHD occurs when the donor's T cells (the graft) recognize the recipient tissues (the host) as foreign (non-self). GVHD is divided into acute and chronic forms, according to the type of symptoms and signs. Acute GVHD appears in the first months after transplantation affecting the skin, gastrointestinal tract, and liver. Chronic GVHD (cGVHD) usually begins between 3 months and 2 years after alloHSCT and can affect multiple tissues and organs. The pathophysiology of cGVHD is different from acute GVHD and mainly characterized by impaired immune tolerance mechanisms.

cGVHD is the main cause of late mortality unrelated to relapse in long-term survivors of alloHSCT.Its incidence is approximately 50% although it has decreased during the last years, thanks to the introduction of new strategies of prevention. Severe forms of cGVHD have a deleterious impact on patient's quality of life and are associated with an estimated 5-year mortality rate of 30–50%. First-line standard treatment consists on corticosteroids associated or not with calcineurin

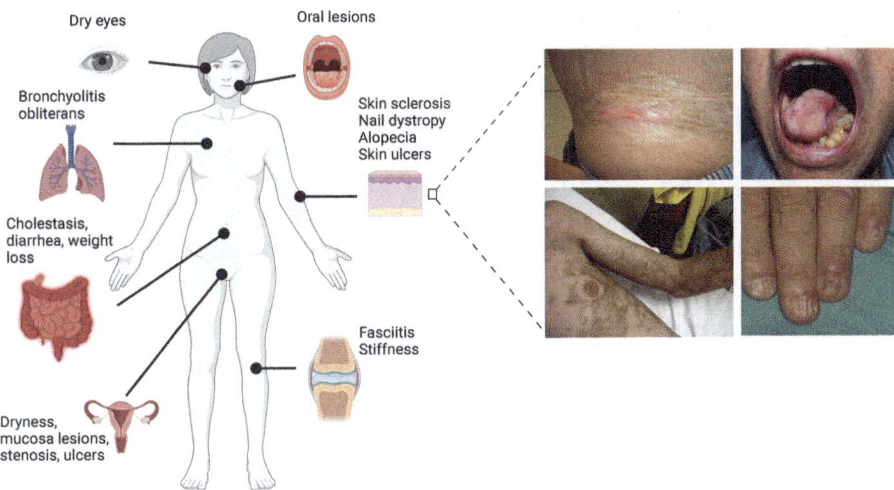

Fig. 2 Chronic graft-versus-host disease: main organs involved (Figures are property of Hospital Clínic of Barcelona and used with permission)

inhibitors and it is successful in about half of patients. Immunosuppressive treatment is usually administered for a prolonged period of time, and it is not uncommon for patients to require treatment for more than 5 years.

cGVHD may involve a single organ or several organs imitating almost any autoimmune disorder [3]. The skin is the most frequently involved organ with different morphology: erythema, maculopapular rash, pruritus, poikiloderma, lichen planus-like, lichen sclerosus-like, morphea-like, deep sclerotic eruptions, hypo- or hyperpigmentation, alopecia, and others (Fig. 2). Moderate and severe forms of cutaneous cGVHD lead to drastic changes in body image that can severely affect the patient psychologically, interfering with self-esteem and personal relationships leading to significant sexual distress [4, 5]. Eyes (keratitis sicca) and oral mucosa (erythema, lichenoid changes, ulcera, sicca syndrome, increase tooth decay and loss) are also frequently affected. Other organs potentially affected by cGVHD are the liver (cholestasis), gastrointestinal tract (dysphagia, nausea and vomiting, diarrhea), lung (bronchiolitis obliterans), joints and fasciae (restricted mobility), and genitals.

Genital cGVHD may occur in males and females although more frequent in the latter. The incidence of genital cGVHD varies from 13 in men [6] to 49% in women [7, 8]. Genital manifestations are often associated with oral manifestations of cGVHD and characterized by lichen planus and/or lichen sclerosus changes. In women, cGVHD may manifest with vaginal dryness and irritation, vulvovaginitis, vaginal synechiae and hematocolpos, ulceration, and fissures. In men, the manifestations consist in irritation of the penis, balanitis, balanoposthitis, narrowing and/or scarring of the urethra, itching or scarring on the penis and scrotum, and phimosis. It is very frequent that patients do not spontaneously report these symptoms, hence the importance of a directed interrogation and a regular gynecological/urological follow-up, especially in patients with manifestations of cGVHD in other organs. Early diagnosis is important to avoid progression to severe forms of genital GVHD.

In women, vaginal cGVHD is a major problem affecting sexual quality of life. Specifically, local morphological and inflammatory changes secondary to cGVHD, vaginal dryness, and dyspareunia have a significant impact on sexual activity. In men, genital cGVHD has been associated with more frequent erectile dysfunction and sexual discontent [6, 9, 10]. Wong et al. found that cGVHD in both genders contributed negatively to sexual dysfunction and dissatisfaction during the 3 years following alloHSCT (lower sexual cognition/fantasy and orgasm in men and sexual arousal and sexual satisfaction in women).

3   Endocrine Dysfunction After AlloHSCT and Its Effects on Sexual Health

Post-transplant endocrine dysfunction is inherent to conditioning chemo/radiotherapy used during alloHSCT. Other factors, such as type of hematologic disease, pre-transplant treatment, development of cGVHD, and prolonged corticosteroid treatment, contribute significantly to its occurrence. Abnormal thyroid function (compensated or overt hypothyroidism, autoimmune thyroid disease) and hypoadrenalism are frequent after transplant. Related symptoms are fatigue, weakness, nausea, changes in weight, which indirectly can affect sexual activity in both, women and men. Gonadal dysfunction is also very usual in these patients [11].

The degree of ovarian damage after transplant depends on the dose and type of chemotherapy/radiotherapy used, and baseline ovarian reserve which in turn is dependent on age and previous treatment. Primary ovarian failure (POF) is a frequent complication of alloHSCT, especially when high-intensity conditioning chemo/radiotherapy is used. Manifestations of POF range from premature menopause to varying degrees of infertility even in very young patients. Premature menopause can lead to vaginal and/or vulvar atrophy, causing continuous discomfort and/or pain, and vaginal dryness during sexual activity, negatively affecting interest and desire. In a recent published study, POF occurred in 74% of the patients, and 86% reported symptoms of hypoestrogenism even in those receiving systemic and/or local hormonal replacement therapy [11]. Changes in sexual life were reported by 76% of the patients, mostly because of low sex drive, the negative impact of infertility problems, physical sequelae, and loss of self-confidence. The desire for pregnancy was also affected in 47% of the patients, mainly due to the fear of relapse of the hematologic disease or its transmission to newborn.

Male patients who received an alloHSCT in childhood or adulthood have impaired testicular, hormonal, and sexual function. Despite the relative chemoresistance and radioresistance of Leydig cells, several studies have reported a markedly high prevalence of hypogonadism (20–30%) that decrease over time [10, 12, 13]. One hypothesis to explain this observation is that patients actually present a functional hypogonadism induced by immediate post-transplant complications (infections, corticosteroids, severe physical stress) that resolves with time. On the other hand, the diagnosis of hypogonadism is difficult in this context since many symptoms (asthenia, depressed mood, decreased libido) are nonspecific and frequent after alloHSCT, regardless of testosterone levels. Zavattaro et al. have reported a high prevalence of erectile dysfunction (72%) with no significant differences between hypogonadal and eugonadal patients after transplant. The same authors showed that 97% of the patients presented spermatogenesis impairment within the first year after transplantation. In the follow-up of these patients, a progressive reduction in FSH level and an increase of inhibin B concentration suggested a gradual recovery of spermatogenesis in the follow-up.

4   Sexual Dysfunction in Women Following AlloHSCT

Compared to men, women report a higher prevalence (50% vs. 80%) and longer post-transplant duration of sexual difficulties [14–16]. Indeed, several prospective studies have shown that men were generally able to return to baseline sexual function after 2–3 years whereas women were less likely to return to baseline even after 5 year or more [6, 17, 18]. Women's sexual health is mainly affected by lack of sexual satisfaction, vaginal dryness, and dyspareunia.

In a recent published study [19], sexual activity and function in adult male and female long-term alloHSCT survivors were compared with non-cancer general population norms. Women were more likely than men to report not being sexually active in the last year after transplant (39% vs. 27%), rates that were higher than in normal controls (19.6%). For both, women and men, older age, not having 4 years of college, having low performance status, and not being in a committed relationship were factors related to sexual inactivity. Main reasons for sexual inactivity in women were the lack of a partner followed by lack of interest in sexual activity. Among sexually active patients, more women than men report low sexual functioning (64% vs. 32%). Women with low sexual function scores had higher prevalence of vaginal dryness, pain or irritation, difficulties with orgasm, and lack of desire. In statistical multivariate analysis, low sexual function scores were associated with low performance status and being in a lower quality, more distressed relationship, more so than being unpartnered. The results of this study suggest that women in particular may benefit from couple-based approaches to enhance feelings of closeness and bolster relationship quality.

5   Sexual Dysfunction in Men Following AlloHSCT

Men's sexual health after alloHSCT is mainly affected by erectile dysfunction, ejaculation and orgasm problems, pain during intercourse, diminished sexual interest, and anxiety about sexual performance dominate [9, 10, 15, 20]. These problems are high prevalent during the first year after transplant, and, in contrast to women, the majority of men experience recovery by 1–3 years. However, in comparison to the general non-cancer population, even 5 years after alloHSCT, some patients continued to report significant worse sexual function [15, 19].

In the study by Syrjala et al., 27% of male recipients of alloHSCT reported not being sexually active in the past year. Sexual inactivity was associated with older age, reduced intensity conditioning, not having 4 years of college, having low performance status, not being in a committed relationship, or were not employed or in school [19]. The main reasons for sexual inactivity were physical issues and lack of interest. Patients with low sexual functioning reported higher rates of difficulties with getting an erection, difficulties to maintaining erections, difficulties with ejaculation, and lack of desire. Worse sexual function was associated with age > 40 and worse performance status. Zavattaro et al. reported that erection dysfunction affected almost 3 out of 4 patients, leading to a significantly higher prevalence than in the general population (72% vs. 12%). It is worth mentioning that erectile dysfunction prevalence did not vary with the time elapsed from alloHSCT. In that study, older age at transplant and cGVHD were found to predict the presence of erectile dysfunction.

Whereas the prevalence of hypogonadism in male patients who received alloHSCT in childhood is well described in the literature, the impact on sexual life in adulthood is less well known. Haavisto et al. reported sexual functions in a group of male adult survivors of childhood alloHSCT and compared the results to a healthy control group. They found that alloHSCT recipients reported less sexual fantasies, poorer orgasms, lower sexual activity with a partner and reduced satisfaction with their sex life, even in the presence of normal erectile functions and a similar frequency of autoerotic acts. Sexual dysfunction was strongly associated with depression, the absence of a life partner, and central nervous system or testicular irradiation.

6 Complexity of Sexual Problems After AlloHSCT

Sexual dysfunction after alloHSCT results from the sum of multiple interrelated factors such as physical difficulties linked to treatments (treatment of underlying hematological disease, transplant conditioning regimen, cGVHD, POF, immunosuppressant, and other drugs), social factors (unemployment, physical isolation, economic difficulties), and psychological factors (depression, anxiety, phobias, mood disorders) (Fig. 3). That underscores the importance of a multidisciplinary approach in order to select appropriate interventions.

Although sexual problems have a strong and negative impact on the quality of life of alloHSCT recipients, they are often underreported by patients themselves and insufficiently addressed by caregivers [15, 16, 21]. Patients and their partners should be informed about the effects that the treatment of the hematological disease and alloHSCT may have on their sex life [22]. Besides, sexual function evaluation should be part of the routine follow-up of alloHSCT survivors [22]. Therefore, it is important that the healthcare providers have the necessary training to properly address these issues. A study by the European Society for Blood and Marrow Transplantation showed that while many alloHSCT survivors experience sexual

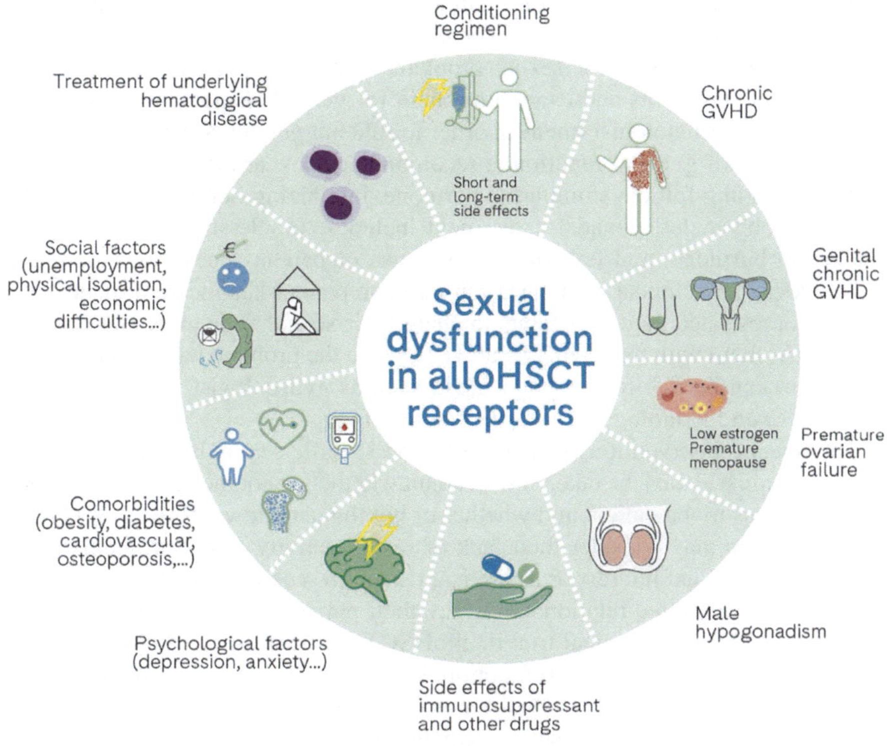

Fig. 3 Factors related to sexual dysfunction after alloHSCT (Figures are property of Hospital Clínic of Barcelona and used with permission)

problems, the majority do not routinely discuss them with their medical doctors or nurses [23]. Embarrassment, or at least a discomfort about discussing sexual concerns, and a lack knowledge and relevant education on the side of the medical staff side, were major barriers for healthcare providers initiating such discussions; the discomfort is such that initiation of discussions on this topic usually originates from the patient [23, 24].

Like patients, partners should be included in the evaluation of post-transplant sexual problems. Yoo et al. compared attitudes about and experiences of sexual activity between alloHSCT survivors and their sexual partners. They observed that survivors gave more importance to sexual activity and tried to discuss sexual activity issues more than their partners. Both male and female survivors had poor agreement with their partners regarding satisfaction with current sexual life and cause of sexual dysfunction. When both survivors and partners thought that adequate sex was important, they were more likely to be sexually active than when both survivors and partners did not. This study highlights the need for providing information and counseling about sexuality both to transplant survivors and partners.

Sexual dysfunction should be included together with other long-term post-transplant complications in the holistic follow-up of alloHSCT survivors. In the post-transplant screening for sexual problems, patients should be asked directly about genital symptoms and examining them for genital changes by gynecologist (women) and dermatologist (men) in order to rule out genital cGVHD. In addition, an assessment of gonadal function is recommended 1 year after transplant for all women including follicle-stimulating hormone, luteinizing hormone, and estradiol levels. Among males, gonadal assessment includes follicle-stimulating hormone, luteinizing hormone, and testosterone. The use of patient-specific questionnaires and booklets, and clinical guidelines can improve patient-healthcare provider communication by encouraging patients to share their sexual symptoms and concerns and discuss them with the medical staff [22]. Once the problem has been identified, the patient can be referred to a specialist, such as gynecologist, urologist, sexual therapist, or endocrinologist, for further management.

Therapeutic interventions should target the specific sexual health needs of the patients. It must always be taken into account whether or not the sexual impairment causes distress to the patient and whether or not the patient wants help [25]. While some survivors may consider their lack of sexual activity as not problematic, for others lack of sexual interest or desire is a reason to seek treatment, particularly if they are in a committed relationship where their partners wish to engage in sexual activity [19]. A recent clinical trial in alloHSCT survivors showed strong efficacy in improving sexual interest and function, suggesting that if lack of interest is distressing, it is treatable [25]. There are non-modifiable factors with a known effect on post-transplant low sexual activity (including age, education, transplant procedures, and the availability of a partner), but also there are others susceptible to be addressed medically or behaviorally such as erectile dysfunction, vaginal dryness, and dyspareunia, as well as relationship quality, treatment-related distress, and depression. Genital changes in women due cGVHD can be treated with topical steroids, topical calcineurin inhibitors, topical estrogen, vaginal dilator therapy and, in some cases, surgical intervention. Vaginal lubricants and moisturizers, and pelvic floor muscle awareness can minimize dryness and pain during sexual activity. Systemic hormonal therapy is also recommended in women aged <40 years regardless of symptoms. Male patients with genital cGVHD also benefit from topical steroids and calcineurin inhibitors. In the case of sexual problems due to hypogonadism and erectile dysfunction, testosterone and phosphodiesterase type 5 inhibitors can improve sexual function. Many drugs commonly used in the treatment of post-transplant complications (corticosteroids, antidepressants, opioids, anxiolytics, antihypertensive drugs) may contribute to sexual dysfunction due to their negative effect on libido, arousal and orgasm, and vaginal dryness. Consequently, it is important to review this aspect and reduce polypharmacy as much as possible to reduce sexual side effects. Low libido could be improved in both women and men through sexual counseling after potentially related medical conditions are evaluated and treated. The support of psychologists, sex therapists, and social workers is also essential for the global management of alloHSCT survivors.

7 Conclusions

Sexual problems are a frequent complication of alloHSCT, often underreported, and occur more prevalently in women than in men. Five years after transplant, patients still report sexual dysfunction. Sexual disorders have a strong and negative impact on the quality of life of transplant patients. Therefore, assessment of sexual and emotional health should be an integral part of the early and long-term follow-up of alloHSCT survivors. To provide appropriate counseling on sexual health after alloHSCT, healthcare professionals need specific training and understand the epidemiology of sexual dysfunction, associated risk factors, available guidelines and therapeutic tools. A biopsychological approach by a multidisciplinary team is highly recommended to treat the different aspects, physical and emotional, of the sexual life of alloHSCT patients.

References

1. Copelan EA, Chojecki A, Lazarus HM, Avalos BR. Allogeneic hematopoietic cell transplantation; the current renaissance. Blood Rev. 2019;34:34–44.
2. Bhatia S, Francisco L, Carter A, et al. Late mortality after allogeneic hematopoietic cell transplantation and functional status of long-term survivors: report from the Bone Marrow Transplant Survivor Study. Blood. 2007;110:3784–92.
3. Jagasia MH, Greinix HT, Arora M, et al. National Institutes of Health consensus development project on criteria for clinical trials in chronic graft-versus- host disease: I. The 2014 diagnosis and staging working group report. Biol Blood Marrow Transplant. 2015;21:389–401.
4. Gillena MM, Markey CH. A review of research linking body image and sexual well-being. Body Image. 2019;31:294–301.
5. Michael S, Skaczkowski G, Wilson C. Sexual satisfaction and sexual distress after cancer: the role of body image disruption, self-compassion, sexual pain and relationship satisfaction. Psychooncology. 2021;30:1902–9. https://doi.org/10.1002/pon.5755.
6. Mueller SM, Haeusermann P, Rovo A, et al. Genital chronic GVHD in men after hematopoietic stem cell transplantation: a single-center cross-sectional analysis of 155 patients. Biol Blood Marrow Transplant. 2013;19:1574–80.
7. Machado AM, Hamerschlak N, Rodrigues M. Female genital tract chronic graft-versus-host disease: a narrative review. Hematol Transfus Cell Ther. 2019;41:69–75.
8. Zantomio D, Grigg A, MacGregor L, et al. Female genital tract graft-versus-host disease: incidence, risk factors and recommendations for management. Bone Marrow Transplant. 2006;38:567–72.
9. Andreini A, Zampieri N, Costantini C, et al. Chronic graft versus host disease is associated with erectile dysfunction in allogeneic hematopoietic stem cell transplant patients: a single-center experience. Leuk Lymphoma. 2018;59:2719–22.
10. Dyer G, Gilroy N, Bradford J, et al. A survey of fertility and sexual health following allogeneic haematopoietic stem cell transplantation in New South Wales, Australia. Br J Haematol. 2016;172:592–601.
11. Forgeard N, Jestin M, Vexiau D, et al. Sexuality- and fertility-related issues in women after allogeneic hematopoietic stem cell transplantation. Transplant Cell Therapy. 2021;27:432.e1–6.
12. Orio F, Muscogiuri G, Palomba S. Endocrinopathies after allogeneic and autologous transplantation of hematopoietic stem cells. ScientificWorldJournal. 2014;2014:282147. https://doi.org/10.1155/2014/282147.

13. Schneidewind L, Neumann T, Probst KA, et al. Recovery from hypogonadism and male health in adult allogeneic stem cell transplantation. Eur J Haematol. 2018;100:584–91.
14. Humphreys CT, Tallman B, Altmaier EM, et al. Sexual functioning in patients undergoing bone marrow transplantation: a longitudinal study. Bone Marrow Transplant. 2007;39:491–6. https://doi.org/10.1038/sj.bmt.1705613.
15. Syrjala K, Kurland B, Abrams J, et al. Sexual function changes during the 5 years after high-dose treatment and hematopoietic cell transplantation for malignancy, with case-matched controls at 5 years. Blood. 2008;111:989–96.
16. Wong FL, Francisco L, Togawa K, et al. Longitudinal trajectory of sexual functioning after hematopoietic cell transplantation: impact of chronic graft-versus-host disease and total body irradiation. Blood. 2013;122:3973–81.
17. Hirsch P, Leclerc M, Rybojad M, et al. Female genital chronic graft-versus-host disease: importance of early diagnosis to avoid severe complications. Transplantation. 2012;93:1265–9.
18. Thygesen KH, Schjodt I, Jarden M. The impact of hematopoietic stem cell transplantation on sexuality: a systematic review of the literature. Bone Marrow Transplant. 2012;47:716–24.
19. Syrjala K, Schoemans H, Yi JC, et al. Sexual functioning in long-term survivors of hematopoietic cell transplantation. Transplant Cell Ther. 2021;27:80.e1–80.e12. https://doi.org/10.1016/j.bbmt.2020.09.027.
20. Claessens J, Beerendonk C, Schattenberg A. Quality of life, reproduction and sexuality after stem cell transplantation with partially T-cell-depleted grafts and after conditioning with a regimen including Total body irradiation. Bone Marrow Transplant. 2006;37:831–6.
21. Douglas JM, Fenton KA. Understanding sexual health and its role in more effective prevention programs. Public Health Rep. 2013;128:1–4.
22. Eeltink CM, Incrocci L, Verdonck-de Leeuw IM, Zweegman S. Recommended patient information sheet on the impact of haematopoietic cell transplantation on sexual functioning and sexuality. Ecancermedicalscience. 2019;13:987–94.
23. Eeltink CM, Witte BI, Stringer J, et al. Health-care professionals' perspective on discussing sexual issues in adult patients after haematopoietic cell transplantation. Bone Marrow Transplant. 2018;53(3):235–45.
24. Dyer K, das Nair R. Why don't healthcare professionals talk about sex? A systematic review of recent qualitative studies conducted in the United Kingdom. J Sex Med. 2013;10(11):2658–70.
25. El-Jawahri A, Fishman SR, Vanderklish J, et al. Pilot study of a multimodal intervention to enhance sexual function in survivors of hematopoietic stem cell transplantation. Cancer. 2018;124:2438–46.

Sexual Function in Breast Cancer and Sexual Health

Camil Castelo-Branco and Eduard Mension

1   Introduction

Breast cancer (BC) is the most prevalent cancer among females worldwide. In 2020, there were 2.3 million women diagnosed with BC, and according to current statistics, at the end of 2020, there were 7.8 million women alive who were diagnosed with breast cancer in the past 5 years [1]. Furthermore, approximately one in eight women will be diagnosed with BC during their lifetime. On the other hand, breast cancer (BC) in men is a rare entity, occurring in approximately 1% of men and representing between 0.5 and 1% of all BC in both genders.

During the last decades, thanks to improvement in BC treatments, survival rates of BC have increased significantly, and new challenges are emerging to handle Breast Cancer Survivors (BCS). Nowadays, BCS do not only seek to remain free of disease, but there is a demand to do it preserving their quality of life. Therefore, there is a need to focus not only on the survival of the patients, but also on their long-term quality of life.

C. Castelo-Branco (✉)
Gynecological Department, Clinical Institute of Gynecology, Obstetrics and Neonatology, Hospital Clinic de Barcelona, Barcelona, Spain

Clinical Sexology Working Group, Hospital Clinic de Barcelona, Barcelona, Spain

Surgery and Medical-Surgical Specialties, Faculty of Medicine and Health Sciences, Universitat de Barcelona (UB), Barcelona, Spain

Institut d'Investigacions Biomèdiques August Pi i Sunyer, Barcelona, Spain
e-mail: ccastelo@clinic.cat

E. Mension
Gynecological Department, Clinical Institute of Gynecology, Obstetrics and Neonatology, Hospital Clinic de Barcelona, Barcelona, Spain

Institut d'Investigacions Biomèdiques August Pi i Sunyer, Barcelona, Spain
e-mail: mension@clinic.cat

Evidence shows that BCS have the highest rates of lost disability-adjusted life years (DALYs) among all types of cancer [1], being sexual dysfunction (SD) one of the main causes [2]. The World Health Organization (WHO) describes sexual health as a positive and respectful approach to sexuality and sexual relationships, as well as the possibility of having pleasurable and safe sexual experiences, free of coercion, discrimination, and violence. A healthy sexual function includes sexual activity, free of pain and discomfort, as well as a sexual response with no psychological difficulty experiencing desire, arousal, and orgasm.

According to Diagnostic and Statistical Manual of Mental Disorders (DSM)-V, women can be diagnosed of SD when having persistent symptoms (at least 6 months) that cause a marked personal disturbance and a serious impairment in their sexual lives. However, for this definition to be complete, it should be considered that SD extends beyond physical symptoms, having serious consequences regarding the psychological health of patients and their sexual quality of life.

The prevalence of SD in BC survivors oscillates between 40% and 80% [3–9], clearly higher compared to healthy women [8–9], and persisting over time, affecting the quality of life of patients through many years [8, 9–12].

The main symptoms of SD reported by BC survivors include difficulties in arousal or excitation [3, 5, 9, 14], decreased sexual desire [3–5, 9, 14, 15], insufficient lubrication [3–5, 9, 14], and dyspareunia [3, 9, 13, 14].

Although being a frequent problem among BC patients, SD is not usually discussed in the clinical practice [16, 17] since health care providers often feel uncomfortable asking sexual-related issues to patients [17] and furthermore, they do not always have received a proper formation on this field [9, 17]. In addition, patients tend to feel embarrassed to discuss sexual concerns during BC related visits [18]. Often, BCS feel that their health care providers are not properly prepared to treat SD issues. As a result, sexual counselling is not usually provided to BC patients and SD remains being an underdiagnosed and undertreated issue for these women [16, 17].

2 Sexual Disfunction in Breast Cancer Survivors

SD in BC survivors is a multifactorial entity severely influenced by the disease itself, as well as, by the secondary effects of treatments of BC (Fig. 1) [2, 5, 9, 14, 17]. It is to note that specific cancer-related causes of SD for BC survivors were found and divided into those related to locoregional strategies (surgery, radiotherapy), those related to systemic treatments (chemotherapy, endocrine therapy), and those related to sociocultural differences among patients.

(a) Biological: direct disruption in the body image, especially among those women undergoing a mastectomy [4, 6, 14, 16, 17]. Radiation therapy can also cause locoregional alterations in the breast, such as pain, discomfort, skin lesions, or loss of flexibility. Chemotherapy sometimes leads to ovarian failure, asthenia, and alopecia, among others. Endocrine that causes menopause-related symptoms among patients [2–6, 14, 17] and among them genitourinary syndrome of menopause appears to be directly related to SD in BCS.

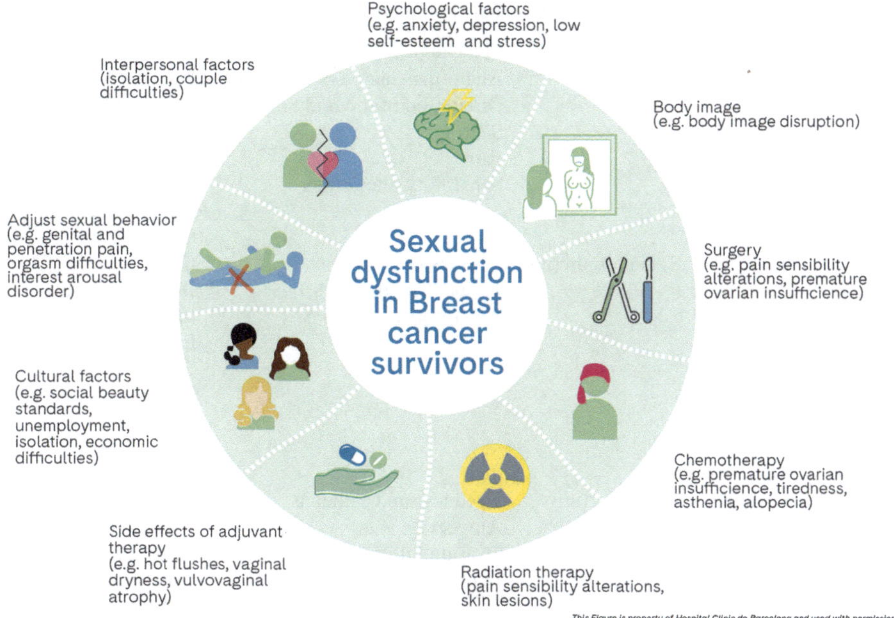

Fig. 1 Main determinants of sexual dysfunction among breast cancer survivors

(b) Psychological: Achieving sexual satisfaction for women does not rely exclusively on physical aspects, but also on psychological responses [17, 19, 20]. Evidence shows that mental health status is poorer in women and men experiencing SD [8, 9]. SD in women also causes patients to feel body shame and to feel unattractive and undesired by their partners, as well as a feeling of rejection by those [20]. Additionally, there have been reported changes in the sense of sexual self [13]. Both BC diagnosis and SD could act as potential stressors for women and men, causing an impairment in their global health status and even a negative impact on the effect of BC treatments and the progression of the disease [21]. The fact of suffering a BC itself can cause mental health disruptions, such as depression, anxiety, or emotional distress [6, 8, 9].

(c) Sociocultural: breasts are considered in most cultures as symbols of female sexuality and sexual identity [6, 8, 16, 17].

(d) Interpersonal: BCS partners can also be affected by SD. Partners can change their attitudes during sexual practice to avoid causing any physical harm to women [20], presenting SD.

The potential causes of SD in BC survivors are summarized in Table 1.

Table 1 Summarize of main causes of Sexual Dysfunction in Breast Cancer survivors

Potential cause of SD		Mechanisms	Authors describing
Locorregional treatments	Surgery	Anatomic change of the breast	Panjari (2011)
		Disruption of the body image	Bartula (2013)
		Scaring	Sadovsky (2010)
		Pain	Gandhi (2019)
		Sensibility alterations	Hungr (2017)
			Boquiren (2016)
			Candy (2016)
	Radiation therapy	Skin lesions	Cobo (2018)
		Tissue discomfort	Boswell (2015)
		Sensibility alterations	Seav (2015)
		Pain	Panjari (2011)
			Sadovsky (2010)
			Ljungman (2018)
			Gandhi (2019)
			Hungr (2017)
			Boquiren (2016)
Systemic treatments	Chemotherapy	Tiredness and asthenia	Cobo (2018)
		Alopecia	Boswell (2015)
		Ovarian failure	Seav (2015)
		Decreased libido	Panjari (2011)
			Sadovsky (2010)
			Ljungman (2018)
			Gandhi (2019)
			Hungr (2017)
			Boquiren (2016)
			Candy (2016)
	Endocrine therapy	Hot flushes	Cobo (2018)
		Vaginal dryness	Boswell (2015)
		Penetration pain	Seav (2015)
		Vulvovaginal atrophy	Panjari (2011)
		Decreased libido	Sadovsky (2010)
			Ljungman (2018)
			Gandhi (2019)
			Hungr (2017)
			Boquiren (2016)
Psychological aspects		Sexualization of the breasts	Bartula (2013)
		The breast as a symbol of feminity	Gandhi (2019)
		Social beauty standards	Langellier (1998)
			Hungr (2017)
			Boquiren (2016)

SD sexual dysfunction modified from Castillo H. et Al [22]

3   Treatment Options

Nowadays, various treatments have been suggested to manage SD in BCS [22]. However, a standardized treatment has still not been established to specifically address SD in BC survivors. Broadly speaking, the treatments available should be managed from a biopsychosocial model and can be summarized into four categories: local treatments, systemic treatments, physical therapies, and educational interventions.

3.1   Local Strategies

Local treatments include vaginal-application products, such as moisturizers and lubricants, aimed to reduce the symptoms of SD. The products assessed are: polycarbophil-based moisturizer, compounded testosterone cream, pH balanced lactic acid gel, and vaginal oestrogens [22]. The effects of each of these products are summarized in Table 2. Other local strategies include the use of vibrators [23–25] and laser therapy [26].

Evidence shows that some symptoms of SD improve with local treatments, especially intercourse pain and vaginal dryness. Regarding the use of vaginal oestrogens, even though they have shown to improve the sexual function more effectively than moisturizers, they have also proven to have systemic absorption [27].

Moreover, evidence from studies in healthy women and women with sexual dysfunction for other causes shows that vaginal vibrator use improves various aspects of the sexual function of patients, especially desire, arousal, lubrication, orgasm, and pain [23], and it has been proved to be a useful treatment tool for anorgasmia [23, 24]. The use of a vaginal vibrator is also effective improving genito-pelvic pain and dyspareunia [23, 25]. A recent study in breast cancer survivors under aromatase inhibitors assessing the usefulness of laser therapy in those patents, compared the use of vaginal vibrators plus moisturizers with vaginal laser vs the use of vibrators plus moisturizers with vaginal sham laser, showing a significant improvement in vaginal tissues and sexual function in both arms after the treatments even though those patients which received active laser sessions did not show significant differences with those who received sham sessions [28].

3.2   Systemic Pharmacological Treatments

Transdermic testosterone and antidepressants like venlafaxine, clonidine, and bupropion are the systemic treatments tested to address SD symptoms in BC patients. However, none of these treatment options have shown to be superior to placebo improving SD [22].

3.3   Physical Therapy

The effect of different modalities of physical therapy has been tested in three clinical trials. There have been evaluated the effects of a home-exercise programme [29], a 1-year strength training [30], and general physical training [31] on the symptoms of

SD. Only body image has shown to improve after a 1-year strength training programme. Slight improvements of sexual health have been shown when combining physical activity with cognitive therapy [29]. Also, a discrete improvement in the perception of one's appearance and sexuality are described with a 1-year strength training [30]. Finally, for those women complaining with dyspareunia, pelvic floor muscle training appears to be effective, and a useful intervention in clinical settings [32].

3.4 Educational and Psychotherapeutic Interventions

Some studies have evaluated the use of educational strategies and counselling as a treatment of SD in BC survivors, understanding as sexual counselling the provider of sexuality information during medical visits and targeted psychological sexual therapies undergone by specific formed professionals in the field.

Evidence shows SD improves after educational interventions specifically focused on sexual aspects related to BC [33]. Couple sexual therapy enhancing the communication of SD aspects and cancer has showed improvement of SD as well [34].

Accordingly, SD appear to be not improved when psychological interventions are not focused on sexual concerns [35].

4 Concerns in the Management of Sexual Health in Breast Cancer Survivors

New challenges regarding BCS are appearing since the survival have increased drastically during the last decades. There is a huge demand from BCS to focus on maintaining quality of life and avoid secondary effects related to the provided treatments, such as SD.

Evidence shows that over half of BCS experience SD at some point during the treatment or posttreatment. Sexual dysfunction in BCS present not only a high prevalence, but also a high degree of under-diagnostic in the clinical practice. Sexuality is not usually evaluated during oncological visits; therefore, a great number of women who suffer SD are not diagnosed and thus, not treated.

Patients need to be informed about secondary effects of BC treatments and its possible impact on sexuality. This topic should be easily and openly discussed during visits, and patients may be offered solutions in case they need help or further information.

The authors believe sexual disfunction should be evaluated systematically to all BCS and if possible, in the near term, through a validated scale for BCS.

The importance of having a specific scale for BC patients relies on the fact that BC may affect the sexual life of women in a different way from other cancers. Since BCS are usually treated using antiestrogenic treatments worsening all menopause dimension symptoms, and directly causing a physical alteration in women in a sexuality-social-related organ [16].

An ideal scale would need to include all the dimensions of SD. It should also assess other aspects of sexuality beyond physical symptoms and include psychological aspects of sexual function, understanding sexuality from a holistic point of view, not focusing exclusively on coital relationships and vaginal intercourse. Finally, the scale would need to be brief and practical to complete, as well as offer the possibility to be repeated in different visits in order to evaluate the effectiveness of the treatment or strategies used.

Sexual dysfunction in BCS needs to be understood as the result of the combination of multiple factors: BC is a disease that affects the breasts, which play an essential role in female sexuality and sexual activities, provoking serious impact on the mental health of BC patients and being a common cause of psychological disruption. This disruption has shown to be a constant reminder of the disease, causing women a feeling of insecurity regarding their health status [17]. Furthermore, many women report feeling unattractive and not desirable after BC [9, 17], which is also affected by cultural aspects [17]. In addition, being aware of having SD and self-conscious during sexual activities, can also cause impairments on desire, arousal, and difficulty to connect with the partner and enjoy the sexual relationships. All of these promote, in turn, SD [9, 13, 17].

Furthermore, cancer treatments (surgery, chemotherapy, radiation therapy, endocrine therapy) themselves also have a negative effect in the sexual life of women through physical symptoms such as fatigue, joint pain, penetration pain, lack of lubrication, decreased libido, and difficulties in arousal.

Despite the high prevalence of SD and its consequences, there are still no clear standardized therapeutic strategies for these patients. Considering the multifactorial nature of SD and its impact on various aspects of the quality of life of patients, proper treatment options may result from the combination of pharmacological and psychological strategies.

The use of vaginal moisturizers combined with psychological therapy focused on sexual aspects should be considered. Moreover, including mechanical stimuli (vibrators, dilators) to the local treatment may be of benefit although is still of no common use and should be potential investigation target for the future.

4.1   Male Breast Cancer and Sexuality

Breast cancer (BC) in men is rare and many people are not aware of this disease. It occurs in approximately 1% of men. Of note, there are differences between female and male BC being more frequently hormonal positive tumours (high rate of endocrine therapy) and later diagnosed (7 years older), as well as different impact on psychosexual and quality of life spheres (erectile dysfunction, stigma due to have a "female disease", impaired male role...). Male BC survivors experience substantial sexual symptoms, with less sexual activity in older patients or advanced disease [36]. At least 40% reported "very poor" ability to perform sexually over the previous month [37]. The authors found no differences in sexual scores in men on endocrine therapy compared to those without. So, it suggests that there may be other causes of sexual symptoms and sexual impairment which should be considered from a biopsychosocial point of view also in male population.

Some qualitative studies [38, 39] reported on psychological and sociocultural themes which can affect male BC sexuality as masculinity role, body image, identities, coping responses, and resources or relationships. The authors demonstrate how current approaches to breast cancer serve to isolate men who develop the illness, potentially alienating and emasculating them. Considering this information, pre- and postoperative gender-specific information to alleviate the potential biopsychosocial problems associated with the diagnosis; and provision of appropriate support/counselling services for partners of patients is mandatory.

In a mixed method study [40] through focus groups (qualitative data) and questionnaires (quantitative data) the unmet information needs of male BC population was assessed. Among 77 male BC participants, the most frequent unmet information needs related to acute or late effects of cancer and treatment were about sexuality based on the questionnaires. However, this topic was not identified in the focus group analysis ($n = 12$). Interested in sex (23%), sexual activity with or without intercourse (22%) and sexual enjoyment (17%) were the main sexual needs in the acute phase, compared to those related to late effects as 25% emotionally (embarrassment, loss of libido) and 23% physical (erectile dysfunction) sexual issues.

However, the literature in this topic is scarce as few studies include male patients with BC and fewer address his sexuality. Unfortunately, care and treatment in male population with BC is based on information from women studies. With the aim to be as inclusive as possible, we would like to highlight with these lines some specific data about sexuality of male BC survivors. Further studies are needed to reach quality and tailored sexual information for the male BC population.

5 Conclusions

Sexual dysfunction is a multifactorial condition that affects among 40–80% of BCS, causing a decrease in quality of life of these women.

Despite its prevalence, SD remains underdiagnosed and there is scarce use of SD assessment scales in regular clinical practice. A regular implementation of a validated scale for its proper assessment would be beneficial for diagnosis screening.

Finally, there is no standardized therapeutic strategies to care for SD in BC survivors although, as in many other conditions, the PLISSIT model can act as a reference guide. Therapeutic options should be potential investigation targets for the near future, which may evaluate local treatments (vaginal moisturizers, vibrators) combined with psychological interventions.

Addressing this condition might suppose a step forward to achieve a healthy and satisfactory sexual life and, thus, higher quality of life of millions of women worldwide.

References

1. World Health Organization. Breast cancer. 2022. https://www.who.int/news-room/fact-sheets/detail/breast-cancer. Accessed 6 Apr 2023.
2. Candy B, Jones L, Vickerstaff V, Tookman A, King M. Interventions for sexual dysfunction following treatments for cancer in women. Cochrane Database Syst Rev. 2016;2:CD005540.
3. Cobo-Cuenca AI, Martín-Espinosa NM, Sampietro-Crespo A, Rodríguez-Borrego MA, Carmona-Torres JM. SD in Spanish women with breast cancer. PLoS One. 2018;13:e0203151.
4. Panjari M, Bell RJ, Davis SR. Sexual function after breast cancer. J Sex Med. 2011;8:294–302.
5. Ljungman L, Ahlgren J, Petersson L, Flynn KE, Weinfurt K, Gorman JR, et al. Sexual dysfunction and reproductive concerns in young women with breast cancer: type, prevalence, and predictors of problems. Psycho-Oncology. 2018;27:2770–7.
6. Gandhi C, Butler E, Pesek S, Kwait R, Edmonson D, Raker C, et al. Sexual dysfunction in breast cancer survivors. Am J Clin Oncol. 2019;42:500–6.
7. Goldfarb SB, Dickler M, Sit L, Fruscione M, Barz T, Atkinson T, et al. Sexual dysfunction in women with breast cancer: prevalence and severity. J Clin Oncol. 2009;27:9558.
8. Raggio GA, Butryn ML, Arigo D, Mikorski R, Palmer SC. Prevalence and correlates of sexual morbidity in long-term breast cancer survivors. Psychol Health. 2014;29:632–50.
9. Boquiren VM, Esplen MJ, Wong J, Toner B, Warner E, Malik N. Sexual functioning in breast cancer survivors experiencing body image disturbance. Psycho-Oncology. 2016;25:66–76.
10. Ganz PA, Rowland JH, Desmond K, Meyerowitz BE, Wyatt GE. Life after breast cancer: understanding women's health-related quality of life and sexual functioning. J Clin Oncol. 1998;16:501–14.
11. Bloom JR, Stewart SL, Oakley-Girvan I, Banks PJ, Shema S. Quality of life of younger breast cancer survivors: persistence of problems and sense of Well-being. Psycho-Oncology. 2012;21:655–65.
12. Kornblith AB, Powell M, Regan MM, Bennett S, Krasner C, Moy B, et al. Long-term psychosocial adjustment of older vs younger survivors of breast and endometrial cancer. Psycho-Oncology. 2007;16:895–903.
13. Ussher JM, Perz J, Gilbert E. Perceived causes and consequences of sexual changes after cancer for women and men: a mixed method study. BMC Cancer. 2015;15:268.
14. Sadovsky R, Basson R, Krychman M, Morales AM, Schover L, Wang R, et al. Cancer and sexual problems. Journal of Sexual Medicine. 2010;7:349–73.
15. Biglia N, Moggio G, Peano E, Sgandurra P, Ponzone R, Nappi RE, et al. Effects of surgical and adjuvant therapies for breast cancer on sexuality, cognitive functions, and body weight. J Sex Med. 2010;7:1891–900.
16. Bartula I, Sherman KA. Screening for SD in women diagnosed with breast cancer: systematic review and recommendations. Breast Cancer Res Treat. 2013;141:173–85.
17. Hungr C, Sanchez-Varela V, Bober SL. Self-image and sexuality issues among young women with breast cancer: practical recommendations. Revista de Investigacion Clinica. 2017;69:114–22.
18. Bachmann GA, Leiblum SR, Grill J. Brief sexual inquiry in gynecologic practice. Obstet Gynecol. 1989;73:425–7.
19. Bowsfield ML, Cobb RJ. Sexual anxiety mediates dyadic associations between body satisfaction and sexual quality in mixed-sex couples. Arch Sex Behav. 2021;50:2603–19.
20. Henson H. Breast cancer and sexuality. Sex Disabil. 2002;20:261–75.
21. Eckerling A, Ricon-Becker I, Sorski L, Sandbank E, Ben-Eliyahu S. Stress and cancer: mechanisms, significance and future directions. Nat Rev Cancer. 2021;21:767–85.
22. Castillo H, Mension E, Cebrecos I, Anglès SC-B, C. Sexual function in breast cancer patients: a review of the literature. Clin Exp Obstet Gynecol. 2022;49(6):134.
23. Rullo JE, Lorenz T, Ziegelmann MJ, Meihofer L, Herbenick D, Faubion SS. Genital vibration for sexual function and enhancement: a review of evidence. Sex Relatsh Ther. 2018;33:263–74.

24. Laan E, Rellini AH, Barnes T. Standard operating procedures for female orgasmic disorder: consensus of the International Society for Sexual Medicine. J Sex Med. 2013;10:74–34.

25. Bakker RM, Vermeer WM, Creutzberg CL, Mens JW, Nout RA, Ter Kuile MM. Qualitative accounts of patients' determinants of vaginal dilator use after pelvic radiotherapy. J Sex Med. 2015;12:764–73.

26. Mension E, Alonso I, Tortajada M, Matas I, Gómez S, Ribera L, et al. Vaginal laser therapy for genitourinary syndrome of menopause—systematic review. Maturitas. 2022;156:37–59.

27. Mension E, Alonso I, Castelo-Branco C. Genitourinary syndrome of menopause: current treatment options in breast cancer survivors - systematic review. Maturitas. 2021;143:47–58.

28. Mension E, Alonso I, Anglès-Acedo S, et al. Effect of fractional carbon dioxide vs sham laser on sexual function in survivors of breast cancer receiving aromatase inhibitors for genitourinary syndrome of menopause: the LIGHT randomized clinical trial. JAMA Netw Open. 2023;6(2):e2255697.

29. Duijts SF, Stolk-Vos AC, Oldenburg HS, van Beurden M, Aaronson NK. Characteristics of breast cancer patients who experience menopausal transition due to treatment. Climacteric. 2011;14:362–8.

30. Speck RM, Gross CR, Hormes JM, Ahmed RL, Lytle LA, Hwang W, et al. Changes in the body image and relationship scale following a 1-year strength training trial for breast cancer survivors with or at risk for lymphedema. Breast Cancer Res Treat. 2010;121:421–30.

31. Berglund G, Bolund C, Gustafsson UL, Sjödén PO. One-year follow-up of the 'Starting again' group rehabilitation programme for cancer patients. Eur J Cancer. 1994;30A:1744–51.

32. Juraskova I, Jarvis S, Mok K, Peate M, Meiser B, Cheah BC, Mireskandari S, Friedlander M. The acceptability, feasibility, and efficacy (phase I/II study) of the OVERcome (olive oil, vaginal exercise, and moisturize R) intervention to improve dyspareunia and alleviate sexual problems in women with breast cancer. J Sex Med. 2013;10(10):2549–58.

33. Anderson DJ, Seib C, McCarthy AL, Yates P, Porter-Steele J, McGuire A, et al. Facilitating lifestyle changes to manage menopausal symptoms in women with breast cancer: a randomized controlled pilot trial of the pink Women's wellness program. Menopause. 2015;22:937–45.

34. Baucom DH, Porter LS, Kirby JS, Gremore TM, Wiesenthal N, Aldridge W, et al. A couple-based intervention for female breast cancer. Psycho-Oncology. 2009;18:276–83.

35. Salonen P, Tarkka MT, Kellokumpu-Lehtinen PL, Koivisto AM, Aalto P, Kaunonen M. Effect of social support on changes in quality of life in early breast cancer patients: a longitudinal study. Scand J Caring Sci. 2013;27:396–405.

36. Schröder CP, van Leeuwen-Stok E, Cardoso F, Linderholm B, Poncet C, Wolff AC, Bjelic-Radisic V, Werutsky G, Abreu MH, Bozovic-Spasojevic I, den Hoed I, Honkoop AH, Los M, Leone JP, Russell NS, Smilde TJ, van der Velden AWG, Van Poznak C, Vleugel MM, Yung RL, Coens C, Giordano SH, Ruddy KJ. Quality of life in male breast cancer: prospective study of the international male breast cancer program (EORTC10085/TBCRC029/BIG2-07/NABCG). Oncologist. 2023;28(10):e877–83.

37. Ruddy KJ, Giobbie-Hurder A, Giordano SH, et al. Quality of life and symptoms in male breast cancer survivors. Breast. 2013;22(2):197–9.

38. Quincey K, Williamson I, Winstanley S. Marginalised malignancies': a qualitative synthesis of men's accounts of living with breast cancer. Soc Sci Med. 2016;149:17–25.

39. France L, Michie S, Barrett-Lee P, Brain K, Harper P, Gray J. Male cancer: a qualitative study of male breast cancer. Breast. 2000;9(6):343–8.

40. Bootsma TI, Duijveman P, Pijpe A, Scheelings PC, Witkamp AJ, Bleiker EMA. Unmet information needs of men with breast cancer and health professionals. Psychooncology. 2020;29(5):851–60.

Autoimmune and Rheumatic Diseases and Sexuality

José Alfredo Gómez-Puerta, José Luis Callejas-Rubio, and Gerard Espinosa

1   Introduction

Autoimmune and rheumatic diseases are a group of chronic conditions that can affect people of all ages and genders, and they have a significant impact on individuals' daily lives. These diseases, including among others fibromyalgia, rheumatoid arthritis, spondyloarthropathies, systemic lupus erythematosus, Sjögren's syndrome, systemic sclerosis, and systemic vasculitis are characterized by chronic inflammation and immune system dysfunction that can result in joint and tissue damage, pain, and disability.

In addition to the physical symptoms, autoimmune and rheumatic diseases can also impact patients' sexual health and quality of life. Sexual health has been defined as the state of physical, emotional, mental, and social well-being in relation to sexuality, and it is influenced by the anatomical, psychological, social, and pathological characteristics of each individual [1]. Sexual dysfunction (SD) defined as a persistent or recurring inability to achieve or maintain sexual satisfaction is a common problem among individuals with these conditions. In a recent systematic review and meta-analysis including 68 studies and 5457 females diagnosed with systemic autoimmune diseases, the overall prevalence of SD was 63%. Across the different

J. A. Gómez-Puerta
Department of Rheumatology, Clinical Institute of Medical and Surgical Specialties, Hospital Clinic de Barcelona, Barcelona, Spain
e-mail: jagomez@clinic.cat

J. L. Callejas-Rubio
Systemic Autoimmune Diseases Unit, Department of Internal Medicine, Hospital San Cecilio, Granada, Spain

G. Espinosa (✉)
Department of Autoimmune Diseases, Clinical Institute of Medicine and Dermatology, Hospital Clínic de Barcelona, Barcelona, Spain
e-mail: gespino@clinic.cat

systemic autoimmune diseases, women with Sjögren's syndrome and systemic sclerosis reported the highest levels of SD (74% and 69%, respectively) [2]. In a recent study including 124 sexually active men diagnosed with systemic lupus erythematosus, 22 of them (18%) answered positively when asked if they believed they had sexual dysfunction. Interestingly, sexual function was impaired, independently of disease activity, chronic disease damage, or pharmacological treatment [3].

In autoimmune and rheumatic diseases, SD can be caused by a variety of factors including disease activity, chronic pain, fatigue, and medication side effects. These factors are summarized in Fig. 1. It is well-known that glucocorticoids may have side effects with great impact on sexual function, due to change in body image, as well as leading to depression and psychosis. Furthermore, several drugs such as tricyclic antidepressants and serotonin reuptake inhibitors used to treat fibromyalgia, a frequent comorbid condition associated to autoimmune diseases, may also have an impact on SD, since may lead to a significant decrease of libido.

Despite the high prevalence of SD in patients with autoimmune and rheumatic diseases, this topic is often overlooked in clinical practice. Nevertheless, sexual functioning remains a neglected area of quality of life in patients affected by autoimmune and rheumatic diseases [4]. This is well demonstrated by a survey conducted a few years ago in which the results revealed that only 12% of patients visited by rheumatologists in routine clinical practice was screened for sexual activity [5]. Among others, different barriers prevent an open communication on

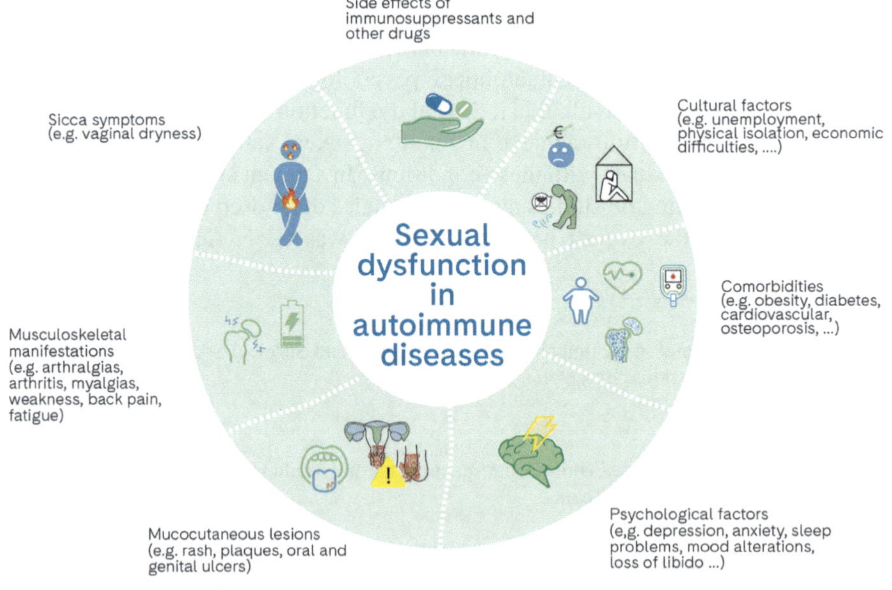

Fig. 1 Factors causing sexual dysfunction in patients with rheumatic and autoimmune diseases

reproduction issues, such as not adequate skills, lack of training, and lack of access to specialized services. There are evidence indicating that physicians and other health professionals might not feel comfortable discussing sexuality with their patients because they have not been trained in these issues [6]. In addition, counseling is often considered to be time-consuming into the limited time frame of an outpatient evaluation.

The impact of SD on patients' quality of life is not well recognized, and it is often underdiagnosed and undertreated. Patients may feel embarrassed or ashamed to bring up the topic with their healthcare providers, and healthcare providers may not feel comfortable discussing sexual health concerns or may not have the necessary training to address them effectively. This lack of communication and awareness can result in a significant gap in care for patients with autoimmune and rheumatic diseases, leading to decreased satisfaction with care and poorer health outcomes. As a result, SD may go untreated, leading to further negative impacts on patients' quality of life and psychological well-being.

According to the results of a recent systematic review, there is a lack of sufficient evidence to recommend a certain management strategy for SD in females with autoimmune and rheumatic diseases [7]. Although the impact of the different therapeutic interventions is not well-known, beyond the control of inflammation of the underlying disease and pain, non-pharmacological therapies such as psychotherapy, physical exercise, and local measures for dry symptoms such as lubricant creams, among others, are useful strategies. However, no definite conclusions can be drawn due to the important limitations of the available literature.

This chapter will focus on sexual health in patients with autoimmune and rheumatic diseases. It will explore the prevalence, causes, and treatment of sexual dysfunction in this population.

2   Fibromyalgia

Fibromyalgia (FM) is a chronic condition characterized by diffuse pain and tenderness of muscles, tendons, and joints without detectable inflammation. FM is not associated with structural deformities but is commonly accompanied by systemic symptoms such as fatigue, non-reparative sleep, intestinal problems, and cognitive-mood symptoms among others [8].

FM is a complex syndrome involving many different factors that can severely impact and disrupt a person's daily life including sexual activity. Several studies have shown that people with FM experience various SD, such as decreased libido, difficulty achieving or maintaining an erection, vaginal dryness, and pain during intercourse [9, 10]. The reasons behind this relationship are not fully understood, but it is thought that the pain and fatigue associated with FM may interfere with sexual function by affecting mood, reducing physical activity, and altering the levels of certain hormones.

A recent Brazilian study evaluated sexual performance by Female Sexual Function Index (FSFI) in 726 FM patients and 858 paired controls [8]. In general, all studies domains were worse in patients with FM vs. controls. Age, menopause, degree of musculoskeletal pain, and underlying psychiatric illness were associated with lower scores.

Treatment options for SD in fibromyalgia include addressing underlying physical and psychological issues, using medications to manage symptoms including selective serotonin reuptake inhibitors, for example, fluoxetine, muscle relaxants, for example, cyclobenzaprine or analgesics such as Tramadol and incorporating sexual counseling and education into a comprehensive treatment plan.

3   Rheumatoid Arthritis

Rheumatoid arthritis (RA) is a chronic autoimmune disorder affecting predominantly female patients in middle age (40–60 years) that can lead without treatment to joint destruction and disability. RA not only involves joint structures but also is related to extra-articular manifestations such as interstitial lung disease, subcutaneous nodules, and sicca syndrome among others. Patients suffering from RA not only have inflammatory symptoms related to synovitis, pain, stiffness sicca symptoms, and fatigue but also a wide variety of psychological symptoms including depression, sleep problems, body dysmorphia among others, which can lead to SD.

The impact of RA on sexual life is well recognized. In studies, sexual problems appear to affect 30–70% of RA patients [11]. SD in RA patients can manifest in various ways, such as decreased libido, problems with sexual satisfaction, difficulty achieving or maintaining an erection, vaginal dryness, and pain during intercourse among others. Various factors, such as physical, social, or psychological problems, are susceptible influencing sexuality. Some of the medications used to treat RA can also contribute to sexual dysfunction. In a recent study in patients with RA, the prevalence of female sexual dysfunction was 49.3% and was associated with younger age, fatigue, mental distress, and HAQ score [11]. A Colombian study that included a big cohort of patients with RA, described some differences among female and male patients in SD symptoms. The orgasmic decrease was more common in male patients, while dyspareunia was more common among female patients [12]. Therefore, people with RA need to discuss their sexual health concerns with their healthcare provider and explore available treatment options, which may include medications, therapy, or other interventions to improve sexual function and overall well-being.

The Quality of Life and Sexuality in Rheumatology (Qualisex) questionnaire is a tool that can be used to assess the impact of RA on a patient's sexual health and quality of life. The Qualisex questionnaire is a validated instrument that can help healthcare professionals assess the extent to which RA is affecting a patient's sexual function and overall well-being. It includes ten questions that cover different aspects of sexual health, such as sexual desire, arousal, lubrication, orgasm, and satisfaction. It also includes questions about the emotional and social impact of RA on sexual function. Patients can complete the questionnaire anonymously and in private, which can help them feel more comfortable discussing sensitive issues related to sexual health [13]. Qualisex has been validated in various languages including English, French, and Spanish, among others, proving to be a highly useful and reliable tool.

Some previous studies conducted in the pre-biological era reported a higher prevalence of erectile dysfunction in male patients with RA. A more recent study conducted in Olmsted County (USA) evaluated the risk factors related with erectile dysfunction in a cohort of 260 RA patients and 260 age-matched male controls [14]. Men with RA did not have a significantly different rate of erectile dysfunction compared to their age-matched comparators.

No major concerns have been reported about RA treatment and the higher risk of SD. In general, both conventional disease-modifying antirheumatic drugs (DMARD) and biological DMARD (bDMARD) are safe treatments regarding sexuality side effects. Only a few cases with loss of libido/impotence after methotrexate have been reported in the literature, especially in males.

4   Spondyloarthropathies

Spondyloarthritis (SpA) is a group of inflammatory rheumatic diseases that primarily affect the axial skeleton and the peripheral joints. The term spondyloarthropathies encompass several different conditions, including ankylosing spondylitis (AS), psoriatic arthritis (PsA), reactive arthritis, and enteropathic arthritis [15]. These conditions share some common clinical features, such as inflammation, pain, and stiffness in the joints and surrounding tissues, as well as a predisposition to spinal involvement.

SpA can lead to various degrees of functional disability, which can significantly impact a person's quality of life. Functional disability refers to the limitations or restrictions a person may experience in carrying out everyday activities. This can include difficulties with mobility, range of motion, and completing tasks that require physical exertion.

One of the primary symptoms of spondyloarthropathies is chronic pain, which can be felt in the joints, back, and other areas of the body. In addition to pain, spondyloarthropathies can also cause stiffness in the joints and spine. This stiffness can limit a person's range of motion, making it difficult to perform certain movements or activities including sexual activity [15].

In a single-center study conducted in Turkey, 98 women with SpA (axial SpA) were compared with 99 controls. No differences were found between clinical characteristics including age, gravida, and parity, previous births among others. The FSFI and quality of life SF-36 scores were significantly lower, and Hospital Anxiety and Depression Scale (HADS) scores were significantly higher in the SpA patients than in the controls. Clitoral and labial atrophy and speculum pain scores were significantly higher in the SpA group [16].

In PsA and psoriasis, sexual function for both men and women is decreased compared with the control group regardless of whether or not associated with their depressive status. Usually, those patients who had a good response to bDMARD have a clear improvement in FSFI, reflecting the relationship with personal perception of sexual health.

5 Juvenile Idiopathic Arthritis

Juvenile idiopathic arthritis (JIA) is a chronic condition that affects children and adolescents. It is an autoimmune disorder that causes joint inflammation and can lead to pain, stiffness, and swelling. While arthritis can have a significant impact on a patient's physical health, it can also affect their sexual Health [17].

Sexual problems are common in patients with JIA. Pain and fatigue associated with the condition can cause difficulties with sexual desire and arousal. Joint stiffness and limited mobility can make it challenging to engage in sexual activity comfortably. Additionally, the use of medication to manage arthritis symptoms may have side effects that affect sexual function.

For young adults, sexual health is an essential aspect of their overall well-being. Therefore, addressing sexual problems in patients with JIA is crucial to their quality of life. It is essential to speak with a healthcare professional, who can offer support and advice on how to manage sexual problems [17].

In a case-control study assessed sexuality in 32 patients with polyarticular juvenile arthritis and 120 healthy controls using a self-administered male sexual evaluation questionnaire (MESQ) as exploratory tool reported no differences in terms of masturbation, regular sex intercourse, desire, and satisfaction rates among groups [18]. However, patients with JIA reported more frequently joint pain during intercourse.

6 Systemic Lupus Erythematosus

Systemic Lupus Erythematosus (SLE) can exert detrimental influences on different aspects of patients' life, leading to an impairment of psychological health (e.g., depression and low self-esteem), health-related quality of life, and sexual function [19].

Over the last years, various studies have addressed the relationship between SLE and SD, demonstrating that SLE was associated with an increased risk of SD in both males and females [20–23] ranging from 15% to 86% [20–23]. A systematic review and meta-analysis of observational studies concluded a nearly two-fold increased risk of SD among subjects with SLE compared with healthy individuals [22]. Women with SLE had a lower desire, lubrication, and orgasm compared with controls [20]. The results of these studies show that female SLE patients have a lower total FSFI score, compared with healthy controls, which means that SLE exerts some influence on women's sexual function.

The reasons for SD are probably multifactorial and comprises disease-related factors as well as medication, and hormonal, psychological, and cultural factors.

Physical symptoms, medical management, and disease activity measured by SLE disease activity index (SLEDAI) were associated with a lower desire and total scores of the FSFI.

The psychological consequences of chronic illness often play a more critical role in the development of SD and therefore should not be neglected. Patients with SLE often have a lower quality of life, higher level of depression and anxiety, and more negative attitudes towards their body image. A significant difference in sexual function between SLE women and healthy group was observed applying a demographic questionnaire, the Depression, Anxiety, and Stress Scales-21 Items (DASS-21), and the FSFI. The difference remained significant after controlling for confounding factors (stress, depression, anxiety). Moreover, the effect of SLE on the sexual function had a significant correlation with age, life status, number and age of children, economic status, menstruation, duration of marriage, age at diagnosis, disease duration and activity, stress, anxiety, and depression [21]. Zhang L et al. [24] reported that fatigue, studied by the multidimensional fatigue questionnaire, was an important potential risk factors of female sexual problems in SLE women.

SLE patients often had a higher level of estrogen but a lower level of testosterone and dehydroepiandrosterone, and it is recognized that the androgenic status could be related with sexual function including sexual desire and satisfaction.

Glucocorticoid agents and non-steroidal anti-inflammatory drugs (NSAID) involved in the treatment of SLE might also negatively impair sexual function and sexual satisfaction [22]. Glucocorticoids cause Cushing's syndrome and exert an inhibitory effect on sex hormones resulting in persistently low sexual desire.

The risk of SD is higher in men with SLE than in the general population (12–68% in SLE patients compared to 0–22% in healthy controls), and this risk is higher compared to females with SLE [22]. Numerous publications have described the negative effects that SLE has on erectile function, libido, anthropometric measurements, ejaculation, sperm quality, and reproductive hormone levels [3]. The main conclusion of this study was that the simple question: "Do you think you have sexual dysfunction?" had a high predictive value to detect patients with worse sexual function. Therefore, clinicians should be considering this question in all man patient with SLE in each periodic assessment.

Treatment in case of having some degree of SD should include both pharmacological and non-pharmacological interventions like lifestyle modifications, such as smoking cessation, weight-loss and exercise, and behavioral therapy [7]. There are not specific studies about the effect of medical treatment of erectile dysfunction in lupus; probably, the treatment should be the same as that the erectile dysfunction associated to other comorbidities according to the updated guidelines on male sexual dysfunction [25].

7　Sjögren Syndrome

Women with primary Sjögren Syndrome (pSS) have significantly more SD compared with healthy controls, with a prevalence reported of 32–56% [26] and is influenced by physical as well as psychological consequences of the disease, such as pain, fatigue, stiffness, functional impairment, depression, anxiety, negative body image, reduced libido, hormonal imbalance, and side effects from treatments. Genital symptoms, such as vulvar and vaginal dryness, dyspareunia, itching, genital pain, increased susceptibility to infection, and dysuria are reported to contribute to SD.

A recent meta-analysis found that women with SS had significantly poorer sexual function than healthy controls, with disruptions observed in levels of desire, arousal, lubrication, orgasm, sexual satisfaction, and pain experienced during vaginal penetration (dyspareunia) [27].

Dyspareunia has been reported in 61% of patients with pSS and vaginal dryness in 52%, both having a great impact on quality of life. The pathobiology of dyspareunia has not yet been clarified. A possible explanation may be the local inflammation of vaginal mucosa, pelvic floor dysfunction, vaginal or cervical atrophy, severity of vaginal dryness, and lower levels of sexual hormones (estrogen and testosterone).

Regarding genital atrophy, Gözüküçük M et al. [28] observed that vaginal, labial, clitoral, and cervical atrophy, and speculum pain scores were significantly higher among women with pSS with a significant correlation between all the domain scores of FSFI and gynecological examination. Women with pSS had worse results in PFDI-20 (Pelvic Floor Disease Inventory), PFIQ-7 (Pelvic Floor Impact Questionnaire), and FSFI scores than healthy control group.

Considering treatments, the use of moisturizers and lubricants with local estrogens is generally considered the gold standard for vulvovaginal atrophy [29]. Aesthetics treatment that utilizes energy-based treatments and other non-invasive modalities as CO_2 and Erbium YAG lasers, radiofrequency, high-intensity-focused electromagnetic energy, hyaluronic acid injection, platelet-rich plasma, and silicone thread treatments might be an option for selected patients.

8   Systemic Sclerosis

Systemic sclerosis (SSc) is a chronic autoimmune disease characterized by endothelial dysfunction, microvascular damage, and fibrosis of the skin and internal organs. A recent systematic review showed that the risk of SD in women with SSc was higher (69%) than in the general population [2].

For males, the erectile dysfunction seems to be a main manifestation of SD, and it has been related to vascular, fibrotic, neurological, and psychological factors. Some studies using the 5-Item International Index for Erectile Function (IIEF-5) have showed a significant high prevalence of erectile dysfunction in male SSc patients. Neither the presence or absence of abnormal capillaroscopy findings nor the subdivision into early, active, and late patterns is associated with coexistent erectile dysfunction in SSc [30].

For females with SSc, SD may be embodied in sexual desire, arousal, lubrication, orgasm, and sexual satisfaction disorders, and sexual pain due to physical and mental reasons [30]. The prevalence of SD in SSc females varies from 46.7% to 86.6% [31]. Vaginal tightness, dryness, ulcerations, or fissures, constricted introitus, small-sized uterus, menstrual changes, dyspareunia, and marked decline in orgasmic function and desire have been reported in SSc women with SD. They often experience discomfort or pain during intercourse attributable to vaginal tightness and dryness. SSc women have reduced clitoral blood flow compared with healthy controls and a negative correlation exists between clitoral blood flow and all domains of the FSFI except for desire.

Clinical features of SSc such as Raynaud's phenomenon, microstomia, joint contractures, gastrointestinal manifestations, fatigue, and ulcers also contribute to pain and physical discomfort, which also affects sexual satisfaction. Other symptoms, such as stiffness, reduced capacity for exercise and muscle weakness may disturb the sex lives of patients. All these factors may impair female sexual functions to some degree.

Although there is limited evidence on topical creams to consider them an effective therapy in patients with SSc, local creams may improve dyspareunia in females with SSc. According to the results of the meta-analysis [7], tadalafil did not result in a statistically significant improvement of SD in females with Raynaud's phenomenon secondary to SSc based on the FSFI. Overall, phosphodiesterase-5A inhibitors (PD5-I) have been also investigated as treatment for erectile dysfunction and, although SSc patients have poor response to on-demand administration, daily fixed doses may be effective.

9   Inflammatory Myopathies

Inflammatory myopathies (IM) including dermatomyositis (DM), polymyositis (PM), and antisynthetase syndrome (ASS) are rare autoimmune diseases characterized by inflammation of the muscles, skin, and other organs and can cause muscle weakness, fatigue, and joint pain.

These conditions can cause a wide range of physical and psychological symptoms, including SD. Patients may experience feelings of shame, embarrassment, and frustration, which can lead to social isolation and relationship problems. The prevalence of some degree of SD in these patients ranges from 20% to 60% [32]. Overall, patients with DM were more likely to report SD than patients with PM [32]. A cross-sectional study compared sexual function in patients with IM to age–/sex-matched healthy controls and determine the potential impact of clinical features on sexual function. The patients and healthy controls completed seven well-established and validated questionnaires assessing sexual health and function (FSFI, Brief Index of Sexual Function for Women, Sexual Function Questionnaire, Sexual Quality of Life Questionnaire–Female, IIEF, Male Sexual Health Questionnaire, Sexual Quality of Life Questionnaire–Male). Interestingly, the prevalence of sexual dysfunction in IM was 59% in women (vs. 40% in healthy controls) and 64% (vs. 9% in healthy controls) in men. In addition, decreased sexual function was associated with muscle weakness, disability, physical inactivity, fatigue, depression, and decreased quality of life [33].

The causes of sexual dysfunction in patients with IM are multifactorial. The physical symptoms of these conditions, such as muscle weakness, joint pain, fatigue, and skin rashes, can make sexual activity difficult or uncomfortable. These symptoms can affect physical activity, including sexual activity. In patients with DM, skin involvement can lead to sexual dysfunction. Skin rashes and ulcers in the genital area can cause pain and discomfort during sexual activity vaginal dryness and vaginal stenosis can also occur, making sexual intercourse difficult or painful. In ASS patients, interstitial lung disease and dyspnea can limit physical activity, including sexual activity.

It is important to keep in mind that the psychological impact of these conditions can also contribute to sexual dysfunction. Patients may experience feelings of anxiety, depression, stress, and low self-esteem, which can impact their sexual function and desire. In addition, the medications used to treat these conditions can also contribute to sexual dysfunction.

The treatment of sexual dysfunction in patients with IM can be challenging due to the multifactorial nature of the problem, the lack of validated assessment tools, and the limited treatment options available. Treatment may involve managing symptoms such as pain and fatigue, adjusting medications, and addressing psychological factors. It is important to develop an individualized treatment plan that considers the patient's specific symptoms and underlying medical conditions. This may involve a multidisciplinary approach that includes input from specialists such as rheumatologists, urologists, gynecologists, and sex therapists.

There are several approaches that can be considered. Medications that are commonly used to treat erectile dysfunction, such as PD5-I may be effective in some patients with IM. However, these treatments may not be appropriate for all patients, particularly those who are taking nitrates for cardiovascular disease or who have certain medical conditions such as severe liver or kidney disease. Hormone therapy, such as testosterone replacement therapy or estrogen replacement therapy, may be appropriate for some patients with IM who have low levels of these hormones. However, hormone therapy can have potential side effects, and it is important to carefully weigh the risks and benefits of this approach. Physical therapy can be helpful in improving muscle strength and mobility, which can in turn improve sexual function. Exercises that target the pelvic floor muscles, such as Kegel exercises, may be particularly helpful for patients with pelvic floor dysfunction. Psychotherapy, such as cognitive behavioral therapy or sex therapy, can be helpful in addressing the psychological and emotional factors that can contribute to sexual dysfunction. This approach may be particularly helpful for patients who are experiencing anxiety, depression, or relationship issues. Lifestyle modifications, such as quitting smoking, losing weight, and reducing alcohol consumption, can be helpful in improving overall health and may also improve sexual function.

10   Behçet's Disease

Behçet's disease (BD) is a chronic autoinflammatory disorder that can affect multiple organs in the body, including the genital tract. SD is a common problem in patients with BD for many different organic and psychological reasons and can significantly impact the quality of life of affected individuals.

The prevalence of sexual dysfunction in patients with BD varies widely depending on the study population and the definition of SD used. Some studies have reported that up to 70% of male patients with BD experience some form of SD, while others have reported a lower prevalence of around 30% without differences among two sexes. Compared with the control group, female BD patients had more complications in terms of satisfaction, avoidance, vaginismus, and orgasm fields, while men for impotence, premature ejaculation, and satisfaction [34].

The causes of sexual dysfunction in patients with BD are not well understood and are likely multifactorial. Some potential causes include inflammation, mucocutaneous involvement, and scarring of the genital tissue, damage to the vascular and nervous systems, hormonal imbalances, and the high frequency of psychiatric involvement and psychological factors such as depression and anxiety [35]. Additionally, the medications used to treat BD such as glucocorticoids and other treatments can also contribute to SD, as many of them have side effects that can impact sexual function.

Male patients with BD reported high levels of erectile dysfunction, and it seems more frequently associated with alteration of the psychological status. Female SD is also common in the cohorts studied and significantly associated with depression rather than to active organic manifestations, such as genital ulcers. Therefore, overall, both genders of BD patients are affected by SD and equally experienced a significant correlation between SD and depression [36].

Erectile dysfunction is the most common form of SD present in up to 55% of male patients with BD which was not statistical different from the healthy control group [35]. It is thought to be caused by both physical and psychological factors, including damage to the vascular and nervous systems, depression, and anxiety. Treatment options for erectile dysfunction in BD include PD5-I, vacuum devices, and penile injections.

Dyspareunia is a common problem in female patients with BD. It is thought to be caused by inflammation and scarring of the vaginal tissue, which can make intercourse painful. Treatment options for dyspareunia in BD include topical estrogen therapy, local anesthetics, and cognitive-behavioral therapy.

Decreased libido is another common problem seen in both male and female patients with BD. It is thought to be caused by a combination of physical and psychological factors, including hormonal imbalances, medication side effects, and depression. Treatment options for decreased libido in BD include hormone replacement therapy, psychotherapy, and antidepressant medications.

Orgasmic dysfunction is a less common form of SD seen in patients with BD. It is thought to be caused by damage to the nervous system and psychological factors such as anxiety and depression. Treatment options for orgasmic dysfunction in BD include psychotherapy and conventional medication.

11   Conclusion

It is important for healthcare providers to recognize the impact of autoimmune and rheumatic diseases on patients' sexual health and to address these concerns proactively. This requires a comprehensive approach that includes a thorough assessment of sexual function, identification of contributing factors, and appropriate management strategies. Addressing sexual health concerns can improve patients' overall quality of life, satisfaction with care, and health outcomes. Collaboration with other healthcare providers, such as sex therapists and physical therapists, may also be necessary to develop a comprehensive approach to addressing sexual dysfunction in these patients.

References

1. Parish SJ, Cottler-Casanova S, Clayton AH. The evolution of the female sexual disorder/dysfunction definitions, nomenclature, and classifications: a review of DSM, ICSM, ISSWSH, and ICD. Sex Med Rev. 2021;9:36–56.
2. Minopoulou M, Pyrgidis N, Tishkov M, Sokolakis I, Banoitopoulos P, Kefas A, Doumas M, Hatzichristodoulou G, Dimitroulas T. Sexual dysfunction in women with systemic autoimmune rheumatic disorders: a systematic review and meta-analysis. Rheumatology. 2023;62:1021–30.
3. Campos-Guzmán J, Valdez-López M, Govea-Peláez S, Aguirre-Aguilar E, Perez-Garcia LF, van Mulligen E, et al. Determinants of sexual function in male patients with systemic lupus erythematosus. Lupus. 2022;31:1211–7.
4. Østensen M. Sexual and reproductive health in rheumatic disease. Nat Rev Rheumatol. 2017;13:485–93.
5. Tristano AG. The impact of rheumatic diseases on sexual function. Rheumatol Int. 2009;29:853–60.
6. Nahata L, Ziniel SI, Garvey KC, Yu RN, Cohen LE. Fertility and sexual function: a gap in training in pediatric endocrinology. J Pediatr Endocrinol Metab. 2017;30:3–10.
7. Baniotopoulos P, Pyrgidis N, Minopoulou I, Tishukov M, Sokolakis I, Hatzichristodoulou G, Dimitroulas Y. Treatment of sexual dysfunction in women with systemic autoimmune rheumatic disorders: a systematic review. Sex Med Rev. 2022;10:520–8.
8. Bair MJ, Krebs EE. Fibromyalgia. Ann Intern Med. 2020;172:ITC33–48.
9. Mutti GW, de Quadros M, Cremonez LP, Spricigo D, Skare T, Nisihara R. Fibromyalgia and sexual performance: a cross-sectional study in 726 Brazilian patients. Rheumatol Int. 2021;41:1471–7.
10. Van Overmeire R, Vesentini L, Vanclooster S, Muysewinkel E, Bilsen J. Sexual desire, depressive symptoms and medication use among women with fibromyalgia in flanders. Sex Med. 2022;10:100457.
11. Saad RB, Fazaa A, Rouached L, Miladi S, Ouenniche K, Souabni L, Kassab S, Chekili S, Abdelghani KB, Laatar A. Sexual dysfunction and its determinants in women with rheumatoid arthritis. Z Rheumatol. 2021;80:373–8.

12. Santos-Moreno P, Castro CA, Villarreal L, Buitrago D. Prevalence of sexual disorders in patients with rheumatoid arthritis and associated factors. Sex Med. 2020;8:510–6.
13. Gossec L, Solano C, Paternotte S, Beauvais C, Gaudin P, von Krause G, Sordet C, Perdriger A. Elaboration and validation of a questionnaire (Qualisex) to assess the impact of rheumatoid arthritis on sexuality with patient involvement. Clin Exp Rheumatol. 2012;30:505–13.
14. Wilton KM, Achenbach SJ, Davis JM 3rd, Myasoedova E, Matteson EL, Crowson CS. Erectile dysfunction and cardiovascular risk in men with rheumatoid arthritis: a population-based cohort study. J Rheumatol. 2021;48:1641–7.
15. Molto A, Gossec L, Meghnathi B, Landewé RBM, van der Heijde D, Atagunduz P, Elzorkany BK, Akkoc N, Kiltz U, Gu J, Wei JCC, Dougados M, ASAS-FLARE study group. An assessment in SpondyloArthritis international society (ASAS)-endorsed definition of clinically important worsening in axial spondyloarthritis based on ASDAS. Ann Rheum Dis. 2018;77:124–7.
16. Gözüküçük M, Türkyilmaz E, Küçükşahin O, Erten Ş, Üstün Y, Yavuz AF. Effects of ankylosing spondylitis and non-radiographic axial spondyloarthropathy on female sexual functions. Clin Exp Rheumatol. 2022;40:967–74.
17. Martini A, Lovell DJ, Albani S, Brunner HI, Hyrich KL, Thompson SD, Ruperto N. Juvenile idiopathic arthritis. Nat Rev Dis Primers. 2022;8:5.
18. de Avila Lima Souza L, Gallinaro AL, Abdo CH, Kowalski SC, Suehiro RM, da Silva CA, Goldenstein-Schainberg C. Effect of musculoskeletal pain on sexuality of male adolescents and adults with juvenile idiopathic arthritis. J Rheumatol. 2009;36:1337–42.
19. Trieste L, Cannizzo S, Palla I, Triulzi I, Turchetti G. State of the art and future directions in assessing the quality of life in rare and complex connective tissue and musculoskeletal diseases. Front Med (Lausanne). 2022;9:986218.
20. García Morales M, Callejas Rubio JI, Peralta-Ramírez MI, Henares Romero LJ, Ríos Fernández R, et al. Impaired sexual function in women with systemic lupus erythematosus: a cross-sectional study. Lupus. 2013;22:987–95.
21. Moghadam ZB, Rezaei E, Faezi ST, Zareian A, Ibrahim FM, Ibrahim MM. Prevalence of sexual dysfunction in women with systemic lupus erythematosus and its related factors. Reumatologia. 2019;57:19–26.
22. Jin Z, Yang C, Xiao C, Wang Z, Zhang S, Ren J. Systemic lupus erythematosus and risk of sexual dysfunction: a systematic review and meta-analysis. Lupus. 2021;30:238–47.
23. Liu M, Dou J, Wang Q. The effect of systemic lupus erythematosus on sexual function in women: an updated meta-analysis based on cross-sectional studies. Adv Rheumatol. 2022;62:24.
24. Zhang L, Wu B, Ye J. Fatigue have impact on the sexual problems in Chinese females with systemic lupus erythematosus. BMC Womens Health. 2022;22:266.
25. Salonia A, Bettocchi C, Boeri L, Capogrosso P, Carvalho J, Cilesiz NC, et al. EAU working group on male sexual and reproductive health. European Association of Urology guidelines on sexual and reproductive Health-2021 update: male sexual dysfunction. Eur Urol. 2021;80:333–57.
26. van Nimwegen JF, Arends S, van Zuiden GS, Vissink A, Kroese FG, Bootsma H. The impact of primary Sjögren's syndrome on female sexual function. Rheumatology (Oxford). 2015;54:1286–93.
27. Al-Ezzi M, Tappuni AR, Khan KS. The impact of Sjögren's syndrome on the quality of sexual life of female patients in the UK: a controlled analysis. Rheumatol Int. 2022;42:1423–9.
28. Gözüküçük M, Türkyilmaz E, Küçükşahin O, Erten Ş, Üstün Y, Yavuz AF. Effects of primary Sjögren's syndrome on female genitalia and sexual functions. Clin Exp Rheumatol. 2021;39 Suppl 133(6):66–72.
29. Sarmento ACA, Kamilos MF, Costa APF, Vieira-Baptista P, Eleutério J Jr, Gonçalves AK. Use of moisturizers and lubricants for vulvovaginal atrophy. Front Reprod Health. 2021;3:781353.
30. Keck AD, Foocharoen C, Rosato E, Smith V, Allanore Y, Distler O, et al. Nailfold capillary abnormalities in erectile dysfunction of systemic sclerosis: a EUSTAR group analysis. Rheumatology (Oxford). 2014;53:639–43.

31. Gao R, Qing P, Sun X, Zeng X, Hu X, Zhang S, Yang Y, Qin L. Prevalence of sexual dysfunction in people with systemic sclerosis and the associated risk factors: a systematic review. Sex Med. 2021;9:100392.
32. de Souza FHC, de Araujo DB, Silva CA, Miossi R, Najjar Abdo CH, Bonfa E, Shinjo SK. Analysis of sexual function of patients with dermatomyositis and polymyositis through self-administered questionnaires: a cross-sectional study. Rev Bras Reumatol Engl Ed. 2017;57:134–40.
33. Hermankova B, Spiritovic M, Oreska S, Storkanova H, Vencovsky HMJ, Klein MKM, Pavelka K, Senolt L, Tomcık M. Sexual function in patients with idiopathic inflammatory myopathies: a cross-sectional study. Rheumatology. 2021;60:5060–72.
34. Talarico R, Elefante E, Parma A, Taponeco F, Simoncini T, Mosca M. Sexual dysfunction in Behçet's syndrome. Rheumatol Int. 2020;40:9–15.
35. Saur SJ, Schlögl A, Schmalen T, Krittian S, Pecher AC, Henes M, Xenitidis T, Henes J. Sexual dysfunction and depression in Behçet's disease in comparison to healthy controls. Rheumatol Int. 2022;42:121–6.
36. Talarico R, Palagini L, Elefante E, Ferro F, Tani C, Gemignani A, Bombardieri S, Mosca M. Behçet's syndrome and psychiatric involvement: is it a primary or secondary feature of the disease? Clin Exp Rheumatol. 2018;36(6 Suppl 115):125–8.

Chronic Respiratory Diseases and Sexual Function

Ana M. Ramirez and Isabel Blanco

1   Introduction

Sexuality accompanies us throughout our entire lives and is an integral part of human expression. It is also a central aspect of a person's quality of life and reflects their level of social, psychological, and physical well-being. Additionally, individual variations of sexuality further contribute to its complexity. Sexual health is a state of physical, emotional, mental, and social well-being related to sexuality; it is not merely the absence of disease, dysfunction, or discomfort. Sexual health requires a positive and respectful approach to sexuality and sexual relationships, as well as the possibility of obtaining pleasure and safe sexual experiences, free from coercion, discrimination, and violence. In order to achieve and maintain sexual health, the sexual rights of all individuals must be respected, protected, and fulfilled [1]. Sexuality will be experienced differently at each stage of life, and it does not always have to be centered on sexual intercourse and/or partnership.

Sexual activity is associated with levels of health [2]; thus, a positive relationship exists between health and good sexual quality of life, frequency, and interest in sex [3]. The full development of sexuality depends on the satisfaction of basic human needs such as the desire for contact, emotional intimacy, pleasure, and, in addition, through sexuality, we satisfy biological, communicative, affective, social, and cultural needs [4].

The problems related to sexual health have to do with sexual orientation and gender identity, relationships, and pleasure although they also include disorders or dysfunctions such as those that have to do with desire (inhibition or decrease of

A. M. Ramirez · I. Blanco (✉)
Pulmonary Hypertension Unit, Hospital Clínic de Barcelona, Barcelona, Spain

Institut d'Investigacions Biomèdiques August Pi i Sunyer, Barcelona, Spain
e-mail: aramirez@clinic.cat; iblanco2@clinic.cat

C. Castelo-Branco, S. Anglès Acedo (eds.), *Medical Disorders and Sexual Health*, Trends in Andrology and Sexual Medicine,
https://doi.org/10.1007/978-3-031-55080-5_20

desire), the sexual aversion, sexually transmitted infections and their adverse consequences, unwanted pregnancy and abortion, sexual violence, harmful practices (including female genital mutilation), also the dysfunctions of each sex such as vaginismus, dyspareunia, or lack of lubrication in women or erectile dysfunction or premature ejaculation in men [5–7].

There are multiple factors that can cause sexual health problems in patients with chronic respiratory diseases. In general, we can talk about aging with its physical and hormonal changes, the onset of diseases and/or comorbidities associated with them, mental or emotional disorders, and some medications for certain conditions. In respiratory diseases, the symptoms of these diseases such as dyspnea, coughing, and fatigue are connected to sexual dysfunction. Moreover, the use of devices to improve health status such as the use of oxygen therapy in patients with resting or exertional hypoxemia, which is also recommended during sexual intercourse, can negatively impact body image and influence sexual health. Non-invasive mechanical ventilation such as CPAP (continuous positive airway pressure) or BiPAP (Bipressure airway positive) in patients with obstructive sleep apnea syndrome (OSA) or those with neuromuscular or thoracic cage problems, or infusion devices for medication delivery through permanently catheters in patients with pulmonary arterial hypertension (PAH) are evident examples of hoe technology origins disruption of sexual function [8–10]. (Fig. 1).

Some male patients may consult their doctor for impaired sexual function, mainly for erectile dysfunction (ED); its onset can be a "sentinel symptom," an early

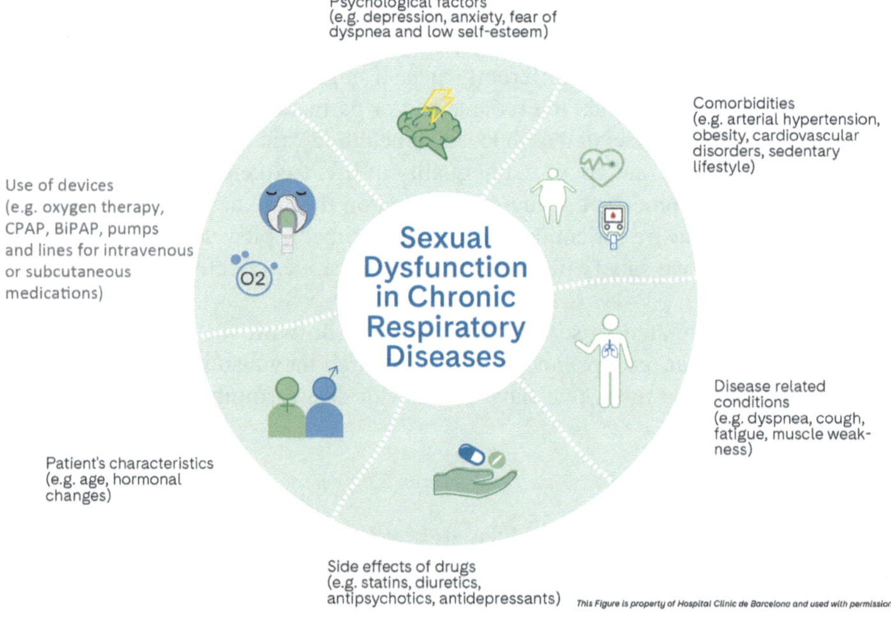

Fig. 1 Sexual dysfunction in chronic respiratory diseases

predictor of cardiovascular events, respiratory and other various chronic diseases, and various chronic diseases such as arterial hypertension or diabetes [11–13], which in women could manifest as a lack of vaginal lubrication, pain during sexual intercourse, and the inability to reach orgasm [14].

In women, hormonal changes due to age and the symptoms caused during menopause negatively impact the quality of sleep, causing sleep disorders. Additionally, sexual function and satisfaction can be affected during this period. Data from the Study of Women's Health Across the Nation demonstrates agreement with the symptomatic triangle of menopause, which includes sleep disorders, depressive state, and sexual problems, concluding that fewer hours of sleep lead to more symptoms related to sexual problems [15].

On the other hand, drugs such as statins and fibrates, used for high blood pressure, can cause decreased libido and erectile dysfunction, and interfere with ejaculation in men; in women, they can cause vaginal dryness and difficulty reaching orgasm in both sexes. Some diuretics can make sexual arousal more difficult, and antidepressants can cause problems in all areas of sexual function. All antipsychotics block dopamine and increase levels of the hormone prolactin, which can cause erectile dysfunction, decreased libido, and difficulties in reaching orgasm; antidepressants block the action of acetylcholine and could cause problems in all areas of sexual function, and benzodiazepines can decrease sexual interest and arousal in both men and women, which can also lead to underlying problems such as pain during sexual intercourse, erectile dysfunction, and ejaculation problems. Some studies have shown that these medications can lower testosterone levels, which can reduce sexual desire and interfere with arousal (erectile dysfunction in men and lubrication problems in women) and may affect the ability to reach orgasm. Some studies on sleep apnea in women did not link the severity of sleep apnea with different sexual problems, but they did associate sexual health problems with the use of psychotropic drugs [15]. Mental disorders, such as depression or emotional disorders such as anxiety, distress, or anticipatory fear of exertional dyspnea are also associated with sexual health problems, which can cause sexual dissatisfaction or decreased sexual appetite [16].

2 Chronic Obstructive Diseases

Patients with chronic diseases also experience limitations in sexual health that impact their quality of life [5–7, 11] and may reflect their physical, psychological, and social well-being. Different studies confirm sexual dysfunction in different spheres of patients with respiratory disease [12, 13], which may lead to decrease sexual interest, sexual function, and testosterone levels, and this may have consequences on the rhythm, frequency, and position of sexual practice [10]. The physical requirements of sexual activity could cause an exacerbation of the underlying respiratory disease although for some authors only sexual arousal is sufficient to trigger or worsen previous suffering. It has been described that sexual intercourse can trigger a severe exacerbation that requires emergency care, hospitalization, or even assisted ventilation. In addition, anticipation of dyspnea can affect patients' behavior of, as they frequently self-limit physical activity to avoid exacerbations [5, 17]. In general, sexual dysfunction occurs more frequently in patients with respiratory diseases than in healthy population, such as those with asthma [11, 12].

Regarding the common symptoms of respiratory diseases: dyspnea is a distressing and debilitating symptom present in all respiratory diseases, with functional consequences including activity limitation and reduced exercise tolerance [7]; exertional dyspnea is often one of the earliest and most disabling problems for patients with lung or heart disease seeking medical attention, and it also tends to worsen as the disease progresses, thus it is a symptom that should be recorded and evaluated [16, 17]. In addition, the anticipation of dyspnea itself can have a significant effect on patients' emotions and behavior, as patients often self-limit physical activity to avoid what has become the hallmark symptom of chronic obstructive pulmonary disease (COPD) [7]. Other symptoms such as cough, muscle weakness, fear of dyspnea, or difficulty breathing also force patients to avoid physical activity, which has negative consequences for their health, such as loss of muscle mass and quality of life [5, 18].

Experiencing dyspnea, cough, dry mouth, feeling of irritability, and concern about the onset of symptoms before or during sexual activity, as well as depression or anxiety, may trigger a loss of libido. This, in turn, can lead to feelings of shame, lower self-esteem, and depression in many patients [5, 7, 19, 20], as well as difficulties with sexual interest or activity.

The symptoms that characterize COPD, such as exertional dyspnea and fatigue, have a negative impact on the quality of life (QoL) of patients and restrict physical activity in daily life [21]. In addition, the majority of male patients suffer from erectile dysfunction (ED), causing a negative impact on sexual relations. It seems that sexuality deteriorates as COPD worsens, but this is an aspect that has been poorly investigated [20, 22, 23]. Both male and female asthmatic individuals present significant sexual dysfunction, which has a multifactorial origin involving several parameters such as symptom severity, the presence of asthma-related comorbidities like rhinitis, or some psychological problems or dysfunctions [24]. In patients with bronchiectasis, persistent cough can be an unpleasant symptom that can affect their sexual life [24]. In those who suffer from obstructive sleep apnea (OSA), particularly those with intermittent nocturnal hypoxemia, it is associated with erectile dysfunction (ED) in males, while in females, OSA appears to be associated with the use of psychotropic drugs, which can influence their sexual life. People with pulmonary arterial hypertension (PAH) experience fatigue, shortness of breath, palpitations, and chest pain that even limit their daily activities. PAH is a chronic and debilitating disease with a higher prevalence rate in women than in men, and it occurs at an early age. Despite it has been observed that it can also impact sexual health, sexuality is not extensively studied in relation to PAH [5–9]. Furthermore, in other diseases such as cystic fibrosis, sexuality has always been studied in relation to reproductive life [25].

Consulting the literature related to the topic, we have found that the information on the impact of respiratory symptoms on sexual activity is scarce, and in general, published studies focus primary on the male population, often underestimating women's dissatisfaction [24, 26]. Some research conducted on patients with COPD, dissatisfied with their sexual life indicates that they have used specific medications to improve sexual performance and short-acting bronchodilators before sexual activity. Others mentioned having to adapt to compensate for the decrease in their tolerance for physical activity. Some patients stated that sexual dysfunction had never been discussed by their physicians (general practitioners or pulmonologists). Despite the high incidence of sexual dissatisfaction among COPD patients, only 6% reported having discussed sexuality with a specialist [7]. Others expressed a desire for specialized consultation with a sexologist, and a few were open to virtual consultations.

In patients with OSA, the sensation of dyspnea is also frequent, and body image is also influenced in sexual activity. However, its potential impact on sexual function has not been well analyzed. In some studies, evaluating sexual function in men with OSA, worse scores were observed in the questionnaire assessing erectile and orgasmic function, as well as higher sexual distress compared to the control group [27–29]. Long-term continuous positive airway pressure (CPAP) treatment in male patients with OSA and nocturnal hypoxemia may improve sexual function related to erectile dysfunction, suggesting a certain degree of reversibility [30, 31]. In women with untreated OSA, sexual function was not affected by the syndrome itself but rather by the presence of psychotropic drugs used for other conditions, which may act as predisposing factors for sexual dysfunction [32, 33].

3   Cystic Fibrosis

The life expectancy of patients with cystic fibrosis (CF) is continuously increasing, thanks to advancements in treatments. However, women with CF still face several unaddressed health concerns. These understudied issues leave women with numerous unanswered questions regarding the management of their sexual and reproductive health. As individuals with CF live longer and experience improved quality of life, there is a growing awareness of the importance of addressing these aspects of care. Multiple studies are currently underway to shed light on these issues that have been relatively neglected in research thus far [34–37], generally the results of some studies conclude that CF patients do not have adequate information for the decision-making process related to sexual and reproductive choices.

4   Pulmonary Hypertension

Pulmonary arterial hypertension (PAH) is a chronic disease characterized by elevated pulmonary artery pressure that causes shortness of breath, fatigue, and decreased functional capacity with progressive limitations in physical activity and quality of life related to health (HRQoL). Deficits in HRQoL may extend beyond the traditional domains of physical activity, psychological health, and emotional well-being to sexual health and function. Sexual health includes a sense of self-esteem, attractiveness and personal competence, and absence of sexual dysfunction [9], and although it is an important dimension of quality of life, little is known about sexual health and quality of life related to sexual health (Sexual HRQoL) in PAH. The impact of PAH on Sexual HRQoL is not well understood, and Sexual HRQoL has not been studied, nor has the impact of PAH therapies on sexual health and intimacy been studied.

After the diagnosis of PAH, individuals may experience a decrease in the frequency of sexual intercourse. They may also develop fear of engaging in sexual activities due to cardiopulmonary symptoms. Participants in studies have reported implementing compensatory strategies or behaviors during and around sexual encounters. For instance, they mentioned changing positions during sexual intercourse to alleviate breathing difficulties. Some participants even mentioned removing their oxygen supply to avoid interrupting intimacy. Complex medical treatments for PAH can sometimes involve continuous and home-based parenteral therapies, which may contribute to symptoms of anxiety and depression [7, 8, 38, 39]. However, some studies have indicated that patients with PAH may face unrecognized challenges in this regard, particularly in relation to parenteral prostacyclin therapies. Concerns related to catheter dislodgement, treatment discontinuation, and pump displacement can arise for both the patient and their sexual partner. Some participants using subcutaneous prostanoids might even discontinue treatment during sexual activity. Additionally, patients may experience feelings of guilt regarding the impact of their disease on their sexual partners and relationships. Low self-esteem due to changes in body image related to the use of a pump, oxygen tube, or weight gain may also be present. However, these findings are inconclusive, and further research is needed to expand our understanding in this field [40, 41].

5   SARS-CoV2 Infection

In relation to the recent Sars-Cov2 pandemic, the literature suggests that the period of confinement would have affected sexual activity and sexual desire throughout the world, possibly due to higher levels of stress, movement restrictions in confinement conditions and changes in the quality of relationships, and in patients with Sars-Cov2 infection, several studies confirm multiple complications after infection, including men's sexual health, which is caused by both physical and psychological factors. However, studies focusing on long-term effects among recovered patients are still lacking although a high prevalence of ED and the diagnosis of major depression have been shown during acute infection [42, 43].

Studies have shown that during the pandemic and in the period of confinement, women suffered more anxiety and depression and a greater risk of difficulties in sexual functioning and sexual dissatisfaction than men, in addition to greater reduced sexual activity. Other studies that reviewed sexual activity in women who were hospitalized for covid concluded that the frequency of sexual contact and female sexual satisfaction decreased after being infected with COVID-19 [44, 45].

6   Barriers

There are difficulties for studying sexuality in respiratory patients. Firstly, detecting sexual dysfunction (SD) through health-related quality of life questionnaires could be interesting to explore more specific aspects if potential sexual dysfunction is detected. This includes problems that arise in any phase of the human sexual response (desire, arousal, orgasm) that hinder or impair the development of a satisfactory sexuality. However, most health-related quality of life questionnaires do not generally include aspects of sexuality. For example, the SF-36 questionnaire is a generic health status profile applicable to both patients and the general population. It is one of the most commonly used generic instruments in descriptive studies measuring the impact on health-related quality of life in patients and for evaluating therapeutic interventions. However, the SF-36 does not encompass certain health concepts such as sleep disorders, cognitive function, family function, or sexual function.

On the other hand, there is limited use of standardized measurement instruments to assess sexual function, and these instruments focus on very specific aspects of sexuality. Additionally, there are no specific questionnaires for respiratory patients. Health-related quality of life questionnaires do not assess sexual function, and it seems interesting to include the assessment of sexuality as part of routine activity within both generic and specific health-related quality of life questionnaires. Most specific questionnaires for measuring sexual health are often limited to a single gender, a specific gender with a partner, or a suspected specific sexual dysfunction [46]. For all these reasons, we report a list of questionnaires where sexual health is evaluated (Table 1).

Table 1 Instruments to measure or assess sexual function

Instrument	Areas assessed	Population	Attributes
Questionnaire	Object of study	Characteristics	Items and time to response
Female Sexual Function Index **(FSFI)**	Women's sexual functioning: Desire, arousal, lubrication, orgasm, satisfaction	Sexually active women	19 items Response time 15 min
Brief Index of Sexual Functioning for Women **(BISF-W)**	Dimensions of sexual functioning: Thoughts/desires, arousal, frequency of sexual activity, receptivity/initiation, pleasure/orgasm, relationship satisfaction, problems affecting sexual function	Women	22 items; self-report Most items rated on Likert scale Response time 15–20 min
Elements of Desire Questionnaire **(EDQ)**	Intensity of sexual desire, thoughts/fantasies about sex, and receptiveness to sexual requests	Women	Nine items PRO Questionnaire
Sexual health and female sexual dysfunctions **(SyDSF-AP)**	Female sexual function and its correlation with the life cycle, socio-family situation and state of health	Women	21 items
Women's sexual function evaluation questionnaire **(FSM)**	Sexual activity Questions that help to know issues such as the frequency of sexual activity, the existence of a partner or Sexual Dysfunction in the respondent or their partner	Women with sexual activity with a partner o no, any age and sexual orientation	Self-administered scale 14 items that are answered using the Likert scale An opening question of the questionnaire
Female Sexual Dysfunction Scale-Revised **(FSDS-R)**		Women who suffering from hypoactive sexual desire disorder	13 items
Female Sexual Distress Scale-Desire/Arousal/Orgasm **(SDS-DAO)**		Women	13 items Likert scale Includes two new items that ask women to rate their level of distress related to arousal and orgasm
Female Sexual Encounter Profile-Revised **(FSEP-R)**	To assess sexual encounters, including initiation, level of desire, satisfaction with arousal, lubrication, arousal, ability to achieve orgasm, and satisfaction with the sexual encounter	Female	Ten items

(continued)

Table 1 (continued)

Instrument	Areas assessed	Population	Attributes
Questionnaire	Object of study	Characteristics	Items and time to response
Suspected erectile dysfunction (**SQUED**)	Evaluates the fundamental concepts of the definition of ED: ability to achieve an erection, ability to maintain it and satisfaction with the sexual relationship	Men over the age of 18 with suspected erectile dysfunction	
Brief Male Sexual Function Inventory (**BMSFI**)	Four functional domains: drive, erection, ejaculation, problem with sexual function; and sexual satisfaction	Men	Ten items
Index of Erectile Function (**ILEF**) Or abbreviated version (**ILEF-5**)	Función eréctil, orgasmo, deseo sexual, satisfacción con el acto sexual y satisfacción sexual general	Men	15 items Short versión five items
Changes in Sexual Functioning Questionnaire (**CSFQ**) and Changes in Sexual Functioning-Short Form (**CSFQ-SF**)	Sexual function in all domains of the sexual response cycle Subscales: Dimensions of pleasure, desire/frequency, desire/interest, arousal/excitement, orgasm/completion, and phases of sexual functioning (desire, arousal, orgasm)	Women and men	CSFQ: females, 35 items; males, 36 items CSFQ-SF: 14 items for each of the female and male versions5-Point Likert scale, from "never or no enjoyment" to "every day or always" may be scored on the three phases of sexual response: Desire, arousal, orgasm/completion Response time for CSFQ, 15–20 min; CSFQ-SF appropriate for clinical setting, with response time of 4–5 min
Massachusetts General Hospital Sexual Functioning (**MGHSFQ**)	Sexual interest, ability to be aroused, ability to achieve orgasm, ability to achieve and maintain an erection, and overall sexual satisfaction	Women and men	Five items

(continued)

Table 1 (continued)

Instrument	Areas assessed	Population	Attributes
Questionnaire	Object of study	Characteristics	Items and time to response
Derogatis Interview for Sexual Functioning (**DISF**) and Derogatis Interview for Sexual Functioning—Self-Report (**DISF-SR**)	Patient's perception of overall current sexual functioning five domains: Sexual cognition/fantasy, sexual arousal, sexual behavior/experience, orgasm, sexual drive/relationship	Women and men	26 items Composite score Gender-specific versions Likert scale Time 15–20 min
Arizona Sexual Experience Scale (**ASEX**)	Sexual function Sexual drive, arousal, vaginal lubrication/penile erection, ability to reach orgasm, satisfaction with orgasm	Women and Men	Five items, male and female
Golombok Rust Inventory of Sexual Satisfaction (**GRISS**)	Adult population	Women and men. In adults	31 items Only one dimension: sexual satisfaction
Multidimensional Body Self Relations Questionnaire (**MBSRQ**)		Women and men	Inventory of 45 items that evaluates the aspects of attitude
(Index of Sexual Satisfaction of Hudson, Harrison and Crosscup en 1981) (**ISS**)	Degree of sexual satisfaction with the partner within a relationship	Women and men with partner	Composed of 25 items Likert-type scale from 1 (never) to 5 (always)
Quality-of-Life for Respiratory Illness Questionnaire (**QoL-RIQ Q**)	Evaluation of the quality of life in the respiratory patient	Respiratory patient	

7 Practical Recommendations

In conclusion, based on the information provided, we believe that patients and/or their partners should be provided with information on ways to improve their overall physical functioning. It is crucial to discuss the numerous pharmacological and non-pharmacological methods available to maintain a healthy sexual life, as it is fundamental for maintaining quality of life. General recommendations and lifestyle habits regarding sexual health should be offered during pulmonology consultations. This includes discussing the appropriate timing for sexual activity, suggesting optimal positions, and providing measures that can enhance well-being. Additionally, studies should be conducted to evaluate sexual health as an integral aspect of a patient's life, as it is necessary for maintaining good quality of life in all dimensions.

8   Conclusions

In general, male sexual health problems are often associated with physical symptoms such as erectile dysfunction and premature ejaculation, while studies in women provide data on symptomatology that disrupts sexual health and is related to emotional or psychological issues. Furthermore, the approach to sexual health often focuses on reproductive health in certain conditions affecting young women. However, there are many other factors that can affect women's sexual well-being throughout their lives, such as female orgasmic disorder, female sexual arousal/interest disorder, and genito-pelvic pain/penetration disorder. These conditions have a negative impact on quality of life but are often under-evaluated. Additionally, there are limitations in the studies conducted to date, such as the frequent grouping of multiple types of sexual dysfunctions in randomized clinical trials. Further research is needed to advance the development of treatments for female sexual dysfunctions and to promote female sexual health.

In conclusion, sexual health is not routinely addressed during follow-up visits and remains a poorly studied aspect in patients with chronic respiratory diseases. The study of sexual health is often associated with the evaluation of interventions aimed at improving a specific health condition. This could be attributed to the lack of confidence or specialized training among healthcare professionals, the discomfort of doctors, patients, and their families in discussing these topics, and patients' reluctance to share intimate details about their relationships and sexual lives. Cultural sensitivities also contribute to the fact that sexual activity is still considered a taboo subject and is not adequately addressed.

References

1. La salud sexual y su relación con la salud reproductiva: un enfoque operativo.
2. Waite LJ, Laumann EO, Das A, Schumm LP. Sexuality: measures of partnerships, practices, attitudes, and problems in the National Social Life, Health, and Aging Study. J Gerontol B Psychol Sci Soc Sci. 2009;64 Suppl 1(Suppl 1):i56–66. https://doi.org/10.1093/geronb/gbp038. Epub 2009 Jun 4.
3. Lindau ST, Tang H, Gomero A, Vable A, Huang ES, Drum ML, Qato DM, Chin MH. Sexuality among middle-aged and older adults with diagnosed and undiagnosed diabetes: a national, population-based study. Diabetes Care. 2010;33(10):2202–10. https://doi.org/10.2337/dc10-0524. Epub 2010 Aug 27.
4. Arrington R, Cofrancesco J, Wu AW. Questionnaires to measure sexual quality of life. Qual Life Res. 2004;13(10):1643–58. https://doi.org/10.1007/s11136-004-7625-z.
5. Dubé B-P, Vermeulen F, Laveneziana P. Exertional Dyspnoea in chronic respiratory diseases: from physiology to clinical application. Arch Bronconeumol (English Edition). 2017;53(2):62–70.
6. Zaneva M, Philpott A, Singh A, Larsson G, Gonsalves L. What is the added value of incorporating pleasure in sexual health interventions? A systematic review and meta-analysis. PLoS One. 2022;17(2):e0261034. https://doi.org/10.1371/journal.pone.0261034.
7. Zysman M, Rubenstein J, Le Guillou F, Colson RMH, Pochulu C, Grassion L, Escamilla R, Piperno D, Pon J, Khan S, Raherison-Semjen C. COPD burden on sexual well-being. Respir Res. 2020;21(1):311. https://doi.org/10.1186/s12931-020-01572-0.

8. Salonia A, Capogrosso P, Clementi MC, Castagna G, Damiano R, Montorsi F. Is erectile dysfunction a reliable indicator of general health status in men? Arab J Urol. 2013;11(3):203–11. https://doi.org/10.1016/j.aju.2013.07.008. Epub 2013 Sep 14

9. Schönhofer B. Sexualität bei Patienten mit beeinträchtigter Atmung [Sexuality in patients with restricted breathing]. Med Klin (Munich). 2002;97(6):344–9. https://doi.org/10.1007/s00063-002-1163-7.

10. Fletcher EC, Martín RJ. Disfunción sexual e impotencia eréctil en la enfermedad pulmonar obstructiva crónica. Cofre. 1982;81:413.

11. Goodell TT. Sexuality in chronic lung disease. Nurs Clin North Am. 2007;42(4):631–8; viii. https://doi.org/10.1016/j.cnur.2007.08.003.

12. Panel de desarrollo de consenso de los NIH sobre la impotencia. Impotencia. JAMA. 1993;270:83–90.

13. Theander K, Hasselgren M, Luhr K, Eckerblad J, Unosson M, Karlsson I. Symptoms and impact of symptoms on function and health in patients with chronic obstructive pulmonary disease and chronic heart failure in primary health care. Int J Chron Obstruct Pulmon Dis. 2014;9:785–94. https://doi.org/10.2147/COPD.S62563.

14. Winkley K, Kristensen C, Fosbury J. Sexual health and function in women with diabetes. Diabet Med. 2021;38(11):e14644. https://doi.org/10.1111/dme.14644. Epub 2021 Aug 1.

15. Janssen I, Powell LH, Crawford S, Lasley B, Sutton-Tyrrell K. Menopause and the metabolic syndrome: the study of women's health across the nation. Arch Intern Med. 2008;168(14):1568–75. https://doi.org/10.1001/archinte.168.14.1568.

16. Jones PW, Watz H, Wouters EF, Cazzola M. COPD: the patient perspective. Int J Chron Obstruct Pulmon Dis. 2016;11 Spec Iss:13–20. https://doi.org/10.2147/COPD.S85977.

17. Dubé B-P, Vermeulen F, Laveneziana P. Exertional dyspnoea in chronic respiratory diseases: from physiology to clinical application. Arch Bronconeumol. 2017;53(2):62–70. https://doi.org/10.1016/j.arbres.2016.09.005.

18. Lauretti S, Cardaci V, Barrese F, Calzetta L. Chronic obstructive pulmonary disease (COPD) and erectile dysfunction (ED): results of the BRED observational study. Arch Italiano Urol Androl. 2016;88(3):165–70. https://doi.org/10.4081/aiua.2016.3.165.

19. Kupryś-Lipińska I, Kuna P. Impact of chronic obstructive pulmonary disease (COPD) on patient's life and his family. Pneumonol Alergol Pol. 2014;82(2):82–95. https://doi.org/10.5603/PiAP.2014.0014.

20. Farver-Vestergaard I, Frederiksen Y, Zachariae R, Rubio-Rask S, Løkke A. Sexual health in COPD: a systematic review and meta-analysis. Int J Chron Obstruct Pulmon Dis. 2022;17:297–315. https://doi.org/10.2147/COPD.S347578.

21. Decramer M, Janssens W. Enfermedad pulmonar obstructiva crónica y comorbilidades. Lanceta Respir Med. 2013;1(1):73–83.

22. Gunaydin Y, Kiliç Z, Zincir H, et al. The effect of dyspnea and fatigue on sexual life marital satisfaction in individuals with chronic obstructive pulmonary disease. Sex Disabil. 2022;40:153–65. https://doi.org/10.1007/s11195-022-09725-3.

23. Curgian LM, Gronkiewicz CA. Enhancing sexual performance in COPD. Nurse Pract. 1988;13(2):34–5, 38.

24. Dias M, Oliveira MJ, Oliveira P, Ladeira I, Lima R, Guimarães M. Does any association exist between chronic obstructive pulmonary disease and erectile dysfunction? The DECODED study. Rev Port Pneumol (2006). 2017;23(5):259–65. https://doi.org/10.1016/j.rppnen.2017.04.005. Epub 2017 Jun 16.

25. Frayman KB, Sawyer SM. Sexual and reproductive health in cystic fibrosis: a lifecourse perspective. Lancet Respir Med. 2015;3(1):70–86. https://doi.org/10.1016/S2213-2600(14)70231-0. Epub 2014 Dec 17.

26. Borgmann M, Linnemann T, Schönhofer B, Ott SR, Bernardy K, Stammberger U, Vedder V, Bals R, Köllner V, Hamacher J. Krankheitserleben, Partnerschaft und Sexualität bei Patienten mit COPD [Experience of disease, relationship and sexuality in patients with COPD]. Z Psychosom Med Psychother. 2019;65(3):257–71. https://doi.org/10.13109/zptm.2019.65.3.257.

27. Rubio-Rask SE, Farver-Vestergaard I, Hilberg O, Løkke A. Sexual health communication in COPD: the role, contents and design of patient information leaflets. Chron Respir Dis. 2021;18:14799731211020322. https://doi.org/10.1177/14799731211020322.

28. Campos JGS, Villegas JR, Galo AP, Malanda NM, Rivero JLG, Sierra CP, Salmones MG, Galán CC, Molina ES, Plaza V, Erquicia SP. Impacto del asma en la vida sexual de los pacientes. Un estudio de casos y controles. Arch Bronconeumol. 2017;53(12):667–74. https://doi.org/10.1016/j.arbres.2017.05.011.

29. Skoczyński S, Nowosielski K, Minarowski Ł, Brożek G, Oraczewska A, Glinka K, Ficek K, Kotulska B, Tobiczyk E, Skomro R, Mróz R, Barczyk A. May dyspnea sensation influence the sexual function in men with obstructive sleep apnea syndrome? A prospective control study. Sex Med. 2019;7(3):303–10. https://doi.org/10.1016/j.esxm.2019.06.005. Epub 2019 Jul 18.

30. Stannek T, Hürny C, Schoch OD, Bucher T, Münzer T. Factors affecting self-reported sexuality in men with obstructive sleep apnea syndrome. J Sex Med. 2009;6(12):3415–24. https://doi.org/10.1111/j.1743-6109.2009.01486.x. Epub 2009 Sep 14.

31. Mostafa RM, Kamel NM, Elsayed EM, Saad HM. Assessment of sexual functions in male patients with obstructive sleep apnea. Am J Otolaryngol. 2021;42(2):102899. https://doi.org/10.1016/j.amjoto.2020.102899. Epub 2021 Jan 5.

32. Kling JM, Manson JE, Naughton MJ, Temkit M, Sullivan SD, Gower EW, Hale L, Weitlauf JC, Nowakowski S, Crandall CJ. Association of sleep disturbance and sexual function in postmenopausal women. Menopause. 2017;24(6):604–12. https://doi.org/10.1097/GME.0000000000000824.

33. Petersen M, Kristensen E, Berg S, Giraldi A, Midgren B. Sexual function in female patients with obstructive sleep apnea. J Sex Med. 2011;8(9):2560–8. https://doi.org/10.1111/j.1743-6109.2011.02358.x. Epub 2011 Jun 23.

34. Sawyer SM, Tully MA, Colin AA. Salud reproductiva y sexual en hombres con fibrosis quística: un caso para la educación y capacitación de profesionales de la salud. J Salud del Adolescente. 2001;28(1):36–40. https://doi.org/10.1016/s1054-139x(00)00172-5.

35. Jain R, Kazmerski TM, Aitken ML, West N, Wilson A, Bozkanat KM, Montemayor K, von Berg K, Sjoberg J, Poranski M, Taylor-Cousar JL. Challenges faced by women with cystic fibrosis. Clin Chest Med. 2021;42(3):517–30. https://doi.org/10.1016/j.ccm.2021.04.010.

36. Norris E, Phillips S, Butler C, James K. Sex and relationships education for individuals with cystic fibrosis: a service-based approach. Sex Disabil. 2018;36(4):363–76. https://doi.org/10.1007/s11195-018-9535-y. Epub 2018 Oct 22.

37. Gage LA. What deficits in sexual and reproductive health knowledge exist among women with cystic fibrosis? A systematic review. Health Soc Work. 2012;37(1):29–36. https://doi.org/10.1093/hsw/hls003.

38. Banerjee D, Vargas SE, Guthrie KM, Wickham BM, Allahua M, Whittenhall ME, Palmisciano AJ, Ventetuolo CE. Sexual health and health-related quality of life among women with pulmonary arterial hypertension. Pulm Circ. 2018;8(4):2045894018788277. https://doi.org/10.1177/2045894018788277.

39. Yee DC, Banerjee D, Vargas SE, Allahua M, Whittenhall ME, Perry N, Ventetuolo CE, Guthrie KM. Sexual health-related quality of life in women with pulmonary arterial hypertension: compensating for loss. Ann Am Thorac Soc. 2022;19(7):1122–9. https://doi.org/10.1513/AnnalsATS.202106-692OC.

40. Cipolletta S, Ravasio G, Bussotti M. Sexual and reproductive health in women with pulmonary hypertension: a qualitative study. Arch Sex Behav. 2022;51(3):1647–57. https://doi.org/10.1007/s10508-022-02284-w. Epub 2022 Feb 14.

41. Al-Naamani N. Let's talk about sex: sexual health in pulmonary arterial hypertension. Ann Am Thorac Soc. 2022;19(7):1097–9. https://doi.org/10.1513/AnnalsATS.202204-322ED.

42. Tan PL. Changes in frequency and patterns of marital sexual activity during COVID-19: evidence from longitudinal data prior to, during and after lockdown in Singapore. J Sex Med. 2022;19(2):188–200. https://doi.org/10.1016/j.jsxm.2021.12.004. Epub 2021 Dec 13.

43. Harirugsakul K, Wainipitapong S, Phannajit J, Paitoonpong L, Tantiwongse K. Erectile dysfunction after COVID-19 recovery: a follow-up study. PLoS One. 2022;17(10):e0276429. https://doi.org/10.1371/journal.pone.0276429.
44. Hernández Figaredo P, García Gutiérrez L. Impact of the COVID-19 pandemic on human sexual activity. Rev Hum Med. 2022;22(1). Epub 06 Apr 2022.
45. Masoudi M, Maasoumi R, Bragazzi NL. Effects of the COVID-19 pandemic on sexual functioning and activity: a systematic review and meta-analysis. BMC Public Health. 2022;22(1):189. https://doi.org/10.1186/s12889-021-12390-4.
46. Gemma V, Montse F, Luis R, Pablo R, Gaietà P-M, Quintana JM, et al. El Cuestionario de Salud SF-36 español: una década de experiencia y nuevos desarrollos. Gac Sanit. 2005;19(2):135.

Sexual Health and Hypertension

Miquel Camafort, Felicia A. Hanzu, and Esteban Poch

1   Introduction

Sexual health and several reproductive disorders have been associated with hypertension and cardiovascular risk. Primary hypertension is considered a major public health problem since it affects more than 25% of the general population. Sexual dysfunction in hypertension has been focused on males and specifically on erectile

M. Camafort
Hypertension Unit, Department of Internal Medicine, Clinical Institute of Medicine and Dermatology, Hospital Clínic de Barcelona, Barcelona, Spain

Medicine Department, Faculty of Medicine and Health Sciences, Universitat de Barcelona (UB), Barcelona, Spain

F. A. Hanzu
Endocrinology and Nutrition Department, Clinical Institute of Digestive and Metabolic Diseases, Hospital Clínic de Barcelona, Barcelona, Spain

Medicine Department, Faculty of Medicine and Health Sciences, Universitat de Barcelona (UB), Barcelona, Spain

Institut d'Investigacions Biomèdiques August Pi i Sunyer, Barcelona, Spain
e-mail: fhanzu@clinic.cat

E. Poch (✉)
Nephrology Department, Clinical Institute of Nephrology and Urology, Hospital Clinic de Barcelona, Barcelona, Spain

Surgery and Medical-Surgical Specialties, Faculty of Medicine and Health Sciences, Universitat de Barcelona (UB), Barcelona, Spain
e-mail: epoch@clinic.cat

C. Castelo-Branco, S. Anglès Acedo (eds.), *Medical Disorders and Sexual Health*, Trends in Andrology and Sexual Medicine,
https://doi.org/10.1007/978-3-031-55080-5_21

dysfunction, leaving female sexual dysfunction an ignored issue. The importance of sexual dysfunction surpasses the issue of quality of life. Since it is currently considered to be of vascular origin in the majority of patients, due to atherosclerotic lesions in sexual organs, it is associated with higher rates of hypertension and other cardiovascular risk factors or associated diseases. In this sense, erectile dysfunction can predict future cardiovascular disease in asymptomatic patients [1]. In addition, antihypertensive therapy has been associated with sexual dysfunction, thus affecting patient's compliance. There is evidence that sexual dysfunction in hypertension often precedes initiation of antihypertensive treatment, which depending on the type of drug can either improve or worsen it.

The physiological effects of sexual hormones not only affect reproductive functions, but also affect other nonreproductive tissues and systems. Particularly, the cardiovascular system has been shown to be affected by disturbances of sexual hormones. On the one hand, testosterone deficiency has been associated not only with hypertension, but also with dyslipidemia and type II diabetes. The effects of testosterone by itself on these disorders has been difficult to dissect from aging, which is a strong determinant of cardiometabolic disease. However, analysis in young populations have demonstrated an independent role of testosterone deficiency [2]. However, the cardiometabolic benefits of hormone replacement therapy are still debated.

On the other hand, perimenopause is a known risk factor for hypertension and cardiovascular disease [3], the role of sexual hormones deficiency as a contributing factor independent of age demonstrated in population with early menopause or premature ovarian insufficiency. The physiological factors involved affect vascular function, through the renin-angiotensin system, inflammation, and oxidative stress. However, the cardiovascular protective effects of hormone replacement therapy have been questioned [4].

Collectively, the link between sexual function and hypertension, besides organ dysfunction through inflammation or endothelial dysfunction, also implicates factors such as psychological status, cultural factors, and patient's characteristics (age, menopause, etc.) (Fig. 1).

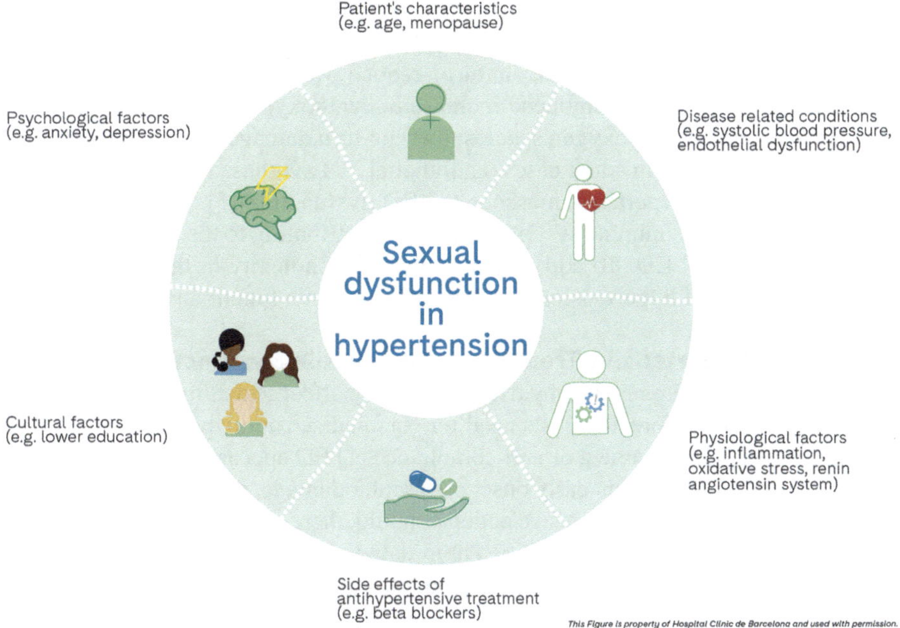

Fig. 1 Sexual dysfunction in hypertension

2 Sexual Life, Hypertension, and Cardiovascular Risk

2.1 Erectile Dysfunction and Hypertension

2.1.1 Introduction

Erectile dysfunction (ED) is a prevalent condition. In fact, its prevalence, worldwide ranges from 3 to 76.5% globally. ED is significantly linked to age as its prevalence increases from 5% at age 40 to 15% at 70 years. Other risk factors include heart diseases, diabetes mellitus, hypertension (HT), psychological factors, certain drugs, and smoking [5].

The prevalence of ED has been shown to be 58.3% in hypertensive patients, and therefore considerably higher than the prevalence of ED in the general population [6]. On the other hand, in patients with ED, HT is the most commonly associated comorbidity. Non-dipping HT is known to be linked to poor cardiac outcomes and in patients with ED, the non-dipper pattern was associated with poorer erectile function when HT was newly diagnosed. The severity of ED dysfunction is, also, an independent marker for non-dipping HT [7].

2.1.2 Pathophysiology

There is a notable relationship between HT and ED due, probably, to common pathophysiological ways, endothelial dysfunction, and/or dysregulation of the vascular and cavernous smooth muscle. There are complex neurovascular mechanisms underlying normal erectile function. These include neurochemical stimulation and end-organ responses (vasculature and penile body), needed for erection initiation and maintenance [8]. The signaling mechanisms involved in the pathophysiology of HT and ED are well connected, as both conditions are linked to an enhancement in pro-contractile pathways, which, in turn, reduce vascular compliance. Another mechanism is hypertension-induced increase in cyclooxygenase activity that leads to an increase in reactive oxygen species; these in turn damage endothelial cells and disrupt their function. In some cases, endothelial NO synthase (eNOS) gene variations may relate to hypertension-associated ED dysfunction [5]. Furthermore, evidence shows that the immune system is actively contributing to the pathophysiology of hypertension and ED. To add another layer of complexity in this interplay, the pharmacotherapy of hypertension can also affect erectile function [9].

2.1.3 Antihypertensive Treatment and Erectile Dysfunction

Antihypertensive treatment can, by itself, negatively affect sexual function increasing or causing ED. Therefore, there is a need for personalized antihypertensive treatment in order to avoid abandonment or non-compliance [1] ED appears shortly after hypertensions onset, suggesting an early onset of vascular damage, and the need for a more aggressive HT control. Hypertensive patients should, therefore, be adequately advised, and antihypertensive treatment modified or initiated, ensuring the confusing effects of the medications are minimized as much as possible and that modifications have begun with changes in the patient's lifestyle [1]. Among the various parameters leading to poor adherence, medication adverse events seem to be the prevailing cause of treatment discontinuation. Antihypertensive drugs of several types can decrease blood pressure in a comparable way, but they have different effects on ED. Overall, our knowledge about the impact of the different antihypertensive drugs on the development of ED is currently based either on small clinical studies or sub-analyses of large studies with inherent limitations. Alpha-blocking or alpha/beta-blocking drugs and guanidine derivatives are more likely to cause ED than calcium channel-blocking drugs, angiotensin-converting enzyme inhibitors, or diuretics [6]. β-blockers are a class of drugs commonly used in the management of hypertension. However, β-blockers use has been associated with various adverse events, among which, ED is a prevalent one. Older studies have shown contradictory findings, which however may be attributed to methodological errors related with the assessment of erectile function. More recent studies, however, unveiled the negative impact of this drug category on erectile function. Nebivolol presents a unique mode of action through enhanced nitric oxide bioavailability that may be associated with benefits on erectile function. Indeed, studies of nebivolol have shown improvement in erectile function, suggesting that nebivolol is the only exception in this class of drugs in terms of erectile function [10]. Larger and completed randomized controlled trials would be needed to confirm whether nebivolol reduces the incidence of ED compared to other β-blockers and independently of endothelial function, especially irrespective of age, and whether switching from other β-blockers to nebivolol might still improve erectile function [11].

Alpha-blockers are believed to have the potential to interfere with corporal smooth muscle constriction. Rare problems with emission and ejaculation have also been reported. Thiazide diuretics are also linked with ED in some studies. As a class, calcium channel blockers are associated with a low incidence of ED. As angiotensin-converting enzyme inhibitors have no effect on the sympathetic nervous system, the incidence of sexual dysfunction should be minimal [12].

2.1.4 Approach of Erectile Dysfunction Associated to Hypertension

Aggressive control of the above risk factors—along with lifestyle modification is recommended to improve symptoms of ED and reduce cardiovascular risk. Phosphodiesterase-5 (PDE5) inhibitors stay the first-choice treatment for ED in ischemic heart disease patients, and they have been shown to be safe and effective. However, PDE5 inhibitors can potentiate the hypotensive effect of nitrates so concomitant administration of sildenafil and nitrates is contraindicated. Gene and stem cell therapy are being investigated as future therapies for ED [5]. Hypertension, in most cases, can be controlled with antihypertensive agents, which are often associated with undesirable side effects, including ED. The relationship between antihypertensive medications and ED has been extensively studied, largely because it might affect the adherence to the prescribed therapy regimen resulting in poor management of blood pressure. Therefore, it is necessary to review which antihypertensive drugs are more suitable for patients with ED. [8]. Noteworthy, the literature is not cohesive, and conflicting findings have been reported. Thus, further studies are needed to clarify the impact antihypertensive drugs in erectile function [6]. This topic, the use of antihypertensive drugs, is of particular interest because drugs used to treat ED target the enzyme PDE5, and therefore, rely on endogenous NO production. While PDE5 inhibitors have been shown to be a safe pharmacological approach in hypertensive patients taking antihypertensive drugs, as we discussed above, these patients have reduced availability of NO, and so, they might not fully receive help from the use of PDE5 inhibitors. In fact, PDE5 inhibitors are ineffective for approximately 30% of the cases, and the presence of comorbid conditions, such as hypertension, negatively affects the drug outcomes. Undoubtedly, the management of hypertension and ED is a double-edged sword challenge in the clinical setting where physicians have to balance between best blood pressure control and patient compliance while preserving the quality of life of sexually active patients [9].

The first step of disease management is to find the underlying aetiology, including vasculogenic, endocrinologic, neurologic, drug-related, psychologic, or mixed causes as well as end-organ disease. Levels of testosterone and other related hormones (prolactin, follicular-stimulating hormone, luteinizing hormone, estrogen, etc.) and penile Doppler examination may aid in the differential diagnosis of ED [8]. Recurrent ulcers and/or gangrene at *glans penis* show the presence of severe pelvic arterial occlusive disease. Yet the majority of patients with pelvic arterial insufficiency-related ED do not develop recognizable changes in the morphology of penis. Erectile dysfunction severity can be objectively measured using the International Index of Erectile Function 5 (IIEF-5) questionnaire or complete IIEF-9. The validated IIEF-5 questionnaire evaluates self-reported indicators of male sexual function, encompassing erectile strength, orgasm, desire, satisfaction with intercourse, and overall satisfaction. In clinical trial settings, a difference in the IIEF-5 score of ≥ 4 is considered a minimal clinically crucial difference [8].

Randomized clinical trials have shown that lifestyle modification supplied clinical benefit for improving ED. Smoking cessation, weight reduction and maintenance, regular physical exercise, moderation of alcohol consumption, and dietary changes are the common lifestyle modification measures to reduce hypertension, risk of ED, and risk of hypertension-related cardiovascular complications. A Mediterranean diet is helpful for patients with ED and hypertension. Moderation of alcohol and salt consumption should also be recommended [8]. Treatment of ED requires lifestyle modification, reduction of comorbid vascular risk factors, and treatment of organic or psychosexual dysfunction with either pharmacotherapy alone (PDE5 inhibitors sildenafil, tadalafil, vardenafil, and avanafil) or in combination with psychosexual therapy. PDE5 inhibitors are known for their efficacy, ease of use, and favorable side-effect profile. A key factor associated with successful PDE5 inhibitor therapy is the instruction and counseling on proper use, including the onset of action of the drug and taking medication on an empty stomach. However, the use of PDE5 inhibitors is contraindicated in men taking nitrates. PDE5 inhibitors should be used cautiously in hypertensive patients receiving an alpha-adrenergic blocker due to an increased risk of hypotension. According to earlier studies, approximately 50% of ED patients showed a poor response to PDE5 inhibitors or had a contraindication to their use. Alternatively, they are instructed to use a vacuum constriction device, receive an intra-penile injection of prostaglandin [13], or undergo implantation of a penile prosthesis. Endovascular therapy is still considered a choice in the context of clinical studies, even though the clinical safety and efficacy data of endovascular therapy for arteriogenic ED is reassuring [8].

2.1.5 Remaining Gaps in Knowledge

Nevertheless, there are still some gaps in our knowledge. The exact prevalence of ED in patients with hypertension, potential geographic, social, and cultural variations, the association of erectile dysfunction with demographic factors, comorbidities, and the various forms of target organ damage in patients with hypertension need to be further investigated. The impact of erectile dysfunction on quality of life of the individual patient with hypertension and the impact of psychological factors (anxiety, depression) on the association between erectile dysfunction and arterial hypertension are not adequately clarified. Therefore, a large, prospective, multicenter, randomized clinical trial is needed to evaluate the effect of first-choice drugs (ARBs, angiotensin-converting enzyme inhibitors, calcium channel blockers, diuretics, and beta-blockers) along with alpha-blockers on erectile function. Importantly, the effect of erectile dysfunction diagnosis or management as a mean of medication adherence and best regulation of blood pressure could strengthen and expand the clinical role of recognition of erectile dysfunction by several different specialties. Finally, the implementation rates of these suggestions in real life are largely unknown. ED in patients with hypertension seems to remain under-appreciated, under-recognized, and under-treated.

2.2 Sexual Dysfunction and Hypertension in Women

Although high blood pressure is known to be associated with sexual dysfunction, this phenomenon has been little studied in females and has received little intervention in clinical practice. A recent study has evaluated 157 women (from 56.4 years) with a diagnosis of arterial hypertension, through the Female Sexual Function Index (FSFI) and the Hospital Anxiety and Depression Scale (HADS). High rates of sexual dysfunction were detected in the women evaluated, and this dysfunction was in all domains as follows: desire (68.2%), excitement (68.2%), lubrication (41.1%), orgasm (55.4%), satisfaction (66.42%), and pain (56.1%). Elevated rates of symptoms of anxiety (43.3%) and depression (26.8%) were also found in this study. Nevertheless, in the present study, such symptoms showed no relationship with sexual dysfunction levels for any of the domains assessed. The authors conclude that hypertensive patients show an elevated presence of sexual dysfunction, as well as anxious and depressive symptoms. Although the literature on female sexuality shows influences of these symptoms on sexual function, this study did not find such a relationship in the studied population [14].

A recent systematic review included articles evaluating the prevalence of sexual dysfunction in women and/or comparing sexual dysfunction between hypertensive and non-hypertensive women. Studies were excluded if they evaluated patients with secondary hypertension, examined sexual dysfunction caused by drugs, did not distinguish by gender, or included patients with hypertension and other comorbidities/pathologies. Five articles were included in the meta-analysis (1057 hypertensive and 715 normotensive). The prevalence of sexual dysfunction in articles varied from 14.1 to 90.1%. In the meta-analysis of the sexual dysfunction, the relative risk between hypertensive and normotensive women was found to be significant and with a high heterogeneity, the pooled results revealed a significant risk ratio of 1.81 (95% CI 1.10–2.97, $p < 0.05$). The relative risk for hypertensive women showed an association with age ($b = 0.0333$, $p < 0.0001$). In summary, the authors found that the studies analyzed presented significant limitations in relation to method and a small sample size. Consequently, the meta-analysis was highly heterogeneous and reinforced the need for further research in this area [15].

3 Male Hypogonadism, Hypertension, Cardiovascular Risk, and Sexual Health

3.1 Low Testosterone and Cardiovascular Risk

Cardiovascular disease (CVD) is a leading cause of death in men and most forms of CV diseases including high blood pressure are higher in men than in age-matched premenopausal women. Androgen receptors are present on myocytes, smooth vascular and endothelial cells and testosterone can potentially present beneficial or deleterious effects at cardiovascular level. What's more an antagonistic, Janus like sex-dependent effect of testosterone on CV system has been questioned, as women after menopause with higher testosterone level and polycystic ovary syndrome patients are prone to cardiovascular and metabolic pathologies [16–18].

At mechanistic level experiments in vitro and in various animal models have shown that testosterone inhibits calcium channels, improves endothelial function, and decreases vascular reactivity inducing vasodilatation, an increased blood flow and decreasing QT interval. At the same time, testosterone is an anabolic hormone that promotes muscle mass, intra-abdominal and subcutaneous fat loss, and insulin sensitivity [16, 17].

Anyway, exercise training generates an equal effect for improving aerobic fitness, muscular strength, and total and visceral fat mass in middle age low-normal adult men with low-normal serum testosterone concentrations and adding testosterone treatment to exercise did not provide any additive benefit for these variables [19, 20].

In addition, testosterone can remodel lipids and endothelial adherence profile by decreasing HDL-cholesterol and increasing cell adhesion molecules and thrombocyte aggregation. The effect on thrombosis is neutral as it increased both thrombotic and antithrombotic factors. Moreover, it promotes sodium retention and therefore edema formation [16, 17, 21].

Testosterone stimulates erythropoiesis increasing erythropoietin and bone marrow erythropoietic progenitors. This increases hematocrit, with a greater increase in older men than younger adults [16, 22, 23].

3.2 Low Testosterone and High Blood Pressure (BP)

Due to the great variability of hypogonadal spectrum associated to low endogenous testosterone levels, starting from established primary and secondary hypogonadism to adult late onset testosterone deficiency, observational studies often yield contradictory results on cardiovascular and metabolic outcomes [18–20, 22, 24–31].

As mentioned, declines in testosterone levels with age or gonadal dysfunction are associated with deleterious effects on metabolic function empowering metabolic syndrome features like dyslipidemia, hyperglycemia, insulin resistance, and the development of T2D and are increasing cardiovascular deaths and overall mortality [16, 21–23, 25].

The relationship between testosterone and BP is complex and paradoxical. Testosterone can activate the vasodilator and vasoconstrictor pathways, but it is primarily prohypertensive and is more likely to induce vasoconstriction, sodium retention, and cardiac hypertrophy. In animal models of hypertension, castration decrease BP [2, 16, 17].

Testosterone circulates bound to sex hormone-binding globulin (SHBG), and free testosterone is considered an equivalent of testosterone's biological activity. With advancing age SHBG increases, while free testosterone decreases more rapidly than total testosterone due to the unresponsiveness of the gonadal Leydig cells to luteinizing hormone stimulation with age. Therefore, the age-related decrease in testosterone level has been implicated as a possible explanation for the increased risk of hypertension, which is a predisposing factor for the future incidence of CVD [2, 16, 17].

Reduced SHBG level has been also reported to be the predictor of metabolic syndrome and T2D [25].

Regarding observational studies, an inverse relationship of endogenous testosterone with BP and cardiovascular risk has been reported, while some find no association after adjustment for body mass index. Low free testosterone and higher LH levels have been independently associated with abdominal aortic aneurysm in older men [26]. What's more primary hypogonadism has been reported to be a risk marker for major cardiovascular diseases in men with severe hypertension [20]. Remarkably, chronic kidney disease (CKD) major hormonal-associated disturbance is considered testosterone deficiency and low testosterone levels have been associated with an increased CV mortality in CKD.

Established hypogonadism is therefore a risk marker for prevalent hypertension at least in older men.

3.3 Testosterone Replacement Therapy and Hypertension

Hypertension or high blood pressure (BP) is a disorder that affects nearly half of the adult population. High BP affects multiple tissues within the body and can lead to severe cardiovascular events, including myocardial infarct, stroke, chronic renal disease, and retinopathy.

Hormonal testosterone replacement treatment (HTRT) has been approved since the 1950s for men with "classical" hypogonadism and specific and well-recognized hypothalamic, pituitary, or gonadal conditions leading to establish deficiency of endogenous testosterone. The modes of testosterone supplementation are intramuscular injections, subcutaneous pellets, percutaneous methods-patches and gels and very recently oral and subcutaneous depot formulations [16, 29].

On the contrary, there is still controversy about the beneficial or deleterious cardiometabolic effect of testosterone treatment of men with age-related low levels of testosterone and age-dependent-hypogonadism. The falling-off in testosterone level with aging may be an adaptive response, as a marker of underlying comorbidities. Consequently, exogenous HTRT may interrupt the whole-body homeostasis leading to cardiometabolic and vascular effect [22, 23, 27, 30, 32].

HTRT in older men with low testosterone was associated with small reductions in cholesterol and insulin but not with other glucose markers, markers of inflammation or fibrinolysis, or troponin and did not result in a significant difference in the rates of change in either common carotid artery intima-media thickness or coronary artery calcium nor did it improve overall sexual function or health-related quality of life [22, 23].

When analyzing results in a cohort of patients who underwent coronary angiography and present with low levels of testosterone, the use of testosterone therapy was associated with increased risk of adverse outcomes [33]. while when used in patients with no CV disease there are no adverse ones [31].

In this line, evidence regarding 24 h BP evolution under testosterone replacement therapy is low. Very recently, 24 BP monitoring was performed in the trials of the last two approved testosterone formulations, respectively, of oral (testosterone undecanoate) and subcutaneous (testosterone enanthate) testosterone showed an increase by at least 4 mmHg. This increase, although low, has been shown to have a significant impact on longitudinal CV outcome, myocardial infarction, and stroke. An observational study suggests that oral and subcutaneous testosterone preparate increase 24 h BP and attenuate exercise induce decrease in BP [29].

While awaiting results from double-blind placebo-controlled CV outcomes trials on monitoring of BP from other testosterone products, for the moment this late introduced formulations are contraindicated for age-related hypogonadism of adult men not related to established classical hypogonadal patients [17, 29, 34].

Therefore, for those men whose hematocrit rose by >6%, BP increases were of greater clinical relevance. Hence, hematocrit can be indicative in predicting the development of BP increases on testosterone therapy. Testosterone could promote platelet aggregation, coronary plaque formation, and affected salt and water retention, endothelium inflammation, or through other mechanisms that might make some men susceptible to adverse CVD outcomes. Interestingly, despite this known effects on sodium retention, a recent published metanalysis suggest the safety of HTRT, in patients with hypogonadism and severe cardiac insufficiency (class NYHA II and III) [28]. What's more, HRTH in patients with chronic kidney disease and associated hypogonadism improves BP control, hematocrit, and inflammation [35].

Altogether are indicated that HTRT must be prescribed taking in account cardiometabolic and vascular risk. Therefore, as stipulated in the hypogonadism guideline HRTH is not recommended in elevated hematocrit, untreated severe obstructive sleep apnea, uncontrolled heart failure, myocardial infarction or stroke within the last 6 months, or thrombophilia. Moreover, mid-normal range testosterone levels are recommended as treatment target with any of the testosterone formulations, taking into consideration patient preference, pharmacokinetics, formulation-specific adverse effects, treatment burden, and costs [16].

Resuming, the relationship between male hypogonadism, hypertension, cardiovascular risk, and sexual health is complex, and treatment indication should be individualized based on medical history and symptoms. Nevertheless, the long-term effects of HTRT on cardiovascular outcomes are still not fully understood, and more investigation is needed in this field.

4 Female Gonadal Function, Hypertension, and Sexual Health

4.1 Perimenopausal and Postmenopausal Periods

There is clear evidence that blood pressure increases with age in both men and women, but the age-related increases are accelerated in women with respect to men, mainly in postmenopausal women [36]. Although this age-related increment in blood pressure may be multifactorial, the importance of gender or sex hormones in the development of hypertension has been a long-debated issue [3] Both cross-sectional and longitudinal studies have demonstrated a relationship between menopause and blood pressure that is independent of age, body mass index, and hormone replacement therapy [36, 37]. This increase in blood pressure was restricted to women with peri and menopause and limited to systolic blood pressure [37]. These differences appear to be observed both in natural menopause and surgically induced menopause. On the other hand, some studies have questioned the influence of menopause in front of age or body mass index in the development of hypertension [38, 39], the differences probably due to differences in the population studied and the study design. Several studies have demonstrated that the prevalence of hypertension in postmenopausal women is higher than in men [40]. The National Health and Nutrition Examination Survey IV study demonstrated that women were more likely to have uncontrolled hypertension than men, despite the use of similar antihypertensive drug use among gender [38]. In addition, postmenopausal women are more prone to exhibit a nocturnal non-dipping pattern of blood pressure, i.e., absent physiological reduction of nocturnal blood pressure in 24 h monitoring [39]; this pattern has been associated to a greater extent of target organ damage in hypertension, which is greater in women than in men [39]. All this evidence suggests a gender-specific effect in the development of hypertension in the postmenopausal women.

There are several factors contributing to hypertension in postmenopausal women. First, the role of changes in the estrogen/androgen ratio has been advocated as a cause of postmenopausal hypertension and cardiovascular disease. Although hormone replacement therapy has been shown to reduce blood pressure in the short and mid-term, there appears to be no effect in the long term [41]. In addition, hormone replacement therapy has no effect in the prevention of primary or secondary cardiovascular disease [4].

From the mechanistic point of view, the loss of estrogens has been shown to contribute to endothelial dysfunction, which is common in patients with hypertension. Even in normotensive postmenopausal women, endothelial dysfunction is predictive of future hypertension. Estrogens stimulate the synthesis, release and availability of nitric oxide, and the reduced level of this mediator may explain endothelial dysfunction in low-estrogen states [42]. However, it seems that estrogen administration improves endothelial dysfunction only in young women with menopause, highlighting the effects of aging in the development of both endothelial dysfunction and hypertension [42]. Another possible target of estrogen is the renin-angiotensin system, which seems to be suppressed by sex hormones. However, clinical studies have been unable to show relation to blood pressure or cardiovascular disease [3]. Other factors associated with postmenopausal hypertension but probably mainly related to aging are arterial stiffness, oxidative stress, salt sensitivity, and obesity [42].

Menopause is often associated with sexual dysfunction, but its specific contribution in patients with or without hypertension has not been explored. A study evaluating sexually active women aged 48–55 years at a menopausal clinic found that 20% of normotensive women, 38% of women with untreated hypertension, and 27% of women with treated hypertension reported sexual dysfunction [43]. Age is an important predictor of sexual dysfunction among hypertensive women [44], and therefore the relative contribution of menopause and hypertension to sexual dysfunction has not been quantified. In addition, most studies relating hypertension with sexual dysfunction have been performed in aged women [43, 45].

4.2   Primary Ovarian Insufficiency and Infertility

Primary ovary insufficiency is a type of ovarian dysfunction produced by causes within the ovary which can be due to genetic defects, chemotherapy, radiotherapy, or surgery. It has been shown that this condition leads to a higher cardiovascular mortality, specifically when it occurs before age 45 years [46]. Although overall mortality was higher in women who did not have estrogen therapy until they were aged 45 years or more, the role of hormone replacement therapy on cardiovascular protection is still controversial.

Premature ovarian insufficiency consist of the loss of ovarian activity before the age of 40 years is characterized by menstrual disturbances for at least 4 months, low estradiol, and increased gonadotrophin levels [47]. Premature ovarian insufficiency has been associated with increased risk for cardiovascular disease, including arterial hypertension [47]. Women with premature ovarian failure before 40 years of age also exhibit endothelial dysfunction compared to age-matched cycling women, and hormone replacement therapy for 6 months reversed the endothelial dysfunction [48].

On the contrary, a cross-sectional analysis of a cohort of self-reported infertility or any fertility treatment was not associated to a higher risk of hypertension, unless the infertility was associated with tubal disease [49]. Since tubal disease may be linked to sexually transmitted diseases, its association with hypertension could be accounted for unidentified socioeconomic factor or chronic inflammation.

The association between infertility and sexual dysfunction can be reciprocal. The inability to conceive often translates to anger during the sexual relationship between couples. In women, the lack of sexual desire, arousal, and sexual pain disorders are the most prevalent sexual dysfunction [50] reported in infertility clinics. Sexual health assessment is an important part of the evaluation of infertility since sexual dysfunction can be both a cause and consequence of infertility.

4.3   Oral Contraceptives Users

The use of oral contraceptives is associated with a mild elevation of blood pressure in most women, but the development of established hypertension affects around 5% of them [51]. Newer preparations with low estrogen and progestogen content seem to be safer, with the progestogen-only pill having no effect on BP. In a metanalysis including 24 studies with 270,284 participants, the duration of oral contraceptive use was positively associated with the risk of developing hypertension, increasing by 13% for every 5 years of oral contraceptive use [51].

The mechanism implicated in this relationship are poorly understood, but very likely is mediated by the combination of several mediators, which include, activation the renin angiotensin system, endothelial dysfunction, and inflammation [51].

Because of this association and plausibility, it is advised to screen for hypertension and monitor hypertensive women under contraceptive medications. Progestogen-only contraceptives would be preferred in hypertensive women.

With respect to sexual health, there is some evidence suggesting that contraceptive medications can be associated with hypoactive sexual desire disorders, mainly to their effects in lowering androgen levels or action. On the contrary, there are studies that have demonstrated no effects of oral contraceptive medications in sexual desire. A metanalysis published in 2013 analyzed 36 studies involving 13,673 women of which 8422 were oral contraceptive users [52]. Eighty-five percent reported either an increase or no change in libido and 15% reported a decrease. Even though contraceptives produced a reduction in testosterone, this seemed to affect sexual desire in a reduced number of women. Psychosocial, cultural, and other relational factors, as well as idiosyncrasy seem to have greater influence on sexual desire. The study concluded that contraceptives with very low-estrogen content were more prone to be associated with reduction of libido. Cyproterone acetate (CPA) is the most potent antiandrogenic progestin, followed by dienogest, drospirenone, and chlormadinone acetate. Nomegestrol acetate and medrogestone also exert some antiandrogenic properties and are similar to chlormadinone acetate in antiandrogenic potency. All these molecules are common in contraceptive pills and while androgens act positively on libido in women, antiandrogenic properties of these progestins may have a negative effect.

References

1. Diosdado-Figueiredo M, Balboa-Barreiro V, Pértega-Diaz S, Seoane-Pillado T, Pita-Fernández S, Chantada-Abal V. Erectile dysfunction in patients with arterial hypertension. Cardiovascular risk and impact on their quality of life. Med Clin (Barc). 2019;152:209–15.
2. Stallone JN, Oloyo AK. Cardiovascular and metabolic actions of the androgens: is testosterone a Janus-faced molecule? Biochem Pharmacol. 2023;208:115347. https://pubmed.ncbi.nlm.nih.gov/36395900/.
3. Coylewright M, Reckelhoff JF, Ouyang P. Menopause and hypertension: an age-old debate. Hypertension. 2008;51(4 PART 2 SUPPL):952–9.
4. Grady D, Herrington D, Bittner V, Blumenthal R, Davidson M, Hlatky M, Hsia J, Hulley S, Herd A, Hsia JWNHRG. Cardiovascular disease outcomes during 6.8 years of hormone therapy: heart and estrogen/progestin replacement study follow-up (HERS II). JAMA J Am Med Assoc. 2002;288(1):49–57.
5. Ibrahim A, Ali M, Kiernan TJ, Stack AG. Erectile dysfunction and ischaemic heart disease. Eur Cardiol Rev. 2018;13(2):98–103.
6. Aguilera-Alvarez VH, Mohammed BK, Fatima A, Patel A, Patel A, Gyabaah FN, et al. The role and efficacy of coenzyme Q10 in the management of erectile dysfunction in a hypertensive male: an interventional study. Cureus. 2021;13:e17937.
7. Yildirim U, Karakayali M, Uslu M, Ezer M, Erihan IB, Artac I, et al. Association between international index of erectile function-5 scores and circadian patterns of newly diagnosed hypertension in erectile dysfunction patients. Andrologia. 2022;54(11):e14622.
8. Wang TD, Lee CK, Chia YC, Tsoi K, Buranakitjaroen P, Chen CH, et al. Hypertension and erectile dysfunction: the role of endovascular therapy in Asia. J Clin Hypertens. 2021;23:481–8.
9. De Oliveira AA, Nunes KP. Hypertension and erectile dysfunction: breaking down the challenges. Am J Hypertens. 2021;34:134–42.
10. Manolis A, Doumas M, Ferri C, Mancia G. Erectile dysfunction and adherence to antihypertensive therapy: focus on β-blockers. Eur J Internal Med. 2020;81:1–6.
11. de Simone G, Mancusi C. Erectile dysfunction and arterial hypertension: still looking for a scapegoat. Eur J Internal Med. 2020;81:22–3.
12. Blumentals WA, Brown RR, Gomez-Caminero A. Antihypertensive treatment and erectile dysfunction in a cohort of type II diabetes patients. Int J Impot Res. 2003;15(5):314–7.
13. McMahon CG. Current diagnosis and management of erectile dysfunction. Med J Aust. 2019;210:469–76.
14. Nascimento ER, Maia ACO, Nardi AE, Silva AC. Sexual dysfunction in arterial hypertension women: the role of depression and anxiety. J Affect Disord. 2015;181:96–100.
15. Santana LM, Perin L, Lunelli R, Inácio JFS, Rodrigues CG, Eibel B, et al. Sexual dysfunction in women with hypertension: a systematic review and meta-analysis. Curr Hypertens Rep. 2019;21:35.
16. Bhasin S, Brito JP, Cunningham GR, Hayes FJ, Hodis HN, Matsumoto AM, et al. Testosterone therapy in men with hypogonadism: an Endocrine Society clinical practice guideline. J Clin Endocrinol Metab. 2018;103(5):1715–44. https://pubmed.ncbi.nlm.nih.gov/29562364/.

17. Nguyen CP, Hirsch M, Kaul S, Woods C, Joffe HV. Testosterone therapy for the treatment of age-related hypogonadism: risks with uncertain benefits. Androg Clin Res Ther. 2021;2(1):56–60. https://pubmed.ncbi.nlm.nih.gov/34041509/.

18. Fan C, Wei D, Wang L, Liu P, Fan K, Nie L, et al. The association of serum testosterone with dyslipidemia is mediated by obesity: the Henan rural cohort study. J Endocrinol Investig. 2023;46(4):679. https://pubmed.ncbi.nlm.nih.gov/36219315/.

19. Chasland LC, Green DJ, Schlaich MP, Maiorana AJ, Cooke BR, Cox KL, et al. Effects of testosterone treatment, with and without exercise training, on ambulatory blood pressure in middle-aged and older men. Clin Endocrinol. 2021;95(1):176–86. https://pubmed.ncbi.nlm.nih.gov/33580564/.

20. Qu M, Feng C, Wang X, Gu Y, Shang X, Zhou Y, et al. Association of Serum Testosterone and Luteinizing Hormone with Blood Pressure and risk of cardiovascular disease in middle-aged and elderly men. J Am Heart Assoc. 2021;10(7):e019559. https://pubmed.ncbi.nlm.nih.gov/33739129/.

21. Mohler ER, Ellenberg SS, Lewis CE, Wenger NK, Budoff MJ, Lewis MR, et al. The effect of testosterone on cardiovascular biomarkers in the testosterone trials. J Clin Endocrinol Metab. 2018;103(2):681–8. https://pubmed.ncbi.nlm.nih.gov/29253154/.

22. Basaria S, Harman SM, Travison TG, Hodis H, Tsitouras P, Budoff M, et al. Effects of testosterone administration for 3 years on subclinical atherosclerosis progression in older men with low or low-Normal testosterone levels: a randomized clinical trial. JAMA. 2015;314(6):570–81. https://pubmed.ncbi.nlm.nih.gov/26262795/.

23. Snyder PJ, Bhasin S, Cunningham GR, Matsumoto AM, Stephens-Shields AJ, Cauley JA, et al. Effects of testosterone treatment in older men. N Engl J Med. 2016;374(7):611–24. https://pubmed.ncbi.nlm.nih.gov/26886521/.

24. Mäkinen J, Järvisalo MJ, Pöllänen P, Perheentupa A, Irjala K, Koskenvuo M, et al. Increased carotid atherosclerosis in andropausal middle-aged men. J Am Coll Cardiol. 2005;45(10):1603–8. https://pubmed.ncbi.nlm.nih.gov/15893174/.

25. Fukui M, Soh J, Tanaka M, Kitagawa Y, Hasegawa G, Yoshikawa T, et al. Low serum testosterone concentration in middle-aged men with type 2 diabetes. Endocr J. 2007;54(6):871–7. https://pubmed.ncbi.nlm.nih.gov/17998764/.

26. Yeap BB, Hyde Z, Norman PE, Paul Chubb SA, Golledge J. Associations of total testosterone, sex hormone-binding globulin, calculated free testosterone, and luteinizing hormone with prevalence of abdominal aortic aneurysm in older men. J Clin Endocrinol Metab. 2010;95(3):1123–30. https://pubmed.ncbi.nlm.nih.gov/20061425/.

27. Chasland LC, Yeap BB, Maiorana AJ, Chan YX, Maslen BA, Cooke BR, et al. Testosterone and exercise: effects on fitness, body composition, and strength in middle-to-older aged men with low-normal serum testosterone levels. Am J Physiol Heart Circ Physiol. 2021;320(5):H1985–98. https://pubmed.ncbi.nlm.nih.gov/33739155/.

28. Cannarella R, Barbagallo F, Crafa A, Mongioì LM, Aversa A, Greco E, et al. Testosterone replacement therapy in hypogonadal male patients with hypogonadism and heart failure: a meta-analysis of randomized controlled studies. Minerva Urol Nephrol. 2022;74(4):418–27. https://pubmed.ncbi.nlm.nih.gov/33781026/.

29. White WB, Dobs A, Carson C, DelConte A, Khera M, Miner M, et al. Effects of a novel oral testosterone undecanoate on ambulatory blood pressure in hypogonadal men. J Cardiovasc Pharmacol Ther. 2021;26(6):630–7. https://pubmed.ncbi.nlm.nih.gov/34191621/.

30. Mangolim AS, de Andrade Rodrigues Brito L, dos Santos Nunes-Nogueira V. Effectiveness of testosterone replacement in men with obesity: a systematic review and meta-analysis. Eur J Endocrinol. 2021;186(1):123–35. https://pubmed.ncbi.nlm.nih.gov/34738915/.

31. Shores MM, Walsh TJ, Korpak A, Krakauer C, Forsberg CW, Fox AE, et al. Association between testosterone treatment and risk of incident cardiovascular events among US male veterans with low testosterone levels and multiple medical comorbidities. J Am Heart Assoc. 2021;10(17):e020562. https://pubmed.ncbi.nlm.nih.gov/34423650/.

32. Galbiati FF, Goldman AL, Gattu A, Guzelce EC, Bhasin S. Benefits and risks of testosterone treatment of older men with hypogonadism. Urol Clin North Am. 2022;49(4):593–602. https://pubmed.ncbi.nlm.nih.gov/36309416/.

33. Vigen R, O'Donnell CI, Barón AE, Grunwald GK, Maddox TM, Bradley SM, et al. Association of testosterone therapy with mortality, myocardial infarction, and stroke in men with low testosterone levels. JAMA. 2013;310(17):1829–36. https://pubmed.ncbi.nlm.nih.gov/24193080/.

34. Bhasin S, Lincoff AM, Basaria S, Bauer DC, Boden WE, Cunningham GR, et al. Effects of long-term testosterone treatment on cardiovascular outcomes in men with hypogonadism: rationale and design of the TRAVERSE study. Am Heart J. 2022;245:41–50. https://pubmed.ncbi.nlm.nih.gov/34871580/.

35. Romejko K, Rymarz A, Sadownik H, Niemczyk S. Testosterone deficiency as one of the major endocrine disorders in chronic kidney disease. Nutrients. 2022;14(16):3438. https://pubmed.ncbi.nlm.nih.gov/36014945/.

36. Staessen J, Bulpitt JC, Fagard R, Lijnen PAA. The influence of menopause on blood pressure. J Hum Hypertens. 1989;3(6):427–33.

37. Staessen JA, Ginocchio G, Thijs LFL. Conventional and ambulatory blood pressure and menopause in a prospective population study. J Hum Hypertens. 1997;11(8):507–14.

38. Casiglia E, d'Este D, Ginocchio G, Colangeli G, Onesto C, Tramontin P, Ambrosio GBPA. Lack of influence of menopause on blood pressure and cardiovascular risk profile: a 16-year longitudinal study concerning a cohort of 568 women. J Hypertens. 1996;14(6):729–36.

39. Luoto R, Sharrett AR, Schreiner P, Sorlie PD, Arnett DES. Blood pressure and menopausal transition: the atherosclerosis risk in communities study (1987-95). J Hypertens. 2000;18(1):27–33.

40. Ong KL, Tso AWK, Lam KSL, Cheung BMY. Gender difference in blood pressure control and cardiovascular risk factors in Americans with diagnosed hypertension. Hypertension. 2008;51(4 PART 2 SUPPL):1142–8.

41. Prelevic GM, Kwong P, Byrne DJ, Jagroop IA, Ginsburg J, Mikhailidis DP. A cross-sectional study of the effects of hormone replacement therapy on the cardiovascular disease risk profile in healthy postmenopausal women. Fertil Steril. 2002;77(5):945–51.

42. Yanes LL, Reckelhoff JF. Postmenopausal hypertension. Am J Hypertens. 2011;24(7):740–9.

43. Foy CG, Newman JC, Berlowitz DR, Russell LP, Kimmel PL, Wadley VG, et al. Blood pressure, sexual activity, and dysfunction in women with hypertension: baseline findings from the systolic blood pressure intervention trial (SPRINT). J Sexual Med. 2016;13(9):1333–46.

44. Doumas M, Douma S. Sexual dysfunction in essential hypertension: myth or reality? J Clin Hypertens (Greenwich). 2006;8(4):269–74.

45. Manolis A, Doumas M. Sexual dysfunction: the "prima ballerina" of hypertension-related quality-of-life complications. J Hypertens. 2008;26(11):2074–84.

46. De Vos M, Devroey P, Fauser BC. Primary ovarian insufficiency. Lancet. 2010;376(9744):911–21.

47. Webber L, Davies M, Anderson R, Bartlett J, Braat D, Cartwright B, et al. ESHRE guideline: management of women with premature ovarian insufficiency. Hum Reprod. 2016;31(5):926–37.

48. Kalantaridou SN, Naka KK, Papanikolaou E, Kazakos N, Kravariti M, Calis KA, et al. Impaired endothelial function in young women with premature ovarian failure: normalization with hormone therapy. J Clin Endocrinol Metab. 2004;89(8):3907–13.

49. Farland LV, Grodstein F, Srouji SS, Forman JP, Rich-Edwards J, Chavarro JE, et al. Infertility, fertility treatment, and risk of hypertension. Fertil Steril. 2015;104(2):391–7.

50. Berger MH, Messore M, Pastuszak AW, Ramasamy R. Association between infertility and sexual dysfunction in men and women. Sex Med Rev. 2016;4(4):353–65.

51. Liu H, Yao J, Wang W, Zhang D. Association between duration of oral contraceptive use and risk of hypertension: a meta-analysis. J Clin Hypertens. 2017;19(10):1032–41.

52. Pastor Z, Holla K, Chmel R. The influence of combined oral contraceptives on female sexual desire: a systematic review. Eur J Contracep Reprod Health Care. 2013;18(1):27–43.

Sexuality and Cardiac Disease

Adelina Doltra

A. Doltra (✉)
Non-invasive Cardiac Imaging Section, Clinical Institute of Cardiovascular Medicine, Hospital Clínic de Barcelona, Barcelona, Spain

Clinical Sexology Working Group, Hospital Clinic de Barcelona, Barcelona, Spain
e-mail: adoltra@clinic.cat

Abbreviations

CAD	Coronary artery disease
CHD	Congenital heart disease
ED	Erectile dysfunction
HF	Heart failure
ICD	Implantable cardioverter-defibrillator
MI	Myocardial infarction
PDE5i	Phosphodiesterase-5 inhibitors
SCD	Sudden cardiac death

1 Introduction

Sexual well-being is of paramount importance for patients with cardiovascular disease, and healthcare providers, particularly cardiologists, should play an active role in providing sexual counseling. Studies have shown that sexual counseling is often neglected in cardiology clinics, despite guidelines recommending its routine practice. By recognizing the significance of sexual well-being and integrating sexual counseling into routine care, healthcare professionals can improve the overall care and outcomes of patients with cardiovascular disease. In this chapter, we will discuss the importance of sexual counseling, the effect of cardiovascular medications on sexual function, cardiovascular responses during sexual activity, and provide recommendations regarding sexual activity in different cardiac conditions.

2   Importance of Sexual Well-Being in Patients with Cardiovascular Disease and the Role of Cardiologists

Despite guidelines from both European and American cardiology societies recommending sexual counseling for cardiovascular patients [1, 2], studies show that it is not routinely practiced in most cardiology clinics. A multicentric study conducted with patients 1 month after myocardial infarction (MI) revealed that only 12% of women and 19% of men received information regarding sexual activity, and the information provided often included restrictions not supported by evidence [3]. The study also found that female gender and older age were independently associated with not receiving sexual counseling from physicians. A similar study conducted with patients after MI [4] reported that only a minority of patients received sexual counseling before being discharged from the hospital (47% of men and 34% of women, $p < 0.001$ for gender differences). Importantly, patients who did not receive instructions about sex were more likely to report a loss of sexual activity, as indicated by multivariate analysis for both women and men. Other works have also demonstrated an association between the lack of counseling and a decrease in sexual activity [5].

While several factors contribute to the lack of communication about sexual matters between physicians and patients, one of the primary reasons appears to be reluctance on the part of healthcare professionals. Surveys have shown that more than 90% of patients agree that it is appropriate for a physician to discuss sexual concerns, and the majority feel comfortable having such discussions [5]. Additionally, close to 90% of patients who did receive sexual counseling reported being either completely satisfied or mostly satisfied with their doctor's recommendations [5]. Conversely, some data suggest that doctors may feel discomfort or lack confidence in addressing sexual issues. A survey among Iranian cardiologists found that only 10.6% reported frequently or always assessing sexual problems with their patients, and only 33% felt confident in their knowledge in this area [6]. In another study involving American and Spanish cardiologists, patients initiated discussions about sex in most cases [5].

Randomized data comparing the receipt of sexual counseling versus not receiving it is limited, mostly focusing on men in small studies. One study randomized 92 male patients undergoing cardiac rehabilitation after acute coronary syndrome or bypass surgery to either sexual therapy (in addition to cardiac rehabilitation) or cardiac rehabilitation alone. The group assigned to sexual therapy experienced an earlier resumption of sexual activity and an improvement in its quality [7].

Based on the available evidence, sexual counseling should be considered crucial for cardiac patients, both women and men, and healthcare providers should play an active role in providing it. Numerous studies from around the world have highlighted the neglect of sexual counseling by healthcare professionals, underscoring the need for training in this area. Consequently, both American and European scientific societies [1, 2] agree that patients with cardiovascular disease and their partners should have the opportunity to discuss sexual issues with their healthcare providers (ESC recommendation level IC). Furthermore, cardiovascular healthcare professionals would benefit from training in sexual assessment, communication, and counseling (ESC recommendation level IC). Information provided to patients should include a review of medications, potential risks related to sexual activity, warning signs, and specific recommendations depending on the diagnosis, as discussed in the current work. Scientific societies have also developed information documents for patients [8].

3   Cardiovascular Medication and Sexual Function

Some cardiovascular drugs have been associated with sexual dysfunction although the extent of this association and whether the symptoms can be solely attributed to medication effects is not clear. Other factors such as psychological issues, cardiac disease itself, or comorbid conditions may also contribute. Therefore, providing information to patients is crucial.

While many studies have investigated this topic, several suffer from methodological issues, and randomized controlled trials are lacking. Furthermore, women are underrepresented [9]. Therefore, caution should be exercised when drawing conclusions.

A review of 15 studies involving over 35,000 patients found a small but significant increase in sexual dysfunction with beta-blockers (approximately one additional case for every 199 patients treated per year) [10]. However, some authors have found that the increase in sexual dysfunction is reported primarily by patients who were aware of the potential side effects of the medication (nocebo effect) and could be reversed with placebo [11]. In contrast, nebivolol has been shown to have a positive impact on erectile dysfunction, possibly due to its higher selectivity for ß1 receptors and its endothelial nitric oxide vasodilatory effects [12, 13].

Thiazides have also been linked to sexual dysfunction, and patients can be switched to loop diuretics if they develop sexual dysfunction due to this medication. Similarly, spironolactone may cause antiandrogen side effects, including erectile dysfunction (ED) and reduced libido, in which case it can be substituted with eplerenone [1]. Spironolactone induces also gynecomastia, which can impact body image perception in males.

Neither angiotensin-converting enzyme inhibitors (ACEIs) nor angiotensin receptor blockers (ARBs) have a negative impact on sexual function, and some authors even suggest a potential benefit of ARBs by improving endothelial function in ED [14].

Statins are often thought to be associated with worsening sexual function [13], but the available evidence demonstrates a neutral or even positive effect. A meta-analysis of six randomized controlled trials found no significant difference in erectile function between statins and placebo, and even an improvement in patients taking statins plus sildenafil (compared to patients taking placebo + sildenafil) [15]. It is likely that the sexual dysfunction observed in patients on statins is due to their underlying arterial disease rather than the statins themselves.

While some authors have hypothesized potential ejaculatory dysfunction due to calcium channel blockers [13], most studies have shown a neutral effect on sexual function [9].

Scientific societies [1, 2] agree that cardiovascular drugs should not be withheld due to concerns about sexual function, as evidence in this regard is conflicting and these medications offer clear benefits in symptoms and survival in cardiac diseases. Both societies also agree that in cases of sexual dysfunction, other potential causes such as underlying vascular or cardiac disease, anxiety, depression, or comorbidities should be investigated (Fig. 1).

In cases of ED, treatment with phosphodiesterase-5 inhibitors (PDE5i) has been proven safe in patients with stable cardiac diseases. Recent observational data even suggests a lower risk of death in men with stable coronary artery disease treated with PDE5i compared to alprostadil treatment [16]. However, the concomitant use of nitrates and PDE5i is contraindicated due to the potentially dangerous reduction in blood pressure they may cause. In patients experiencing chest pain, nitrates should not be administered until at least 24 h after the last dose [1]. Healthcare workers should inquire about PDE5 inhibitor use when evaluating patients

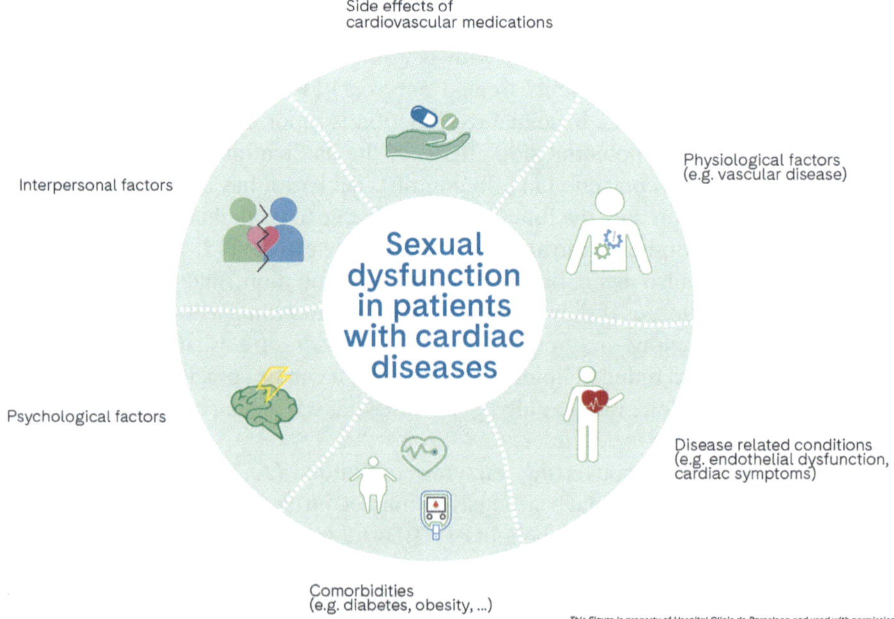

Fig. 1 Factors related to sexual dysfunction in patients with cardiac diseases

presenting with chest pain to avoid the administration of nitrates in combination with these medications.

Finally, due to their potential hypotensive effect, caution is advised when using PDE5i in patients with severe aortic stenosis or obstructive hypertrophic cardiomyopathy [1].

4 General Recommendations for the Cardiovascular Patient

4.1 Cardiovascular Responses to Sexual Activity

Several studies, primarily conducted in men who are either healthy or have coronary artery disease, have examined the cardiovascular changes that occur during sexual activity. During foreplay and arousal, a mild increase in systolic and diastolic blood pressure and heart rate is observed, with a further increase during orgasm. Both blood pressure and heart rate return to baseline levels shortly afterward. Additionally, sexual intercourse leads to a modest increase in oxygen consumption, which is only sustained for a short duration. Importantly, these changes are not significantly different from those observed during other daily activities [1, 17, 18].

Although there is considerable individual variability and differences based on specific sexual activities, most authors agree that the cardiovascular workload during sexual activity is comparable to mild to moderate physical activity or three to five metabolic equivalents (METS) [1, 17, 18].

4.2 Is There a Significant Cardiovascular Risk Associated with Sexual Activity?

Sexual activity is associated with a small but significant increase in the risk of cardiovascular events, and may trigger MI, arrhythmia, or sudden cardiac death (SCD) in susceptible individuals. However, despite this association, the absolute risk of events is small due to infrequent exposure to sexual activity and its transient effects [1, 18, 19]. The estimated absolute risk of MI associated with 1 h of sexual activity per week is 2–3 per 10,000 person-years, and the absolute risk of sudden death is <1 per 10,000 person-years [1, 19]. More recent data confirms that sexual activity (both solo-sex or partnered-sex) triggers MI in a very small proportion of patients [20].

A meta-analysis of studies investigating the association between sexual activity and MI found an increased risk of MI during sexual activity (RR = 2.70; 95% CI, 1.48–4.91) [19]. Furthermore, some studies have shown that this risk is higher in sedentary patients compared to physically active individuals [21], highlighting the importance of encouraging patients to lead physically active lives.

Regarding SCD, there is some evidence that extramarital sexual activity or engaging in sexual activity in an unfamiliar setting may be associated with an increased risk of SCD. In a forensic study conducted over a 25-year period, deaths occurring during sexual intercourse were predominantly recorded in men, and 75% of these cases involved individuals engaged in extramarital relationships [22]. Excessive alcohol or food consumption may have acted as additional stressors in some cases [18]. A recent report investigating SCD in a younger population (mean age 38 years) found a higher proportion of women (35%), and sudden arrhythmic death syndrome and cardiomyopathies were the predominant underlying causes [23].

In light of the above, scientific cardiology societies agree that sexual activity is reasonable in patients who tolerate low to moderate physical activity or can exercise ≥3–5 METS without cardiovascular symptoms or ECG abnormalities [1, 2]. In cases where exercise tolerance cannot be ascertained or the risk is unclear, an exercise test can be useful. Conversely, patients with unstable, decompensated, or severe symptomatic cardiovascular disease should defer sexual activity until their condition is stabilized (level of recommendation IIIC for both guidelines).

Patients should be informed about the level of risk associated with sexual activity and be educated about warning signs. They should also be encouraged to report any symptoms experienced during sexual activity. If cardiovascular symptoms are triggered by sexual activity, patients should defer sexual activity until their condition is properly managed.

Finally, it is advisable to inform patients that physical exercise is associated with a decreased risk of cardiovascular events.

5 Sexual Health in Cardiovascular Diseases

5.1 Coronary Artery Disease and Myocardial Infarction

Coronary artery disease (CAD) has been reported to be associated with a decrease in sexual activity based on population-based data, both in women and men [24]. Similarly, the diagnosis of myocardial infarction (MI) is also linked to a decrease in sexual activity in the year following the MI [4, 5], with approximately 50% of patients experiencing a reduction in sexual activity and more than 10% reporting no sexual activity [4]. Importantly, as mentioned earlier, the lack of discussion with a physician about sex was found to be predictive of a delay in resuming sexual activity. A recent study showed that maintaining or increasing sexual activity frequency was inversely associated with all-cause mortality [25]. Furthermore, sexual dysfunction is common in both women and men with CAD. A recent study reported a prevalence of ED of 57.8% among patients with early-onset CAD, and this was associated with the severity of coronary atherosclerosis. Interestingly, coronary revascularization appeared to improve ED although this effect was observed only in patients without beta-blocker treatment [26]. In women, the most commonly described sexual problems are lack of interest and trouble with lubrication (39% and 22% in one study—(5)). Some data suggest a decreased sexual function in partners of MI patients [27].

As discussed earlier, the risks associated with sexual activity are very low if the patient can tolerate mild to moderate exercise (or ≥3–5 METs) without experiencing ischemia. A study with stable CAD patients found no cases of coital angina in patients with a normal exercise test [28], emphasizing the role of exercise testing in CAD.

Therefore, sexual activity can be resumed 1 week after MI, provided the patient can tolerate mild to moderate physical exercise [1, 2]. Patients with stable CAD should undergo an initial assessment of risk: cases of mild, stable angina are considered low risk, whereas patients with unstable or refractory angina are considered high risk, and sexual activity should be deferred until their condition stabilizes. Exercise testing can be useful in patients with unclear exercise tolerance.

Patients who have undergone complete revascularization through percutaneous coronary intervention (PCI) may typically resume sexual activity within a few days, assuming there are no vascular access complications [1]. In cases of incomplete revascularization, it may be advisable to check symptoms or exercise tolerance before resuming sexual activity.

5.2   Cardiac Surgery

Similarly to CAD patients, individuals undergoing cardiac surgery may often not receive sufficient information regarding sexual activity, which can lead to a decrease in sexual activity after surgery [29]. Initial randomized data suggest that adding sexual therapy to cardiac rehabilitation may improve sexual activity in patients after coronary bypass graft [7].

In addition to the general recommendations, the integrity of the sternotomy should be considered in sexual counseling. In general, it is reasonable to resume sexual activity 6 to 8 weeks after standard coronary or non-coronary open-heart surgery, provided that sternotomy complications are ruled out [1, 2]. In the early stages after surgery, it is advisable to avoid sexual positions that put strain on the sternum.

In recent years, there has been an increase in minimal-access cardiac surgery and robot-assisted surgery. In these cases, resumption of sexual activity may be possible earlier than with conventional sternotomy. A study including only men undergoing mitral valve surgery found that a total endoscopic approach was associated with a lower rate of postoperative sexual dysfunction [30].

5.3   Heart Failure and Heart Transplantation

Sexual dysfunction is highly prevalent in patients with heart failure (HF), with rates ranging from 60 to 87% [31]. The most commonly encountered problems are reduced lubrication in women and ED in men [31]. The prevalence of sexual dysfunction may also vary during the course of the disease, with more than one-quarter of patients without problems after hospital discharge developing them over time [32].

Regarding heart transplantation, data is limited, with a small study finding a prevalence of sexual dysfunction of 61% in this subset of patients [33]. Another small report found a lower prevalence of dysfunction, with heart transplant patients reporting higher satisfaction with their sex life compared to those with a left ventricular assist device [34].

In patients with HF, the risk associated with sexual activity is determined by their exercise tolerance. Patients classified as New York Heart Association (NYHA) class I-II are at a low risk for sex-triggered events compared to individuals in NYHA classes III-IV, for whom sexual activity should be deferred until their condition is stabilized [1, 2, 31].

Some data suggest that sexual dysfunction may improve after cardiac resynchronization therapy implantation, along with an improvement in exercise capacity [35].

5.4 Arrhythmia and Implantable Cardioverter Defibrillators

Although sexual activity can occasionally induce heart rhythm abnormalities, the risk of SCD during sexual activity is rare, with a recent study reporting a frequency of 0.2% of all SCD cases [23]. Current guidelines agree that the risk of malignant arrhythmias is low in stable patients who tolerate moderate physical activity [1, 2].

In one of the few studies investigating this topic, ventricular ectopic activity (but not life-threatening arrhythmias) was detected in more than half of men with CAD [36]. Another study including men with an implantable cardioverter-defibrillator (ICD) showed a high prevalence of ED (70%), reduced interest in sex (83%), and orgasmic dysfunction (58%) [37].

As with patients with HF and CAD, if moderate exercise does not trigger symptoms such as arrhythmia or ICD discharge (in the case of patients with an ICD), sexual activity is generally considered safe [1, 2]. Sex is also considered safe in well-controlled supraventricular arrhythmias and in patients with an ICD implanted for primary prevention. However, patients and their partners may have concerns about the potential for an ICD shock during sex or causing harm to their partner [38]. These concerns should be addressed by healthcare providers.

Conversely, sexual activity should be deferred until stabilization in cases of uncontrolled supraventricular or ventricular arrhythmias, as well as in patients receiving multiple ICD shocks [1].

5.5 Congenital Heart Disease

Research suggests that individuals with congenital heart disease (CHD) often have concerns about engaging in sexual activity and report low levels of sexual enjoyment, with women being more insecure about it than men. Interestingly, the degree of sexual problems experienced is not necessarily related to the severity of the heart defect. However, individuals with a worse NYHA class tend to report lower levels of sexual enjoyment and arousal, as well as more concerns about sexual activity [39].

A recent report studying 37 sexually active men with Fontan circulation found that 24% of them experienced ED, mostly of mild severity. The Fontan cohort also reported decreased levels of sexual desire and satisfaction [40].

It is important to note that the CHD population is typically younger than other cardiac conditions discussed in this chapter. Therefore, in addition to the general recommendations mentioned earlier (tolerance to mild to moderate physical exercise and optimizing treatment in cases of decompensation), access to contraception and the avoidance of unwanted pregnancies should also be considered, particularly for individuals at high risk of pregnancy-related cardiovascular complications [1]. A large study of women with CHD found that over 40% of them had not received counseling about contraception or been informed about the risks associated with pregnancy. Additionally, one in five women was using a contraceptive method that was contraindicated for their condition [41].

6   Gaps of Knowledge

Despite the significant impact of sexual health on overall quality of life, there is limited evidence available for most of the topics discussed in this chapter. International guidelines have not been updated since 2013, and many of the recommendations included in these guidelines have a Level of Evidence B or C, emphasizing the need for further research in this important area.

There is a notable issue of underrepresentation in the available studies, particularly with regard to women, older individuals, and patients in the LGBTQIA+ community. As mentioned earlier, women are less likely to receive sexual counseling at discharge [3], and they may also be less inclined to discuss their sexual concerns with healthcare practitioners [42]. Additionally, recent reports have highlighted the overall poorer cardiovascular health among members of the LGBTQIA+ community [43]. Therefore, it is crucial to increase their representation in future research in order to provide tailored counseling and support.

7   Conclusions

Sexual counseling is crucial for cardiovascular patients, but it is often neglected in clinical practice. Healthcare professionals should be trained in sexual assessment, communication, and counseling. Although some cardiovascular medications can cause sexual dysfunction, they are far from the main cause of dysfunction in this group of patients, and other physical or psychological causes should be ruled out. The absolute risk of cardiovascular events linked to sexual activity is low. Patients should be educated about the risks and encouraged to lead physically active lives. Sexual activity should be considered safe if mild to moderate physical exercise is tolerated. Conversely, in decompensated pathologies, sexual activity should be deferred until stabilization. Exercise testing can be useful in cases where patient exercise tolerance is unclear. There is a need for further research, especially including groups underrepresented in previous studies.

References

1. Levine GN, Steinke EE, Bakaeen FG, et al. Sexual activity and cardiovascular disease. Circulation. 2012;125:1058–72.
2. Steinke EE, Jaarsma T, Barnason SA, et al. Sexual counselling for individuals with cardiovascular disease and their partners. Eur Heart J. 2013;34:3217–35.
3. Lindau ST, Abramsohn EM, Bueno H, et al. Sexual activity and counseling in the first month after acute myocardial infarction among younger adults in the United States and Spain. Circulation. 2014;130:2302–9.
4. Lindau ST, Abramsohn E, Gosch K, et al. Patterns and loss of sexual activity in the year following hospitalization for acute myocardial infarction (a United States National Multisite Observational Study). Am J Cardiol. 2012;109:1439–44.
5. Lindau ST, Abramsohn E, Bueno H, et al. Sexual activity and function in the year after an acute myocardial infarction among younger women and men in the United States and Spain. JAMA Cardiol. 2016;1:754.
6. Salehian R, Khodaeifar F, Naserbakht M, Meybodi A. Attitudes and performance of cardiologists toward sexual issues in cardiovascular patients. Sex. Med. 2017;5:e44–53.
7. Klein R, Bar-on E, Klein J, Benbenishty R. The impact of sexual therapy on patients after cardiac events participating in a cardiac rehabilitation program. Eur J Cardiovasc Prev Rehabil. 2007;14:672–8.
8. Rosman L, Cahill JM, McCammon SL, Sears SF. Sexual health concerns in patients with cardiovascular disease. Circulation. 2014;129:e313–6.
9. La Torre A, Giupponi G, Duffy D, Conca A, Catanzariti D. Sexual dysfunction related to drugs: a critical review. Part IV: Cardiovascular drugs. Pharmacopsychiatry. 2014;48:1–6.
10. Ko DT, Hebert PR, Coffey CS, Sedrakyan A, Curtis JP, Krumholz HM. β-Blocker therapy and symptoms of depression, fatigue, and sexual dysfunction. JAMA. 2002;288:351.
11. Silvestri A, Galetta P, Cerquetani E, et al. Report of erectile dysfunction after therapy with beta-blockers is related to patient knowledge of side effects and is reversed by placebo. Eur Heart J. 2003;24:1928–32.
12. Brixius K, Middeke M, Lichtenthal A, Jahn E, Schwinger RHG. NITRIC OXIDE, ERECTILE DYSFUNCTION AND BETA-BLOCKER TREATMENT (MR NOED STUDY): BENEFIT OF NEBIVOLOL VERSUS METOPROLOL IN HYPERTENSIVE MEN. Clin Exp Pharmacol Physiol. 2007;34:327–31.
13. Kaplan-Marans E, Sandozi A, Martinez M, Lee J, Schulman A, Khurgin J. Medications Most commonly associated with erectile dysfunction: evaluation of the Food and Drug Administration National Pharmacovigilance Database. Sex Med. 2022;10:–100543.
14. Shindel A, Kishore S, Lue T. Drugs designed to improve endothelial function: effects on erectile dysfunction. Curr Pharm Des. 2008;14:3758–67.
15. Cui Y, Zong H, Yan H, Zhang Y. The effect of statins on erectile dysfunction: a systematic review and meta-analysis. J Sex Med. 2014;11:1367–75.
16. Andersson DP, Landucci L, Lagerros YT, et al. Association of Phosphodiesterase-5 inhibitors versus Alprostadil with survival in men with coronary artery disease. J Am Coll Cardiol. 2021;77:1535–50.
17. Cheitlin MD. Sexual activity and cardiac risk. Am J Cardiol. 2005;96:24–8.
18. Drory Y. Sexual activity and cardiovascular risk. Eur Hear J Suppl. 2002;4:H13–8.
19. Dahabreh IJ, Paulus JK. Association of Episodic Physical and Sexual Activity with Triggering of acute cardiac events. JAMA. 2011;305:1225.
20. Rothenbacher D, Dallmeier D, Mons U, Rosamond W, Koenig W, Brenner H. Sexual activity patterns before myocardial infarction and risk of subsequent cardiovascular adverse events. J Am Coll Cardiol. 2015;66:1516–7.

21. Moller J, Ahlbom A, Hulting J, et al. Sexual activity as a trigger of myocardial infarction. A case-crossover analysis in the Stockholm Heart Epidemiology Programme (SHEEP). Heart. 2001;86:387–90.
22. Parzeller M, Raschka C, Bratzke H. Sudden cardiovascular death in correlation with sexual activity—results of a medicolegal postmortem study from 1972–1998. Eur Heart J. 2001;22:610–1.
23. Finocchiaro G, Westaby J, Behr ER, Papadakis M, Sharma S, Sheppard MN. Association of Sexual Intercourse with Sudden Cardiac Death in young individuals in the United Kingdom. JAMA Cardiol. 2022;7:358.
24. Steptoe A, Jackson SE, Wardle J. Sexual activity and concerns in people with coronary heart disease from a population-based study. Heart. 2016;102:1095–9.
25. Cohen G, Nevo D, Hasin T, Benyamini Y, Goldbourt U, Gerber Y. Resumption of sexual activity after acute myocardial infarction and long-term survival. Eur J Prev Cardiol. 2022;29:304–11.
26. Dai Y, Mei Z, Zhang S, et al. Sexual dysfunction and the impact of Beta-blockers in young males with coronary artery disease. Front Cardiovasc Med. 2021;8:8.
27. Arenhall E, Eriksson M, Nilsson U, Steinke EE, Fridlund B. Decreased sexual function in partners after patients' first-time myocardial infarction. Eur J Cardiovasc Nurs. 2018;17:521–6.
28. Drory Y, Shapira I, Fisman EZ, Pines A. Myocardial ischemia during sexual activity in patients with coronary artery disease. Am J Cardiol. 1995;75:835–7.
29. Ghazy T, Haeberle E, Kappert U, et al. Sexual quality of life in men <60 years old after coronary bypass surgery. Heart Surg Forum. 2021;24:E480–6.
30. Yan L, Tang M, Dai X, Chen L, Fang G. Impact of minimally invasive mitral valve surgery on sexual dysfunction in male patients. J Cardiothorac Surg. 2022;17:77.
31. Jaarsma T. Sexual function of patients with heart failure: facts and numbers. ESC Hear Fail. 2017;4:3–7.
32. Hoekstra T, Jaarsma T, Sanderman R, van Veldhuisen DJ, Lesman-Leegte I. Perceived sexual difficulties and associated factors in patients with heart failure. Am Heart J. 2012;163:246–51.
33. Phan A, IsHak WW, Shen B-J, et al. Persistent sexual dysfunction impairs quality of life after cardiac transplantation. J Sex Med. 2010;7:2765–73.
34. Hasin T, Jaarsma T, Murninkas D, et al. Sexual function in patients supported with left ventricular assist device and with heart transplant. ESC Hear Fail. 2014;1:103–9.
35. Vural A, Agacdiken A, Celikyurt U, et al. Effect of cardiac resynchronization therapy on libido and erectile dysfunction. Clin Cardiol. 2011;34:437–41.
36. Drory Y, Fisman EZ, Shapira Y, Pines A. Ventricular arrhythmias during sexual activity in patients with coronary artery disease. Chest. 1996;109:922–4.
37. Palm P, Zwisler A-D, Svendsen JH, Giraldi A, Rasmussen ML, Berg SK. Compromised sexual health among male patients with implantable cardioverter defibrillator: a cross-sectional questionnaire study. Sex Med. 2019;7:169–76.
38. Steinke EE, Gill-Hopple K, Valdez D, Wooster M. Sexual concerns and educational needs after an implantable cardioverter defibrillator. Hear Lung. 2005;34:299–308.
39. Moons P, Van Deyk K, Marquet K, De Bleser L, Budts W, De Geest S. Sexual functioning and congenital heart disease: something to worry about? Int J Cardiol. 2007;121:30–5.
40. Rubenis I, Tran D, Bullock A, et al. Sexual function in men living with a Fontan circulation. Front Pediatr. 2021;9:9.
41. Vigl M, Kaemmerer M, Seifert-Klauss V, et al. Contraception in women with congenital heart disease. Am J Cardiol. 2010;106:1317–21.
42. Fischer S, Bekelman D. Gender differences in sexual interest or activity among adults with symptomatic heart failure. J Palliat Med. 2017;20:890–4.
43. Caceres BA, Streed CG, Corliss HL, et al. Assessing and addressing cardiovascular health in LGBTQ adults: a scientific statement from the American Heart Association. Circulation. 2020;142:e321.

Sexual Health in Post-Stroke Patients

Mònica Serrano, Carla Box, and Inés García-Bouyssou

1   Stroke

In the European Union (EU), cerebrovascular accident (CVA) or stroke is the second leading cause of death and is one of the leading causes of disability in adults. It affects approximately 1.1 million Europeans each year and causes about 440,000 deaths [1]. However, the number of stroke survivors continues to increase and therefore more individuals must learn to cope with the long-term sequalae associated with a stroke.

The World Health Organization (WHO) defines stroke as a clinical syndrome, presumably of vascular etiology, characterized by rapidly developing signs of focal (or global) impairment of brain function, lasting greater than 24 h or that leads to death, without any other apparent cause.

The lack of cerebral blood flow causes a loss in oxygen and glucose supply due to either vascular occlusion (ischemic stroke) or cerebral hemorrhage (hemorrhagic stroke). This lack of blood supply produces changes in the cells' metabolism and

M. Serrano
Clinical Institute of Neurosciences, Hospital Clínic de Barcelona, Barcelona, Spain
e-mail: moserrano@clinic.cat

C. Box (✉)
Clinical Institute of Medical and Surgical Specialties, Hospital Clinic de Barcelona,
Barcelona, Spain

Clinical Sexology Working Group, Hospital Clinic de Barcelona,
Barcelona, Spain
e-mail: cebox@clinic.cat

I. García-Bouyssou
Clinical Institute of Medical and Surgical Specialties, Hospital Clinic de Barcelona,
Barcelona, Spain
e-mail: ingarcia@clinic.cat

© The Author(s), under exclusive license to Springer Nature Switzerland AG 2024
C. Castelo-Branco, S. Anglès Acedo (eds.), *Medical Disorders and Sexual Health*, Trends in Andrology and Sexual Medicine,
https://doi.org/10.1007/978-3-031-55080-5_23

ultimately leads to necrosis and death of neurons in the region of where the stroke occurred. In addition, depending on where the stroke occurs, there will be certain clinical consequences, which may cause severe disability [1]. This is why early treatment is necessary to stop said process and prevent neuronal death. The stroke protocol or code has been implemented in most countries within the last 10–20 years, with the goal of improving early diagnosis and treatment and enhancing understanding of the concept "time is brain." Hence, early diagnosis and treatment are critical for improving survival rates and decreasing long-term morbidity in patients who suffer strokes.

1.1 Clinical Consequences of Stroke

The WHO's International Classification of Functioning, Disability, and Health classifies the effects of diseases such as stroke as those problems related to "bodily functions and structure," "activity," and "participation." Most stroke survivors have residual disabilities, such as hemiparesis, spasticity, post-stroke fatigue, headache, and cognitive dysfunctions such as executive dysfunction and/or memory loss, mood disorders, language disorders such as aphasia and dysarthria, and both urinary and anal incontinence, among others [2]. Complete recovery is only achieved in a small proportion of stroke survivors. These issues appear in the acute phase, and some of them can become chronic. Depending on the location of the stroke, both the symptoms and the complexity of the clinical cases will vary.

2 Correlation Between the Location of the Stroke and Changes in Sexual Function

During an acute stroke, autonomic dysfunction has been observed to occur which can affect the autonomic nervous system, the respiratory, cardiovascular, genitourinary, and sexual systems. Regarding sexual dysfunction, decrease in libido and in coital frequency are common in men, whereas reduction in vaginal lubrication and orgasmic capacity are common among women [3].

Regarding the relationship between sexual dysfunction and anatomical location, it has been seen that the right hemisphere plays an important role in activation/attention of libido and erectile functionality. Right middle cerebral artery strokes produce perceptual neglect (inattention to the left side of the environment), thus interfering with erotic sensations, in addition to hypoesthesia or anesthesia. Lacunar strokes which affect frontolimbic connections can cause hypersexuality. On the other hand, regarding subarachnoid hemorrhages, the presence of blood in the region of the basal cisterns and the third ventricle can cause hypothalamopituitary dysfunction and deficiencies in growth hormone, gonadotrophin, or both [4].

Jung JH et al. [5] described the relationship between the location of the stroke and the subsequent appearance of sexual dysfunctions in men. A survey was conducted on 109 male stroke patients and 109 male control patients of a similar age. A significant decrease in erectile function was observed in the subjects who had suffered a stroke compared to the control group. It was also reported that lesions in the right cerebellum were associated with ejaculation disorders, while lesions in the left basal ganglia were associated with decreased sexual desire. Studies of functional neuroanatomy and brain control of sexual function have found that the limbic system, including the hippocampus, dentate gyrus, and gyrus in relation to the thalamus and hypothalamus, play important roles in emotional changes, memory, and patterns of sexual behavior.

Additionally, Calabrò et al. [6], described the relationship between brain areas and sex-related functions in men, such as the modulation of sexual drive being controlled by the amygdala, septal region, prefrontal cortex, cingulate cortex, and insula; and sexual motivation being triggered by the reward system. Others include relays in erotic stimuli coming from the spinal cord via the thalamus, the awareness of tumescence of erectile organs by the insula and the coordination of autonomic events in sexual behavior being processed by the hypothalamus. Different areas, both cortical and subcortical, seem to influence different aspects of sexual behavior.

Unfortunately, no data about correlation of female sexual function and location of stroke is available.

3   Sexuality in Post-stroke Patients

The WHO defined sexuality in 2006 as a broad concept that can be experienced and expressed in multiple ways through thoughts, fantasies, desires, beliefs, attitudes, values, behaviors, practices, roles, and relationships. Sexuality is an important aspect of quality of life for both cisgender and transgender people. This concept is understood from a biopsychosocial perspective.

The importance of addressing sexuality after stroke has been highlighted in clinical guidelines for stroke rehabilitation and by stroke survivors. However, the literature shows that most professionals, regardless of their profession or geographic location, do not routinely include approaching the patient's sexuality in their clinical practice [7]. This is a major omission and there is an urgent need for change so that stroke survivors receive the best rehabilitation program.

The impairment of sexual function or activity in stroke survivors is common as sexual function may be diminished or in some cases even absent in both genders and partner dissatisfaction is high [8]. In addition to a change in sexual activity, a decrease in sexual satisfaction has also been observed in stroke patients and their partners [9].

It has been described that the sexual dysfunction in these patients has been undertreated by healthcare professionals [7] despite being directly related to quality of life. For sexual health to be attained and maintained, the sexual rights of all persons must be respected, protected, and fulfilled [10].

In a review of qualitative studies about cis-female and cis-male patients and their partners' perspective, without specifying sexual orientation, two main themes emerged: (1) sexuality is silenced in these patients, and (2) despite this silence surrounding sexuality, sexuality itself is not forgotten by the patient [11]. Said review found that the issues that stroke survivors reported included difficulty in communicating during relationships, health professionals not discussing sexuality, sexuality together with disability continuing to be a taboo subject, changes in personal prestroke relationships, changes in the relationship with one's body and resuming sexual intimacy—adaptation and loss [11]. In addition, all of this directly coincides with the clinical consequences of stroke which can alter the relationship between romantic partners and turn the relationship into one of a caregiver and recipient of care [7].

In most cases, sexual frequency decreases following a stroke, with sexual activity declining by as much as 70% the frequency of intercourse after a stroke becoming monthly or even less frequent. In previously sexually active cis-men and cis-women, this in turn causes a reduction in sexual satisfaction, which ranges from 50 to 75% [12]. This sexual dissatisfaction can be a factor that influences the affected person and causes negative physical changes such as changes in sexual arousal, changes in orgasm, as well as lack of lubrication, erection, or ejaculation. In severe strokes, movement difficulties may appear and will influence the positioning of the body and may affect the way of moving during sexual intercourse.

Another aspect to consider in post-stroke patients is the connection between the presence and management of urinary and anal incontinence and sexual functioning. It has been observed that patients with incontinence refuse to have sexual relations with their partners and that this incontinence affects between 40 and 60% of post-stroke patients [13] and these deficits, UI or IA as well as drooling, are considered as unattractive behavior [8].

As for transgender people, the use of cross-sex hormonal therapies (CHT) and gender affirming surgery (GAS) can affect their sexual function such as sexual desire or sexual interest, arousal and ability to reach orgasm. In addition, body image, self-esteem, psychological wellbeing, and sexual anxiety are also aspects to be considered in health and sexual satisfaction [14]. There are no data linking transgender individuals who have suffered a stroke to post-stroke sexual dysfunction.

It is important to consider that there is still a very coitus-centric, binary conception of sexual activity that is studied from a cis-gender perspective. Gender is also a determinant of health, influencing the physical and social environments to which people are exposed, their access to resources that affect their health, their ability to seek health care and receive treatment, and the equity of the research that drives medical advances [15].

4   Factors After a Stroke That Affect Sexual Dysfunction

The alteration of sexual activity or function can be produced by modifications of biological factors and/or by psychosocial factors, such as the reduction or disappearance of sexual desire, arousal, or orgasm (Fig. 1).

4.1   Body Image, Self-Esteem, and Self-Efficacy

The self is a complex concept that involves different areas of the individual. Changes in the post-stroke survivor's body image can have different etiological bases, such as involving perceptual dysfunctions, however, in some cases these bases may not

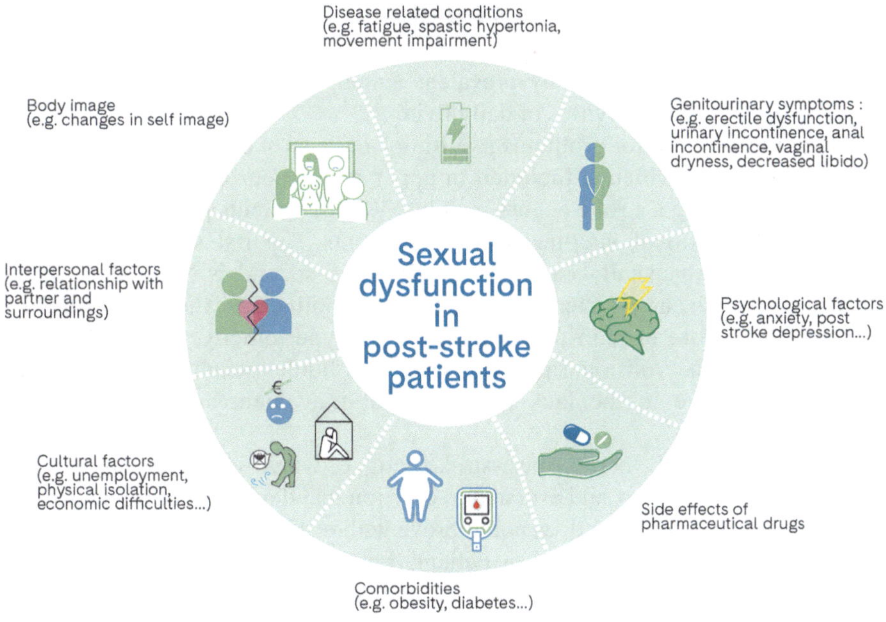

Fig. 1 Sexual dysfunction in post-stroke patients

be primarily perceptual. These body image evaluations have implications for global evaluations of the self and for self-esteem [16]. Self-esteem represents an individual's global self-evaluation or perceived worth as a person. In the case of body image evaluations, there are gender differences, for instance, women have greater difficulty experiencing their bodies positively [17]. Body image and self-esteem may be affected in post-stroke patients.

There is another construct that captures self-evaluation, known as self-concept. This construct represents a collection of evaluative judgments of attributes within discrete or multidimensional domains, such as cognitive competence, social acceptance, and physical appearance, in patients with brain injury. This view of themselves changes negatively, and this can affect mood and participation in rehabilitation. A study showed that patients with acquired brain injury (ABI) (stroke and traumatic brain injury) have lower total self-concept ratings than the control group and it also showed lower self-esteem. Individual item analyses suggested that the ABI survivors rated themselves overall as "undesirable" and doubtful about their own self-worth [18].

Self-efficacy is a psychological construct that has been defined as people's beliefs about their capabilities to produce designated levels of performance that exercise influence over events that affect their lives [18, 19]. In people with stroke, this variable of self-efficacy perception could be relevant for outcomes like quality of life (or perceived health status), depression, activities of the daily living (ADL), and, to a certain extent, physical function [20].

4.2 Spastic Hypertonia and Fatigue

These two symptoms are highly prevalent among post-stroke patients, limiting basic and instrumental activities of daily living.

One of the main motor problems resulting from a stroke is hyper-resistance or spastic hypertonia, which is included in upper motor neuron syndrome criteria. Spasticity following a stroke occurs in about 30% of patients [21] increased tone can have two functional outcomes in stroke patients. The first is hypertonia in the upper limbs which usually causes disability. The second is hypertonia in the lower limbs which can interfere with standing. In both cases, the aim of physical therapy is to restore or gain functionality. This hypertonicity, which cannot be controlled from the volitional point of view, can hinder sexual functioning and sexual activity due to the lack of functional movement and reduced range of motion.

On the other hand, there is post-stroke fatigue, which is the feeling of early exhaustion, lack of energy and aversion to exertion that develops during physical or mental activity and normally does not improve with rest [22]. These symptoms have not been widely studied in post-stroke patients, but the presence of fatigue, decreased sensitivity and post-stroke pain have been associated with decreased interest and sexual function [23].

4.3 Genitourinary Symptoms

4.3.1 Urinary Incontinence

Several studies indicate that the lesion of the frontal lobe, the area in charge of urination, is what can favor the appearance of UI after a stroke. Unfortunately, no data was found regarding UI and sexual dysfunction in post-stroke patients. However, according to the literature, UI has negative impact on sexual function. As stated by a systematic review regarding women's sexual health and UI, it is probable that this affection, directly or indirectly, contributes decisively to the avoidance of women in having sex [24]. In another study, in older population, self-reported UI was associated with impairment in sexual health in women and men, and mainly linked to recent declines in sexual activity and function along with elevated sexual concerns [25].

During the first month post stroke, urinary incontinence (UI) may affect around half of the population of stroke survivors. A significant proportion of stroke survivors, less than half of the population, will still be incontinent at 3 months and just over one-third of stroke survivors will remain incontinent at 12 months post stroke [26]. The disorders experienced may range from urinary retention to complete incontinence. The most common types of problems are an increase in urinary frequency, urinary urgency, and urge incontinence [27].

Improvement is common over time [27], which suggests that problems with continence may be transient in some stroke survivors or amenable to intervention, or both [26].

Due to the lack of studies regarding the impact UI has on sexuality in post-stroke patients, we would recommend further research take place. In the case that UI does occur, it is recommended that it be treated to hopefully contribute to improving sexual function.

4.3.2   Anal Incontinence

Anal incontinence (AI) has also been described as a post-stroke sequela. Brocklehurst et al. found that 23% of both cis-female and cis-male stroke survivors were incontinent during the first year after stroke [28]. These episodes of anal incontinence may last until hospital discharge, but in other cases may persist in time. These episodes and the changes they cause in the patient who suffers from them can affect sexual function. Therefore, carrying out treatment for AI is recommended.

It is important to promote using the toilet rather than using other hygienic materials such as diapers to encourage the patient's autonomy and possibly help prevent or improve UI and AI as well as avoiding self-image problems to an extent when treating in-patients.

4.3.3   Vaginal Dryness

Vaginal mucosa dryness, which is one of the most described symptoms in post-stroke patients with a prevalence of 46% [9], has a negative impact on sexual arousal and sexual satisfaction. Vaginal dryness contributes to a decrease in sexual desire in many cases and even causes pain during intercourse. In addition, suffering a stroke has repercussions in many cases in orgasmic capacity with 55% of post-stroke cis-female patients experiencing this condition [9].

4.3.4   Erectile Dysfunction

Erectile dysfunction is one of the most common sequelae in post-stroke patients. The results of numerous studies show that International Index for Erectile Function-5 (IIEF-5) values reflect moderate/severe erectile dysfunction in this patient population, as well as ejaculation problems [29]. The patient's age also must be considered because there is a significant correlation with the decrease in sexual function, and furthermore, patients with two or more brain lesions have a significant decrease in erectile function compared with patients with one lesion [5].

Moreover, it is important to determine if these patients are taking medications, such as antihypertensive medications that may contribute to erectile dysfunction and some of them (β blockers) can reduce desire as well. They may have other comorbidities, such as diabetes mellitus, which can contribute to sexual dysfunction [9].

4.4   Psychological Aspects After a Stroke That Affect Sexual Dysfunction

There are a number of psychological factors in post-stroke patients that may affect sexual function. The most significant factors include post-stroke depression (PSD), anxiety, fear of rejection by the sexual partner, sleep problems, and fear of suffering another stroke during sexual intercourse. PSD is a frequent neuropsychiatric manifestation that affects one third of stroke survivors [30] and negatively affects the recovery, rehabilitation, and quality of life of patients who suffer from it. It is also related to higher mortality [30]. An observational study described a strong association between depression and post-stroke sexual dysfunction [31]. The tendency of stroke survivors to develop depressive symptoms, anxiety, and other mood disorders can affect sexual behavior. It has also been described that sexual dysfunction or loss of sexual desire after a stroke can contribute to the appearance of depression as well as a loss of self-esteem. The causes of changes in mood appear to be related to difficulties in performing activities of daily living. The severity of neurological deficits decreased sexual intercourse frequency when compared to patients with milder deficits [32].

5   Sexuality Assessment Tools in Post-stroke Patients

Sexual function or sexual activity is a broad and complex aspect of life that is difficult to evaluate. In general, according to the literature, post-stroke sexuality is mainly evaluated using quantitative methods [33]. These quantitative methods include: (1) global questionnaires used for these particular patients which also include sexual function items or, (2) questionnaires designed to assess sexuality such as the Female Sexual Function Index (FSFI), IIEF, among others. Qualitative methods such as interviews or open-ended questionnaires can also be useful.

5.1   Questionnaires for Post-stroke Patients

In the case of post-stroke patients, some questionnaires are used to assess different aspects of quality of life which also include some items that mention sexual function or sexual activity in all genders such as the Quality of Life Index—Stroke Version, the Stroke Impact Scale and the Canadian Occupational Performance Measure.

5.2   Sexual Function Questionnaires

Within the sexual health questionnaires, some options are included for specific genders (FSFI, IIEF…) in addition to questionnaires that can be used for all genders (CSFQ-14), see Table 1.

After a thorough review of the literature on the topic of sexuality, a significant finding was that women's sexuality is not studied nearly as frequently as is men's sexuality. In a systematic review presented in 2021, it was observed that gender-specific questionnaires are used six times more for men than for women [33]. According to the literature, women are less represented than men in studies regarding post-stroke sexuality [34–37].

Table 1 Sexuality assessment scales in post-stroke patients

Sexuality assessment scales in post-stroke patients
Post-stroke questionnaires
The quality of life index—stroke version
The stroke impact scale
The Canadian occupational performance measure
Sexual function questionnaires
Women
Female sexual function index-19 (FSFI-19)
Female sexual function index-9 (FSFI-9)
Men
International index for erectile function-15 (IIEF-15)
International index for erectile function-5 (IIEF-5)
Female and male version
Change in sexual functioning questionnaire short form (CSFQ-14)
Derogatis sexual functioning inventory (DSFI)
Arizona sexual experience scale (ASEX)
Sexual inhibition/sexual excitation scale (SIS/SES)
Eleven questions about sexual functioning (ESF)
Not gender-specific
Sexual beliefs and information questionnaire (SBIQ)
Index of sexual satisfaction (ISS)
Quality of sexual function scale (QSF)
Post-stroke patients' partner
Quality of sexual function scale (QSF)

5.3 Structured Interviews or Specifically Designed Questionnaires

Qualitative methods, such as structured interviews and open-ended questionnaires, are also useful strategies for assessing post-stroke sexuality. It is recommended that interview questions be designed to cover the issues related to sexuality found to be most affected following a stroke. One option for ensuring that all pertinent topics are addressed would be to use the topics presented by Monga et al. as a guide in developing interview questions. These topics include attitudes towards sexuality, fear of impotence, fear that sexual intercourse will cause a stroke, the ability to talk about sexuality, and a lack of desire to engage in sexual behaviors [34].

5.4 Function and Sexual Activity in Post-stroke Patients' Partners

In most standardized questionnaires, the sexual health of the stroke survivor's partner is not considered, despite being an important contributing factor for why the couple may experience sexual health issues. Therefore, it is also recommended that the Quality of Sexual Function Scale [37] be used to address the partner's point of view because it is the only standardized and non-gender specific tool found that includes this assessment [37].

In conclusion, it is vital that research tools specifically addressing post-stroke sexuality be developed and validated in order to fill the void of validated tools on this topic. Providing healthcare professionals with validated tools will enable them to better assess their stroke patients' and their partners' sexual health needs and determine how best to optimize their care.

6 Role of Healthcare Professionals: Barriers and Limitations in Clinical Practice, Transdisciplinarity

Currently, several international guidelines recommend assessment and treatment of sexual function after stroke. These guidelines are mostly based on consensus and do not address either the types of interventions to be performed or their efficacy [38]. Health education and counseling on sexual activity in post-stroke patients should be addressed by healthcare professionals both at the time of discharge from hospital (acute phase) and in the rehabilitation process (chronic phase). Unfortunately, sexual health is often overlooked although it is of great importance to patients and those with whom they share significant relationships [39]. Such counseling and support should be provided to both the person who has suffered the stroke and their sexual partner(s) and should be initiated by healthcare professionals. Although healthcare professionals recognize the importance of having conversations about sexual health, it is often a difficult experience, especially for those who have not been trained to have these challenging conversations.

A qualitative study carried out by Mellor et al. in which 30 stroke professionals were asked about discussing sexuality with stroke patients reported a number of barriers addressing sexuality, such as lack of motivation, lack of training, organizational constraints, and lack of skills needed to address sexual wellbeing routinely after stroke [40]. Furthermore, in a letter to the editor by Calabrò et al., he described the fact that physicians believe that sexuality is not as important as the injury or illness itself [39].

There is clearly a need for greater awareness among healthcare professionals of the sexual wellbeing of stroke patients. Training is first needed to increase healthcare professionals' awareness of how critical sexuality is to stroke patients' overall health and wellbeing. Once the significance of this issue is understood, ongoing training is required to prepare healthcare professionals to safely and compassionately treat sexual dysfunction and promote sexual wellbeing in this patient population. It is also important to develop communication skills in order to first acknowledge feelings of discomfort in addressing these issues and then learn to adopt a proactive, objective, and compassionate approach, including obtaining consent to raise more sensitive issues as well as providing privacy, time, and an appropriate environment [40].

7 Interventions to Address Sexual Dysfunction in Post-stroke Patients

The recommendation is that sexual health should be addressed during the sub-acute and chronic phases after the stroke; in collaboration with professionals specializing in sexology and sexual health and that the health personnel who treat these patients should receive the necessary training to have the essential knowledge, skills, and abilities to effectively help these patients [39].

Although women have poorer outcomes and are more likely to die after a cerebrovascular event, they are still underrepresented in clinical trials, and this is mirrored by the lack of sex-tailored therapies. A greater effort is needed in the future to ensure improved treatment and quality of life for both sexes.

7.1   Pharmacological Interventions

There are several pharmacological interventions which may be used to address sexual health issues following a stroke. Pharmacological interventions to treat erectile dysfunction include phosphodiesterase-5 inhibitors (e.g., sildenafil, tadalafil, or vardenafil), intracavernosal injections and intraurethral suppositories by increasing blood flow to the penis to achieve and maintain erection. Hormonal treatments, such as testosterone injections may be administered to improve libido and erectile function in men [35]. However, there are no data on how effective these medications are in improving sexual dysfunction after stroke. There are no recommendations regarding when to start pharmacological treatment in men and no general pharmacological recommendations for women.

7.2   Non-pharmacological Intervention

Regarding the physical aspects of sexual activity, as with many other activities that the patient will perform, where there may be limitations of mobility, endurance, pain, or even lack of sensation, it is recommended that modifications or adaptations be made, if necessary. Preferred variations in frequency, type of activity or postures should also be considered. It is recommended that both the patient and their partner be guided in seeking intimacy and pleasure in both coital relations, especially in patients with pain during penetration or erectile dysfunction, as well as in other forms of intimate contact, such as exploring their sexuality from other points of view. This may involve exploring other parts of the body and in different facilitating postures to cover items directly related to sexual function such as arousal, erection, and orgasm.

Healthcare professionals must learn to recognize and question patients in the areas of sexual function: desire, arousal, and orgasm, and expectations of both the affected person and their partner, if there is one, so they can then be referred to healthcare professionals with an expertise in sexual therapy with whom they can carry out therapy.

The role of healthcare professionals with expertise in clinical sexology should be to help the patient resume their sexual life, as they would do with any other daily activity. For this purpose, it is recommended to use the PLISSIT model which is a tool that was developed in the 1970s to assess and manage sexual concerns. This emphasizes the role of giving permission in all steps: permission, limited information, specific suggestions, and intensive therapy (PLISSIT) [35]. In the PLISSIT, the progression from one step to the other is followed in a linear mode and the limitation is getting no feedback from the patients in each of the model's steps. On the other hand, an extended version of the original model, called EX-PLISSIT is done following a cyclic form. This model extends the original one by emphasizing the Permission step during all the different stages so that interaction between healthcare professionals and patients is improved, giving the individuals the opportunity to ask questions or explain their concerns [41].

The topic should be approached gently and respectfully, asking pertinent questions so that the patient feels that they have permission to talk about their concerns and explain them to their healthcare provider, receive information that will benefit them in terms of their sexual health as well as suggestions for their specific case and intensive therapy.

Pelvic floor physiotherapy should be included to treat patients presenting with pelvic pain, genital pain, or other symptoms listed above such as urinary or anal incontinence. Targeted pelvic floor muscle training can sometimes be helpful in treating sexual dysfunction and pelvic floor symptomatology in these patients [35].

As discussed throughout the chapter, many studies refer to the physical limitations that result in functional limitation when it comes to sexual intercourse [3, 5, 6, 9, 13, 28, 29, 42]. One of the approaches promoted by neuro-physiotherapy that has been well supported in the literature task-oriented learning [2]. This is why it might be relevant to train by means of therapeutic physical exercise positions in which the patient is comfortable for sexual practice, such as physiotherapy for bed mobility, as is also done in gait rehabilitation. On the other hand, the importance of sensory information for motor functioning must be considered, as sensory input plays a fundamental role in motor recovery. Another possible objective within the framework of rehabilitation could be to help these patients re-familiarize themselves and feel comfortable with their bodies.

Lifestyle factors have been found to play a key role in sexual health of post-stroke patients. What has been associated with erectile dysfunction in men is the presence of modifiable cardiovascular risk factors. It is therefore important to intervene in lifestyle changes, which include recommended weight, consumption of a healthy diet such as the Mediterranean or plant-based diet, aerobic exercise at least 150 min a week and smoking cessation [43].

As discussed above, sexual dysfunction in post-stroke patients is multifactorial and therefore treatment strategies should be multimodal, encompassing a multidisciplinary team of healthcare professionals and should include treating the primary healthcare problems that may be contributing to sexual dysfunction, such as mobility issues, post-stroke fatigue, and lifestyle as well as various comorbidities.

8   Conclusion

Changes in sexual function, activity, and rehabilitation in post-stroke patients are under-studied. These changes that may occur after such an episode on a personal level as well as in the stroke survivor's relationships are often significant. They can be affected by physical limitations and changes as well as decrease in self-esteem and can even produce changes in roles between family members or partners (e.g., change from partner to caregiver).

Models such as PLISSIT or EX-PLISSIT that put consent at the center of the therapy can help us to establish this conversation with stroke patients. It is important to educate both the patient and their sexual partner about the possible consequences of stroke on their future sexuality and intimacy, and to teach them to ask for help when they may need it. Specialized sexual health care provided by a sexologist, physiotherapist, psychologist, etc. should be a right for all patients suffering from sexual dysfunction.

In the course of writing this chapter, we have noted how limited literature on sexual dysfunction after stroke is. This fact is even more evident when we try to answer questions exclusively related to women (sexuality, motherhood, and menstruation) or the LGBTQIA+ collective. This is why we believe it is vitally important to continue researching sexual dysfunction after stroke in all the areas we have described in this chapter, adding a gender perspective and including sexual and gender diversity.

References

1. Wafa HA, Wolfe CDA, Emmett E, Roth GA, Johnson CO, Wang Y. Burden of stroke in Europe: thirty-year projections of incidence, prevalence, deaths, and disability-adjusted life years. Stroke. 2020;51(8):2418–27.
2. Langhorne P, Coupar F, Pollock A. Motor recovery after stroke: a systematic review. Lancet Neurol. 2009;8:741–54.
3. Korpelainen JT, Sotaniemi KA, Myllylä VV. Autonomic nervous system disorders in stroke. Clin Auton Res. 1999;9(6):325–33.
4. Park JH, Ovbiagele B, Feng W. Stroke and sexual dysfunction—a narrative review. J Neurol Sci. 2015;350(1–2):7–13.
5. Jung JH, Kam SC, Choi SM, Jae SU, Lee SH, Hyun JS. Sexual dysfunction in male stroke patients: correlation between brain lesions and sexual function. Urology. 2008;71(1):99–103.
6. Calabrò RS, Cacciola A, Bruschetta D, Milardi D, Quattrini F, Sciarrone F, et al. Neuroanatomy and function of human sexual behavior: a neglected or unknown issue? Brain Behav. 2019;9(12):e01389.
7. Low MA, Power E, McGrath M. Sexuality after stroke: exploring knowledge, attitudes, comfort and behaviours of rehabilitation professionals. Ann Phys Rehabil Med. 2022;65(2):101547.
8. Rees PM, Fowler CJ, Maas CP. Sexual function in men and women with neurological disorders. Lancet. 2007;369(9560):512–25.
9. Korpelainen JT, Nieminen P, Myllylä VV. Sexual functioning among stroke patients and their spouses. Stroke. 1999;30(4):715–9.
10. WHO. Defining sexual health: report of a technical consultation on sexual health, 2002;28–31. Geneva: World Health Organization; 2006.
11. McGrath M, Lever S, McCluskey A, Power E. How is sexuality after stroke experienced by stroke survivors and partners of stroke survivors? A systematic review of qualitative studies. Clin Rehabil. 2019;33:293–303.
12. Cheung RTF. Sexual functioning in Chinese stroke patients with mild or no disability. Cerebrovasc Dis. 2002;14(2):122–8.
13. Barrett JA. Bladder and bowel problems after stroke. Rev Clin Gerontol. 2002;12:253–67.
14. Getahun D, Nash R, Flanders WD, Baird TC, Becerra-Culqui TA, Cromwell L, et al. Cross-sex hormones and acute cardiovascular events in transgender persons. Ann Intern Med. 2018;169(4):205.

15. Beery AK, Zucker I. Sex bias in neuroscience and biomedical research. Neurosci Biobehav Rev. 2011;35:565–72.
16. Keppel CC, Crowe SF. Changes to body image and self-esteem following stroke in young adults. Neuropsychol Rehabil. 2000;10(1):15–31.
17. Rosenberg M, Schooler C, Schoenbach C, Rosenberg F. Global self-esteem and specific self-esteem: different concepts, different outcomes. Am Sociol Rev. 1995;60(1):141.
18. Ponsford J, Kelly A, Couchman G. Self-concept and self-esteem after acquired brain injury: a control group comparison. Brain Inj. 2014;28(2):146–54.
19. Bandura A. Encyclopedia of mental health, vol. 4. Academic Press; 1994.
20. Jones F, Riazi A. Self-efficacy and self-management after stroke: a systematic review. Disabil Rehabil. 2011;33(10):797–810.
21. Thibaut A, Chatelle C, Ziegler E, Bruno MA, Laureys S, Gosseries O. Spasticity after stroke: physiology, assessment and treatment. Brain Inj. 2013;27:1093–105.
22. Staub F, Bogousslavsky J. Fatigue after stroke: a major but neglected issue. Cerebrovasc Dis. 2001;12(2):75–81.
23. Nilsson MI, Fugl-Meyer K, von Koch L, Ytterberg C. Experiences of sexuality six years after stroke: a qualitative study. J Sexual Med. 2017;14(6):797–803.
24. Pinheiro Sobreira Bezerra LR, Britto DF, Ribeiro Frota IP, Lira do Nascimento S, Morais Brilhante AV, Lucena SV, et al. The impact of urinary incontinence on sexual function: a systematic review. Sex. Med Rev. 2020;8(3):393–402.
25. Lee DM, Tetley J, Pendleton N. Urinary incontinence and sexual health in a population sample of older people. BJU Int. 2018;122(2):300–8.
26. Thomas L, Barrett J, Cross S, French B, Leathley M, Legg L, et al. Prevention and treatment of urinary incontinence after stroke in adults. In: Cochrane database of systematic reviews. Chichester, UK: John Wiley & Sons, Ltd; 2003.
27. Marinkovic SP, Badlani G. Voiding and sexual dysfunction after cerebrovascular accidents. J Urol. 2001;165(2):359–70.
28. Brocklehurst JC, Andrews K, Richards B, Laycock PJ. Incidence and correlates of incontinence in stroke patients. J Am Geriatr Soc. 1985;33(8):540–2.
29. Dusenbury W, Palm Johansen P, Mosack V, Steinke EE. Determinants of sexual function and dysfunction in men and women with stroke: a systematic review. Int J Clin Pract. 2017;71(7):e12969.
30. Castilla-Guerra L, Fernandez Moreno M d C, Esparrago-Llorca G, Colmenero-Camacho MA. Pharmacological management of post-stroke depression. Expert Rev Neurother. 2020;20:157–66.
31. Steinke EE, Jaarsma T, Barnason SA, Byrne M, Doherty S, Dougherty CM, et al. Sexual counseling for individuals with cardiovascular disease and their partners: a consensus document from the American Heart Association and the ESC council on cardiovascular nursing and allied professions (CCNAP). Circulation. 2013;128(18):2075–96.
32. Moon KJ, Chung ML, Hwang SY. The perceived marital intimacy of spouses directly influences the rehabilitation motivation of hospitalized stroke survivors. Clin Nurs Res. 2021;30(4):502–10.
33. Auger LP, Grondin M, Aubertin M, Marois A, Filiatrault J, Rochette A. Interventions used by allied health professionals in sexual rehabilitation after stroke: a systematic review. Top Stroke Rehabil. 2021;28(8):557–72.
34. Monga TN, Lawson JS, Inglis J. Sexual dysfunction in stroke patients. Arch Phys Med Rehabil. 1986;67(1):19–22.
35. Stratton H, Sansom J, Brown-Major A, Anderson P, Ng L. Interventions for sexual dysfunction following stroke. Cochrane Database Syst Rev. 2020;2020:CD011189.
36. Lever S, Pryor J. The impact of stroke on female sexuality. Disabil Rehabil. 2017;39(20):2011–20.
37. Heinemann LAJ, Potthoff P, Heinemann K, Pauls A, Ahlers CJ, Saad F. Scale for quality of sexual function (QSF) as an outcome measure for both genders? J Sex Med. 2005;2(1):82–95.
38. Ng L, Sansom J, Zhang NY, Khan F. Interventions for sexual dysfunction following stroke. Cochrane Database Syst Rev. 2014;2014:CD011189.

39. Calabrò RS, Bramanti P. Post-stroke sexual dysfunction: an overlooked and under-addressed problem. Disabil Rehabil. 2014;36(3):263–4.
40. Mellor RM, Greenfield SM, Dowswell G, Sheppard JP, Quinn T, McManus RJ. Health care professionals' views on discussing sexual wellbeing with patients who have had a stroke: a qualitative study. PLoS One. 2013;8(10):e78802.
41. Taylor B, Davis S. Using the extended PLISSIT model to address sexual healthcare needs. Nurs Stand. 2006;21(11):35–40.
42. Frigerio M, Barba M, Cola A, Braga A, Celardo A, Munno GM, et al. Quality of life, psychological wellbeing, and sexuality in women with urinary incontinence—where are we now: a narrative review. Medicina (Lithuania). 2022;58(4):525.
43. Ostfeld RJ, Allen KE, Aspry K, Brandt EJ, Spitz A, Liberman J, et al. Vasculogenic erectile dysfunction: the impact of diet and lifestyle. Am J Med. 2021;134:310–6.

Multiple Sclerosis and Sexual Dysfunction

Maria Sepúlveda Gázquez

1   Introduction

Multiple sclerosis (MS) is a demyelinating inflammatory and neurodegenerative disease of the central nervous system (CNS) that commonly affects young people. Clinical disease is characterized by acute episodes (relapses) of inflammatory activity (relapsing-remitting MS), although one-third of the MS patients will develop progressive and persistent symptoms without superimposed relapses, and even 10% of the patients will suffer progressive symptoms from the onset (progressive MS forms). It is a predominantly immune-mediated disease, but the underlying cause and pathologic mechanisms are not well established. No curative treatments are available. Different immunomodulating and/or immunosuppressive treatments focused on neuroinflammation have been discovered and approved for relapsing MS during the last 30 years. These treatments are considered to have a limited impact on neurodegeneration, which is the main mechanism of progression of disability in MS.

MS affects patients worldwide, and its prevalence ranges from 50 to 300 cases per 100,000 inhabitants [1]. Relapsing MS forms have a female: male sex ratio of 3:1 and the onset age are around the third decade of life, when the patients are normally sexually active and with most of them planning to build a family. Clinical manifestations of the disease include visual loss, extra-ocular movement disorders, dysarthria, paresthesia, loss of sensation, weakness, spasticity, ataxia, and bladder dysfunction. Sexual dysfunction (SD), because of the variated physical symptoms of the disease, is also a common complaint in people with MS (pwMS) although often unreported or underassessed and thus undermanaged. MS patients can also suffer psychological

M. Sepúlveda Gázquez (✉)
Neuroimmunology and Multiple Sclerosis Unit, Neurology Department, Clinical Institute of Neurosciences, Hospital Clinic de Barcelona, Barcelona, Spain

Clinical Sexology Working Group, Hospital Clinic de Barcelona, Barcelona, Spain
e-mail: msepulve@clinic.cat

symptoms that can affect their sexual function. Communication about sexuality is not a usual part of the routine neurological visit, and most of time, it would be necessary an interdisciplinary care. It has been estimated that up to 90% of pwMS reported to have never discussed sexuality issues with their treating neurologist [2].

Some studies have showed that pwMS can suffer sexual disorders even on early stages, when physical disability is mild [3]. This, together with the repercussion that a disturbed sexual function may cause in the quality of life, urges for an early identification and management of SD in this disease.

2   Characteristics of Sexual Dysfunction in People with MS

There are several studies which have reported SD prevalence in pwMS [2–13]. Most of them are cross-sectional studies, with the limitation that implies such design for controlling confusing indicators. Few case-control [12] and follow-up studies [13] have also been conducted. The most frequent assessment method used for the diagnosis of SD has been self-reported with patients or using self-administered questionnaires.

The prevalence of SD in women with MS has been reported ranging from 17 to 95% [4] and in men, from 31 to 92% [5]. This wide range could be explained in part for the heterogeneity of the study population and because there isn't a consistent definition in the literature for the diagnosis of SD. Some studies have shown that the proportion of SD in pwMS is higher than in the general population [2, 4, 5].

Sexual dysfunction can arise at any time in the disease. One study reported that one-third of newly diagnosed women complaint about SD despite no major neurological impairment [3]. The most frequent symptoms of SD in men with MS are erectile dysfunction (50–75%), ejaculatory dysfunction (50%), reduced libido (39%), and anorgasmia (37%) [2, 14]. In contrast, women's most common presentations of SD in MS are reduced libido (31–64%), problems with arousal and vaginal lubrication (33–52%) and failure to orgasm (37–38%) [2, 14].

3   Etiology of Sexual Dysfunction in People with MS

Different causes have been involved in the etiology of SD in MS. SD can appear at the different forms of the disease, with growing prevalence as the disease progresses. The growing physical impairment, but also psychological factors and side effects of different drugs contribute to increase the rates of SD in MS. Besides, SD symptoms quite often are associated with long-term urogenital impairment.

For SD in pwMS, it has been suggested that different levels of contributing factors exist, and have been defined as primary, secondary, and tertiary causes [2, 14] (see Fig. 1). In a cross-sectional study which included 93 pwMS, from 43 patients reporting SD, 37% were classified as suffering from secondary causes, 29% primary, and 19% tertiary causes [8], although in the majority of the MS patients, SD will present as a combination of primary, secondary, and tertiary causes.

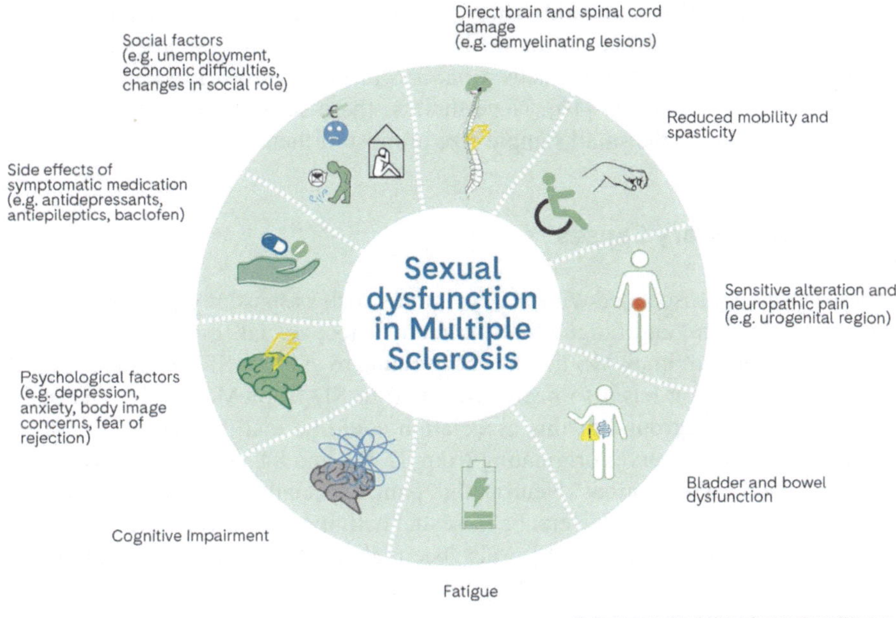

Fig. 1 Contributing factors to sexual dysfunction in multiple sclerosis

3.1 Primary Causes

Primary causes are associated with the direct neurological damage caused by the demyelinating lesions affecting the neural pathways in the brain and spinal cord that control sexual function. They include sensitive alterations (paresthesia, numbness) but also loss of libido, decreased lubrication, and erectile dysfunction.

Peripheral control of sexual functions involves somatic, thoracolumbar sympathetic (Th10-L2), and sacral parasympathetic (S2–4) efferent neurons although sexual responses are modulated by cerebral descending excitatory and inhibitory control over the pelvic innervations. The motor and sensory somatic control is via the pudendal nerve, and the components of the autonomic system are via the pelvic nerve (sacral parasympathetic) and hypogastric nerve (thoracolumbar sympathetic). Somatic afferent (motor) pathway is essential for initiation of the pelvic floor muscles contractions. Afferent (sensory) pathway is involved in sensory innervations of the genitalia and contribute to sexual interpretation of genital stimulation. Psychogenic erection and vaginal lubrication are mediated via the sympathetic fibers in conjunction with the parasympathetic, whereas reflex erection and vaginal lubrication are mediated by the parasympathetic nervous system. Ejaculation requires coordination of the sympathetic and parasympathetic spinal centers in addition to the somatic nervous system via the pudendal nerve [15]. In men with MS, spinal cord lesions are a major cause of erectile dysfunction [14].

A functional MRI brain study showed that impaired female sexual arousal was associated with MS lesions in the occipital region [16]. Other studies highlighted limbic and paralimbic regions activation, and in men with MS, brainstem lesions correlate with anorgasmia [16]. Nevertheless, these results should be interpreted with caution, due to the small sample size of most of them.

3.2 Secondary Causes

These causes are associated with MS symptoms such as spasticity, pain, bladder and bowel dysfunction, and fatigue that indirectly affect sexual response. Fatigue is a common complaint in pwMS that has been found to amplify SD in both sexes [10]. Bladder dysfunction has also been associated to SD in pwMS [6, 7]. The pathophysiological background of this association could be that the sexual response is under the control of nerves originating from S2, S3, and S4 spinal levels, which also provide bladder innervations. Neuropathic pain, especially affecting the urogenital regions, would produce interference in sexual activity. Reduced mobility and spasticity and its increase over time have also been related to changes of sexual functioning in patients with MS [13]. Pelvic floor muscle weakness and reduced genital sensitivity have correlated with orgasmic quality in women with advanced MS [13].

3.3 Tertiary Causes

Finally, tertiary causes include changes in social roles, mood disorders, demoralization, interpersonal difficulties, body image concerns, fear of rejection, cognitive impairment, and others. Among mood disorders, depression and anxiety are frequent comorbidities in pwMS with a prevalence ranging from 27 to 54% [2]. Some studies have demonstrated depression and fatigue as factors with profound influence on patient's sexual life [6, 9, 10]. In a study with 93 MS patients, depression was an independent prognostic factor for changes in sexual function over 6 years [13]. More than 50% of pwMS will suffer cognitive impairment. Cognitively impaired MS patients participate in fewer social activities and report more SD, than patients without cognitive deficit [2].

3.4 Medications as Contributory Factors for SD in pwMS

Several medications prescribed in MS patients to ameliorate different symptoms can interfere sexual function. Selective serotonin-reuptake inhibitors (SSRI), used frequently to treat anxiety and depression, can affect different areas of sexual function in both sexes, including loss of libido, anorgasmia, and impaired ejaculation. The incidence of SSRI-associated SD varies between 30% and 50% [14]. Other relevant medications include 5-alpha-reductase inhibitors (e.g., finasteride), retinoids (e.g., isotretinoin), alpha-blockers (e.g., prazosin, tamsulosin), and different classes of antihypertensives (e.g., beta-blockers, thiazide) [2, 14] (see Table 1).

Table 1. Symptomatic medications frequently used in MS patients that affect sexual function

Medication	Dmax Indication	Effect on sexual function
Baclofen	75–125 mg/day Spasticity	Erectile dysfunction
Dantrolene	200–400 mg/day Spasticity	Decreased libido, erectile dysfunction, retrograde ejaculation
Gabapentin	900–3600 mg/day Pain, spasticity	Erectile dysfunction, decreased libido, anorgasmia
Pregabalin	150–300 mg/day Pain	Erectile dysfunction, decreased libido, anorgasmia
Carbamazepine	200–400 mg/day Pain	Erectile dysfunction, decreased libido, anorgasmia
SSRI		
Paroxetine Sertraline	20 mg/day 50–100 mg/day Depression	Decreased libido, anorgasmia, impaired ejaculation
Duloxetine	60–120 mg/day Pain, depression	Decreased libido, erectile dysfunction, impaired ejaculation
Venlafaxine	75–375 mg/day Depression	Erectile dysfunction, anorgasmia
Amantadine	100-200 mg/day Fatigue	Decreased libido
Antimuscarinics		
Oxibutinine Tolterodine Solifenacine	15–20 mg/day 4 mg/day 10 mg/day Urinary incontinence, overactive bladder	Vaginal dryness

SSRI selective serotonin reuptake inhibitors

Some immunosuppressants, such as cyclophosphamide, could induce premature ovarian insufficiency. The gradual introduction in the last years of new highly effective MS modifying therapies has led to an increasingly exceptional use of cyclophosphamide.

4   Factors Associated with SD in MS

There has been identified different factors related to SD in pwMS: advanced age, lower educational level, longer disease duration, suffering a progressive MS form, greater neurological disability, fatigue, urinary problems, and worse cognitive function [6–11, 13, 14].

One study with 162 patients with MS who completed the Multiple Sclerosis Intimacy and Sexuality Questionnaire-19 showed that patients with and without SD did not differ in median income, age, sex, race, marital status, and use of MS drugs but fatigue and pain scores were significantly worse in those with SD [6]. Mood disorders such as depression, anxiety has been related with MS in a reciprocal manner, thus mood disorders were found to be associated with developing SD in pwMS [10], whereas some studies have suggested SD as a trigger for depression in pwMS. Depression affects desire, arousal, and the ability to orgasm. Use of antidepressant medication and history of behavioral consultations were higher in those with sexual dysfunction [6]. So, depression and anxiety should be screened in pwMS reporting SD.

A cross-sectional study conducted on 300 women with MS, revealed that there was a significant higher probability of an SD among patients with MS and a high fatigue score. The scores of the different dimensions of sexual function were found to have inverse and significant correlations with age, fatigue, and the duration of marriage [9]. Other cross-sectional study of 93 pwMS where SD assessed also with MSISQ-19, found disability (a score of 4 in the expanded disability status scale) as a strong risk factor for SD [OR, 18.1 (95% CI, 3.3–31.4)]. In this study, depression was univariately associated with SD, but statistical significance was lost in the multivariate model. Thus, this study concluded that screening for SD becomes particularly relevant in patients with growing disability [8].

4.1   Sexual Dysfunction and Quality of Life in People with MS

Quality of life (assessed throughout the MS-specific quality of life questionnaire, MS quality of life-54, physical and mental composite—MSQoL-54) in different studies has been found to be significantly poorer in pwMS and SD [7, 9]. In a study with 300 women with MS, mean score of the combined physical and mental health aspects of quality of life (MSQoL-54) was lower in the group of women with MS and SD compared to those without SD, and the difference between the two groups was statistically significant [9].

4.2   Sexual Dysfunction in Sexual Minorities with MS

MS patients identified as sexual and gender minorities (SGM—lesbian, gay, bisexual transgender, queer/questioning, intersexual, or asexual) have also reported lower mean satisfaction scores in the domain of sexual health in comparison to other health domains. SGM patients with MS face additional challenges when accessing quality medical care due to factors such as social discrimination, homophobia, and transphobia, lack of culturally competent healthcare and structural disparities. Discrimination at healthcare setting may led patients to avoid seeking medical care because fear of discrimination. MS symptoms can also make it harder to socialize and date due to the stigmatization of the disease. In a study conducted at San Francisco MS Center through the National MS Society, a web-based survey was proposed to those patients with MS who self-identified as owing to a sexual minority, to identify clinical and social needs in this clinical population [17]. Twenty-six patients answered the survey, mean age 50.2 (SD 10.6) years; gender identity: women (46%) men (38%) and genderqueer, transgender, or other (15%); sexual orientation: gay/lesbian/bisexual (35%), pansexual/queer (27%), questioning (23%), or other identity (15%). The overall satisfaction with MS care was high and most of them felt that their SGM status did not affect their MS care, but still 30% did report feeling uncomfortable discussing their SGM identities with their clinician. Participants reported lower participation in SGM community because of fatigue, immobility, and stigmatization of disease as primary factors; 32% stated they would like to see more representation, inclusivity, and openness from their doctors and office spaces and 28% noted they wanted more support groups for SGM individuals with disabilities or chronic illness, and greater representation of SGM people in MS pamphlets and educational seminars.

In SGM patients with MS, it would be important to stimulate their inclusivity and representation in the clinical practice (most of the sexual questionnaires used to examine sexual function in MS have been tested almost exclusively with heterosexual samples), as well as more gender inclusive terms in the health records and the creation of SGM-specific MS support groups.

5 Diagnosis of Sexual Dysfunction in People with MS

Many times, at the routine neurological visit, presence of sexual problems is not investigated because other neurological symptoms are given more priority, or directly sexual problems are not even addressed. Different factors have been related to this absence of sexual health approach; sometimes the presence of family or friends in the consultation room is an impeding factor; other sexual issues are not enquired during the conversation due to lack of knowledge in the field from the healthcare professional; others, due to an inadequate time during the appointment. So, to initiate a proper discussion about sexual difficulties, patient should feel comfortable. If it is possible, clinicians should give the opportunity for the patient to be seen alone in a confidential environment, using questions of SD as part of a holistic approach to managing MS and encouraging patients to divulge sensitive topics that may be perceived as embarrassing. Asking patients to complete an SD questionnaire before entering the consultation room can also be a helpful tool [2, 14].

Evaluation of SD in pwMS requires a comprehensive sexual history and examination. Laboratory tests could be performed only if organic pathology is suspected. Afterwards, information and education related to the sexual problem and potential contributing factors along with their management should be discussed with patient and/or with his/her partner. Finally, discussion on the therapeutic intervention and patient's follow-up take place.

5.1 History

Sexual history should identify sexual problems, contributing factors and patients or couples' treatment goals. It is important to define the problem and specific etiology of SD (primary, secondary, tertiary causes, and/or medication adverse event); it is also of great importance to identify potential risk factors and to assess the impact of SD on the patient's life. It can be helpful to ask first about bladder and bowel complaints, before stating possible sexual problems. It is necessary to collect information about the onset and time course of SD in relation to MS and its relapses; questions about the sexual desire, about difficulties in sexual arousal and to achieve orgasm; in men, if they can get and keep an erection. In women, it is important to inquiry about obstetric and gynecological history and menstrual status [14].

Some questionnaires have been developed to capture most of these aspects [18]. The most relevant are listed in Table 2 and include the above-mentioned MS Intimacy and Sexuality Questionnaire-19 (MSISQ-19), the International Index of Erectile Function (IIEF-15), the Female Sexual Function Index (FSFI), Sexual Satisfaction Scale (SSS), or the Arizona Sexual Experience Scale.

In men, one of the most important symptoms about sexual dysfunction is erectile dysfunction. It is important to inquire about onset and duration of erectile problems and quality of erections, whether the problem is with achieving or maintaining an erection (or both), and erections achieved in different situations (such as through self-stimulation (masturbation), with a partner and morning erections). As Neurogenic erectile dysfunction is a diagnosis of exclusion, it is important to exclude other causes as vasculogenic, urological, endocrine, and psychogenic factors. In women, endocrine and psychogenic factors can also contribute to SD. Gynecological causes as pain during penetrative intercourse or vaginal dryness may be relevant on the SD [14].

In order to address properly SD in MS, a multidisciplinary team integrated by urologists, gynecologists, psychiatrists, psychologists, social workers, physical therapists, nurses, apart from neurologists is necessary. MS patients with a suspected underlying disorder affecting sexual health may require referral to an appropriate specialist.

5.2 Examination

General physical inspection and basic cardiovascular assessment can be feasibly incorporated to screen for underlying endocrine or vasculogenic factors. Performing a urogenital examination, while desirable, may not be practical for all patients because most neurologists are unfamiliar with performing a focused urogenital or pelvic examination. In those cases, it seems reasonable to derivate to urologist and/or gynecologist.

5.3 Investigations

If a neurogenic cause is strongly suspected, then laboratory testing is usually not necessary. Any tests should be performed if risk factors and comorbidities are present, aiming to identify reversible or modifiable causes. Blood test includes measurement of glycated hemoglobin and lipid profile in patients with high cardiovascular risk, as erectile dysfunction in men and arousal/lubrication disorders in women, can be an early manifestation of atherosclerosis. Checking serum testosterone

Table 2 Questionnaires used for sexual evaluation in MS patients

Scale		What evaluates	Which sex it applies	Structure	Content	Scoring—interpretation
FSFI	Female Sexual Function Index	Sexual function over the last 4 weeks	Females	19 items Likert scale (1–5)	Domains: sexual desire, arousal, lubrication, orgasm, satisfaction, pain	Score 2–36 $SD \leq 26.55$ Higher scores indicate better sexual function
MSISQ-19	Multiple Sclerosis Intimacy and Sexuality Questionnaire	Influence of MS symptoms on sexual function over the last 6 months	Females and males	19 items Likert scale (1–5) 1 (symptom never occurs) to 5 (constant symptoms)	Five questions inquiring about primary causes of SD Nine questions about secondary causes of SD Five questions about tertiary causes of SD	Score 19–95 High scores indicate higher levels of SD
MSISQ15	Multiple Sclerosis Intimacy and Sexuality Questionnaire	Influence of MS symptoms on sexual function over the last 6 months	Females and males	15 items Likert scale (1–5)	Five questions inquiring about primary causes of SD Five questions about secondary causes of SD Five questions about tertiary causes of SD	Score 15–75 High scores indicate higher levels of SD
SSFS	Szasz Sexual Functioning Scale	Sexual function and their impact on quality of life	Females and males	Five items	Five groups depending of the level of sexual activity and impact in quality of life: 0, sexually active as before and/or not experiencing sexual problems; 1, sexually less active than before, and/or now experiencing some sexual problems but not concerned; 2, sexually less active than before and/or now experiencing some sexual problems and concerned; 3, sexually inactive but still concerned; and 4, sexually inactive and not concerned (given up)	Score > 0 is considered dysfunction

Table 2 (continued)

Scale		What evaluates	Which sex it applies	Structure	Content	Scoring—interpretation
SEA-MS-F	Sexual Expectations Evaluation in Women with Multiple Sclerosis	Expectations of the treatment of SD in MS	Females	Eight items Likert scale 0–4 (0 = no expectation to 4 = very high expectation)	Three domains (eight questions): 1. General expectations regarding sexuality 2. Specific expectations In sexual function 3. Patient goals for the treatment of SD	Score 0–32
IIEF-15	International Index of Erectile Function	Clinical follow-up of erectile dysfunction	Males	15 items	Five domains: Erectile function, orgasm, sexual desire, sexual satisfaction, global satisfaction	Score 0–75 Scores less than 25 are considered erectile dysfunction, scoring was rated from 1 to 30, 26 to 30 as normal
ASES	Arizona Sexual Experience Scale	Sexual function over the last 1 week	Females and males	Five items Likert scale 1–6	Five items: sex drive, arousal, vaginal lubrication/penile erection, ability to reach orgasm, and satisfaction from orgasm	Score 5–30 Higher scores indicating more sexual dysfunction
FSDS	Female Sexual Distress Scale	Problems concerning women sexuality and how often those problems have caused distress during the past 30 days	Females	13 items Likert scale 0–4 (0 = never to 4 = extreme)	13 items	Score 0–52 Score of ≥11 effectively discriminates between women with SD and no SD
SSS	Sexual Satisfaction Scale	Indicator of overall sexual adjustment	Females and males	Four items	Four items Degree of satisfaction with: (1) physically expressing affection; (2) variety of sexual activities engaged in; (3) sexual relationship in general and (4) perceived level of satisfaction experienced by the partner within the relationship	Score 4–24 Higher score shows higher sexual dissatisfaction

SD sexual dysfunction

concentration in patients with erectile dysfunction may not be essential in MS if a neurogenic cause is likely. Morning serum total testosterone should be tested in patients with clinically suspected hypogonadism or if first-line treatment of erectile dysfunction is unsuccessful [14].

6   Management of Sexual Dysfunction in People with MS

A proper evaluation of SD in MS implies the involvement of a team of healthcare professionals, in order to address not only the physical but the psychosocial components of SD. This multidisciplinary approach is important to restore the patient's sexual function and to achieve a holistic approach with the most effective therapeutic result.

The PLISSIT model [19] is one of the most used models in sexual counseling and assessment and consists of four levels of intervention: permission, limited information, specific suggestion, and intensive therapy. During the first level of this model, patients are "given permission" to discuss about their sexual experience in a safe and comfortable environment. During the second level, health practitioners provide patients with "limited information" related to sex and their concerns, the impact of the disease on their sexual expectations and the effects of treatment on sexual function. At the third level, patients receive "specific suggestions" about each person's individual needs, and finally, at the last level, some of the patients who need more intervention are provided with "intensive therapy," and they are referred to the relevant specialists. The use of PLISSIT model has reported improvement in different domains of SD in pwMS. A randomized controlled trial study conducted in 62 married women with MS showed a significant improvement of sexual quality of life (Sexual Quality of Life-Female questionnaire) in the experimental group better than the control group 2 weeks and 2 months after the intervention. Women in the experimental group participated in four face-to-face individual training and counseling sessions, which lasted 45–75 min per session and one session per week [20]. Other randomized clinical trial carried out in 88 married women with MS, obtained a significant increase in the mean score of the total Female Sexual Function Index score in different timepoint evaluations of the experimental group of patients that followed the PLISSIT model [21].

Regarding pharmacological treatments, unfortunately, MS disease-modifying therapies have not demonstrated a significant role in improving SD in MS patients. Oral phosphodiesterase type-5 inhibitors (sildenafil citrate, tadalafil) have been shown to be effective improving erectile function in male patients with MS, and both drugs are considered the first-line choice in patients with MS with erectile dysfunction [2, 14, 22]. Use of these drugs in women with MS and SD has obtained controversial results. In one study, limited effects were shown with improvement only in lubrication whereas, in another trial, sildenafil resulted effective [2, 14]. For the treatment of erectile dysfunction, dopamine receptor agonist (sublingual apomorphine) and intracavernosal injection of vasodilatory agents (alprostadil and papaverine) have also been tested. Other possibilities for certain patients comprise vacuum constriction devices or penile implants.

Genital hypersensitivity in both men and women with MS can be addressed with medication for neuropathic pain as anticonvulsants, antidepressants, and topical local anesthetics. In those cases of MS women with reduced lubrication, water-soluble vaginal lubricants and estrogen administered with methyl-testosterone may improve vaginal lubrication. Use of vibrator may be an option in those cases of women with MS and difficulties to intercourse [2, 14].

Some non-pharmacological interventions can be helpful in achieve an improvement in the desire and orgasm parameters of female patients, such as pelvic floor exercises alone or in combination with neuromuscular electric stimulation [22]. Yoga technique showed significant beneficial results in sexual satisfaction in a study with 60 female patients with clinically definite MS (yoga training and exercises for 3 months, 8 sessions per month) compared with a control group. Pre- and poststudy evaluations of the effects were measured using the MSQoL-24 Questionnaire. After the 3-month mark, there was a significant statistical difference in the case group participants [23].

Fatigue is another important factor to be address. Those patients suffering disabling fatigue can try strategies of energy conservation. Since a decline in energy occurred in the afternoon and evening, sexual activity earlier during the day could be suggested [14]. Amantadine, modafinil, and methylphenidate are drugs that could improve fatigue. Patients suffering spasticity may benefit from finding more comfortable positions as well as by using pillows and muscle-relaxing activities (massage and stretching exercises). Alternatively, patients may take drugs, such as baclofen, tizanidine, or benzodiazepines, prior to sexual intercourse [2].

Management of bladder dysfunction has been demonstrated to improve sexual function in MS patients. In one interventional study in 41 females with MS with refractory overactive bladder symptoms and 21 continent MS females as control group, the administration of onabotulinum toxin A via intradetrusor injections in the first group significantly improved not only their bladder symptoms but also their sexual function (desire, arousal, lubrication, orgasm, and satisfaction) 6 months after the injection [24]. Patients using intermittent self-catheterization are encouraged to empty the bladder before sexual activity [2].

Finally, addressing psychological and neuropsychological factors in pwMS and SD may be crucial. It is important to review patient medications due to the potential side effects of some medications on sexual functioning. Antidepressants, especially selective serotonin-reuptake inhibitors, may cause delayed ejaculation, absent or delayed orgasm, and reduced sexual desire; therefore, careful assessment of the risk–benefit ratio of each drug must be considered and consider cognitive behavioral therapy as an effective alternative treatment instead of antidepressants.

Sexual counseling, psychotherapy, and education showed significant improvements in affective and problem-solving communication, marital satisfaction, and sexual satisfaction in a pilot study conducted in nine couples (MS patients and their spouses) [14].

7 Conclusion

In conclusion, SD is highly prevalent in both females and males with MS. Assessment and treatment of SD in pwMS should be part of the neurologist's routine assessment. Knowing that sexual dysfunction affects all aspects of the quality of life in these patients, results of high importance to assess the influence of MS-related symptoms on sexual issues and to identify those patients at risk of suffering SD to implement early and proper treatment. Management of SD in MS should involve a multidisciplinary team of healthcare professionals and should be comprehensive because the symptoms could be somatic, psychological, or related to social problems.

References

1. Yamout BI, Alroughani R. Multiple Sclerosis. Semin Neurol. 2018;38(2):212–25.
2. Drulovic J, Kisic-Tepavcevic D, Pekmezovic T. Epidemiology, diagnosis, and management of sexual dysfunction in multiple sclerosis. Acta Neurol Belg. 2020;120:791–7.
3. Tzortzis V, Skriapas K, Hadjigeorgiou G, et al. Sexual dysfunction in newly diagnosed multiple sclerosis women. Mult Scler. 2008;14:561–3.
4. Dunya CP, Tulek Z, Uchiyama T, et al. Systematic review of the prevalence, symptomatology and management options of sexual dysfunction in women with multiple sclerosis. Neurourol Urodyn. 2020;39:83–95.
5. Dastoorpoor M, Zamanian M, Moradzadeh R, et al. Prevalence of sexual dysfunction in men with multiple sclerosis: a systematic review and meta-analysis. Syst Rev. 2021;10:10.
6. Domingo S, Kinzy T, Thompson N, et al. Factors associated with sexual dysfunction in individuals with multiple sclerosis: implications for assessment and treatment. Int J MS Care. 2018;20(4):191–7.
7. Tepavcevic TK, Kostic J, Basuroski ID, et al. The impact of sexual dysfunction on the quality of life measured by MSQoL-54 in patients with multiple sclerosis. Mult Scler. 2008;14:1131–6.
8. Altmann P, Leutmezer F, Leithner K, et al. Predisposing factors for sexual dysfunction in multiple sclerosis. Front Neurol. 2021;12:618370.
9. Nazari F, Shaygannejad V, Mohammadi Sichani M, et al. Sexual dysfunction in women with multiple sclerosis: prevalence and impact on quality of life. BMC Urol. 2020;20(1):15.
10. Young CA, Tennant A, TONiC Study Group. Sexual functioning in multiple sclerosis: relationships with depression, fatigue and physical function. Mult Scler. 2017;23(9):1268–75.
11. Marck CH, Jelinek P, Weiland TJ, et al. Sexual function in multiple sclerosis and associations with demographic, disease and lifestyle characteristics: an international cross-sectional study. BMC Neurol. 2016;16(1):210.
12. Zorzon M, Zivadinov R, Bosco A, et al. Sexual dysfunction in multiple sclerosis: a case–control study. I. Frequency and comparison of groups. Mult Scler. 1999;5:418–27.
13. Kisic-Tepavcevic D, Pekmezovic T, Trajkovic G, et al. Sexual dysfunction in multiple sclerosis: a 6-year follow-up study. J Neurol Sci. 2015;358:317–23.
14. Li V, Haslam C, Pakzad M, et al. A practical approach to assessing and managing sexual dysfunction in multiple sclerosis. Pract Neurol. 2020;20:122–32.
15. Krassioukov A, Stacy E. Neural control and physiology of sexual function: effect of spinal cord injury. Top Spinal Cord Inj Rehabil. 2017;23(1):1–10.

16. Winder K, Linker RA, Seifert F, et al. Neuroanatomic correlates of female sexual dysfunction in multiple sclerosis. Ann Neurol. 2016;80:490–8.
17. Anderson A, Dierkhising J, Rush G, et al. Experiences of sexual and gender minority people living with multiple sclerosis in northern California: an exploratory study. Mult Scler Relat Disord. 2021;55:103214.
18. Gaviria-Carrillo PA, Ortiz-Salas KP, Rueda-Vergara GA, et al. Tools for comprehensive evaluation of sexual function in patients with multiple sclerosis. Neurologia. 2023;38:197–205.
19. Taylor B, Davis S. The extended PLISSIT model for addressing the sexual wellbeing of individuals with an acquired disability or chronic illness. Sex Disabil. 2007;25:135–9.
20. Kazemi Z, Mousavi MS, Etemadifar M. The effect of counseling based on the PLISSIT model on sexual quality of life of married women with multiple sclerosis referring to MS center in 2019: a randomized, controlled trial. Arch Womens Ment Health. 2021;24:437–44.
21. Khakbazan Z, Daneshfar F, Behboodi-Moghadam Z, et al. The effectiveness of the permission, limited information, specific suggestions, intensive therapy (PLISSIT) model based sexual counseling on the sexual function of women with multiple sclerosis who are sexually active. Mult Scler Relat Disord. 2016;8:113–9.
22. Giannopapas V, Kitsos D, Tsogka A, et al. Sexual dysfunction therapeutic approaches in patients with multiple sclerosis: a systematic review. Neurol Sci. 2023;44:873–80.
23. Najafidoulatabad S, Mohebbi Z, Nooryan K. Yoga effects on physical activity and sexual satisfaction among the Iranian women with multiple sclerosis: a randomized controlled trial. Afr J Tradit Complement Altern Med. 2014;23(115):78–82.
24. Giannantoni A, Gubbiotti M, Rossi de Vermandois JA, et al. Effects of onabotulinum toxin a intradetrusor injections on urinary symptoms and sexual life in women affected by multiple sclerosis: a prospective controlled study. J Neurol Neurophysiol. 2017;8:3.

Headache and Sexual Dysfunction

Marta Torres-Ferrús and Alicia Alpuente

1   Introduction

Although secondary headache disorders need to be recognized, the most common ones are primary headache disorders (migraine, tension-type headache, and cluster headache). Often, these conditions are lifelong [1]. While there are regional differences, headache disorders affect people of all sexes, ages, races, income levels, and geographical areas. The significant public-health concern of headache disorders arises from their causal association with personal and societal burdens, including pain, disability, diminished quality of life, and financial costs [1].

Sexual dysfunction refers to difficulties that occur during the sexual cycle and prevent individuals from experiencing satisfaction from sexual activity. Risk factors for sexual dysfunction in both women and men include biological, psychological, and sociocultural factors [2]. Sexual dysfunction is a prevalent symptom in many chronic neurological disorders [3–5] as well as in pain syndromes [6, 7]. The pathophysiology of sexual dysfunction is multifactorial, with several factors contributing directly or indirectly, such as primary nervous system injury, other symptoms like fatigue, pain, mood-related disorders, or medication side effects [8].

Patients with headache disorders such as migraine or cluster headache may be at risk for sexual dysfunction due to their chronic neurological and pain conditions that are often comorbid with mood disorders. Additionally, pharmacological treatments used to treat and prevent headache may have potential side effects on sexual function.

M. Torres-Ferrús (✉) · A. Alpuente
Headache Clinic, Neurology Department, Vall d'Hebron University Hospital, Barcelona, Spain
e-mail: marta.torres@vallhebron.cat; alicia.alpuente@vallhebron.cat

377

2 Impact of Primary Headache Disorders on Sexual Performance

2.1 Migraine

Migraine is a prevalent neurological disorder defined by the presence of recurrent episodic headache attacks and neurological-associated symptoms. Typically, migraine attacks last from 4 to 72 h and patients experience unilateral cephalic pain of a pulsating quality and moderate or severe intensity, which can be intensified by movement or exercise, leading to avoidance of physical activity. Accompanying symptoms include at least one of the following: sensitivity to light or sound (photophobia or phonophobia), nausea, and/or vomiting. Classically, two forms have been described: migraine without aura and migraine with aura, consisting of transitory neurological symptoms (most common visual, sensitive, or speech disturbances) that usually precede the pain phase [9]. Recurrent attacks of intense headache and accompanying symptoms impact daily functioning.

Migraine affects an estimated 12% of the population and is one of the ten leading causes of global disability, especially in young adults [10]. Prevalence and headache-related disability peak is between 30 and 50 years old [11], so migraine has a significant impact during the most demanding years of life affecting all spheres of personal, social, work, or sexual life [12, 13].

Migraine is a predominantly female disorder, as prevalence in women is nearly threefold higher than in men. Moreover, menarche, menstruation, pregnancy, and menopause as well as the use of oral contraceptives and menopausal hormone therapy may influence migraine occurrence. Until puberty, migraine affects both sexes equally. After the menarche, there is an increasing prevalence of migraine in women. There is still limited data on migraine prevalence in gender minorities [14]. The mechanism for the gender difference in migraine is not clear even though endogenous sex steroids are considered to play a relevant role [15].

The prevalence of sexual dysfunction among migraine patients ranges between 30 and 40% for females [16, 17] and 20–60% for male patients [18, 19]. Whether there are differences in prevalence of sexual dysfunction in migraine patients compared to non-headache patients, some studies have demonstrated an increased prevalence of sexual dysfunction in headache and migraine patients than in the general population [16, 20, 21]. However, other studies have failed to find differences between headache patients and controls regarding sexual activity, desire, or satisfaction although sexual pain disorder might be more frequent [17, 22] and do not appear to be less satisfied with sex [16].

Risk factors for sexual dysfunction in migraine patients do not seem to differ from general risk factors for sexual dysfunction as older age, female gender, menopause, and the presence depression [23]. Nonetheless, we have to keep in mind that migraine and particularly chronic migraine is a chronic disorder frequently comorbid with psychiatric disorders as well as cardiovascular risk factors and other pain disorders [24, 25] also affecting sexual performance, what makes migraine patients a very sensitive population to suffer from sexual dysfunction. Concomitant depression increases the risk of sexual dysfunction, and even in the absence of a clinical depression, negative mood has been found to impair sexual function [4, 26]. Though it might be hypothesized that sexual dysfunction is more prevalent among patients with more severe migraine phenotypes (frequent and severe attacks), many studies have failed to find association between sexual dysfunction and headache frequency [16, 20, 23, 27].

Migraine pain typically worsen with physical exercise, and around 50% of migraine patients may avoid sexual intercourse due to fear of triggering or worsening a migraine attack [23]. However, sexual activity during a headache is not an uncommon behavior, and it may even relieve or stop a migraine attack in up to 73% of male and 58% of female migraine patients [23, 28].

The goal of pharmacotherapy for migraine is to control symptoms and minimize the impact of the disorder on each patient's life and lifestyle. Patients require analgesic drugs for the attack, and when attacks are frequent or poorly controlled, prophylactic medication can reduce the number or intensity of attacks together with headache-related disability [29]. Several medications used to prevent migraines may cause sexual dysfunction and decreased sex drive for both men and women, and these effects may occur during and in between migraine episodes. Between 25 and 45% of patients who start a preventive treatment report sexual adverse events and seem more frequent in patients treated with antidepressants or neuromodulators [23, 30]. Although sexual side effects are not usually spontaneously reported, the majority of patients tolerate them well [30]. Beta blockers (such as propranolol and metoprolol) have detrimental effects on erectile function in men, while newer drugs as nebivolol or candesartan seem to have either neutral or even beneficial effects. The effect on sexual performance in women remains considerably understudied [31]. Venlafaxine, an antidepressant frequently used for migraine prevention, has been reported to have a high risk of sexual dysfunction, while amitriptyline may have a better profile [32]. Topiramate can cause anorgasmia in women and erectile dysfunction in men [32]. Sexual adverse events for Flunarizine and newer migraine preventive drugs as botulinum toxin or CGRP-targeted therapies have not been reported.

The possibility of sexual dysfunction associated with medications should be openly discussed with the patient prior to starting the medication. The physician should always consider starting the patient on a medication with a lower probability of associated sexual dysfunction, especially in sexually active patients, and monitor sexual functioning during the treatment [33].

Given the significant impact that sexual dysfunction can have on the quality of life of patients, ensuring accurate screening and diagnosis of sexual dysfunction in individuals with migraine can potentially lead to a change in therapeutic approaches and ultimately improve their overall quality of life. Cognitive-behavioral therapy and sex therapy have often been recommended as management strategies for sexual dysfunction. However, currently, there is a lack of literature available to support their efficacy specifically in migraine patients. While intuitively these therapeutic modalities may seem beneficial, further research is needed to determine their effectiveness in improving sexual dysfunction in individuals with migraine [33].

2.2   Tension-Type Headache

Tension-type headache is usually mild or moderate, with a generalized pressure or tightness sensation, and lack specific associated symptoms [9]. Tension-type headache is the most common headache disorder, affecting over 70% of the population, though the prevalence varies significantly worldwide [1]. Tension-type headache affects three women to every two men presenting highly variable course, often starting in the teenage years and peaking in the 30 s [1].

Both female and male tension-type headache patients experience sexual problems in several aspects of sexuality compared to controls, including sex drive, arousal, penile erection/vaginal lubrication, the ability to reach orgasm and orgasmic satisfaction [16, 18]. In females with tension-type headache, sexual function has been studied using Female Sexual Function Index and Female Sexual Distress Scale, showing lower scores in the patient group compared to healthy controls [20, 34]. Similarly to migraine, it has been observed that tension-type headache patients differ somewhat in their difficulties within certain domains of sexuality, and this does not seem to be related to headache characteristics, which suggests that other variables may play a role [34]. The relationship between tension-type headaches and psychiatric disorders that might also cause sexual dysfunction is particularly interesting but still not clear. Male tension-type headache patients more frequently sowed erectile dysfunction compared to the control group, without a direct relationship with depression scores, suggesting that other complex and heterogeneous factors may exist, causing the development of sexual dysfunction along with the effect of chronic disease and pain [18]. Further studies focusing on the relationship between sexual problems and comorbid conditions such as anxiety and depression, in migraine and tension headache patients are essential.

When physicians come across patients with sexual dysfunction, it is crucial to offer support and inquire about how they can best assist in restoring optimal sexual function. By creating an open and nonjudgmental environment, healthcare providers can encourage patients to discuss their concerns openly and honestly. This allows for a comprehensive understanding of the specific challenges they are facing and enables the development of personalized treatment plans to address their needs and goals effectively.

2.3   Cluster Headache

Cluster headache is a rare primary headache disorder characterized by severe unilateral short headache attacks accompanied by ipsilateral trigeminal-autonomic symptoms (conjunctival injection, lacrimation, nasal congestion and/or rhinorrhea, eyelid edema, forehead and facial sweating, and miosis and/or ptosis) or/and agitation. Typically, headache attacks occurs in clusters or bouts (periods in which patients can have up to eight attacks in a day) and headache-free periods without headache [9].

Unlike other frequent primary headaches such as migraine and tension-type headache, cluster headache is more frequent in men than in women [35]. Men with migraine and cluster headache more often suffer from symptoms consistent with clinical androgen deficiency as decreased libido and number of morning erections than males without a primary headache disorder [36]. A study that compared the presence of erectile dysfunction in male patients with low frequency episodic migraine, cluster headache in asymptomatic period (without active pharmacological treatment) and controls found that 43% of cluster headache patients presented some degree of erectile dysfunction. Cluster headache patients also showed a higher frequency of erectile dysfunction and lower sexual satisfaction than non-headache patients [37].

During a headache attack, patients feel restless and agitated, and often, physical activity can relieve pain [35]. There are anecdotal cases of patients with cluster headache whose attacks remitted completely after orgasm [38, 39]. In cluster headache, male patients benefit more from sexual activity than female patients and use sexual activity as an active therapeutic tool [28]. Some theories suggest that endorphin excretion or hypothalamic activation during orgasm as the possible underlying mechanism [38]. However, sexual intercourse has also been reported to trigger cluster headache attacks [39] and compared with migraine, significantly less patients with cluster headache reported an improvement with sexual activity [28]. The higher pain intensity and shorter attack duration of cluster compared to migraine attack may influence the reported outcomes.

Limited available data suggesting that calcium channel antagonist verapamil, the first-line preventive treatment for cluster headache, do not have detrimental effect on sexual function [40]. On the other hand, lithium and topiramate, may reduce sexual thoughts and desire, worsen erectile function in males or anorgasmia in female patients and reduce sexual satisfaction [32, 41].

2.4 Primary Headache Associated with Sexual Activity

Primary headache associated with sexual activity is characterized by at least two episodes of headache precipitated by sexual activity alone. The pain in the head increases in intensity with increasing sexual arousal, and/or it has an abrupt explosive intensity just before or with orgasm [9]. The headache is typically bilateral and occipital with an explosive and throbbing sensation [42]. Although the prevalence of headache triggered by sexual activity is estimated to be 1–1.6%, it is probably underdiagnosed and underreported, with a male preponderance [42]. Intercourse is the most frequently reported sexual act causing headache, followed by masturbation [42]. The pathophysiology remains unclear, but may include the hyper-sympathetic response during sexual arousal and orgasm and an impairment of the cerebrovascular vasodilator reserve [43].

A comprehensive neuroimaging study is necessary to distinguish primary headache associated with sexual activity from secondary causes, especially subarachnoid hemorrhage and reversible cerebral vasoconstriction syndrome [44].

Although most patients with primary headache associated with sexual activity have a self-limited course, studies have shown that up to 40% have a chronic course lasting more than a year. Thus, specific instructions may be needed for these patients to cope with future attacks, such as maintaining a passive sexual role or keeping the neck lower than the trunk [42]. Preemptive therapy with indomethacin or triptans before intercourse can be effective in preventing headache associated with sexual activity. Some patients have shown good response to betablockers, nimodipine or topiramate, but the evidence from randomized controlled trials is still lacking [42].

Although primary headache associated with sexual activity is considered a benign condition, it can be very distressing for both patient and partner, with the development of fears around sexual activity and orgasm, affecting immediate and long-term sexual satisfaction. Patients may develop patterns of impaired sexual arousal or secondary sexual avoidance behaviors. Therefore, patients must be given the opportunity to talk about sexual fears in an ongoing way, especially in chronic patients [45].

3 Headache Attributed to Drugs Used in Sexual Medicine

Headache is a common side effect of many medications, including those used to enhance sexual function in all phases of the sexual response cycle from desire to orgasm.

3.1 Phosphodiesterase-5 (PDE-5) Inhibitors

Drugs used for pulmonary hypertension or erectile dysfunction can induce headache in healthy individuals and migraine-like headache in patients with migraine. PDE-5 inhibitors work by increasing the intracellular level of cGMP causing smooth muscle cell relaxation or neuronal stimulation. In experimental provocation studies, compounds increasing the concentration of cGMP (nitric oxide donors and sildenafil) have consistently induced migraine-like headache in patients with migraine without aura [46].

PDE-5 inhibitor-induced headache is defined as any headache developed within 5 h of taking the PDE-5 inhibitor. Headache is usually tension-type-like and resolves spontaneously within 72 h. However, in individuals with a history of migraine, the use of PDE inhibitors may provoke migraine-like headache [9]. Considering the lifetime prevalence of migraine in the general population and given the migraine-inducing effects of sildenafil and possibly also of the other PDE-5 inhibitors, migraine patients should be made aware of the risk of inducing a migraine attack. The most short lasting PDE-5 inhibitors (avanafil, vardenafil, or sildenafil) in the lowest doses should be used first [47].

3.2   Hormone Therapy

Significant sex differences exist in prevalence and clinical presentation of primary headaches. These gender differences suggest that both male and female sex hormones could have an influence on the course of primary headaches [48]. The role of sex hormones has been studied most profoundly in migraine, suggesting that migraine is influenced by the fluctuating hormonal status, as well as the use of oral contraceptives and menopause hormone therapy.

Oral contraceptives have been associated with both migraine and non-migraine headaches and has been related to estrogen use (develops or worsens within 3 months of commencing exogenous hormones) or withdrawal (typically during the free-pill week) [9]. Possible contraceptive strategies to reduce headache include extended-cycle combined hormonal contraception, progesterone-only contraception, or new generation hormone combinations that include estradiol valerate, estradiol hemihydrate, and estetrol and different progestins [48]. Tamoxifen, a selective estrogen receptor modulator used in breast cancer treatment among other indications has been suggested as a possible treatment for menstrual migraine, but it can also cause headache [49]. Menopause hormone therapy used to ease climax symptoms during menopausal transition can provoke new onset or worsening of pre-existent migraine. Non-oral routes seem preferable over oral variants as constant blood hormones levels are maintained stably and avoid liver first pass [50]. However, hormone therapy should be stopped in case of a new onset or worsening of migraine with aura, transitory ischemic attack, or other vascular pathology [48]. Along with female sex hormones, male sex hormones like testosterone might have an influence on the course of headache disorders although the exact effect or pathophysiological mechanisms are unknown [48].

While it is expected that hormone therapy will affect migraine in transgender people, the data are limited, suggesting that the prevalence of migraine is increased in transgender women treated with estrogen and is reduced in transgender men treated with testosterone [51]. It is important to maintain steady levels of estrogen and testosterone, often best accomplished with non-oral formulations. If migraine does occur, it should be managed according to guidelines with additional consideration of reducing the impact of hormone therapy [51].

4   Sexual and Gender Considerations in Headache

Most headache studies collect data on sex or gender in binary formulations, which limits our understanding of the epidemiology, pathophysiology, and sexual impact of headaches in sexual and gender minority populations.

Although the literature on sexual orientation and headaches is scarce, data from national US health survey showed that prevalence of headache or migraine was higher among bisexual women, followed by lesbians, bisexual men, heterosexual women, gay men, and heterosexual men [52]. Another one study showed that gay and bisexual men had 50% higher odds of migraine compared to heterosexual men [53]. However, differences in age and factors reflecting the social determinants of health between groups should also be considered.

Significant sex differences exist in migraine, affecting three times more women than men, particularly during the reproductive years. The difference is considered to be due to the additional effects of estrogen in women [15]. While it is to be expected that hormone therapy will affect migraine in transgender people, the data are extremely limited. One study found the prevalence of migraine in transwomen was comparable to prevalence in cisgender women [54]. There are no prevalence data for migraine before and after hormone therapy, but an Italian study in transgender women found an increase in headache following the use of feminizing hormones and suggests that testosterone therapy can reduce headache [55]. On the other hand, psychiatric comorbidities such as anxiety, depression, and stress can affect migraine frequency and severity in cisgender individuals. Although there are no specific studies, stigma and discrimination can affect health outcomes in the transgender and gender-diverse community and exacerbate migraine and other primary headache disorders [56].

New-onset headache in transgender patients should be carefully evaluated for secondary causes. Evaluation should exclude prolactinoma and meningioma (associated to androgen blockers use in transgender women) and polycythemia (associated to testosterone therapy in transgender men). If aura starts for the first time, transient ischemic attacks should be excluded [51].

5 Conclusions

Patients with headache disorders, such as migraine or cluster headache, are at risk of experiencing sexual dysfunction due to the chronic nature of these neurological conditions, which often coexist with pain and mood disorders. Furthermore, pharmacological treatments used for headache prevention may potentially have adverse effects on sexual function. The physician should always consider choosing medication with a lower probability of associated sexual dysfunction, especially in sexually active patients, and monitor and discuss sexual functioning during the treatment in an open and nonjudgmental environment. Also, it is important to inform migraine patients about the potential risk of inducing migraine attacks or worsening the frequency of migraines when using hormonal therapy or PDE-5 inhibitors. When acute headache is triggered by sexual activity should be carefully evaluated to identify any underlying secondary causes. Further research is needed to expand our knowledge in these areas, including sexual and gender minority populations (Fig. 1).

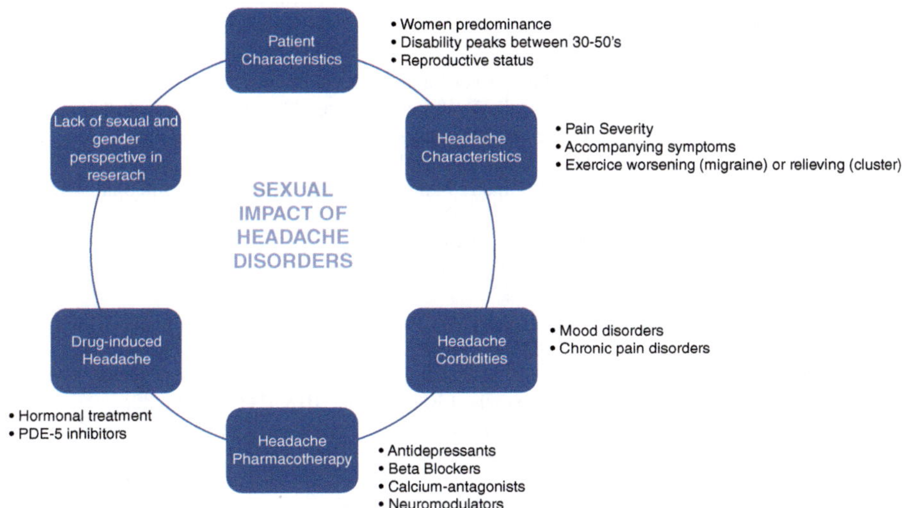

Fig. 1 Factors influencing sexual performance in headache patients

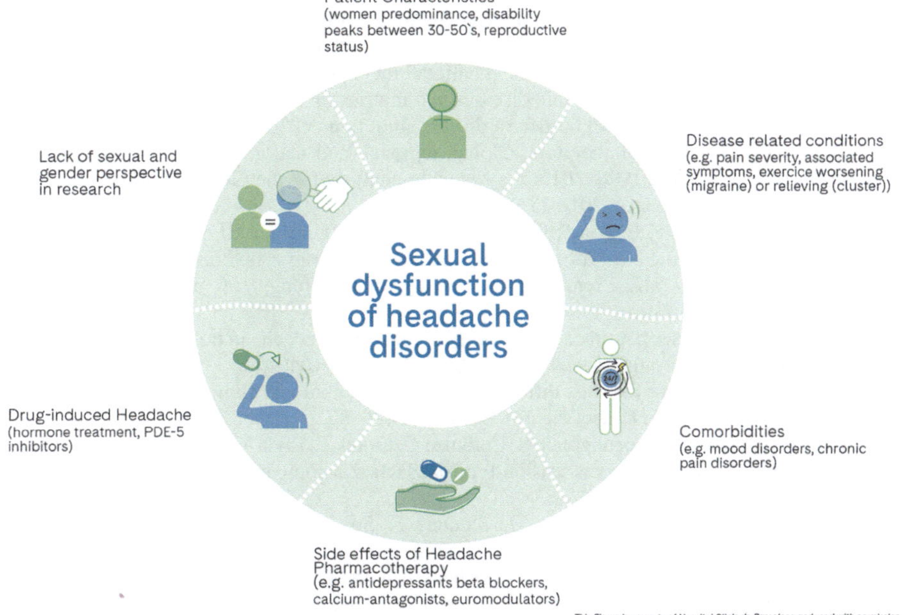

Fig. 2 Sexual Dysfunction of headache disorders

References

1. Martelletti P, Steiner TJ, editors. Handbook of headache. 2011.
2. McCabe MP, Sharlip ID, Lewis R, Atalla E, Balon R, Fisher AD, et al. Risk factors for sexual dysfunction among women and men: a consensus statement from the fourth international consultation on sexual medicine 2015. J Sex Med. 2016;13(2):153–67.
3. Rathore C, Henning OJ, Luef G, Radhakrishnan K. Sexual dysfunction in people with epilepsy. Epilepsy Behav. 2019;100(Pt A):106495.
4. Hartmann U, Philippsohn S, Heiser K, Ruffer-Hesse C. Low sexual desire in midlife and older women: personality factors, psychosocial development, present sexuality. Menopause. 2004;11(6 Pt 2):726–40.
5. Buhmann C, Dogac S, Vettorazzi E, Hidding U, Gerloff C, Jürgens TP. The impact of Parkinson disease on patients' sexuality and relationship. J Neural Transm. 2017;124(8):983–96.
6. Zhao S, Li E, Wang J, Luo L, Luo J, Zhao Z. Rheumatoid arthritis and risk of sexual dysfunction: a systematic review and Metaanalysis. J Rheumatol. 2018;45(10):1375–82.
7. Besiroglu MDH, Dursun MDM. The association between fibromyalgia and female sexual dysfunction: a systematic review and meta-analysis of observational studies. Int J Impot Res. 2019;31(4):288–97.
8. Basson R, Rees P, Wang R, Montejo AL, Incrocci L. Sexual function in chronic illness. J Sex Med. 2010;7(1 PART 2):374–88.
9. Headache Classification Committee of the International Headache Society. The international classification of headache disorders, 3rd edition. Cephalalgia. 2018;38(1):1–211.
10. Vos T, Barber RM, Bell B, Bertozzi-Villa A, Biryukov S, Bolliger I, Charlson F, Davis A, Degenhardt L, Dicker D, Duan L, Erskine H, Feigin VL, Ferrari AJ, Fitzmaurice C, Fleming T, Graetz N, Guinovart C, Haagsma J, Hansen GM, Hanson SW, Heuton KR, Higashi MC. Europe PMC funders group global, regional, and national incidence, prevalence, and years lived with disability for 301 acute and chronic diseases and injuries in 188 countries, 1990–2013: a systematic analysis for the global burden of disease stud. Lancet. 2015;386(9995):743–800.
11. GBD 2016 Headache Collaborators. Global, regional, and national burden of migraine and tension-type headache, 1990–2016: a systematic analysis for the Global Burden of Disease Study 2016. Lancet Neurol. 2018;17:954–76.
12. Diamond M, Freitag F, Lipton RB, Stewart WF, Reed ML, Bigal ME. Migraine prevalence, disease burden, and the need for preventive therapy. Neurology. 2007;68(5):343–9.
13. Lipton RB, Bigal ME. Ten lessons on the epidemiology of migraine. Headache. 2007;47(SUPPL. 1):2–9.
14. Hranilovich JA, Kaiser EA, Pace A, Barber M, Ziplow J. Headache in transgender and gender-diverse patients: a narrative review. Headache. 2021;61(7):1040–50.
15. Vetvik KG, MacGregor EA. Sex differences in the epidemiology, clinical features, and pathophysiology of migraine. Lancet Neurol. 2017;16(1):76–87.
16. Bestepe E, Cabalar M, Kucukgoncu S, Calikusu C, Ornek F, Yayla V, et al. Sexual dysfunction in women with migraine versus tension-type headaches: a comparative study. Int J Impot Res. 2011;23(3):122–7.
17. Del Bene E, Conti C, Poggioni M, Sicuteri F. Sexuality and headache. Adv Neurol. 1982;33:209–14.
18. Aksoy D, Solmaz V, Cevik B, Gencten Y, Erdemir F, Kurt SG. The evaluation of sexual dysfunction in male patients with migraine and tension type headache. J Headache Pain. 2013;14(1):1.
19. Wu S-H, Chuang E, Chuang T-Y, Lin C-L, Lin M-C, Yen D-J, et al. A Nationwide population-based cohort study of migraine and organic-psychogenic erectile dysfunction. Medicine (Baltimore). 2016;95(10):–e3065.
20. Nappi RE, Terreno E, Tassorelli C, Sances G, Allena M, Guaschino E, et al. Sexual function and distress in women treated for primary headaches in a tertiary university center. J Sex Med. 2012;9(3):761–9.
21. Bond DS, Pavlović JM, Lipton RB, Graham Thomas J, Digre KB, Roth J, et al. Sexual dysfunction in women with migraine and overweight/obesity: relative frequency and association with migraine severity. Headache. 2017;57(3):417–27.

22. Ifergane G, Ben-Zion IZ, Plakht Y, Regev K, Wirguin I. Not only headache: higher degree of sexual pain symptoms among migraine sufferers. J Headache Pain. 2008;9(2):113–7.
23. Torres-Ferrus M, López-Veloso AC, Gonzalez-Quintanilla V, González-García N, Díaz de Teran J, Gago-Veiga A, et al. The MIGREX study: prevalence and risk factors of sexual dysfunction among migraine patients. Neurologia (Engl Ed). 2021;38:541–9.
24. Buse DC, Manack A, Serrano D, Turkel C, Lipton RB. Sociodemographic and comorbidity profiles of chronic migraine and episodic migraine sufferers. J Neurol Neurosurg Psychiatry. 2010;81(4):428–32.
25. Torres-Ferrús M, Quintana M, Fernandez-Morales J, Alvarez-Sabin J, Pozo-Rosich P. When does chronic migraine strike? A clinical comparison of migraine according to the headache days suffered per month. Cephalalgia. 2017;37(2):104–13.
26. Mitchell KR, Mercer CH, Ploubidis GB, Jones KG, Datta J, Field N, et al. Sexual function in Britain: findings from the third National Survey of sexual attitudes and lifestyles (Natsal-3). Lancet (London, England). 2013;382(9907):1817–29.
27. Maizels M, Burchette R. Somatic symptoms in headache patients: the influence of headache diagnosis, frequency, and comorbidity. Headache. 2004;44(10):983–93.
28. Hambach A, Evers S, Summ O, Husstedt IW, Frese A. The impact of sexual activity on idiopathic headaches: an observational study. Cephalalgia. 2013;33(6):384–9.
29. Tepper SJ, Tepper DE, editors. The cleveland clinic manual of headache therapy. New York; 2011.
30. Domínguez E, Ruiz L, Hernández MS, Muñoz I, Ruiz-piñero M, Uribe F, et al. Disfunción sexual en pacientes migrañosos que reciben tratamiento preventivo: identificación mediante dos tests de cribado. Rev Neurol. 2015;60(1):10–6.
31. Manolis A, Doumas M. Antihypertensive treatment and sexual dysfunction. Curr Hypertens Rep. 2012;14(4):285–92.
32. Rothmore J. Antidepressant-induced sexual dysfunction. Med J Aust. 2020;212(7):329–34.
33. Balon R. The textbook of clinical sexual medicine. Springer; 2017.
34. Solmaz V, Ceviz A, Aksoy D, Cevik B, Kurt S, Gencten Y, et al. Sexual dysfunction in women with migraine and tension-type headaches. Int J Impot Res. 2016;28(6):201–4. https://doi.org/10.1038/ijir.2016.22.
35. May A, Schwedt TJ, Magis D, Pozo-Rosich P, Evers S, Wang S. Cluster headache. Nat Rev. 2015;4:135–48.
36. Verhagen IE, Brandt RB, Kruitbosch CMA, MaassenVanDenBrink A, Fronczek R, Terwindt GM. Clinical symptoms of androgen deficiency in men with migraine or cluster headache: a cross-sectional cohort study. J Headache Pain. 2021;22(1):1–9.
37. Bellosta-Diago E, Velázquez-Benito A, Viloria-Alebesque A, Iñíguez-Martínez C, Santos-Lasaosa S. Estudio de la función sexual en la migraña y la cefalea en racimos. Rev Neurol. 2016;62(11):487–92.
38. Gotkine M, Steiner I, Biran I. Now dear, I have a headache! Immediate improvement of cluster headaches after sexual activity. J Neurol Neurosurg Psychiatry. 2006;77:1296.
39. Maliszewski M, Diamond S, Freitag FG. Sexual headaches occurring in cluster headache patients. Clin J Pain. 1989;5(1):45–7.
40. Nicolai MPJ, Liem SS, Both S, Pelger RCM, Putter H, Schalij MJ, et al. A review of the positive and negative effects of cardiovascular drugs on sexual function: a proposed table for use in clinical practice. Netherlands Hear J. 2014;22(1):11–9.
41. Elnazer HY, Sampson A, Baldwin D. Lithium and sexual dysfunction: an under-researched area. Hum Psychopharmacol. 2015;30(2):66–9.
42. Lin PT, Chen SP, Wang SJ. Update on primary headache associated with sexual activity and primary thunderclap headache. Cephalalgia. 2023;43(3):033310242211486.
43. Evers S, Schmidt O, Frese A, Husstedt I-W, Ringelstein EB. The cerebral hemodynamics of headache associated with sexual activity. Pain. 2003;102(1–2):73–8.
44. Lin P-T, Wang Y-F, Fuh J-L, Lirng J-F, Ling Y-H, Chen S-P, et al. Diagnosis and classification of headache associated with sexual activity using a composite algorithm: a cohort study. Cephalalgia. 2021;41(14):1447–57.

45. Redelman MJ. What if the "sexual headache" is not a joke? Br J Med Pract. 2010;3(1):13–6.
46. Butt JH, Eddelien S, H, Kruuse C. The headache and aura-inducing effects of sildenafil in patients with migraine with aura. Cephalalgia. 2022;42(10):984–92.
47. Evans RW, Kruuse C. Phosphodiesterase-5 inhibitors and migraine. Headache. 2004;44(9):925–6.
48. Delaruelle Z, Ivanova TA, Khan S, Negro A, Ornello R, Raffaelli B. Male and female sex hormones in primary headaches. J Headache Pain. 2018;7:1–12.
49. Maggioni F, Palmieri A, Tropea M, Zanchin G. Influence of physiologic hormonal modification and of hormonal treatment in a patient with a history of migraine with aura. J Headache Pain. 2008;9(2):129–31.
50. MacGregor A. Effects of oral and transdermal estrogen replacement on migraine. Cephalalgia. 1999;19:124–5.
51. MacGregor EA, van den Brink AM. Gender and migraine. In: Transgender and migraine. Springer; 2019. p. 113–27.
52. Heslin KC. Explaining disparities in severe headache and migraine among sexual minority adults in the United States, 2013-2018. J Nerv Ment Dis. 2020;208(11):876–83.
53. Hammond NG, Stinchcombe A. Health behaviors and social determinants of migraine in a Canadian population-based sample of adults aged 45-85 years: findings from the CLSA. Headache. 2019;59(9):1547–64.
54. Pringsheim T, Gooren L. Migraine prevalence in male to female transsexuals on hormone therapy. Neurology. 2004;63(3):593–4.
55. Aloisi AM, Bachiocco V, Costantino A, Stefani R, Ceccarelli I, Bertaccini A, et al. Cross-sex hormone administration changes pain in transsexual women and men. Pain. 2007;132(Suppl):S60–7.
56. Pace A, Barber M, Ziplow J, Hranilovich JA, Kaiser EA. Gender minority stress, psychiatric comorbidities, and the experience of migraine in transgender and gender-diverse individuals: a narrative review. Curr Pain Headache Rep. 2021;25(12):82.

Anxiety and Sexual Disorders

Antoni Martin Moreno and Sílvia Pastells Pujol

1   Introduction

1.1   Definition of Anxiety

Anxiety is an emotional response that is part of human existence, all people feel a moderate degree of it and it is considered an adaptive response.

In the context of stress or danger, these reactions are normal. However, some people feel extremely anxious about activities of daily living, which can lead to distress and significant impairment in normal activity.

In general, the term anxiety refers to the combination of physical and mental manifestations related to the anticipation of future, indefinable and/or unpredictable dangers. The most notable characteristic of anxiety is its anticipatory nature, with the ability to anticipate the supposed danger or threat and this gives it an important functional value.

In the late 1960s, anxiety began to be understood as a behavior pattern characterized by subjective feelings of tension, cognitions, and physiological arousal. It is, therefore, a multidimensional construct made up of three components (cognitive, physiological, and motor) which interact with each other. Bodily aspects are characterized by a high degree of activation of the autonomic nervous system: palpitations, rapid and shallow breathing, choking, sweating, tremor, muscle tension, etc.; and maladaptive behaviors: paralysis, avoidance behaviors, flight behaviors, etc. that can alter the sexual response and cause sexual dysfunctions.

A. Martin Moreno (✉) S. Pastells Pujol
Sexology Clinic, Barcelona, Spain
e-mail: 15143amm@comb.cat; silviapastells@copc.cat

After the 1960s, cognitive variables provided a greater understanding of how anxiety works. Lazarus, Beck, and Meichenbaum's formulations stress the importance of cognitive processes, which appear between the reception of the potentially aversive signal and the possible anxiety response. From this approach, the person perceives the situation, evaluates it, and interprets its implications; if the result of this evaluation is threatening, then an anxiety reaction will start, also modulated by other cognitive processes. It is also in this context of threatening cognitive appraisal that the interaction between anxiety and sexual function probably occurs.

1.2   Definition of Sexual Dysfunction

Sexual dysfunctions are a heterogeneous group of disorders, characterized by a clinically significant impairment in the person's ability to respond sexually or experience sexual pleasure. Not all sexual difficulties need to be diagnosed as dysfunction (e.g., a lack of knowledge regarding effective stimulation may prevent arousal or orgasm). In the evaluation of sexual dysfunction, several factors must be considered: (1) couple factors; (2) relationship factors; (3) individual vulnerability factors, comorbidity, and stress factors; (4) cultural or religious factors, and (5) medical factors relevant to prognosis, course, or treatment. A sexual difficulty is diagnosed as dysfunction when the DSM-V criteria are met [1].

- Female Sexual Dysfunctions: Female Sexual Interest/Arousal Disorder, Female Orgasmic Disorder, Genito-Pelvic Pain/Penetration Disorder
- Male Sexual Dysfunctions: Male hypoactive sexual desire disorder, Erectile disorder, Premature ejaculation, Delayed ejaculation

In each case, the diagnostic criteria include both impaired function and clinically relevant levels of personal distress (i.e., worry, frustration, shame) regarding the impairment. Not always in the same sexual deterioration there is the same affectation in the quality of sexual life. In fact, the association between sexual function and broadly defined subjective sexual well-being appears to be quite variable [2]. For more insights into these aspects, the reader is referred to the chapters on Sexuality across lifespan (Women and men vulnerabilities).

2   Possible Links Between Anxiety and Sexual Dysfunction

Anxiety could play an important role in the pathogenesis and maintenance of sexual dysfunctions. This co-presence is very common in clinical practice: patients with sexual dysfunctions often present with anxiety and, in many cases, it is not clear what the primary disorder is. On the other hand, for many patients with an anxiety disorder, sexual dysfunction may be a persistent disturbance.

According to the Cognitive-Behavioral Therapy (CBT) model, emotions such as anxiety are understood through the interplay of three factors: physiological sensations (e.g., increased heart rate and sweating), cognition (e.g., beliefs and interpretations associated with the feared stimuli), and behavior (e.g., avoidance, safety behaviors, and hypervigilance). We also consider "anxiety" as an emotional process that is triggered within a context. It is noteworthy that a person may experience anxiety during sexual interactions for fear of not pleasing their partner or that their partner will not perform adequately; there is also a fear of contracting sexually transmitted infections during an unprotected interaction or may feel anxious for fear of being caught engaging in sexual activity [3].

Anxiety can be induced by different stressors: conflicts in the relationship, problems in the social and work environment, affective problems and stress, low self-esteem, depression, sexual inhibition, consequences of sexual abuse in childhood, religious or cultural taboos, result of sexual preferences, fear of pregnancy and sexually transmitted diseases, neurosis, psychosis, erroneous sexual beliefs, consequence (or cause) of other sexual disorders. With all this, anxiety can distract from erotic stimuli and impair sexual arousal, mainly through a greater sympathetic tone. The neurobiological expression of anxiety is complex, but it mainly involves a release of adrenergic substances (epinephrine and norepinephrine). Sympathetic dominance is also negatively involved in the arousal and orgasmic phases and can interfere with sexual desire [4].

Despite the consequences that anxiety would have on sexual response, its effects on sexual arousal can vary. There are studies that question the bidirectional causal relationship between anxiety and sexual dysfunction. Although it is recognized that sex and anxiety are antipodal emotions, there is no reason to believe that anxiety disorders are caused by underlying sexual problems or that sexual problems are maintained by anxiety. Emotions can be discriminated according to whether they prepare us for the approach or for the avoidance/flight. Therefore, anxiety and sexual arousal represent opposite ends of a continuum: anxiety promotes avoidance while sexual arousal promotes closeness. The function of anxious avoidance and sexual approach are identical from an evolutionary perspective: to optimize the chances that the subjects' genes will be conserved in the gene pool [5].

Along the same lines, Kempeneers and Barbier proposed that anxiety might enhance attention to sexual cues, such that people may misinterpret anxious arousal as sexual arousal, thus enhancing the arousal response. This misinterpretation could be explained through cognitive and physiological mechanisms such that bodily sensations present during sexual arousal and anxiety overlap; for example, increased heart rate, sweating, or racing thoughts [6].

The review by Kane et al. indicates that anxiety can sometimes inhibit, facilitate, or have no effect on sexual arousal, as measured through genital arousal or through self-reported sexual arousal. These disconcerting findings do not fully support existing clinical models that suggest anxiety is at the root of sexual dysfunction, as the interactions between anxiety and potential sexual dysfunction appear more complex. Therefore, the findings highlight the need to re-examine the utility and mechanisms of action of anxiety-focused interventions for sexual dysfunction. Future research would benefit from studies that aim to explore the question of why and how anxiety has a variable effect on sexual arousal rather than simply anxiety having an effect on sexual arousal. Experimental research examining the impact of individual differences in beliefs about anxiety (e.g., anxiety sensitivity) and sex (e.g., sexual inhibition, sexual arousal, fear of penetration) may be a fruitful avenue to answer this important question and pave the way for more targeted and effective cognitive interventions [7].

3 Cognitive and Behavioral Aspects of Anxiety in Sexual Dysfunction

In their research on the cognitive aspects of sexual dysfunction, Tavares, Moura, and Nobre have highlighted the importance of distraction from erotic cues. The distraction derived from automatic thoughts regarding failure to perform and the hypothetical catastrophic consequences of sexual dysfunction impaired sexual function. For example, they have identified common beliefs related to "catastrophizing the partner's reaction to a man's sexual failure" and "catastrophizing the public consequences of sexual failure," as well as automatic thoughts during sexual activity such as "I'm not satisfying my partner." [8].

In addition, sexual expectations about how men and women "should" behave sexually mean that cognitions regarding sexual interactions are wrapped in myths, beliefs, and thoughts that are difficult to fulfill. For example: "I have to hold on (in penetration) until my partner has an orgasm, I have to make them enjoy, if not, I'm a bad lover." A sexual intercourse and heteronormative perspective, based on vaginal penetration, often makes people focus more on goals such as "having to orgasm" or "having to put up with it," above tenderness, sensuality, and self-care and of the other person.

From the perspective of our clinical experience, it is observed that the use of pornography could also influence the increase of both unrealistic expectations about one's own sexual behavior and the increase in concerns about the perception of body image. These concerns would facilitate cognitive distraction during the sexual encounter with the partner.

According to Barlow's model, when sexual function is impaired, and with the intention of avoiding the feared consequences, hypervigilance occurs, generating more automatic negative thoughts, diverting attention from erotic signals, further damaging arousal and maintaining negative affect (i.e., anxiety) regarding sex. Given all this, a habitual behavioral response is the avoidance of sexual relations, which becomes the main factor in maintaining the dysfunction [9] (Fig. 1).

As Corretti and Baldi conclude, anxiety could represent the common pathway through which social, psychological, biological, and moral factors converge to impair sexual response [4].

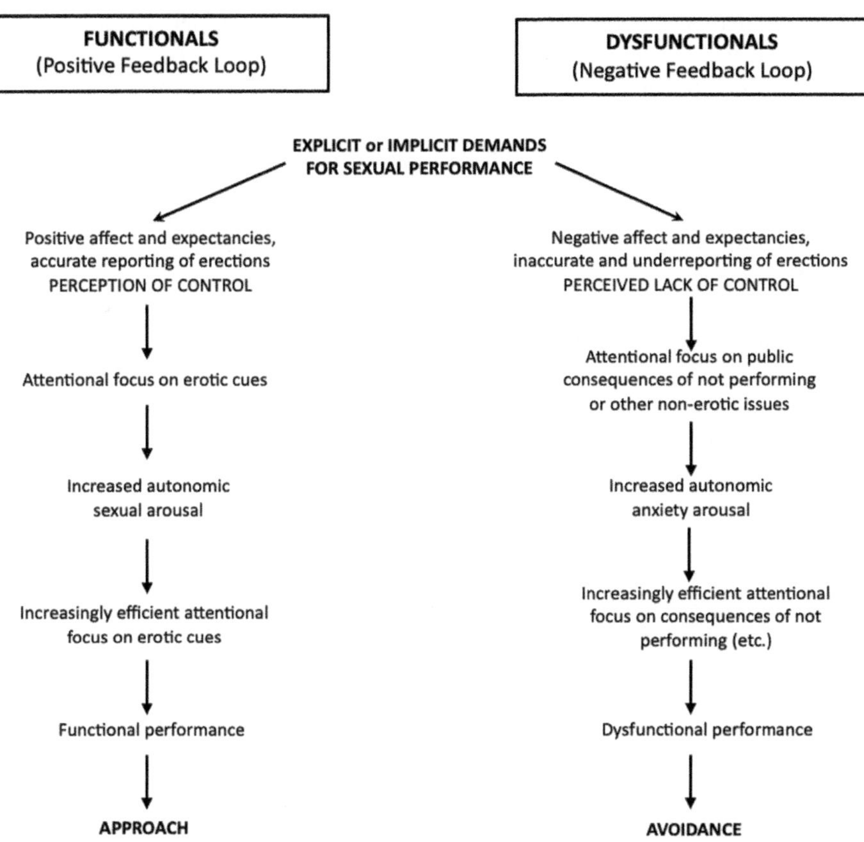

Fig. 1 Model of erectile dysfunction [9]

4 Sexual Performance Anxiety (SPA)

One of the most common expressions of anxiety in sexual dysfunctions is Sexual Performance Anxiety (SPA).

Sexual performance anxiety (SPA) is characterized by excessive concern about one's own sexual performance and one's partner's sexual satisfaction during a sexual relationship. It is one of the most frequent sexual complaints; however, this diagnosis is not recognized for either of the two sexes. SPA was described and treated more than 50 years ago, before modern diagnoses of sexual dysfunction were created, but it remains unrecognized as a diagnosis. Therefore, research on treatment has been minimal. There is no SPA entity in any of the current diagnostic schemes; however, SPA is familiar to most in the field of sexual medicine, usually as one of many factors associated with sexual dysfunction. Sexual performance anxiety may not be recognized at diagnosis, but it can cause, aggravate, or sustain the most common sexual dysfunctions.

People who feel anxiety about sexual performance tend to have idealized expectations about how the sexual encounter should be, there may be a negative vision about the body or some area of the body, and negative thoughts about one or oneself are frequent. If, in addition, this approach to sexuality coincides with stressors such as work or academics, it is easy for SPA to compromise the physiological processes of the sexual response.

SPA affects 9–25% of men and contributes to premature ejaculation and psychogenic erectile dysfunction (ED). SPA affects 6–16% of women and severely inhibits sexual desire. Cognitive-behavioral therapy and mindfulness meditation training have been shown to be effective for PA/SA and are recommended for SPA, but controlled studies are lacking [10].

5   Anxiety and Erectile Dysfunction

From the outset, we must consider the discordance between erection and sexual satisfaction. There are individuals who with an adequate erection do not have satisfactory sexual intercourse, and others who without a full erection have the ability to penetrate and have satisfactory sexual intercourse. In all ED, there is a psychological component, regardless of whether there is an organic cause, hence the importance of multidisciplinarity when investigating and treating this process [11].

ED is a clear example of the consequences of sexual performance anxiety (SPA), already described by Masters and Johnson, and that certain men present after having experienced some erection failure. Given the lived experience, fear and an absolute loss of confidence regarding the next sexual relationship are established. The individual will tend to self-observe the penis, where he will focus all his attention, with the consequent loss of sexual stimulation and loss of attention towards the partner. In these situations, the brain releases a greater amount of norepinephrine; its vasoconstrictor effect on the penile arteries and cavernous tissue may become superior to the vasodilator effect of nitric oxide released in penile nerve endings and vessels in response to sexual stimulation. The consequence is the loss of penile rigidity, thus clearly establishing the important role of the brain in sexual function. The failure of the erection and its dramatic consequences in the sexual relationship with the couple is very "engraved" in the brain and can condition subsequent failures or the avoidance of sexual activity [12].

When SPA is the cause of ED, the person perceives a lack of control, increases their anxiety and tends to avoid sexual encounters. It has been seen that avoiding sexual relations is the variable that is most related to the severity of erectile dysfunction, rather than anticipatory anxiety [13].

6   Anxiety and Female Sexual Interest/Arousal Disorders

Epidemiological studies confirm that anxiety disorders are risk factors for low sexual interest and arousal. Increased sexual arousal activity in the sympathetic nervous system, while increasing genital engorgement in women, implies non-genital sensations that could be misinterpreted as threatening by an anxious woman, thus denying any potential sexual pleasure. Trait anxiety is related to anxiety sensitivity, that is, the fear of the anxiety response itself and the misinterpretation of these sensations: it is therefore postulated that a highly anxious woman is unlikely to experience pleasure from the physical sensations of sexual arousal [14].

7 Anxiety and Orgasmic Difficulties in Women

In addition to desire and arousal, orgasm can also be affected by anxiety. While it is widely accepted that anxious thoughts or feelings disrupt female orgasm, few studies have examined this relationship or attempted to identify specific aspects of anxiety related to impaired orgasm. Most research strongly links aspects of anxiety with orgasmic difficulties [15].

Greater sexual inhibition has been observed among women with orgasmic dysfunction. It is noteworthy that a greater frequency of negative thoughts about their own execution, about the lack of affection from their partner, on body image and/or excessive attention and altruism towards their partner (as well as in cases of delayed ejaculation) have been observed. For orgasm to occur, a focus of attention on erogenous stimuli, positive affect, and pleasure is required.

A review of studies carried out with functional neuroimaging techniques confirm that for orgasm to occur, a significant decrease in regional cerebral blood supply is necessary in some areas (left lateral orbitofrontal cortex, fusiform gyrus, and anterior pole of the temporal lobe) while the brain is activated. Therefore, thoughts about the dangers and fears of letting go of control and being vulnerable would also block orgasm [16].

8 Anxiety and Delayed Ejaculation

We can say that it is a disorder of the male orgasm similar to female orgasmic dysfunction.

Not all cases of delayed ejaculation are related to anxiety although through the clinical history some of them can be explained by the mechanism of performance anxiety.

In the orgasm disorder, the level of sexual arousal may be excellent, but the orgasmic reflex is not activated, nor does the patient detect the premonitory sensations that ejaculation is about to occur. This situation may be due to excessive attention, the person focuses on evaluating the possible change that would be the trigger to ejaculate, the burden increases as time goes by until reaching anxiety levels that finally maintain the ejaculatory block. In other cases, there is a significant inability to concentrate on the erotic encounter, leaving the mind scattered in other ideas that prevent arousal [11].

9   Anxiety and Premature Ejaculation

From a sociological point of view, premature ejaculation was an irrelevant problem until the middle of the twentieth century. In the 1960s, with the sexual revolution, men began to feel responsible for the sexual satisfaction of women. This responsibility, in a sexist context, is the cause of many male sexual dysfunctions, and specifically the fear of not lasting long enough for the woman to reach orgasm, despite the fact that achieving orgasm in women does not depend so much on penetration time as well as other aspects.

There are many definitions of premature ejaculation, as there are currently no single criteria. But the most useful is what the International Academy of Medical Sexology (AISM) defines as "the persistent or recurring condition in which man cannot perceive and/or control the proprioceptive sensations that precede the ejaculatory reflex." And it is this perception of control that is directly correlated with ejaculatory distress.

A study by Kempeneers et al. examined trait anxiety and sexual cognitions in 610 men with premature ejaculation (PE) (DSM-IV-TR criteria) and in 107 partners of these men and compared their scores with normative data. It was concluded that: (a) Men affected by PE are more distressed by the problem than their partners; (b) there is no evidence that trait anxiety levels in individuals with PE are different from those found in the general population; (c) "dysfunctional" sexual cognitions likely play a role in PE, especially with regard to PE-related distress; (d) the different PE subtypes have similar profiles on measures of trait anxiety, sexual anxiety, and sexual cognitions; (e) differences between subtypes are only apparent with respect to feelings of control over ejaculation, with men with acquired or lifelong PE scoring significantly lower than those with a subjective form of the problem [17].

10   Anxiety and Genito-Pelvic Pain/Penetration

Genito-pelvic pain/penetration disorder is characterized by: a) the presence of persistent difficulties with vaginal penetration; b) marked vulvovaginal or pelvic pain during vaginal intercourse or penetration attempts; c) the presence of a marked fear or anxiety of feeling vulvovaginal or pelvic pain during penetration; and d) tension or contraction of the pelvic floor muscles during the attempted vaginal penetration [1].

The pathophysiological factors that regulate this phenomenon are unknown. An interesting hypothesis suggests that there is a strong relationship between anxiety and hypervigilance in patients with anxiety and pain (DS), paying attention to threatening stimuli during sexual intercourse [5, 18].

The best understanding of pain perception has shown that it consists of a complex series of spinal, mesencephalic, and cortical structures. Pain perception can be roughly divided into a lateral somatosensory system involved in discriminating pain location and intensity and a central system that mediates the anticipatory, fearful, and affective quality of pain through limbic structures [19].

Patients with chronic pelvic pain have often been found to have a history of trauma or sexual abuse. Such pain could represent not only a symptom of DS, but also the expression of an anxiety disorder, such as PTSD. In these women, "anxious arousal" is related to sexual pain, reduced subjective arousal, and impaired lubrication [20].

These internal stressors are thought to modulate pain circuitry and be involved in central nervous system sensitization [21].

The resulting damage to self-image and sexual self-confidence and the increased burden of guilt and responsibility for deteriorating relationships due to the inability to have penetrative sex only add to the stress on the woman and keep the vicious cycle going [22].

11   Sexual Dysfunctions in Patients with Anxiety Disorders

Looking at the other side of the picture, sexual difficulties are common in patients affected by anxiety disorders. According to 2020 data from the Spanish Ministry of Health, anxiety as a disorder affects approximately 6.7% of the Spanish population. The review conducted by Szuhany and Simon in 2022 indicates that, at some point in their lives, anxiety disorders will affect approximately 34% of Americans [23]. Anxiety disorders affect 264 million people in the world, being the most important disorder by number of people affected. Taking into account the relevance and prevalence that anxiety disorders and their symptoms have in the world, it is essential to investigate and/or ask about the quality of sexual life of our patients. Sexual dysfunctions are also a frequent difficulty among these patients:

- **Panic anxiety disorder and sexuality**. Sexual aversion disorder is more frequent among these patients. It is believed that sexual aversion disorder could be part of the agoraphobic spectrum [24]. In addition, patients with panic anxiety disorders would have a higher risk of erectile dysfunction and sexual avoidance.
- **Social anxiety disorder** (formerly known as social phobia). The correlation between social anxiety disorder and some sexual disorders is generally accepted, but the specific mechanisms of interaction are still unclear.
  The comorbidity of sexual disorders in patients with social anxiety disorder is estimated to be 30%. Arousal disorders, loss of desire during sexual intercourse, orgasm disorders in both men and women, and high avoidance of sexual intercourse are some of the common difficulties among patients with this anxiety diagnosis [25].
- **Obsessive-Compulsive Disorder (OCD)**. Sexual disorders have a prevalence of 39% in women with OCD, who report high sexual disgust, absence, or very low levels of sexual desire and arousal, anorgasmia, and avoidance of sexual relations. In addition, these patients may show a high deterioration in interpersonal relationships and are perceived as less sensual compared to patients diagnosed with other anxiety disorders. It would therefore seem that OCD would be more detrimental to sexual-affective quality than other anxiety disorders [26].

- **Posttraumatic Stress Disorder (PTSD)**. PTSD affects people's emotional, social, professional, and sexual lives. A prevalence of ED of approximately 69%, orgasm problems, and low levels of sexual satisfaction were observed in male veterans diagnosed with PTSD. Sexual dysfunction following trauma exposure may be mediated by PTSD-related biological, cognitive, and affective processes [27].

12 Treatments Aimed at Anxiety in Sexual Dysfunctions

As we have seen throughout the chapter, the relationship between anxiety and sexual dysfunction is complex because the reciprocal interaction between the two must be considered and, in clinical practice, understanding the cause-effect link in each case requires experience and a multidisciplinary perspective.

There are still no conclusive studies that refer to the different treatment modalities, but Pike's review of the relevant literature during the period 2000–2018 allows us to draw the following conclusions [10]:

- Cognitive-behavioral therapy (CBT), mindfulness training (MBT), and pharmacotherapy with serotonergic anxiolytics (Buspirone ± Testosterone, Trazodone ± Bupropion) show therapeutic potential.
- PDE5 inhibitors appear effective for two performance anxiety-related male sexual dysfunctions: Erectile Dysfunction and Premature Ejaculation.
- Cognitive-behavioral therapy and mindfulness training are effective for performance anxiety (PA) and social anxiety (SA) and are recommended for sexual performance anxiety (SPA), but controlled studies are lacking.

13 Cognitive-Behavioral Treatments Targeted Anxiety in Sexual Dysfunction

CBT has been shown to be effective in the treatment of certain sexual dysfunctions including vaginismus, provoked vestibulodynia, and anorgasmia in women and premature ejaculation and erectile dysfunction in men [28].

Taken together, the results suggest that addressing fears or anxiety related to sex may be beneficial in the treatment of some sexual dysfunctions. However, research on the treatment of other sexual dysfunctions in women and men (e.g., female sexual interest/arousal disorder, hypoactive sexual desire disorder) is limited.

13.1 Treatments Based on Full Attention (Mindfulness)

There are three categories of obstacles to healthy sexual functioning: attention deficit, negative self-judgment cognitions, and anxiety.

Mindfulness-based interventions can address anxiety in sexual contexts by increasing awareness of sexual responses, decreasing judgment towards these responses, and reducing the effect of distractions, for example, by viewing them as mental events that do not necessarily need to be addressed [29].

Besides, lack of interoceptive awareness can inhibit sexual arousal. Silverstein et al. studied the effect of mindfulness training on interoceptive awareness, with participants showing increased awareness of their bodily responses to sexual stimuli (interoceptive awareness) and improvements in attention, self-judgment, and anxiety scores [30].

A systematic review on mindfulness meditation (MBT)-based interventions for sexual dysfunctions indicated that MBT led to improvements in subjectively assessed arousal and desire, sexual satisfaction, and reduced fear related to sexual activity. Moreover, MBT interventions have demonstrated to improve the consistency between subjectively perceived arousal and genital response in women. The research indicated that MBT did not make a significant change in reducing pain during sexual activities. Evidence-based data on the efficacy of MBT in the treatment of male erectile dysfunction was found in one study. Thus, MBT could be used effectively in the treatment of female sexual dysfunction, specifically to improve sexual arousal/desire and satisfaction, and to reduce sexual dysfunction associated with anxiety and negative cognitive schemas [31].

Finally, there is little literature linking MBT to the treatment of male sexual dysfunction. There is a review of 12 investigations that seems to indicate that the practice of mindfulness also favors different variables of male sexuality, such as satisfaction and sexual functioning or genital self-image [32].

13.2   Anxiety, Sexual Disorders, and Psychotropic Drugs

There are people with anxiety disorders who need to take psychotropic drugs. The most common are: benzodiazepines and selective serotonin reuptake inhibitors (SSRIs). Both can facilitate the improvement of anxiety and mood, and therefore, promote the quality of sexual life. But, at the same time, the high incidence of its side effects such as delayed orgasm, inhibition of desire, and sexual arousal are important issues to consider when prescribing medication for anxiety.

14   Conclusions

Studies show conflicting relationships between anxiety and sexual dysfunction.

A low dose of anxiety may not affect sexual response or satisfaction; however, high levels of anxiety inhibit sexual behavior in most people.

One of the most common expressions of anxiety in sexual dysfunctions is sexual performance anxiety (SPA), where negative thoughts about one's own sexual performance predominate, the possible inability to satisfy the partner, the dramatic consequences of this ineffectiveness, together with other cognitive aspects such as a low perception of body image.

Most of the therapeutic strategies are aimed at making attitudes more flexible, learning not to judge oneself, focusing more on the physical sensations of pleasure and not being distracted by anxious thoughts that promote behavioral avoidance with its clear consequences in the perpetuation of dysfunction.

Cognitive-behavioral therapy (CBT) and mindfulness-based therapeutic strategies (MBI) have shown efficacy in reducing the effect of anxious thoughts and learning to connect with erotic sensations without false expectations.

In selected cases, pharmacotherapy may also be indicated within a comprehensive and biopsychosocial treatment of Sexual Disorders.

References

1. American Psychiatric Association, et al. Diagnostic and statistical manual of mental disorders: DSM-5. Washington, DC: American Psychiatric Association; 2013.
2. Stephenson KR, Truong L, Shimazu L. Why is impaired sexual function distressing to men? Consequences of impaired male sexual function and their associations with sexual well-being. J Sex Med. 2018;15:1336–49.
3. Kane L, Dawson SJ, Shaughnessy K, Reissing ED, Ouimet AJ, Ashbaugh AR. A review of experimental research on anxiety and sexual arousal: implications for the treatment of sexual dysfunction using cognitive behavioral therapy. J Exp Psychopathol. 2019;10(2):1–24.
4. Corretti G, Baldi I. The relationship between anxiety disorders and sexual dysfunction. Psychiatr Times. 2007;24(9):16–21.
5. van den Hout M, Barlow D. Attention, arousal and expectancies in anxiety and sexual disorders. J Affect Disord. 2000;61(3):241–56.
6. Kempeneers P, Barbier V. L'influence de l'anxiété sur l'excitation sexuelle: vers une théorie cognitive. Theol Sex. 2008;17(2):66–75.
7. Kane L, et al. A review of experimental research on anxiety and sexual arousal: implications for the treatment of sexual dysfunction using cognitive behavioral therapy. J Exp Psychopathol. 2019;10(2).
8. Tavares I, Moura CV, Nobre PJ. The role of cognitive processing factors in sexual functions and dysfunction in women and men: a systematic review. Sexual Medicine Review. 2020;8(3):403. https://doi.org/10.1016/j.sxmr.2020.03.002.
9. Barlow DH. Causes of sexual dysfunction: the role of anxiety and cognitive interference. J Consult Clin Psychol. 1986;54(2):140.
10. Pyke RE. Sexual performance anxiety. Sexual Med Rev. 2020;8(2):183–90.
11. Cabello F. Manual de sexología y terapia sexual. Madrid: Síntesis; 2010.
12. Pomerol Monseny JM. Disfunción eréctil de origen psicógeno. Arch Español Urol (Ed. impresa). 2010;63(8):599–602.
13. Saito J, et al. Experiential avoidance as a mediator between anticipatory anxiety and the severity of erectile dysfunction. J Sex Med. 2022;19(5):S136–7.
14. Bradford A, Meston CM. The impact of anxiety on sexual arousal in women. Behav Res Ther. 2006;44:1067.
15. Leeners B, Hengartner MP, Rössler W, et al. The role of psychopathological and personality covariates in orgasmic difficulties: a prospective longitudinal evaluation in a cohort of women from age 30 to 50. J Sex Med. 2014;11:2928–37.
16. Stoléru S, Fonteille V, Cornélis C, et al. Functional neu roimaging studies of sexual arousal and orgasm in healthy men and women: a review and meta-analysis. Neurosci Biobehav Rev. 2012;36:1481–509.

17. Kempeneers P, Andrianne R, Cuddy M, Blairy S. Sexual cognitions, trait anxiety, sexual anxiety, and distress in men with different subtypes of premature ejaculation and in their partners. J Sex Marital Ther. 2018;44(4):319–32. https://doi.org/10.1080/0092623X.2017.1405299.
18. Barlow DH. The causes of sexual dysfunction: the role of anxiety and cognitive interference. J Consult Clin Psychol. 1986;54:140–8.
19. Kanda M, Nagamine T, Ikeda A, et al. Primary somatosensory cortex is actively involved in pain processing in human. Brain Res. 2000;853:282–9.
20. Kalmbach DA, Kingsberg SA, Ciesla JA. How changes in depression and anxiety symptoms correspond to variations in female sexual response in a nonclinical sample of young women: a daily diary study. J Sex Med. 2014;11:2915–27.
21. Arpana G, Rapkin AJ, Gill Z, et al. Disease-related differences in resting state networks: a comparison between localized provoked vulvodynia, irritable bowel syndrome, and healthy control subjects. Pain. 2015;156(5):809–19.
22. Basson R. The recurrent pain and sexual sequelae of provoked vestibulodynia: a perpetuating cycle. J Sex Med. 2012;9:2077–92.
23. Szuhany KL, Simon NM. Anxiety disorders: a review. JAMA. 2022;328(24):2431–45. https://doi.org/10.1001/jama.2022.22744.
24. Figueira I, Possidente E, Marques C, Hayes K. Sexual dysfunction: a neglected complication of panic disorder and social phobia. Arch Sex Behav. 2001;30:369–76.
25. Bodinger L, Hermesh H, Aizenberg D, et al. Sexual function and behavior in social phobia. J Clin Psychiatry. 2002;63:874–9.
26. Pozza A, et al. Sexual dysfunction and satisfaction in obsessive compulsive disorder: protocol for a systematic review and meta-analysis. Syst Rev. 2020;9:1–13.
27. Yehuda R, Lehrner A, Rosenbaum TY. PTSD and sexual dysfunction in men and women. J Sex Med. 2015;12(5):1107–19. https://doi.org/10.1111/jsm.12856. Epub 2015 Apr 6.
28. Günzler C, Berner MM. Efficacy of psychosocial interventions in men and women with sexual dysfunctions—a systematic review of controlled clinical trials. J Sex Med. 2012;9(12):3108–25.
29. Brotto LA, Basson R. Group mindfulness-based therapy significantly improves sexual desire in women. Behav Res Ther. 2014;57:43–54.
30. Silverstein RG, Brown A-CH, Roth HD, Britton WB. Effects of mindfulness training on body awareness to sexual stimuli: implications for female sexual dysfunction. Psychosom Med. 2011;73(9):817–25. https://doi.org/10.1097/PSY.0b013e318234e628.
31. Jaderek I, Lew-Starowicz M. A systematic review on mindfulness meditation-based interventions for sexual dysfunctions. J Sex Med. 2019;16(10):1581–96. https://doi.org/10.1016/j.jsxm.2019.07.019.
32. Valderrama Rodríguez MF, Sánchez-Sánchez LC, García-Montes JM, Petisco-Rodríguez C. A scoping review of the influence of mindfulness on Men's sexual activity. Int J Environ Res Public Health. 2023;20(4):3739. https://doi.org/10.3390/ijerph20043739.

Depression and Sexual Health

Anna Giménez Palomo and Antoni Benabarre Hernández

1 Introduction

Depression is considered one of the most disabling mental illnesses. It affects a broad spectrum of populations and is associated with major biopsychosocial disabilities [1].

Depression symptoms include reduced motivation for or reward from engaging in pleasurable activities and may also impair sexual well-being, interfering with intimate relationships. This explains an increased prevalence of sexual dysfunction (SD) in depression compared to general population, estimated approximately twice that of controls (50 vs. 24%) [2].

According to Diagnostic and Statistical Manual for Mental Disorders (DSM-5), SD is a clinically significant disturbance in a person's ability to respond sexually or to experience sexual pleasure, characterized by impairment of one or more phases of sexual function, such as desire, arousal, or orgasm [3]. Sexual dysfunction and depression have a bidirectional relationship, conferring a major burden on patients'

A. Giménez Palomo
Bipolar and Depression Disorders Unit, Psychiatry and Psychology, Clinical Institute of Neurosciences, Hospital Clinic de Barcelona, Barcelona, Spain
e-mail: agimenezp@recerca.clinic.cat

A. Benabarre Hernández (✉)
Bipolar and Depression Disorders Unit, Psychiatry and Psychology, Clinical Institute of Neurosciences, Hospital Clinic de Barcelona, Barcelona, Spain

Centro de Investigación Biomédica en Red de Salud Mental (CIBERSAM), Instituto de Salud Carlos III, Madrid, Spain

Institut d'Investigacions Biomèdiques August Pi i Sunyer, Barcelona, Spain

Medicine Department, Faculty of Medicine and Health Sciences, Universitat de Barcelona (UB), Barcelona, Spain
e-mail: abenaba@clinic.cat

© The Author(s), under exclusive license to Springer Nature Switzerland AG 2024
C. Castelo-Branco, S. Anglès Acedo (eds.), *Medical Disorders and Sexual Health*, Trends in Andrology and Sexual Medicine,
https://doi.org/10.1007/978-3-031-55080-5_27

functionality and quality of life. They share common etiologies, since some hormonal and neurotransmitter disturbances have been shown to be related to the presence of SD among depressed patients [2]. Apart from SD, depression is also associated with lifestyle and behavioral patterns that may contribute to an increased incidence of other conditions, such as metabolic syndrome, which might further exacerbate SD [4].

The most frequently reported sexual problem in untreated depressed patients is reduction in sexual desire (40% of men and 50% of women), followed by difficulties with erection/ejaculation (22% of men) and orgasm (15% of women) [2]. Prevalence of SD has been correlated with increased severity, duration, and recurrence of a depressive episode [5]. According to Hawton's biopsychosocial model, depression may represent not only a predisposing factor, but also a maintenance factor for SD [6].

Even though depression by itself is linked to SD, a great proportion of cases has been associated with the antidepressant pharmacological treatment, which is the most common strategy used for the treatment of depressive episodes given its widely proven efficacy [7]. The complex relationship between depressive disorder, its treatment, and SD becomes a challenge for the identification and management of SD in depressed patients, since it is often difficult to ascertain what is caused by the disease and what is an adverse effect of its treatment.

Given the tendency to the underreport of sexual adverse effects in depression, growing attention to the prevention, assessment and management of antidepressant-induced sexual adverse effects has been paid over the last decades, with the aim to improve sexual functionalities and quality of life while achieving the remission of the depressive symptoms [1, 8].

2 Influence of Depression on Sexual Function

Depressive disorders are typically associated with loss of ability to experience pleasure and social withdrawal, which may affect sexual functioning. The prevalence of SD in depression is around 50% to 70% [9], and loss of interest in sex is the most common sexual difficulty associated with depression [2].

Specifically, loss of libido has been reported to affect 25–75% of depressed patients, and its prevalence appears to be correlated with the depression severity [10]. Decreased desire and arousal have been reported in around 50% of men and women diagnosed with depression [11], but this mood disorder has been also associated with erectile disorder and difficulty reaching orgasm [12].

Differentiating the effect of the depressive disorder from the effect of medications used to treat the disorder can be quite difficult in these cases. Some studies have been performed with the aim to elucidate the influence of depression by itself on sexual difficulties.

An observational study comparing sexual function between adult non-depressed men, treated depressed men, and depressed men who had not received any antidepressant showed no significant differences between treated and untreated men [13].

Unmedicated men and women with depressive disorders showed lower total scores in the Changes in Sexual Functioning Questionnaire (CSFQ) compared to healthy controls [14]. Midlife women with a history of recurrent major depressive disorder were reported to experience less frequent sexual arousal, less physical pleasure, and less emotional satisfaction within their current sexual relationships, even after controlling for medication use, compared with women without depression history or with a single past episode [5].

Dopamine dysregulation is hypothesized to mediate the relation between depression and SD domains. Beside psychological effects, different biological mechanisms have been suggested as implicated in the pathogenesis of erectile dysfunction, such as a vascular dysfunction that affect both brain and cavernous systems, and autonomic overactivity [1].

Studies comparing functional neuroimaging responses between depressed and non-depressed individuals support the previous evidence, since they showed during arousal in depressed men decreased levels of activation in the hypothalamus, thalamus, caudate, and temporal gyri compared with controls, and in depressed women lower activity in the hypothalamus, parahippocampus, and anterior cingulate gyrus. However, evidence on neuroimaging differences during orgasm in depression is still lacking [2].

The above-mentioned evidence indicates that, independently from antidepressant treatment, different areas of sexual health are affected in depressed patients.

3   Effects of Antidepressants on Sexual Function

3.1   Use of Antidepressants in Depressive Disorders

Antidepressants are known for their beneficial effect on mood and anxiety disorders through the modulation of monoaminergic neurotransmission. They have slightly different mechanisms of action and have been associated with SD at some point in both men and women [15].

Most of the commonly prescribed antidepressant drugs are associated with sexual side effects. Sexual adverse effects are independent from their main therapeutic effects on mood disturbances [1]. Rates of SD attributable to antidepressants are approximately 40% [2], even though there is wide variability depending on antidepressant types and the assessment tools used. They usually occur within about 1–3 weeks of initiating a treatment regimen [4] and are associated with 42% of treatment discontinuation in men and 15% in women [4]. They can also worsen the course of the depressive illness, compromise treatment outcome, and affect patients' self-esteem and quality of life [2].

Sexual dysfunction has been mostly described with serotonergic antidepressants. Compared to women, men generally report higher rates of adverse effects in sexual desire and orgasm, whereas women are more likely to report sexual arousal dysfunction, even though rates of problems in sexual desire and orgasm are also common [4].

## 3.2	Mechanism of Action of Antidepressants on Sexual Function

The main neuroanatomic areas that control sexual behavior include the hypothalamus, the limbic system, the medial forebrain bundle, and the ventral tegmentum of the midbrain through a combination of neurogenic, psychogenic, vascular, and hormonal stimuli. A number of neurotransmitters and hormones are responsible for the sexual response [2, 16].

Different mechanisms of action have been associated with determined aspects of sexual function. Specifically, in desire, dopamine, melanocortin, testosterone and estrogen exert a positive influence, while prolactin and serotonin (5-HT) have negative effects. Sexual arousal, which is correlated with erection in men and with genital swelling and lubrification in women, is facilitated by nitric oxide (NO), norepinephrine, melanocortin, testosterone, estrogen, acetylcholine, and dopamine, with negative effects of serotonin. Activation of serotonin systems results in suspension of vasocongestion, thus diminishing arousal mechanisms in genital organs; serotonin activity may also decrease NO function and genital sensation. Orgasm, which is associated with ejaculation, is inhibited by serotonin and facilitated by norepinephrine, dopamine, and NO [2, 16, 17].

The precise mechanisms of action of antidepressant-induced SD remain unclear, since they are complex and different among antidepressants. However, it has been mainly associated with the sexual inhibitory action of serotonin, which inhibits sexual desire, ejaculation, and orgasm, mainly through 5-HT2_A, 5-HT2_C, and 5-HT3 receptor agonism [2, 16]. This explains the fact that antidepressants that raise brain serotonin levels possess a greater tendency to cause sexual side effects compared to those primarily affecting noradrenergic and dopaminergic transmission (Fig. 1) [18]. Specific genetic factors may be also involved in the development of SD [16].

## 3.3	Differential Effects of Antidepressants on Sexual Function

Selective serotonin reuptake inhibitors (SSRIs), including citalopram, escitalopram, sertraline, fluoxetine, paroxetine, and fluvoxamine, are the most commonly used antidepressants [2]. Serotonin and norepinephrine reuptake inhibitors (SNRIs), namely venlafaxine and duloxetine, are the other widely used categories of antidepressants. Tricyclic antidepressants (TCAs) include clomipramine, amitriptyline, imipramine, and nortriptyline, which are generally associated with side effects. Other compounds, such as monoamine oxidase inhibitors (MAOIs), agomelatine, bupropion, mirtazapine, vortioxetine, and trazodone, with different mechanisms of action, are also available as antidepressants [2]. Recently, esketamine has been approved for treatment-resistant depression, with antidepressant effects attributed to its action on the NMDA receptors [19].

The majority of evidence suggests that those antidepressants with greater serotonergic effects are associated with significantly higher rates of treatment-emergent SD than those with predominantly noradrenergic, dopaminergic, or non-monoaminergic effects. Thus, antidepressants can be divided into high-risk

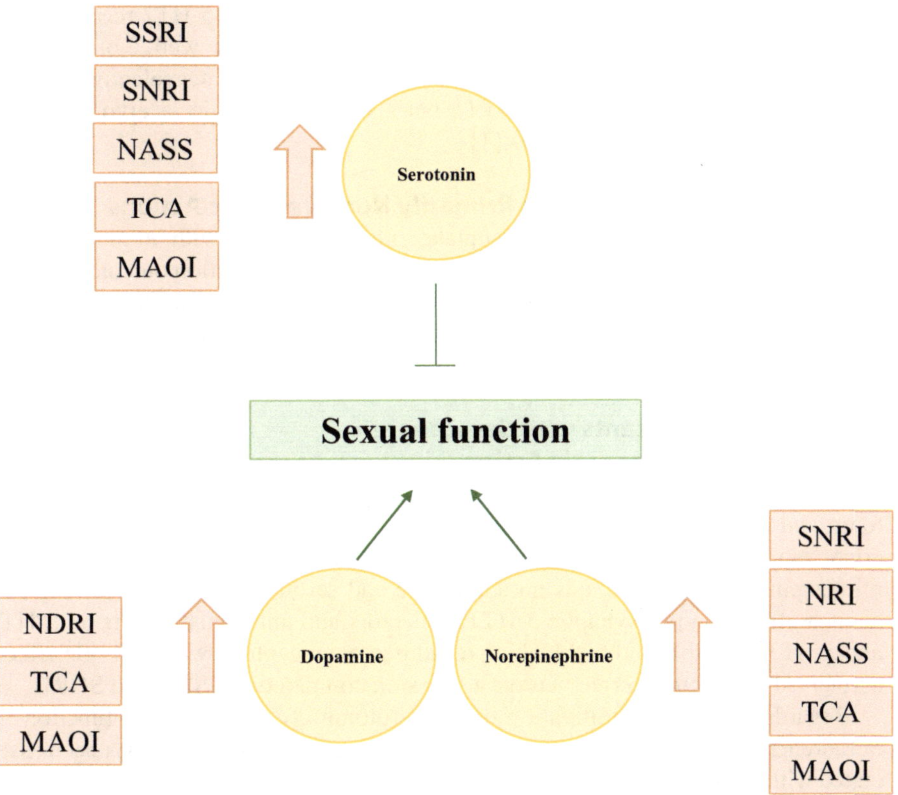

Fig. 1 Impact of different classes of antidepressants on sexual function. Abbreviations: *SSRI* selective serotonin reuptake inhibitor, *SNRI* serotonin and noradrenaline selective reuptake inhibitor, *NASS* noradrenergic and specific serotonergic antidepressant, *TCA* tricyclic antidepressant, *MAOI* monoamine oxidase inhibitor, *NRI* norepinephrine reuptake inhibitor

(SSRIs, SNRIs, TCAs, MAOIs) and low-risk (agomelatine, bupropion, reboxetine, vortioxetine) categories with regard to propensity for antidepressant-induced SD [1].

3.3.1 Antidepressants with Primarily Serotonergic Actions

Selective serotonin reuptake inhibitors (SSRIs), such as citalopram, escitalopram, fluvoxamine, fluoxetine, paroxetine, and sertraline, are the antidepressant group most commonly associated with SD [1], with reports on delayed or absent orgasm/ejaculation, and a reduction in libido and arousal. Up to 70% of patients receiving SSRIs report some form of treatment-emergent SD [2].

Studies report that erectile dysfunction occurs in 10–34% of patients on SSRIs and that anorgasmia is the most common SD, occurring in 30–40% of patients treated with SSRIs [1]. However, in certain conditions such as premature ejaculation, SSRIs can be used as an effective therapy. Comparative studies of SSRIs and recent meta-analyses have generally not identified any statistical difference in their sexual side effect profile between them [1].

These effects seem to be related to the agonist effects on 5-HT2 receptors, but other mechanisms have been postulated to be involved as well. For example, paroxetine-associated SD may be attributed not only to its greater selectivity for the serotonin transporter than other SSRIs, but also to cholinergic receptor blockade and NO synthase inhibiting effects [1].

3.3.2   Antidepressants with Primarily Noradrenergic Actions

Reboxetine is a norepinephrine reuptake inhibitor (NRI) with minimal sexual adverse effects. It has demonstrated superiority in sexual function outcomes in several clinical trials compared with citalopram, paroxetine, and fluoxetine [16]. However, there is insufficient published evidence to state any definitive conclusions.

3.3.3   Antidepressants with Serotonergic
and Noradrenergic Actions

Serotonin and noradrenaline selective reuptake inhibitors (SNRIs), with dual serotonin and norepinephrine action, include venlafaxine, desvenlafaxine, and duloxetine. Noradrenergic and specific serotonergic antidepressants (NASS) include mirtazapine, which stimulates noradrenergic and serotonergic activity through its agonist effects on postsynaptic $5\text{-}HT1_A$ receptors and antagonist effects on 5-HT2 and 5-HT3 receptors and by blocking α_2-adrenergic receptors, with less side effects associated with serotonergic neurotransmission compared to SSRIs and SNRIs.

Regarding SNRIs, a mitigation of the serotonin effects on sexual function by noradrenergic activity has been postulated. For example, venlafaxine has been associated with slightly less risk of orgasm/ejaculation inhibition than SSRIs, but higher than nefazodone, trazodone, mirtazapine, or bupropion [16]. Venlafaxine and desvenlafaxine, its major active metabolite, seem to have lower sexual adverse effects in women compared with men [16].

Advantages of duloxetine compared with SSRIs have also been described, but evidence suggests that SNRIs may only have a short-term advantage over SSRIs [8].

The majority of studies with mirtazapine have suggested a lower incidence of SD compared with other serotonergic antidepressants, such as venlafaxine and SSRIs, which has been associated with the 5-HT2 blockade [16]. The addition of mirtazapine to SSRI therapy has been suggested for the improvement of sexual side effects [16].

3.3.4   Antidepressants with Primarily Dopaminergic Actions

The neuroimaging evidence demonstrates a strong link between orgasm and the ventral tegmental area, caudate and putamen, which are high in dopamine receptors and the neurotransmitter. Thus, dopamine agonists could be particularly useful for ameliorating treatment-emergent SD.

Bupropion is norepinephrine-dopamine reuptake inhibitor (NDRI) antidepressant that has shown not only very low rates of SD (3–14%), but also positive effects on sexual functioning by increasing sexual desire and an improvement in psychosexual function [2].

Strong evidence has shown significantly lower incidence of SD, specifically on libido, arousal, and orgasmic or ejaculatory delay, compared to patients treated with SSRIs and SRNIs [8].

Methylphenidate has demonstrated a significant improvement in overall sexual function, although only for patients who were sexually active at baseline [2], demonstrating that improvements may only be significantly noticeable with patients who maintain sexual functioning.

The addition of bupropion or other dopaminergic agents, such as dextroamphetamine or methylphenidate, during treatment with SSRIs seems to improve sexual side effects. It has been recommended as a first-line strategy used for combating impaired libido, arousal, and orgasm in men and women treated with antidepressants [16].

3.3.5 Tricyclic Antidepressants

Tricyclic antidepressant (TCA) agents act on either the 5-HT or receptors within the central nervous system transporter, and on other additional central nervous receptor systems, with minimal impact on the dopamine system [2].

The prevalence of SD is high with these antidepressants, but the available data is limited. The TCAs have been associated with disturbances in desire, arousal, and orgasm [2]. Being clomipramine the most serotonergic TCA, it seems to cause the greatest disturbance in desire and orgasm, with 41–96% of clomipramine-treated patients reporting SD. This explains the reported efficacy in the treatment of patients with premature ejaculation. In contrast, desipramine and nortriptyline appear to induce lower rates of SD [1].

3.3.6 Monoamine Oxidase Inhibitors

Monoamine oxidase inhibitors (MAOIs) act by preventing the degradation of monoamine neurotransmitters including serotonin, norepinephrine, and dopamine [16]. Irreversible monoamine oxidase inhibitors, including phenelzine, isocarboxazid, and tranylcypromine, are associated with reduced sexual desire, erection difficulties, delayed orgasm, and inhibited ejaculation, likely because they increase serotonin availability [16]. Phenelzine has been associated with delayed ejaculation and failure to ejaculate with higher proportion of delayed orgasm than observed in patients treated with imipramine [8]. Similarly, anorgasmia in females has also been reported to be common with phenelzine, as occurs with isocarboxazid and tranylcypromine [16].

By contrast, moclobemide, a reversible inhibitor of monoamine oxidase A, is associated with a low incidence of SD, having shown 1.9% of incidence compared to 21% in patients on SSRIs, with enhancing effects on sexual desire reported in some cases [2]. However, the available evidence on MAOIs and SD is limited.

3.3.7 Other Antidepressants

Vilazodone, an SSRI and 5-HT1$_A$ partial agonist, and nefazodone, a 5-HT2 antagonist, have shown a very low rate of treatment-emergent SD, with differences mainly in decreased libido and delayed orgasm or ejaculation [20].

Trazodone, a 5-HT2$_A$ antagonist, is an antidepressant widely used in clinical practice. It has also demonstrated lower rates of SD compared to SSRIs, and it seems to increase sexual desire and prolong time to orgasm [16].

Agomelatine, an antidepressant with melatonergic agonist activity (MT1 and MT2) and serotonin 5-HT2$_C$ receptor antagonist activity, appears to be associated with very low rates of sexual side effects [21].

Switching to tianeptine, a selective serotonin uptake enhancer with structural similarities to the TCAs has been suggested as an effective strategy to alleviate SD caused by other antidepressants [16].

Vortioxetine, an antidepressant with a multimodal mechanism of action, has also shown low rates of SD in patients with major depressive disorder. Compared with escitalopram, vortioxetine has shown greater improvements in CSFQ-14 total score, and specifically in pleasure, desire, arousal, and orgasm domains, being both similar in efficacy [22].

Finally, evidence regarding sexual effects of esketamine is still lacking.

4 Effects of Antidepressants on Fertility

Although the direct negative effects of antidepressants on sexual function are well known, there is still insufficient knowledge about their potential impact on the possibility of conception in men and women.

4.1 Impact of Antidepressants on Male Fertility

Moderate-to-severe depressive episodes and psychosocial stress have been associated with lower levels of testosterone, as well as lower sex hormone-binding globulin and DHEA-S, higher secretion of cortisol and prolactin, and lower semen volume and sperm density [15]. A positive association between testosterone levels and sperm motility [23] and a negative association between testosterone levels and impairments in sperm morphology have been described [23].

Associations of antidepressant medications with impaired male fertility and semen parameters have been described in males [15]. Most studies have focused on SSRIs, which have demonstrated a negative impact on semen quality in in vitro, animal and human studies, such as harmful effects on sperm concentration, motility, and morphology [24, 25], as well as increase oxidative stress within reproductive organs. Most of these effects seem to be reversible on cessation of treatment with SSRIs, although this might not be recommended for patients who need these medications to control their depression. An insignificant difference between different SSRIs, including fluoxetine, paroxetine, citalopram, escitalopram and sertraline, has been reported [17].

Evidence is not so consistent in other groups of antidepressants on male fertility parameters. However, it seems that mirtazapine and bupropion may be significantly safer than SSRIs [15].

Given that the existing data are often based on animal studies or human studies with low number of patients [15], it is difficult for clinicians to inform patients on the effect that these medications might have on their fertility. In determined cases, checking a baseline semen analysis and sperm DNA fragmentation might provide some relevant clinical guidance.

4.2 Impact of Antidepressants on Female Fertility

There is controversial data on the potential impact of antidepressants on the possibility of conception [18, 26, 27].

The most commonly prescribed classes of antidepressants increase allopregnanolone, a progesterone derivative considered a neurosteroid that is neuroactive in the brain. Allopregnanolone enhances GABA inhibitory activity, and this suppresses GnRH release, with a decrease in LH and FSH levels and decreased rates of ovulation [26]. Thus, increased allopregnanolone seems to inhibit the pulsatile action of GnRH needed to maintain ovulation, negatively impacting women's ability to conceive.

A prospective study comparing ability to conceive between women with and without history of depression showed similar fecundability. However, symptoms of stress and anxiety have been associated with a reduced success of an in vitro fertilization (IVF) procedure [28, 29].

Other evidence showed that untreated depression in women was not associated with poorer fertility outcomes. One study considering antidepressant use in women without currently active major depression showed it was associated with an increased likelihood of first trimester loss, but there were no significant differences in live birth rates between groups [30].

Antidepressant use in a given cycle, when analyzing cycles individually, has been also associated with a reduced probability of conceiving in that cycle, remaining after adjusting for history of depression [26] (Fig. 2).

Regarding IVF procedures in patients treated with antidepressants, in the case of fluoxetine, it was not associated with adverse effects on IVF parameters, implantation, pregnancy, frequency of miscarriage, and birth rate [31]. Similarly, other evidence in women under IVF procedures found no significant effects of SSRIs on rate of embryonic aneuploidy, implantation rate, clinical pregnancy rate, pregnancy loss rate, and multiple pregnancy rate [27]. Insignificant differences between different SSRIs in IVF outcomes have been reported [30, 32].

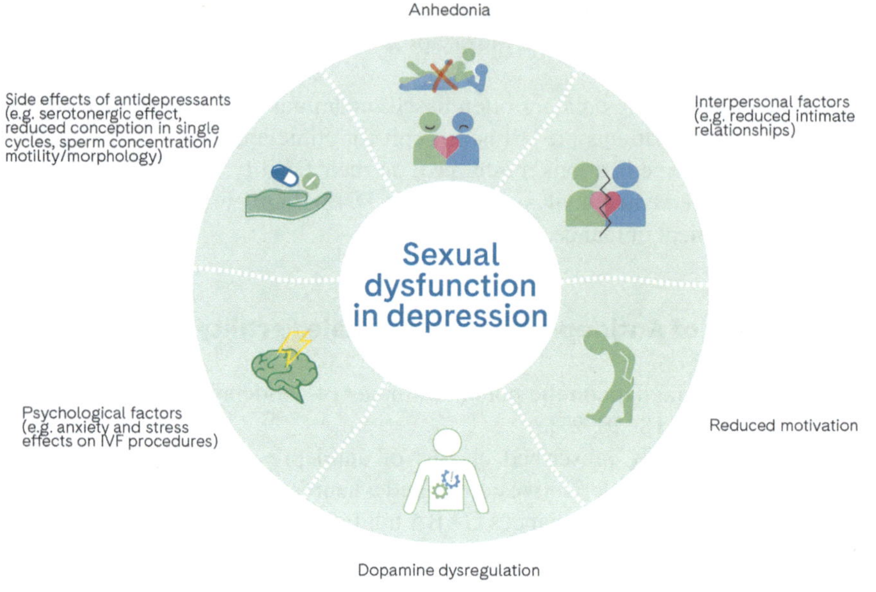

Fig. 2 Summary of sexual adverse effects associated with depression and antidepressant treatments. Abbreviations: *IVF procedures* in vitro fertilization procedures

5   Assessment of Sexual Dysfunction in Depression

5.1   Clinical Assessment

In clinical practice, it may be difficult to determine whether dysfunction is due to depression or is a medication adverse effect. Thus, the assessment of sexual functioning is important before the prescription of an antidepressant and at subsequent visits. Also, the assessment of cardiovascular risk is important for both the diagnosis and management of SD [1].

Educating patients about the potential for sexual adverse sexual effects with pharmacological treatment is important, and also assessing how this problem may impact their compliance, since this information could influence medication choice. Repeated assessments may provide relevant information about either decline in sexual function, which could be due to treatment adverse effects, or improvement, which might be associated with an improvement in depression.

The healthcare professional should determine whether the sexual health issue is distressing or bothersome, and whether any intervention is needed to mitigate this symptom. If the patient reports any sexual impairment, the assessment should address each domain of sexual function. For its detection, direct questioning of the patient and the use of specific instruments are recommended rather than self-reporting [9].

In cases of SD, the presence of comorbidities, the effects of other medications, and possible substance abuse should be explored apart from investigating potential antidepressant-related SD. A comprehensive examination of SD should include the assessment of hormonal profile, especially testosterone and prolactin. In addition, the study of complete blood count, lipid profile, glycemic status, and prostate specific antigen in men should be performed [33].

5.2   Objective Assessment

In order to identify SD, it is important to encourage the use of direct assessment methods aimed to evaluate sexual function before and during antidepressant treatments [2]. The use of standardized questionnaires helps to objectify the assessment of patients and to quantify patients' symptoms. The most commonly used questionnaires include: the Arizona Sexual Experience Scale (self-reported), the Changes in Sexual Functioning Questionnaire (clinician-reported), the Psychotropic-Related Sexual Dysfunction Questionnaire (clinician-reported), and the Sex Effects Scale (either self- or clinician-reported) [2].

6   Interventions on Sexual Health in Patients with Depression

6.1   Management of Sexual Dysfunction

Close monitoring of the potential sexual adverse effects is recommended for optimal care to support treatment adherence and also to consider if any changes or additional strategies are necessary. The aim of managing antidepressant-induced SD is to remove or reduce sexual side effects and to maintain an acceptable control of depressive symptoms at the same time [12]. It is advisable to adopt a biopsychosocial approach to determine all the aspects that can affect both the development and persistence of SD during the follow-up. Clinicians should consider switching to an antidepressant that is less likely to cause SD or add an agent to potentially improve sexual function and promote long-term treatment adherence [12].

There are a number of effective pharmacological and non-pharmacological treatments for antidepressant-induced SD. Before deciding any options with the patient, whose collaboration is necessary, prescribers should first ask which strategies have already been tried, since the patient may already have identified a potentially effective strategy and may need reassurance to continue [4]. Thus, decisions about potential treatments for SD should be individualized and addressed through a shared decision-making process.

The assessment of any potential risk factors might help planning a successful therapeutic strategy. Different treatment strategies should be carefully evaluated considering each patient profile (Fig. 3).

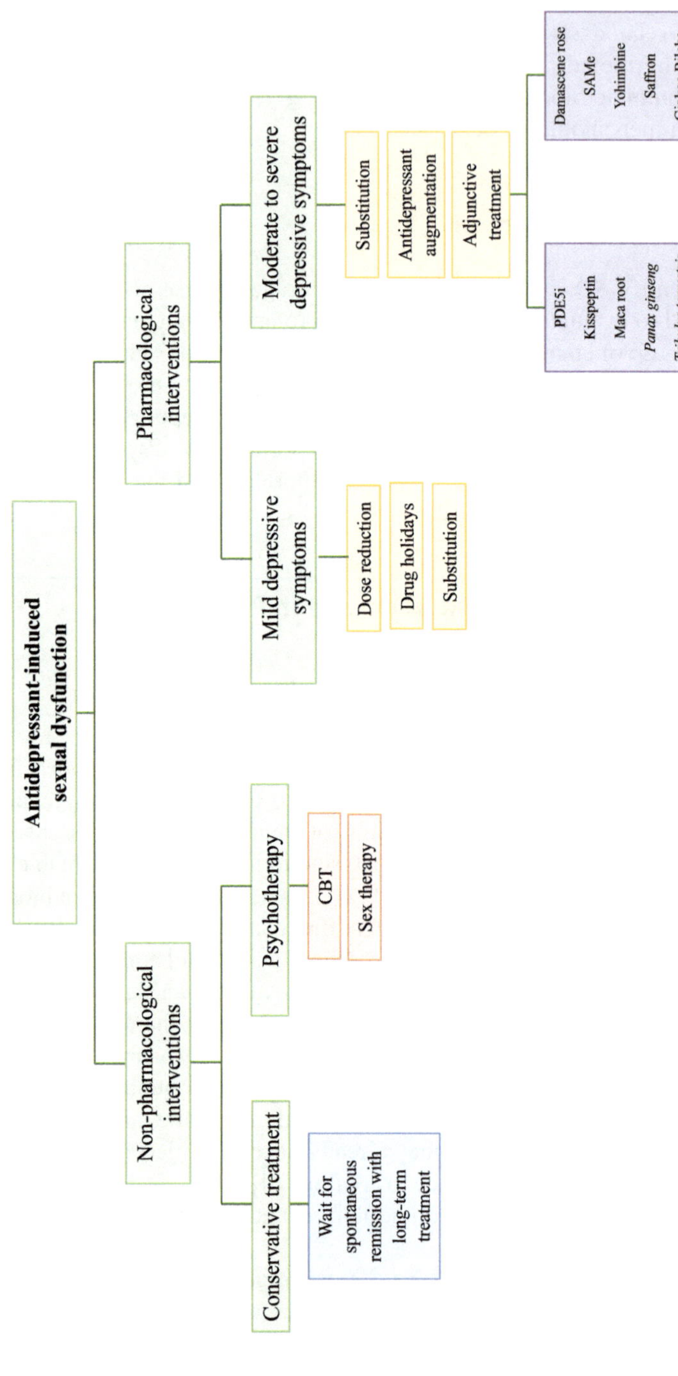

Fig. 3 Potential non-pharmacological and pharmacological interventions for the treatment of antidepressant-induced sexual dysfunction. Abbreviations: *PDE5i* phosphodiesterase 5 inhibitor, *SAMe* S-adenosylmethionine

6.2   Conservative Treatment

Waiting for spontaneous remission of the symptom can be an effective strategy in a small proportion of patients. Nevertheless, since it may take several months for its improvement, it may not be a practical option for the majority of patients [12].

Scheduling sexual activity in accordance with doses of antidepressants could be another possibility in patients taking short half-lives antidepressants, in order to engage in sexual activity when adverse effects are minimized. Lifestyle modifications, such as changing unhealthy dietary habits, smoking cessation, or regular physical exercise could be also beneficial [1].

6.3   Psychotherapy

There is growing evidence that combination of psychotherapy, especially sex therapy or cognitive behavioral therapy, and pharmacotherapy is more effective than one of the interventions alone [16]. The aim of sex therapy is to help patient focus on sensation rather than performance. Cognitive therapy addresses modulating risk factors like stress, performance anxiety, lack of attraction, and relationship issues [16].

6.4   Antidepressant-related Strategies

6.4.1   Antidepressant Selection

Selecting a priori an antidepressant with low incidence of associated SD (e.g., bupropion, mirtazapine, vortioxetine) [4, 8] should be considered particularly in sexually active patients and in those with SD at baseline. However, this option may not be feasible in some circumstances such as, for example, treating patients whose depression has already stabilized with the use of an antidepressant previously prescribed by another professional [4].

6.4.2   Antidepressant Dose Reduction

Reducing the dose or discontinuing the antidepressant is feasible only if the mood disorder is well controlled, since this strategy may entail a considerable risk to relapse of depression [12].

6.4.3   Drug Holidays

A drug holiday (e.g., skipping drug on weekends) is possible with antidepressants with short half-lives in order to improve desire, orgasm, and sexual satisfaction. However, there is a risk of antidepressant withdrawal syndrome with drug discontinuation, which may influence treatment adherence and increase the risk of relapse, being the main reasons why this strategy is not recommended [12].

6.4.4 Antidepressant Substitution

Changing antidepressant to an alternative agent with lower risk of sexual adverse events is a possible option to consider, despite the risk of recurrence of depressive symptoms entailed [12]. Even being a reasonable approach, changing medication needs to be done carefully by monitoring the effectiveness of antidepressant treatment, symptoms of relapse, and potential adverse effects [8].

6.5 Adjunctive Treatment

6.5.1 Antidepressant Augmentation

Augmenting the initial medication with another drug might be useful to maintain effective treatment for depression and also reduce side effects. For instance, there is some evidence supporting the use of high-dose bupropion to offset sexual problems associated with antidepressants, especially SSRIs [34]. Other antidepressant agents that have shown potential efficacy as adjunctive therapy are trazodone, nefazodone, mirtazapine, and vortioxetine [1].

6.5.2 Phosphodiesterase 5 Inhibitors

There is evidence supporting the use of phosphodiesterase type 5 inhibitors (PDE5i) for erectile dysfunction in men receiving antidepressant treatment. They are the most commonly prescribed for antidepressant-induced ED, since they are usually well tolerated [1]. However, further trials are needed to elucidate the safety and tolerability of PDE5i in adjunct with different antidepressants, especially SSRIs.

The addition of PDE5i, as well as the augmentation with other antidepressants with a more tolerable sexual side effect profile, are the strategies that have shown strongest evidence in randomized controlled trials for the management of SD [1].

6.5.3 Other Agents

There are numerous other antidotes that have been reported as successful in alleviating SD associated with antidepressants.

Some of these agents that have shown potential benefits in SD include a partial alpha-noradrenergic antagonist (buspirone), a 5-HT1$_A$ partial agonist (gepirone), serotonin antagonists (cyproheptadine and granisetron), an alpha-adrenergic antagonist (yohimbine), dopaminergic agonists (amantadine, lisuride, bromocriptine), cholinergic enhancers (neostigmine, bethanechol), S-adenosylmethionine, or herbal medicines (Ginkgo biloba, Maca root, *Panax ginseng*, Damascene rose, *Tribulus terrestris*, saffron) [4].

Particularly, Maca root (*Lepidium meyenii*) has been found to improve orgasmic function for women with antidepressant-induced arousal and orgasm dysfunction. In addition, *Tribulus terrestris* and *Panax ginseng* were found to be effective for enhancing sexual arousal and sexual desire compared to placebo in female patients [35]. Ginseng has also shown to reduce hot flashes, menopausal symptoms, and quality of life in menopausal women [16].

Finally, the hormone kisspeptin, a key endogenous activator of the reproductive hormonal axis with additional emerging roles in sexual and emotional behavior, has been studied in women with hypoactive sexual desire disorder (HSDD) in a randomized placebo-controlled clinical trial, showing beneficial effects in sexual function [36].

The selection of an adjunctive treatment should depend on the offending antidepressant, character of the dysfunction, patient's preference, and clinical experience.

7   Sexual Minorities and Depression

Limited data reporting the prevalence of depression and SD is sexual minorities is available. There is evidence indicating that men who have sex with men (MSM) have higher rates of depression and anxiety compared to the rest of male population. There is also a direct correlation between an increase in depression and in antidepressant use and the prevalence of SD among this population. Sexual dysfunction and overall decreased sexual quality of life among MSM can also be attributed to negative body image, internalized stigma, and experiences of discrimination [37].

With regard to gender minorities, there are a limited number of studies on the topic of sexual function and depression. Transgender and non-binary individuals are burdened by poor mental health outcomes, with similar rates between them of depression, anxiety, and suicidal ideation and attempts, which are higher compared to cisgender individuals [38]. This has been associated with high levels of social rejection, such as a lack of support from parents, bullying, increased stigma, and the discrimination experienced. In both male and female transgender individuals, gender-affirming treatments have demonstrated to reduce symptoms of anxiety and depression, to lower perceived and social distress, and to improve quality of life and self-esteem [38]. Non-binary individuals assigned female at birth have shown to report more lifetime traumatic experiences and higher depression scores compared to cisgender sexual minority women [38].

Regarding SD, transgender women have shown a higher prevalence compared to transgender men [39]. Transition procedures such as gender-affirming treatments appear not only to improve depressive symptoms, but also the overall sexual satisfaction in transgender individuals. However, so far, limited evidence is available regarding the effects of depression by itself and by the antidepressant treatments on sexual health in gender minorities.

8   Conclusions

Depression is considered one of the most disabling mental illnesses and is typically associated with loss of ability to experience pleasure and social withdrawal, and also with sexual dysfunction. Even though antidepressants are known for their beneficial effect on mood and anxiety disorders, their mechanisms of action are also associated with sexual dysfunction in both men and women, mainly due to the sexual inhibitory action of serotonin, which inhibits sexual desire, ejaculation, and orgasm. Antidepressants have been also suggested to have a negative impact on male and female fertility, which seems to be reversible. In patients with depression, the assessment of sexual functioning is important before the prescription of an antidepressant, and at subsequent visits, it might alter treatment adherence and patients' quality of life. Non-pharmacological and pharmacological treatment of antidepressant-induced sexual dysfunction, such as switching to a different antidepressant or adding an adjunctive treatment, should be considered through an individualized shared decision-making process.

Acknowledgments Anna Giménez Palomo receives financial support from an educational grant from Spanish Ministry of Health, Instituto De Salud Carlos iii (cm21/00094), and by the European Social Fund Plus (ESF+).

References

1. Bakr AM, El-Sakka AA, El-Sakka AI. Pharmaceutical management of sexual dysfunction in men on antidepressant therapy. Expert Opin Pharmacother. 2022;23:1051–63.
2. Kennedy SH, Rizvi S. Sexual dysfunction, depression, and the impact of antidepressants. J Clin Psychopharmacol. 2009;29:157–64.
3. American Psychiatric Association. Diagnostic and statistical manual of mental disorders. Diagnostic and statistical manual of mental disorders 2013
4. Lorenz T, Rullo J, Faubion S. Antidepressant-induced female sexual dysfunction. Mayo Clin Proc. 2016;91:1280–6.
5. Cyranowski JM, Bromberger J, Youk A, Matthews K, Kravitz HM, Powell LH. Lifetime depression history and sexual function in women at midlife. Arch Sex Behav. 2004;33:539–48.
6. Hawton K, Catalan J. Prognostic factors in sex therapy. Behav Res Ther. 1986;24(4):377–85. https://pubmed.ncbi.nlm.nih.gov/3741303/
7. Segraves RT, Balon R. Antidepressant-induced sexual dysfunction in men. Pharmacol Biochem Behav. 2014;121:132–7.
8. Segraves RT. Sexual dysfunction associated with antidepressant therapy. Urol Clin N Am. 2007;34:575–9.
9. Bonierbale M, Tignol J. The ELIXIR study: evaluation of sexual dysfunction in 4557 depressed patients in France. Curr Med Res Opin. 2003;19(2):114–24.
10. Williams K, Reynolds MF. Sexual dysfunction in major depression. CNS Spectr. 2006;11:19–23.
11. Montejo-Gonalez AL, Llorca G, Izquerdo JA, Ledesma A, Bousono M, Calcedo A, et al. SSRI-induced sexual dysfunction: fluoxetine, paroxetine, sertraline, and fluvoxamine in a prospective, multicenter, and descriptive clinical study of 344 patients. J Sex Marital Therapy. 1997;23:176.
12. Clayton AH, Croft HA, Handiwala L. Antidepressants and sexual dysfunction: mechanisms and clinical implications. Postgrad Med. 2014;126:91–9.
13. Laforgue J, Busnel G, Lauzeille D, Grall-Bronnec M, Cabelguen C, Bulteau S, et al. Evolution of sexual functioning of men through treated and untreated depression. Encéphale. 2022;48(4):383–9.
14. Chen KC, Yeh TL, Lee IH, Chen PS, Huang HC, Yang YK, et al. Age, gender, depression, and sexual dysfunction in Taiwan. J Sex Med. 2009;6(11):3056–62.
15. Beeder LA, Samplaski MK. Effect of antidepressant medications on semen parameters and male fertility. Int J Urol. 2020;27:39–46.
16. La Torre A, Giupponi G, Duffy D, Conca A. Sexual dysfunction related to psychotropic drugs: a critical review—part I: antidepressants. Pharmacopsychiatry. 2013;46(5):191–9.

17. Safarinejad MR. Evaluation of endocrine profile and hypothalamic-pituitary-testis axis in selective serotonin reuptake inhibitor-induced male sexual dysfunction. J Clin Psychopharmacol. 2008;28(4):418–23. https://pubmed.ncbi.nlm.nih.gov/18626269/

18. Milosavljević JZ, Milosavljević MN, Arsenijević PS, Milentijević MN, Stefanović SM. The effects of selective serotonin reuptake inhibitors on male and female fertility: a brief literature review. Int J Psychiatry Clin Pract. 2022;26(1):43–9. https://pubmed.ncbi.nlm.nih.gov/33480810/

19. Garay RP, Zarate CA, Charpeaud T, Citrome L, Correll CU, Hameg A, et al. Investigational drugs in recent clinical trials for treatment-resistant depression. Expert Rev Neurother. 2017;17(6):593–609. https://pubmed.ncbi.nlm.nih.gov/28092469/

20. Clayton AH, Kennedy SH, Edwards JB, Gallipoli S, Reed CR. The effect of vilazodone on sexual function during the treatment of major depressive disorder. J Sex Med. 2013;10(10):2465–76. https://pubmed.ncbi.nlm.nih.gov/23216998/

21. Montejo A, Majadas S, Rizvi SJ, Kennedy SH. The effects of agomelatine on sexual function in depressed patients and healthy volunteers. Hum Psychopharmacol. 2011;26(8):537–42. https://pubmed.ncbi.nlm.nih.gov/22102540/

22. Jacobsen PL, Mahableshwarkar AR, Chen Y, Chrones L, Clayton AH. Effect of vortioxetine vs. escitalopram on sexual functioning in adults with well-treated major depressive disorder experiencing SSRI-induced sexual dysfunction. J Sex Med. 2015;12(10):2036–48. https://pubmed.ncbi.nlm.nih.gov/26331383/

23. Huang I, Jones J, Khorram O. Human seminal plasma nitric oxide: correlation with sperm morphology and testosterone. Med Sci Monit. 2006;12(3):CR103. https://pubmed.ncbi.nlm.nih.gov/16501419/

24. Elnazer HY, Baldwin DS. Treatment with citalopram, but not with agomelatine, adversely affects sperm parameters: a case report and translational review. Acta Neuropsychiatr. 2014;26(2):125–9. https://pubmed.ncbi.nlm.nih.gov/24855891/

25. Tanrikut C, Schlegel PN. Antidepressant-associated changes in semen parameters. Urology. 2007;69(1):185.e5–7. https://pubmed.ncbi.nlm.nih.gov/17270655/

26. Casilla-Lennon MM, Meltzer-Brody S, Steiner AZ. The effect of antidepressants on fertility. Am J Obstet Gynecol. 2016;215(3):314.e1–5. https://pubmed.ncbi.nlm.nih.gov/26827878/

27. Hernandez-Nieto C, Lee J, Nazem T, Gounko D, Copperman A, Sandler B. Embryo aneuploidy is not impacted by selective serotonin reuptake inhibitor exposure. Fertil Steril. 2017;108(6):973–9. https://pubmed.ncbi.nlm.nih.gov/29202974/

28. Csemiczky G, Landgren BM, Collins A. The influence of stress and state anxiety on the outcome of IVF-treatment: psychological and endocrinological assessment of Swedish women entering IVF-treatment. Acta Obstet Gynecol Scand. 2000;79(2):113–8.

29. Verhaak CM, Smeenk JMJ, Evers AWM, Van Minnen A, Kremer JAM, Kraaimaat FW. Predicting emotional response to unsuccessful fertility treatment: a prospective study. J Behav Med. 2005;28(2):181–90. https://pubmed.ncbi.nlm.nih.gov/15957573/

30. Evans-Hoeker EA, Eisenberg E, Diamond MP, Legro RS, Alvero R, Coutifaris C, et al. Major depression, antidepressant use, and male and female fertility. Fertil Steril. 2018;109(5):879–87. https://pubmed.ncbi.nlm.nih.gov/29778387/

31. Serafini P, Lobo DS, Grosman A, Seibel D, Rocha AM, Motta ELA. Fluoxetine treatment for anxiety in women undergoing in vitro fertilization. Int J Gynaecol Obstet. 2009;105(2):136–9. https://pubmed.ncbi.nlm.nih.gov/19201400/

32. Klock SC, Sheinin S, Kazer R, Zhang X. A pilot study of the relationship between selective serotonin reuptake inhibitors and in vitro fertilization outcome. Fertil Steril. 2004;82(4):968–9. https://pubmed.ncbi.nlm.nih.gov/15482784/

33. Simopoulos EF, Trinidad AC. Male erectile dysfunction: integrating psychopharmacology and psychotherapy. Gen Hosp Psychiatry. 2013;35(1):33–8.

34. Taylor MJ, Rudkin L, Bullemor-Day P, Lubin J, Chukwujekwu C, Hawton K. Strategies for managing sexual dysfunction induced by antidepressant medication. Cochrane Database Syst Rev. 2013;2013(5):CD003382. https://pubmed.ncbi.nlm.nih.gov/23728643/

35. Martimbianco ALC, Pacheco RL, Vilarino FL, Latorraca CDOC, Torloni MR, Riera R. Tribulus terrestris for female sexual dysfunction: a systematic review. Rev Bras Ginecol Obstet. 2020;42(7):427–35. https://pubmed.ncbi.nlm.nih.gov/32736394/
36. Thurston L, Hunjan T, Ertl N, Wall MB, Mills EG, Suladze S, et al. Effects of Kisspeptin administration in women with hypoactive sexual desire disorder: a randomized clinical trial. JAMA Netw Open. 2022;5(10):E2236131. https://pubmed.ncbi.nlm.nih.gov/36287566/
37. Cheng PJ. Sexual dysfunction in men who have sex with men. Sex Med Rev. 2022;10(1):130–41.
38. Newcomb ME, Hill R, Buehler K, Ryan DT, Whitton SW, Mustanski B. High burden of mental health problems, substance use, violence, and related psychosocial factors in transgender, non-binary, and gender diverse youth and young adults. Arch Sex Behav. 2020;49(2):645. /pmc/articles/PMC7018588/
39. Mattawanon N, Charoenkwan K, Tangpricha V. Sexual dysfunction in transgender people: a systematic review. Urol Clin North Am. 2021;48(4):437–60. https://pubmed.ncbi.nlm.nih.gov/34602167/

Psychopathy and Sexuality

Francisco Valdesoiro and Fernando Gutiérrez

1   How to Have Sex

Sex is an old issue, dating back to around 1.5 billion years. The evolutionary success of sexual reproduction is attested by its dominant presence in fungi, plants, insects, reptiles, fish, birds, and mammals. However, disseminating genes through sex makes life complex. Beyond the difficulties inherent in surviving to reproductive age, it entails choosing a suitable partner and displaying—or faking—high mate value in order to be chosen in turn. This is not as easy as it sounds, as mutual mate choice is governed by sophisticated decisional algorithms aimed at maximizing reproduction. In fact, a sizable proportion of the individuals of any species fail in this attempt and their genes get lost [1].

Human mating systems are an ancient legacy that we share with our closest relatives, the primates. In polygynous species such as mountain gorillas, males compete violently for the entire harem of females, and only the winning 5% engenders 95% of offspring. Other species, such as bonobos, have multimale-multifemale systems. Their sexual activity is indiscriminate and has, like in humans, non-reproductive functions, namely appeasement, strengthening bonds, or exchanging favors [2]. Still other species, such as gibbons, form stable couples that last several reproductive seasons or even a lifetime. Although monogamy is not preponderant in primates (27%), it is quite common compared with other mammals (3%). However, it is rather named *social monogamy* since strict genetic monogamy—whereby all siblings invariably come from the same male—is virtually nonexistent in nature. On the other hand, monogamous pair bonding does not build on sex, but in love. This is an entirely different mechanism that can be found in some species with immature

F. Valdesoiro · F. Gutiérrez (✉)
Psychiatry and Psychology, Clinical Institute of Neurosciences,
Hospital Clinic de Barcelona, Barcelona, Spain
e-mail: valdesoiro@clinic.cat; fguti@clinic.cat

    421
C. Castelo-Branco, S. Anglès Acedo (eds.), *Medical Disorders and Sexual Health*, Trends in Andrology and Sexual Medicine,
https://doi.org/10.1007/978-3-031-55080-5_28

Table 1 Different types of casual and non-monogamous relationships

Types	Definitions
Situationship	A fusion of "situation" and "relationship," meaning a non-committal romantic or sexual relationship that has not been explicitly defined or labeled and lacks commitment and future projection
Friends with benefits	A relationship which is primarily a friendship, but with occasional sex
Booty-call	Punctual or repeated encounter for the express purpose of having sex
Consensual non-monogamy	Also ethical or responsible nonmonogamy. A range of relational and sexual practices implying more than one partner with the knowledge and explicit acceptance of everyone involved. Includes polyamory, swinging, and open relationships
Polyamory	Consensual non-monogamous relationship in which partners may engage in loving relationships with others outside of a primary dyad
Swinging	The practice by a primary couple of pursuing extradyadic sexual relationships together, often exchanging spouses within a group. Romantic attachment is excluded
Open relationship	The practice in a couple of seeking outside partners independently, with the expectation that this will not interfere with the primary dyad
Polygamy	Culturally sanctioned stable relationship in which a man marries multiple wives (polygyny) or, very infrequently, a woman marries multiple husbands (polyandry)
Infidelity	The act of having a romantic or sexual relationship while in a monogamous relationship without the partners' knowledge and consent
Poaching	The attempt to seduce an already mated individual with the intention to displace their partner

offspring and that, plausibly, has the function of assuring biparental care, keeping the youngster alive until their emancipation [3].

Although mostly monogamous, we humans have a bit of every mating tactic mentioned above, and we are in fact strategic pluralists. This means that we can be promiscuous, celibate, polygynous, (more rarely) polyandrous, or all this sequentially [3], resulting in a wealth of sexual practices and mating systems that differ from each other in the number of people involved as well as in the level of emotional engagement and future prospects (Table 1) [4]. The strategy chosen depends on diverse factors such as physical attractiveness, wealth (in men), age, environmental parasite prevalence, or extrinsic mortality. Importantly, in both humans and non-humans, individuals with different personalities also differ in their sexual strategies, and therefore in their probability of success in the mating game.

2 Psychopathy and Dark Traits

2.1 A Primer

Psychopathy refers to a constellation of interrelated personality traits that are usually organized along two main axes. The *antagonism* axis reflects an interpersonal style that includes selfishness, callousness, low empathy, social dominance, inability to bond with others, and a manipulative, exploitative, and violent attitude toward everyone else without guilt or remorse. The *disinhibition* axis includes an erratic and impulsive disposition, together with need for strong stimulation, intolerance to frustration, discounting of the future, irresponsibility, recklessness, and a parasitic or criminal lifestyle [5].

In functional terms, psychopathy is construed as a hyperactivation of the incentive system, and then an urge for seeking and consuming appetitive stimuli: material goods, social contact, drugs, novelty, power, and, of course, sex. It also entails the hypoactivation of all other motivational brain systems: the alarm, attachment, and control systems [6]. As a result, psychopathic personalities disregard threats, have no close bonds with others, and are poorly equipped to hold back immediate satisfaction in favor of long-term goals.

The prevalence of psychopathy is estimated at 1–3% in the general population, twice as high in men as in women [6]. It also presents some diverging features between the sexes: Whereas men show more overt aggression and antisocial behavior, women manifest greater emotional instability [7]. Psychopathy has its onset in childhood or adolescence and, as witnessed by families, it does not mellow with age, but get worse [8]. At least, this is the case with antagonism, while impulsivity gradually subsides over time.

2.2   Psychopathy and Dark Traits

Psychopathy is neither a unitary nor a well-delimited construct. First, psychopaths are disinhibited, callous, unafraid, or antinormative to various degrees, giving place to differentiated profiles. For example, a distinction is made between subjects with pronounced disinhibition and normal anxiety responses (secondary psychopaths) and those with prevailing antagonistic and unemotional traits (primary psychopaths) [5]. Distinct profiles sometimes lead to diverging life outcomes.

Second, psychopathy is a matter of degree, not of kind. Disinhibition is just an escalation of normal-range traits such as extraversion and recklessness, whereas antagonism is continuous with self-serving and unfriendly dispositions that are unexceptional in the general population. In fact, a total absence of psychopathic traits can cause as many headaches as an excess. At the upper pole of the psychopathy spectrum, we can find sadistic sexual predators that derive pleasure from torture and mutilation [9, 10].

Finally, mental conditions generally show blurred boundaries, so psychopathy overlaps with a range of other socially aversive features that are located in the quadrant formed by high antagonism and disinhibition. The two most important are narcissism and Machiavellianism, with which psychopathy forms the so-called Dark Triad of personality (Table 2). This construct becomes the Dark Tetrad with the addition of sadism. This set of features sharing amorality, egotism, duplicity, and malevolence are jointly referred to as *dark traits*.

Table 2 Personality traits associated with psychopathy

Traits	Definitions
Primary psychopathy	Predominance of the antagonistic features of psychopathy: callousness, manipulative tendencies, instrumentalization of relationships, and lack of empathy, anxiety, or remorse
Secondary psychopathy	Predominance of the disinhibited aspects of psychopathy: impulsivity, reactive aggression, risky behaviors, absence of long-term goals, and low frustration tolerance, with the possibility of accompanying anxiety
Machiavellianism	Manipulativeness, emotional coldness, and deceptiveness. Machiavellian subjects focus on what will be beneficial for themselves with no regard for others. They have a cynical, scornful, and instrumental view of relationships
Narcissism	A sense of entitlement and superiority, dominance, inflated ego, vanity, exhibitionism, self-ascribed grandiosity, and self-sufficiency
Sadism	The tendency to obtain pleasure by causing physical or psychological suffering to others, such as humiliating, subjugating, or exercising cruelty
Social dominance	A preference for social stratification and inequity, and a strong desire to stay in the lead in any interpersonal circumstance and be at the top of the power hierarchy
Anxious attachment	High dependency toward close others, together with worries about being rejected and intrusive or submissive behaviors aimed at obtaining greater commitment from an intimate partner
Extraversion	Normal-range, broad personality domain defined by sociability, assertiveness, activity, positive emotions, impulsivity, spontaneity, and outgoingness
Agreeableness	Normal-range, broad personality domain defined by cooperativeness, politeness, kindness, warmth, altruism, and empathy
Conscientiousness	Normal-range, broad personality domain defined by self-control and self-discipline, hardworking, rule abiding, orderliness, organization, and responsibility

2.3 The Causes of Psychopathy

Psychopathy has proximate and ultimate causes. Unfortunately, all of them are barely known. Proximate causes concern both inherited dispositions and the way they are environmentally calibrated during development. Additive genetic components have been shown to account for about 52% of the variance in psychopathy, whereas unshared (extra-familial) environmental influences explain the remaining 48% [11]. Contrary to common belief, family background and parenting style have little role regarding disinhibition, and no role at all regarding callous-unemotional traits, whose heritability is around 75% [12]. Even so, the developmental aspects of psychopathy are still understudied, and it has been repeatedly pointed out the possible existence of gene-environmental correlations and interactions [6]. Particularly, childhood adversities—parental separation and conflict, maltreatment, deprivation, sexual abuse—are thought to heighten dark traits in adulthood [12]. However, the causal role of environmental hardships may be easily confounded with the effects of heritable traits running in families.

Ultimate causes refer to how psychological mechanisms came to be the way they are throughout evolutionary history. Psychopathy has long been considered a mental disorder, that is, a dysfunction of the brain mechanisms that enable normal protective responses to threats, inhibit self-damaging or antisocial impulses, and generate the affiliative bonds that make social life possible. This view has been called into question on several grounds. First, some psychopathic features do not look like deficits. For example, psychopaths have proved able to feel empathy, but they can deliberately avert attention from the victim's distress to focus on their own goals [13]. Second, diseases rarely confer abilities. Psychopaths are opportunistic exploiters with exceptional skills to deceit, manipulate, and take advantage of others, including the sex terrain. Like many predators, they are also capable of identifying the most vulnerable victims by picking up subtle cues from their gait pattern, a talent that non-psychopaths lack [14]. Finally, an illness is not expected to benefit the carrier and harm the people all around.

In this sense, psychopathy has been alternatively construed as an evolutionarily adaptive strategy based on a parasitic or predatory lifestyle. Exploiting or harming others is often not detrimental for the individual and can constitute an effective—though risky—way of enhancing one's own fitness. In order for this strategy to be successfully implemented, empathy, fear, inhibition, or honesty only get in the way, and need to be downregulated [15]. For example, a developmental trajectory prioritizing immediate rewards, discounting the future, and exploiting others may be beneficial in adverse rearing environments and a winning strategy in adulthood [6, 7, 16]. The evolutionary success of such a strategy has been purported to lie in its promiscuous and uncommitted mating tactics, aimed at maximizing reproductive benefits [17].

3 The Sex Life of Dark Personalities

3.1 Sexual Arousal and Dysfunction

Contrary to many medical conditions, dark traits have not been found to be particularly linked to sexual dysfunction. Instead, they are associated with higher sex drive, more time devoted to thinking about sex, better sexual self-esteem and assertiveness, and decreased anxiety and fear regarding sex. Among dark traits, psychopathy is the strongest predictor of good sexual self-concept and quality of sexual life [18]. Rather are the opposite features, high anxiety and low extraversion, which appear associated—even if weakly—with erectile dysfunction and dyspareunia [19].

There is a flip side, however. First, dark traits negatively correlate with the perceived quality of romantic relationships. Second, if analyzed independently, Machiavellianism does not appear as advantageous regarding sexual motivation and self-esteem as other dark traits. Third, men benefit more than women from these traits [20]. For example, female psychopaths tend to report more lifetime sexual health problems, greater pain during sexual intercourse, a higher number of miscarriages, as well as lower self-esteem and more body shame [21]. Finally, as will be shown shortly, dark traits have countless negative consequences for sexual and romantic relationships, even if these do not exactly fall into the category of dysfunctions (Fig. 1).

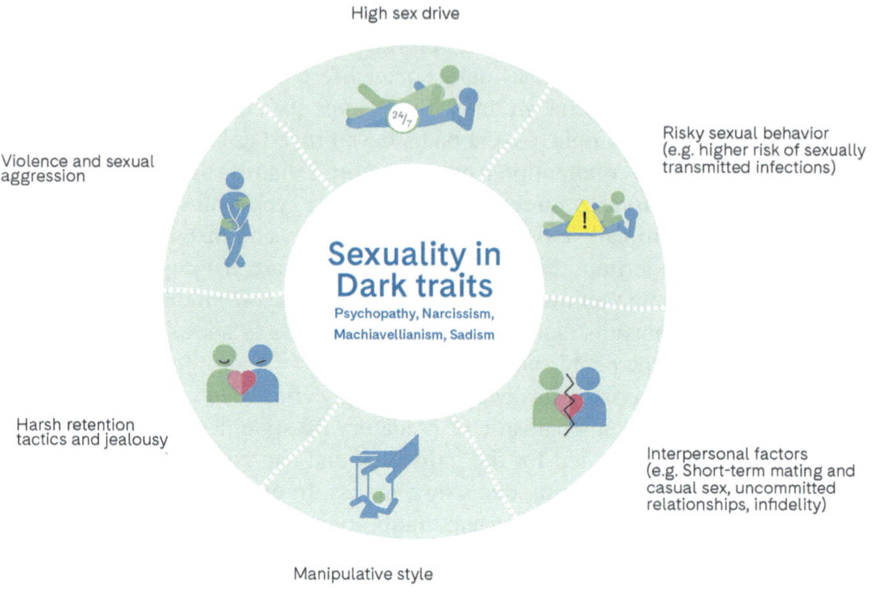

Fig. 1 Sexual and relational correlates of dark traits

3.2 Sexual Interests and Fantasies

Fantasies reveal desires more directly than behavior, as the latter is subject to social sanction, opportunity, mate value, and negotiation with partners. People with dark traits tend to fantasize and consume pornography to a greater extent than the general population. They also fantasize about a wider variety of topics, including unconventional sexual practices such as group sex, bondage, sadomasochism, voyeurism, exhibitionism, frotteurism, transvestism, rape, or pedophilia [22]. Their fantasies more often revolve around anonymous, uncommitted sexual activity without any romantic component, and include elements of control and domination over others. This suggests that their uncommitted and coldhearted sex behavior is not owing to difficulties with close relationships, but is a preference. One exception is that subjects with narcissistic traits more often fantasize about intimate and romantic sexual relationships, due to their greater need to feel special and desired [22]. Although sex fantasies do not necessarily predict deviant sexual behaviors, psychopaths are also more likely to put their fantasies into action [23].

3.3 Risky Sexual Behaviors and Sexual Disgust

Engaging in sexual intercourse with unknown or multiple partners, without protection, or under the influence of alcohol/drugs increases the risk of negative outcomes. Main examples are unwanted pregnancies, sexually transmitted infections (STIs), and sexual assault. Normal-range traits such as high extraversion and low agreeableness are predictors of risky sexual behaviors, whereas conscientiousness is associated with sexual inhibition and fear to performance failure, and thereby is a protective factor [24]. Psychopathy, as an extreme variant of these traits, is expectedly related to increased risks. Particularly, subjects showing traits of impulsivity, irresponsibility, and sensation seeking take more risks across a range of situations and contexts [6]. This association is partly mediated by a lower risk perception [25].

Another conditioning factor in risky sexual practices is disgust sensitivity. Sex entails attraction to the same body parts, products, and odors that most easily can cause aversion, so disgust reactions need to be downregulated by sexual arousal. This is particularly important in the case of casual sex, where intimate contact occurs before sufficient information can be acquired about the sexual history, hygiene, and health status of potential mates. Consistent with this, short-term mating strategies, as well as psychopathic and narcissistic traits, have been found to be associated with decreased sexual disgust. In fact, the lack of sexual disgust has been identified as a mediator between psychopathy and short-term mating [26]. An unusually high threshold (and hence low sensitivity) for disgust may facilitate a more satisfying sex life, greater motivation, more sexual fantasies, a broader range of sexual targets, and less anxiety about sex. The price is more risky practices and a greater likelihood of STIs [21].

A newcomer to the field of risky behaviors are dating applications such as Tinder or Bumble, which have been spreading mainly among younger people as shortcuts to find mates. More men than women recur to dating apps, and their utilization is associated with both the intention of getting casual sex and psychopathic or narcissistic traits [27]. However, motives seem to be gender-differentiated. Among men, its use is chiefly aimed at expanding short-term mating opportunities, regardless of mate value and previous success rate in the mating market. Among women, instead, recourse to Tinder may be compensatory for those with anxious attachment, multiple unsuccessful relationship attempts, and perceptions of being less attractive [20]. Whatever the aim, the use of dating apps is related to a greater number of unprotected sexual encounters, a risk that grows with the duration and frequency of use. Unsurprisingly, the prevalence of STIs is higher among active users of dating apps [25].

Social networks bring other benefits to subjects high in dark traits. They provide new ways to give a false impression of oneself, as well as a quick and easy way to get rid of someone that does not raise interest anymore. For example, they facilitate leaving a conversation with no further explanation (*"ghosting"*), blocking an outgoing partner, or ending a relationship without annoying costs such as grievances, quarrels, or guilt. Terminating an affair through "silent treatment" is more common among people high in psychopathy and Machiavellianism [28].

4 The Romantic Relationships of Dark Personalities

4.1 Quantity Over Quality

Psychopathy and other dark traits have been consistently related to unrestricted sociosexuality. This means that both men and women show earlier sexual debut, increased mate seeking and promiscuity, and greater number of lifetime sexual partners [26]. In line with this, subjects with dark traits preferentially engage in short-term relationships. Casual sex may appear in the form of one-night stands, booty-call relationships, or friends-with-benefits relationships [25].

This association is stronger for the disinhibition component of psychopathy. Disinhibited subjects—and to a lesser extent well-adjusted extraverted subjects—are more likely to get bored quickly, and tend to seek novelty and highly stimulating situations. However, antagonism, narcissism, and Machiavellianism also play a non-trivial role in unrestricted sociosexuality. The selfish and disloyal nature of psychopaths, together with their reluctance to establish human connections, remove barriers to deceiving or abandoning partners, and facilitate a sexual life free of any moral or sentimental constraint [28]. Because of this, subjects with dark personalities more often refuse, withdraw from, or are unable to hold exclusive romantic relationship for a long time. This does not mean that these subjects will never have longer-term relationships. It does mean, however, that when they do, these relationships are more eventful and less placid than the average, and are associated with lower satisfaction and higher divorce rates [16]. Furthermore, the unrestricted sociosexuality of psychopaths must not be confused with nonmonogamy more broadly (Table 1), which can be practiced in a consensual manner and to the satisfaction of all parties, and appears to be unrelated to dark traits [4]. As will be shown below, dark personalities seem better suited for self-serving and capricious versions of nonmonogamy than for ethical polyamory.

The uncommitted sex life of dark personalities has been increasingly understood as an alternative evolutionary strategy, rather than as the side-effect of a mental disorder. This strategy is presumably aimed at outcompeting others in the sexual marketplace, thereby maximizing reproductive success. To this end, it prioritizes quantity over quality of relationships. Indeed, overly impulsive, unempathetic, and narcissistic personalities triple the number of mates compared with normal-range personalities [17] and may also increase the number of offspring, at least in men. Naturally, there is no strategy without costs. These subjects show a decreased interest in caring for their mate and offspring [6, 21], and the resulting instability and discord in the relationship may harm the descent in countless ways. They also have a disproportionate exposure to physical risks and shorter life spans [17]. This tradeoff has been reported in non-human animals too, with bold and aggressive personalities incurring survival costs in return for higher fitness, usually in the form of mating and reproductive success [6, 29]. Furthermore, benefits may be smaller—and costs larger—for women. On the one hand, a promiscuous strategy will not produce in females more than one child per year. On the other, huge intersexual differences exist in the minimum parental investment required: Whereas females should obligately afford the risks of delivery and the energy costs of gestation and rearing, males only need to invest one minute and two milliliters of sperm. This is believed to have selected for greater promiscuity in males and increased choosiness in females throughout the animal kingdom. Finally, it is unclear whether unconstrained sex still is an effective reproductive strategy today. Mixed data on reproductive success suggest that its advantages may have been increasingly offset by contraceptive methods that uncouple sex from reproduction, and by societal and legislative changes that prevent a psychopathic father from getting rid of unwelcome children [21].

4.2   Attraction and Mate Preferences

One may wonder why dark personalities are so successful in the mating terrain, as they seem a rather poor choice for a relationship. This is less problematic for men picking psychopathic-like women. In long-term mating contexts, men are known to target youth and attractiveness over personality. Moreover, when pursuing short-term relationships, men lower their standards in such a way that personality and even physical attractive become irrelevant. Still more, dark traits in potential female partners may rather act as a signal to men about their sexual availability, and then as an attractor [7, 27].

Benefits for women are less obvious. Across cultures, they rather express a preference for kind and reliable men as partners. However, they are not rarely caught by adventurous, arrogant, and hopelessly unreliable ruffians [30], which has been attributed to a number of reasons. First, bold, dominant, and aggressive men are more physically attractive than the community average, though the causes of this association are unclear. Second, dominant and narcissistic individuals also possess universally appealing personality traits such as energy, boldness, social dominance, or self-confidence, which in addition bring with them desirable outcomes such as auspicious economic prospects, popularity, and status. This partly explains why narcissistic men are deemed to have higher mate value than average [26]. Third, dark personalities show accentuated masculine traits: greater stature, broader shoulders, heavier musculature, greater strength, more facial hair, and deeper voices [31]. Women—just as non-human females—have been found to be attracted to these formidable, aggressive, and hypermasculine males in impoverished or hostile environments [7, 16]. This is thought to favor their own survival and that of their offspring when competition for resources becomes harsher, even at the very great cost of partner violence. Fourth, attractive or hypermasculine men are also favored over good-natured men in short-term mating contexts, such as one-night stand relationships, while responsible and kindhearted partners are preferred for long-term relationships [27]. Fifth, women tend to adopt a more promiscuous strategy when entering the fertile window of the menstrual cycle. This is further accompanied by a measurable shift of preferences toward domineering, defiant, quarrelsome, and hypermasculine men, whereas interest in faithful men droops [30]. Finally, both men and women high in dark traits tend to select partners with resembling personality features [7, 16, 26], which is known as assortative mating. This is due to an explicit preference, but also to greater availability, as persons with dark traits are often more willing to initiate a new relationship.

5   Dark Personalities in Conflict

5.1   Infidelity and Poaching

Infidelity is a risky business. Risks include STIs, marital discord or dissolution, harm to the offspring, and (mainly in women) reputational damage, violence, or death [32]. Despite so, 60% of men and 40% of women already in a relationship have made an attempt of extra-pair relationship, and 80% of them have been successful.

Dark traits increase the possibility of extra-pair affairs. Psychopathy in particular, but also adjacent traits such as extraversion, dominance, narcissism, or Machiavellianism, are each one independently related to lower commitment in marital relationships and higher intention to maintain extramarital affairs [32]. Subtle differences have been reported between some of these traits, though this does not modify the general conclusion. For example, infidelities committed by psychopathic personalities commonly lead to relationship dissolution, whereas those committed by Machiavellian subjects—or by women—generally do not, suggesting that the latter are more interested or better able to reduce the potential costs of disloyal behavior [27]. Motives may also differ: Whereas the infidelities of psychopaths rather fall under impulsive sex drives and sensation seeking, narcissistic subjects try to a greater degree to satisfy admiration needs or to accumulate trophy partners [32].

The other side of infidelity is mate poaching (Table 1). Nearly 70% of people in a relationship has received poaching attempts, either for short-term or long-term involvement. Women receive more invitations but make fewer attempts, and are more successful when try. Dark traits predict successful poaching experiences in both sexes. More unexpectedly, they also predict in men a greater risk to have their partner successfully poached by a rival. This may be due to the fact that women commit infidelity not only owing to their own dark traits, but also to analogous traits in their partners. Thus, psychopathic personalities are more likely to both deceive and be deceived [29].

5.2 Harsh Couple Acquisition and Retention Tactics

Couple relationships with psychopathic men or women are bumpier partly because they use abrasive tactics to either gain access to new affairs, negotiate the terms of the relationship, or retaining partners. For example, dark traits are related to the use of more manipulative maneuvers at the beginning of a relationship. These subjects legitimate to a greater extent the use of deception during courtship, and tell more lies. More specifically, psychopaths are more likely to lie for no reason, and to experience more positive emotions associated with lying. Subjects high in Machiavellianism lie more strategically and devote more cognitive effort associated with deception. And narcissists lie more often to gain dominance or popularity [33]. Hoaxes also differ between the sexes in some aspects. In men, they are often aimed at increasing access to sexual partners, e.g., faking more romantic involvement than they actually feel. Women more frequently deceive about their appearance, fake vulnerability, and use seduction or sex instrumentally to please the partner, maintain access to resources, or solve conflicts [33]. A frequently reported form of manipulation is *love bombing*, a pattern of intensive focus on a new partner based on unceasing attention and exaggerated displays of adoration, deliberately intended to create idealization and dependence. Over time, engulfment is alternated with disregard, devaluing comments, and abusive behaviors that reinforce subjugation [34].

Once the relationship with a desired partner is ongoing, people carry out a variety of maneuvers in order to maintain this bond or to deter infidelity or defection, which are called mate retention tactics. These maneuvers are often driven by jealousy. Reactive jealousy, our preset emotional response in front a real or potential relationship threat by a rival, is commonly considered healthy and is in fact positively related to the quality of the relationship. This is also the case with innocuous or benefit-provisioning tactics of mate retention, such as showing affection, paying compliments, buying gifts, or enhancing one's appearance. On the contrary, dark traits are associated with preemptive or possessive jealousy and with the recourse to cost-inflicting mate retention tactics. Among the latter, there are hypervigilance, monopolization of time, verbal pressure, jealousy induction, restraining movement, thwarting social life, blaming, stalking, sexual coercion, menaces of violence, or actual violent retaliation against partner or rivals [29]. Also, subjects with narcissistic and psychopathic traits remain more alert to potential rivals, perceive a greater likelihood of partner's infidelity, and are more predisposed to take vengeance on both the partner and the potential rival [15, 32]. It is difficult to discern, however, whether psychopaths are in fact more jealous, their partners are more likely to double-cross them, or both. For example, it has been found that nonpaternity rates are 2% worldwide for men with high paternity confidence, but are as high as 30% for those who suspect that the biological father is a rival. An additional complexity is that dark personalities are at the same time possessively jealous and unfaithful. This is not unexpected, as securing exclusive access to one's partner while capitalizing on any other mating opportunity seems a winning reproductive strategy.

Finally, subjects with dark personalities solve conflicts in hurtful ways. They often live relationships like a strategic game and specialize in the use of particularly unrespectful and biting movements. These include denigration, destroying property, questioning partner's perception or memory (*"gaslighting"*), shutting down conversations or discontinuing any communication in the case of conflict (*"stonewalling"*), hostile withdrawing, threatening violence, and actual physical violence [34]. Within intimate relationships, physical aggression is equally likely for men and women, but are men who cause the most serious harm. These maneuvers are aimed at producing fear, creating uncertainty about the relationship, increasing dependency, or damaging partners' self-concept.

6 The Darkest Side of Dark Personalities

Although many psychopaths may conduct their lives far away from legal problems, they show as a group a higher rate of criminal behavior than the general population. Despite a low prevalence of around 1–3%, psychopaths carry out 50% of violent crimes [9]. In prison populations, psychopathic offenders had twice as many charges for violent offences as their non-psychopathic counterparts. Psychopathy also is the single most reliable predictor of recidivism regarding sexual assault and homicide [35].

In addition, the crimes committed by psychopaths are of a different nature. Their distinctive sign is not defensive aggression—an emotional response to a perceived menace, like in crimes of passion—but the calm, unemotional violence exerted in pursuit of desired goals. About 93.3% of the homicides committed by psychopaths are carried out in cold blood and with instrumental rather than emotional motives, in contrast with 48.4% for non-psychopathic offenders [15]. Concerning domestic violence, aggressions by male primary psychopaths are more instrumental and indirect, rather resorting to diverse manipulation techniques, while secondary psychopaths, with a prevailing impulsive component, have the highest likelihood of direct physical aggression toward the partner. However, psychopathy is an uncommon condition among perpetrators of femicide [36].

There exists systematic covariation between psychopathy and sexual crimes as well. Psychopaths are consistently overrepresented among rapists. Their prevalence has been found to be one-third for polymorphic (indiscriminate) sexual aggressors, one quarter for sexual aggressors of women, and one in seven for sexual aggressors of children [23]. The presence of psychopathy discriminates single from multiple sexual killers and rapists from sexual murderers, and psychopathic murderers exhibit a significantly higher level of gratuitous and sadistic violence [9, 10].

In the upper extreme of the so-called *scale of evil* [10], there is serial sexual murder, which is chiefly related to callous-unemotional traits. In contrast to the poorly planned and executed assaults by disinhibited psychopaths, antagonistic perpetrators choose deserted crime scenes, more often kill the victim, remove evidence to avoid detection, and are more difficult to identify and convict. The other crucial component of serial murder appears to be severe sexual sadism, a paraphilic disorder in which sexual arousal is triggered by the infliction of pain, suffering, or humiliation on a non-consenting victim, and usually entails extreme sexual violence. Up to 50% of sexual killers are sexually sadistic, and rates are still higher for serial sexual killers. In fact, sex drive is a frequent motivation for serial murder. These homicidal acts are typically fantasy driven rather than instrumental and are conducted in a ritualistic way that includes control and torture; the victims mostly are casual acquaintances or strangers, female, of about the same age and race of the perpetrator, who is almost invariably a male (95%); vaginal penetration occurs in half—and anal in one quarter—of cases; intimate methods of killing requiring close contact are chosen, such as strangulation, stabbing, or beating, whereas firearms are uncommon; post-mortem sexual acts occur in one-third of cases, and mutilation, dismemberment, and biting occur in almost 10% of cases each [10]. Fortunately, the fascination that sexual predators exert is inversely proportional to their epidemiological relevance, as only 20–50 serial killers are estimated to operate in the USA—and probably elsewhere—at any given time, and they are responsible for only 1–2% of annual homicide victims.

7 Conclusions

Psychopathy and dark traits are associated with a better sex life, mainly through increased drive, greater variety and enjoyment, and less anxiety and dysfunction. A thoughtless lifestyle, however, also entails costs to the individual in terms of frenzied romantic lives and health issues, such as a fourfold higher risk of STIs [37]. Psychopaths are not amenable to—and rarely seek—treatment for their traits. They follow unalterable trajectories that will repeatedly require medical attention due to injuries, infections, or drug misuse. But above all, dark personalities produce casualties around them [28]. They pursue selfish social and sexual agendas, utilize and exploit others, and use self-serving, insensitive, duplicitous, and manipulative tactics to get their way. Not unexpectedly, having had a dark partner is a better predictor of posttraumatic stress disorder than childhood abuse [34]. It is therefore people around the psychopath who will be often in need of professional advice, support, and protection.

References

1. Puts D. Human sexual selection. Curr Opin Psychol. 2016;7:28–32. https://doi.org/10.1016/j.copsyc.2015.07.011.
2. Meston CM, Buss DM. Why humans have sex. Arch Sex Behav. 2007;36(4):477–507. https://doi.org/10.1007/s10508-007-9175-2.
3. Gangestad S, Simpson J. The evolution of human mating: trade-offs and strategic pluralism. Behav Brain Sci. 2000;23:573–87. https://doi.org/10.1017/S0140525X0000337X.
4. Scoats R, Campbell C. What do we know about consensual non-monogamy. Curr Opin Psychol. 2022;48:101468. https://doi.org/10.1016/j.copsyc.2022.101468.
5. Patrick CJ. Psychopathy: current knowledge and future directions. Annu Rev Clin Psychol. 2022;18:387–415. https://doi.org/10.1146/annurev-clinpsy-072720-012851.
6. Ene I, Wong K, Salali G. Is it good to be bad? An evolutionary analysis of the adaptive potential of psychopathic traits. Evol Hum Sci. 2022;4:E37. https://doi.org/10.1017/ehs.2022.36.
7. Blanchard AE, Dunn TJ, Sumich A. Borderline personality traits in attractive women and wealthy low attractive men are relatively favoured by the opposite sex. Pers Individ Diff. 2021;169:109964. https://doi.org/10.1016/j.paid.2020.109964.
8. Andersen DM, Veltman E, Sellbom M. Surviving senior psychopathy: informant reports of deceit and antisocial behavior in multiple types of relationships. Int J Offender Ther Comp Criminol. 2022;66(15):1703–25. https://doi.org/10.1177/0306624X211067089.
9. Fox B. Psychopathy and homicide. In: DeLisi M, editor. Routledge international handbook of psychopathy and crime. New York, NY: Routledge; 2018. p. 279–300. https://doi.org/10.4324/9781315111476.
10. Hickey EW, Walters BK, Drislane LE, Palumbo IM, Patrick CJ. Deviance at its darkest: serial murder and psychopathy. In: Patrick CJ, editor. Handbook of psychopathy. New York, NY: Guilford Press; 2018. p. 570–84.
11. Waldman ID, Rhee SH. Genetic and environmental influences on psychopathy and antisocial behavior. In: Patrick CJ, editor. Handbook of psychopathy. New York, NY: Guilford Press; 2018. p. 205–28.
12. Watts AL, Donahue K, Lilienfeld SO, Latzman RD. Gender moderates psychopathic traits' relations with self-reported childhood maltreatment. Pers Individ Diff. 2017;119:175–80. https://doi.org/10.1016/j.paid.2017.07.011.

13. Dutton K. The wisdom of psychopaths: what saints, spies, and serial killers can teach us about success. Toronto, ON: Doubleday Canada; 2012. p. 222.
14. Gillespie SM, Centifanti LC, Brewer G. Psychopathy and sexual violence. In: DeLisi M, editor. Routledge international handbook of psychopathy and crime. New York, NY: Routledge; 2018. p. 413–25. https://doi.org/10.4324/9781315111476.
15. Meloy J, Book A, Hosker-Field A, Methot-Jones T, Roters J. Social, sexual, and violent predation: are psychopathic traits evolutionarily adaptive? Violence Gend. 2018;5:153–65. https://doi.org/10.1089/vio.2018.0012.
16. Burtaverde V. Women high on the dark triad traits are more attracted to narcissistic males if they are oriented to long term mating and had fewer experiences with unfaithful men. Pers Individ Diff. 2021;173:110627. https://doi.org/10.1016/j.paid.2021.110627.
17. Gutiérrez F, Valdesoiro F. The evolution of personality disorders: a review of proposals. Front Psych. 2023;14:1110420. https://doi.org/10.3389/fpsyt.2023.1110420.
18. Steininger B, Pietschnig J. Evidence for the superordinate predictive ability of trait psychopathy: the dark triad and quality of sexual life. Pers Individ Diff. 2022;193:111620. https://doi.org/10.1016/j.paid.2022.111620.
19. Vance G, Zeigler-Hill V, Shackelford TK. Personality and erectile dysfunction in heterosexual romantic relationships: results from men's self-reports and women's partner-reports. Curr Psychol. 2022;42:30800–12. https://doi.org/10.1007/s12144-022-04091-x.
20. Jonason P, Bulyk R. Who uses tinder?: the dark triad traits, attachment, and mate value. Stud Psychol. 2019;19(1):5–15. https://doi.org/10.21697/sp.2019.19.1.01.
21. Carter GL, Lyons M, Brewer G. Lifetime offspring and the dark triad. Pers Individ Diff. 2018;132:79–83. https://doi.org/10.1016/j.paid.2018.05.017.
22. Baughman HM, Jonason PK, Veselka L, Vernon PA. Four shades of sexual fantasies linked to the dark triad. Pers Individ Diff. 2014;67:47–51. https://doi.org/10.1016/j.paid.2014.01.034.
23. Cale J, Burton M. Psychopathy and sexual aggression: a review of empirical research. In: DeLisi M, editor. Routledge international handbook of psychopathy and crime. New York, NY: Routledge; 2018. p. 334–50. https://doi.org/10.4324/9781315111476.
24. Allen MS, Walter EE. Linking big five personality traits to sexuality and sexual health: a meta-analytic review. Psychol Bull. 2018;144(10):1081–110. https://doi.org/10.1037/bul0000157.
25. Flesia L, Fietta V, Foresta C, Monaro M. "What are you looking for?" investigating the association between dating app use and sexual risk behaviors. Sex Med. 2021;9(4):100405. https://doi.org/10.1016/j.esxm.2021.100405.
26. Burtaverde V, Jonason PK, Ene C, Istrate M. On being "dark" and promiscuous: the dark triad traits, mate value, disgust, and sociosexuality. Pers Individ Diff. 2021;168:110255. https://doi.org/10.1016/j.paid.2020.110255.
27. Freyth L, Jonason PK. Overcoming agreeableness: Sociosexuality and the dark triad expanded and revisited. Pers Individ Diff. 2023;203:112009. https://doi.org/10.1016/j.paid.2022.112009.
28. Jonason PK, Kaźmierczak I, Campos AC, Davis MD. Leaving without a word: ghosting and the dark triad traits. Acta Psychol. 2021;220:103425. https://doi.org/10.1016/j.actpsy.2021.103425.
29. Jonason PK, Li NP, Buss DM. The costs and benefits of the dark triad: implications for mate poaching and mate retention tactics. Pers Individ Diff. 2010;48(4):373–8. https://doi.org/10.1016/j.paid.2009.11.003.
30. Durante KM, Griskevicius V, Simpson JA, Cantú SM, Li NP. Ovulation leads women to perceive sexy cads as good dads. J Pers Soc Psychol. 2012;103(2):292–305. https://doi.org/10.1037/a0028498.
31. Rodriguez N, Lukaszewski A. Functional coordination of personality strategies with physical strength and attractiveness: a multi-sample investigation at the HEXACO facet-level. J Res Pers. 2020;89:104040. https://doi.org/10.1016/j.jrp.2020.104040.
32. Alavi M, Kye Mei T, Mehrinezhad SA. The dark triad of personality and infidelity intentions: the moderating role of relationship experience. Pers Individl Diff. 2018;128:49–54. https://doi.org/10.1016/j.paid.2018.02.023.

33. Jonason PK, Lyons M, Baughman HM, Vernon PA. What a tangled web we weave: the dark triad traits and deception. Pers Individ Diff. 2014;70:117–9. https://doi.org/10.1016/j.paid.2014.06.038.
34. Arabi S. Narcissistic and psychopathic traits in romantic partners predict post-traumatic stress disorder symptomology: evidence for unique impact in a large sample. Pers Individ Diff. 2023;201:111942. https://doi.org/10.1016/j.paid.2022.111942.
35. Douglas KS, Vincent GM, Edens JF. Risk for criminal recidivism: the role of psychopathy. In: Patrick CJ, editor. Handbook of psychopathy. New York, NY: Guilford Press; 2018. p. 682–709.
36. Santos-Hermoso J, González-Álvarez JL, López-Ossorio JJ, García-Collantes Á, Alcázar-Córcoles MÁ. Psychopathic femicide: the influence of psychopathy on intimate partner homicide. J Forensic Sci. 2022;67(4):1579–92. https://doi.org/10.1111/1556-4029.15038.
37. Lin YT, Hsu JW, Huang KL, Tsai SJ, Su TP, Li CT, et al. Sexually transmitted infections among adolescents with conduct disorder: a nationwide longitudinal study. Eur Child Adolesc Psychiatry. 2021;2021(30):1187–93. https://doi.org/10.1007/s00787-020-01605-5.

Parkinson and Sexuality

Alessandra Graziottin and Laura Bertolasi

1   Introduction

Parkinson's disease (PD) is a neurodegenerative, chronic, and progressive disorder. It is a prerogative of advanced age, reaching the prevalence of 2.6% after the age of 80. In a very small percentage (3–5%), it can affect young individuals (sometimes younger than 20 years) [1].

From the neuropathological point of view, PD presents two leading features:

1. An accumulation of α-synuclein aggregates inside the nerve cells.
2. A neuronal degeneration at the pars-compacta level of the black substance of the ventral midbrain.

Although the brain areas involved are defined, the underlying pathogenetic mechanism is not yet well understood.

In recent years, the hypothesis that PD has a gastrointestinal onset has gained ground: the lesion or malfunction of the gut wall would allow various pathogens to reach and damage the enteric nervous system and then the damage could reach the central nervous system.

The main consequence will however be a progressive neuronal loss with the degeneration of the circuits of deep nuclei of the brain: the basal ganglia [2]. PD

A. Graziottin (✉)
Center of Gynecology and Medical Sexology, H. San Raffaele Resnati, Milan, Italy

Department of Obstetrics and Gynecology, University of Verona, Verona, Italy

Department of Endocrinology and Metabolic Diseases, Federico II University, Naples, Italy

Alessandra Graziottin Foundation for the Cure and Care of Pain in Women NPO, Milan, Italy
e-mail: a.graziottin@studiograziottin.it

L. Bertolasi
Department of Neurology, University of Verona, Verona, Italy
e-mail: laura.bertolasi@univr.it

becomes clinically evident when 70–80% of motor neurons have already been destroyed. This leads to a major disruption of the fine motor tuning that underlines motor competence.

An immunologic etiology is equally discussed currently, even if the precise phenomenology remains not perfectly understood [3].

Sexual dysfunctions (SD) are the most systematically neglected non-motor symptoms in PD, in spite of their high prevalence [4–8] (Box 1).

Box 1: Sexual Dysfunction in Parkinson Patients: Key Points
- Sexual dysfunctions (SD) are the most neglected non-motor symptoms in Parkinson's disease (PD).
- Prevalence rates of sexual dysfunctions in Parkinson's disease are under-estimated.
- SD were described in about 68% of men, and in around 53% of women.
- Loss of libido is the main sexual concern in both sexes.
- Decreased libido is likely caused by loss of the neurotransmitter dopamine, proper of the pathophysiology of PD [4].
- Prevalence of SD in the form of compulsive sexual behavior is higher in men, by 5.2%, than in women, by 0.5%.
- SDs associated with the use of drugs for PD therapy are reported in 98.1% of cases (Fig. 1).

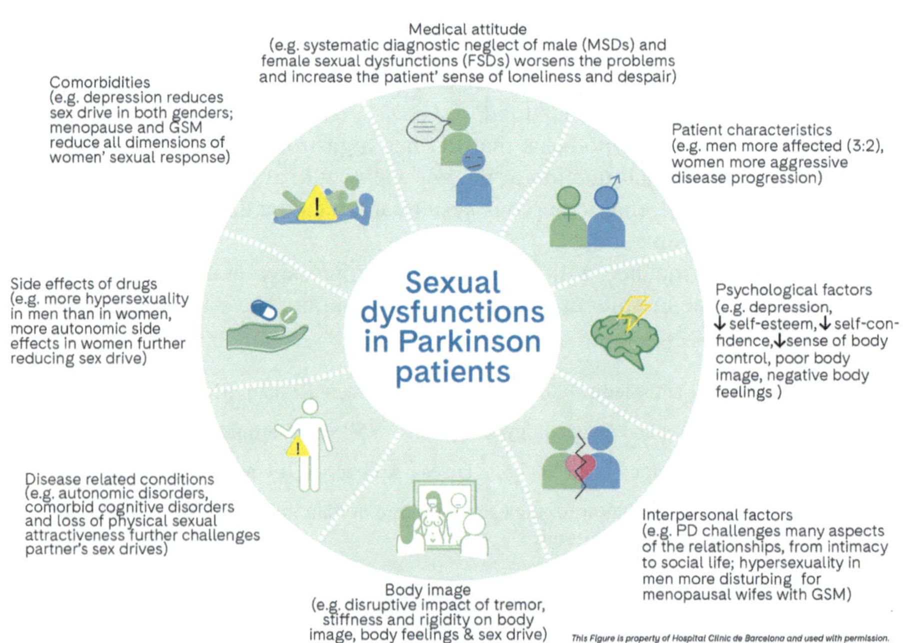

Fig. 1 Sexual dysfunctions in Parkinson patients

Depression, caused by this devastating disease, is a major symptom in PD patients [9] and a major contributor of the loss of sex drive in affected women. It can have a more pervasive effect on different biological component of sexual response when the inhibiting impact of depression on sex drive is amplified both by the menopausal loss of sexual hormones (estrogens and progesterone) and by the age dependent loss of testosterone and dehydroepiandrosterone (DHEA). Please refer to chapters on *"Sexuality across lifespan II: FSD classification and women's vulnerabilities in the reproductive age"* and *"Sexuality across the lifespan III: women's vulnerabilities from early menopause to senescence."*

Of note, recent experimental data suggest that sexual symptoms, still so neglected and under-investigated in PD patients, could be the heralds, the early red-alerts of an impaired dopamine metabolism and of an impending PD [10].

The aim of this chapters is threefold:

1. Analyze the key impact of PD on both male and female sexual function.
2. Describe the impact of PD treatments, and specifically of L-Dopa, on male sexuality, focusing on impulse control disorders, namely hypersexuality, as the female seems to be less affected by this drug.
3. Stress the importance of menopausal hormone therapy (MHT) in reducing the onset and progression of PD in women, while attenuating all the menopausal symptoms that can as well burden and impair the female life and sexual experience.

2 PD: The Leading Features

First described by James Parkinson in 1817 in "An Essay on the Shaking Palsy," it is clinically characterized by key motor symptoms:

- **Tremor:** The most evident clinical manifestation in PD can be reduced until it disappears during voluntary action and is always absent during sleep. Characterized by low frequency (4–6 cycles/s), it is aggravated both by emotional stress and cold. It habitually involves the upper extremities. It often affects one hand with the peculiar *"pill rolling"* pattern, but it can also affect the chin, jaw, and legs. Neck or voice involvement rarely occurs, unlike essential tremor, which is why this element may be useful in differential diagnosis [11, 12].
- **Hypertonia:** Continuous and uniform muscle stiffness, perceived as a constant resistance to passive movement [13]. Generally, uniform throughout the range of movement of the joint, sometimes it is so intense as to generate rhythmic interruptions at a frequency of 4–6 Hz. Hypertonia is accentuated during the execution of voluntary movements with the contralateral limb (Froment's maneuver), as demonstrated by the neurologist Froment in the 1920s of the last century. This maneuver is, in fact, used to perceive the milder forms of rigidity [14].

  In the more advanced stages, when hypertonia is sustained, functional deformities of flexion of the neck and trunk posture (camptocormia) may occur [13].
- **Bradykinesia:** Slowness in movements and reaction times, difficulty planning, starting and executing a certain action [13]. It is the main marker of damage to the basal

ganglia. It is believed that the slowdown in movements derives from a reduced ability of the nuclei of the base to reinforce the cortical mechanisms involved in the preparation and execution of motor commands. From a practical point of view, the deficit correlates with an insufficient recruitment of muscle strength by the patient during the initiation of movement, caused by an undersizing of motor power.

Peculiar expressions of bradykinesia concern the reduction of pendular movements of the upper limbs while walking, freezing, or stopping gait, and alteration of automatic movements such as blinking.

- **Postural instability:** It is often a characteristic manifestation of the most advanced phases of PD and is characterized by the loss of postural reflexes. It is clinically validated by the *pull test,* during which the patient is stimulated by pushing backwards. The test is positive and indicates postural instability if the patient takes two or more steps backwards or if he loses his balance in retropulsion. Postural instability is frequently the cause of falls and fractures [13].

These symptoms may appear at the onset of the disease and combine, at different stages, with the others, or be associated with the so-called non-motor symptoms:

- Behavioral disorders.
- Cognitive impairment.
- Alterations in blood pressure control.
- Neuropsychiatric symptoms (depression, anxiety, hallucinations, dementia).
- Sleep disorders (restless legs syndrome, REM sleep behavior disorders).
- Autonomic dysfunctions (urinary disorders, orthostatic hypotension, sexual dysfunction) and paresthesias.

The presence of on-motor symptoms increases with the severity of the disease. Unlike motor symptoms, they do not respond to dopaminergic therapy. This element has prompted some researchers to explore the potential involvement of alternative neurotransmitter pathways to dopaminergic ones in PD [15].

Their association but, above all, the intensity of the individual manifestations make the disease more serious and invalidating. Women's wording focusing on the disease experience and its impact on their sense of femininity and on their sexual function is reported in Box 2, to give the reader the inner sense of how this devastating neurological disease con impact women's sexuality and couples' intimate life.

Box 2: Parkinson's Disease and Sexuality through the women's Wording

I used to control every aspect of my life, successful and serene. This devastating disease is a bomb from within my body. The impossibility to control the hand tremor humiliates me deeply. It blocks my professional and social life. I detest the sense of compassion and pity that I see in the others' eyes. I'm more and more depressed and isolated. I divorced as my husband felt "socially embarassed" by my disease. I feel ugly, handicapped and sexually invisible....—Francesca

I couldn't believe this disease could be so devastating. The early symptoms began at 48 and they went much worse after the menopause, at 50. Nobody told me that the impact of this disease can be made worse by the loss of sexual hormones. Nor that it could be less aggressive if a woman uses estrogens, after the menopause. I discover it myself. Why neurologist and gynecologist say nothing about a much needed good news? I've been using hormone therapy for a year now, and I feel much much better. I got back my sexual life with my husband and also the Parkinson's drugs seem to work better. Why not sharing at least a good news when everything seems to be destined to go inescapably worse?— Laura

Testosterone cream is a magic drug for me. When you're diagnosed with Parkinson, you go to internet and you feel your life is finished. Every symptom is read as a consequence of the disease. I am 58, I had vaginal dryness, pain at intercourse, and it took ages to have an orgasm. When a healthy friend, menopausal like me, recommended me to go to a gynecologist skilled in hormone therapy and pelvic floor therapy, I was very skeptical. I was wrong! In three months dryness and sexual pain disappeared. And, unexpectedly, the intensity of my clitoral orgasm was gradually back. A miracle. In those moments, I feel healthy again. I can still hope for better days. And my partner is so relieved as well.— Josephine

*My neurologist, a she, suggested music and dance therapy, besides a rigorous treatment with specific PD drugs. She works in team with a gynecologist, who also recommended MHT. After a few months, I realized that when dancing I could be more fluent in my movement and I could do steps that I couldn't do without music. They told me that MHT, music and dance therapy help the brain to play the life music again! These two wonderful young doctors together gave back to me my sense of feminity, at least when I dance: it's like seen a fragment of blue bright sky under the more threatening black clouds… And when I go back home from the dancing evening, sex drives comes happily home with me.—*Marta.

3   Risk and Protective Factors

Age is the main predisposing factor of PD. In this regard, it is not yet known whether the main culprit is chronological age or the aging process. In women, the menopausal loss of estrogen production is associated with an increased risk of developing PD, demonstrating the protective effect of estrogens on dopaminergic function within the black substance [16, 17].

Different researches [18] and a recent meta-analysis [19] confirm the protective role of MHT in reducing by 50% the onset and the progression of PD (Box 3). Inexplicably, this impressive and solid benefit is not routinely presented, neither by

Box 3: Parkinson's Disease in Women. Role of Menopausal Status and Estrogens
- Before 50 years of age, men are more affected by PD than women (1.5:1).
- After the menopause, women's vulnerability to PD increases significantly.
- Women with premature menopause/premature ovarian insufficiency, and who did not take MHT, have a higher risk of developing PD and at a younger age, in comparison to women with menopause at 50 years of age.

> • Menopausal hormone therapy (MHT) has a protective role against PD: more women without PD used post-menopausal estrogen (50%) compared to women with PD (25%) [20].
> • A recent meta-analysis on 21 studies confirms that MHT reduces by 50% the risk of Parkinson in women [19], confirming previous data.

family physicians nor by neurologists, to still healthy menopausal women and menopausal women who have been recently diagnosed with PD.

There are, however, juvenile-onset variants, which have some differences compared to PD onset in old age. Early-onset PD is characterized, not only by more marked motor fluctuations and a higher incidence of dyskinesias, but also by a long course of the disease (26.6 years, compared to 10.2 years in patients with a late-onset) [21].

The relevance of genetics in the pathogenesis of PD is emerging after the identification of monogenic familial parkinsonisms and specific polymorphisms in the context of early-onset variants. A recent meta-analysis has demonstrated the role of genetics in PD, identifying 90 polymorphisms that would explain the hereditary risk of this neurodegenerative disorder. The most frequently encountered polymorphisms involve the genes α-synuclein (also called PARK-1 gene), parkin (PARK-2), ubiquitin hydrolase UCHL1 (Ubiquitin Carboxyl-terminal Hydrolase L1, PARK-5), PINK-1 (PARK-6), DJ-1 (PARK-7), and LRRK2 (PARK-8). It is currently believed that the main genetic mutations underlie a minority of PD cases (about 10%), while in the remaining cases, non-genetic factors could play a crucial role by interacting with susceptibility genes [22]. Sporadic PD is thought to be more likely related to a complex interaction between genetic and environmental factors [23, 24].

In addition, the increased risk of developing PD has been associated with the exposure to industrial or agricultural toxicants, dairy products, a history of melanoma, and brain traumas [25].

The main toxic substances for which a correlation with the pathogenesis of PD has been shown are some solvents (n-hexane, methanol); MPTP, which exerts its damaging effect on dopamine-producing nigrostriatal neurons; paraquat, a commercial herbicide capable of destroying dopaminergic cells; rotenone, a constituent of countless pesticides, which acts by inhibiting complex I associated with the mitochondrial electron transport chain.

Instead, habits such as moderate caffeine consumption (1–3 cups/day), smoking, and performing physical activity have been identified as protective factors [26].

Caffeine, in particular, is predictive of a more advanced age at the onset of this neurodegenerative disorder and a lower severity of motor symptoms. The responsible mechanism is believed to be due to the neuroprotective effect that this alkaloid exerts through an inhibition of MAO-B promoting an increase in dopamine levels at the central level, as well as through an activation of antioxidant signaling pathways [25, 27, 28].

Physical activity seems to reduce the risk of developing PD through the induction of the expression of neuroprotective factors, such as Glial-cell-line-Derived Neurotrophic Factor (GNDF) and Brain Development Neuroprotective Factor (BDNF), by modulating the noradrenergic and serotonergic systems and preventing cholinergic dysfunction [29–31]. Furthermore, irisin, an exercise-induced polypeptide secreted by skeletal muscle, crosses the blood–brain barrier, with a powerful neuroplastic effect on neurons [32]. The irisin-mediated protective role of physical activity on the brain gives new strength to the ancient Latin say «Mens sana in corpore sano» (the brain keeps on being healthy in a healthy body). New evidence supports its specific beneficial role on Parkinson's disease [33].

Cigarette smoke, to be avoided in any case for its damaging effect on different health systems, is however outlined as a protective factor by some studies. Smoking probably exerts this effect through its action on nicotinic receptors at the CNS level or through the increase in the plasma concentration of hydrazine, which is responsible for a reduction in the activity of cerebral MAO-B [34, 35].

Finally, given the probable involvement of neuroinflammatory mechanisms in the neurodegenerative cascade of PD, the use of NSAIDs is considered a potential protective factor. In fact, the activation of microglial cells in patients affected by PD [36] has led to the recognition of neuroinflammation as a probable pathophysiological element of this neurodegenerative disorder [37].

4　　Gender and PD

Past analyses of the etiology of PD focused on finding the mechanisms underlying the degeneration of nigrostriatal dopaminergic cells. The main hypothesized phenomena underlying this neuronal loss are excitotoxicity, neuroinflammation, mitochondrial dysfunction, and altered proteolysis. All factors are closely linked to a common basic element: the oxidative stress, with progressive neuroinflammation and death of dopaminergic neurons.

Gender differences between male and female subjects affected by PD have increasingly been investigated [38].

New hypotheses on the connection between biological sex and disease characteristics emerged, including disease development, phenotype, and progression. Therefore, along with age, genetics, and environmental exposure, sex is credited to be an important factor in the development of PD and in the underlying etiopathogenetic mechanisms [39].

PD affects the male sex more than the female sex, with a ratio of 3:2; however, this relationship is variable according to age, as seen in [40].

The mean age at onset in men is 2 years earlier than in women (51.3 and 53.4 years, respectively) [41].

Although the female gender is less affected, there is a higher mortality rate and a faster progression rate than in the male sex [39].

In the past decades, several studies highlighted phenotypic differences between males and females, which can have a significant meaning in the management and prognosis of PD.

At onset, with regard to motor symptoms, while men tend to present with a bradykinetic-rigid phenotype, women tend to develop a tremor-dominant form more frequently [42]. In addition to such clinical manifestations, a higher level of striatal dopamine uptake in women than in men was noted in the early stages. In fact, a better striatal dopaminergic regulation has been identified in the female sex. However, the underlying mechanism is not yet well understood. It is believed that a possible source of such gender differences may lie in the effect of estrogens on dopaminergic activity and central neuronal connections [43]. In favor of this assumption, the work of Benedetti et al. (2001) highlighted the estrogenic influence on the risk of developing PD. Through a case-control study on 144 patients (72 cases, 72 controls), a direct correlation between endogenous estrogen deficiency (following oophorectomy or hystero-adnexectomy) and the onset of PD emerged [44, 45].

In the context of the more advanced stages of the disease, men show greater alterations in cognitive functions, REM sleep disorders, ADL (Activity of Daily Living) and verbal fluency, as well as a remarkable preponderance of sialorrhea [45].

Women, on the other hand, in the late stages are more affected by deficits of visuospatial functions, with a greater tendency to develop postural instability, dysphagia, dyskinesias, and episodes of wearing off [39].

The high incidence of dyskinesias in women appears to be related to the use of L-dopa: in fact, it is generally assumed that dyskinesias are associated with elevated plasma L-dopa levels. In the female sex, there is a higher bioavailability of L-dopa, due to lower levels of clearance than in the male sex. Furthermore, it should be noted that women often take the same pharmacological dosage as male subjects: but having a lower weight than men, they are treated with a higher amount of L-dopa per kilogram of body weight [46]. Rarely, in fact, appropriate dosage corrections depending on parameters such as body weight are performed. This would increase the risk of developing dyskinetic episodes in female patients [47–49].

In addition, sleep disorders are more common in the male sex than in the female sex, as demonstrated by Yoritaka et al. (2009) [50], and Özekmekçi et al. (2005) [51]: men more frequently report vivid, violent, or dramatic dreams during REM sleep.

Finally, gender also influences exposure to risk and protective factors. In this regard, women have a lower risk profile due to their work contexts which, in most cases, do not involve exposure to solvents, MPTP, herbicides, or pesticides. These substances, as seen above, have been correlated by some studies as potential risk factors for PD [25, 52].

As for the complications associated with PD, anxiety and depression are highlighted in women, while impulse control disorders, such as gambling and hypersexuality, are more frequent in males [46, 53].

With regard to the response to the Deep Brain Stimulation (DBS) procedure, some gender differences are highlighted. Female patients seem to benefit more than men in terms of autonomy in daily activities, thanks to an improvement in motility and cognitive functions. Instead, men, post DBS, present a substantial improvement in posture: in fact, a correction of camptocormia is noted [54].

Significant elements in the analysis of gender differences concern the severity and the progression of the disease, which is more severe and rapidly progressive in males. Males show a faster decline, confirming the study by Kalf et al. [55].

Gender is emerging as well as a qualitative variable both in illness experience and care preferences in PD patients [56], along with further insights on key aspects of therapy that could contribute (also) to a better sexual life if appropriately tailored with a gender perspective [57].

5   Therapy

Nowadays there are effective drugs available to improve the symptoms of PD. However, despite numerous advances in the therapeutic field, we still do not have a therapy aimed at slowing the progression of the disease. The key pathophysiologic weakness preventing a radical disease change remains the fact that PD becomes clinically relevant when up to 80% of dopaminergic neurons have been destroyed. MAO-B inhibitors, dopaminoagonists, and levodopa mainly improve motor symptoms of PD and partially affect non-motor symptoms (NMS) [58].

MAO inhibitors (selegiline and rasagiline) stabilize dopamine levels in the intersynaptic space by prolonging dopaminergic activity. However, they expose to the risk of tyramine-induced hypertension and increased activity of catecholaminergic neurons [59].

Dopaminoagonists act directly on postsynaptic dopaminergic receptors. These drugs require a slow and measured titration period due to their poor tolerability, determined by the appearance of nausea, drowsiness, and impulse control disorders (gambling, hypersexuality, excessive spending, binge eating) [60–62].

Levodopa (L-dopa), a precursor to dopamine, is the gold standard in the treatment of PD. In the majority of patients on therapy with this molecule, there has been a clinically significant benefit [63].

L-dopa administered orally is absorbed in the gastrointestinal tract and reaches the CNS by crossing the blood–brain barrier. Once the pre-synaptic terminals are reached, it is converted into dopamine by enzymes called decarboxylase. L-dopa is commonly given in combination with a decarboxylase inhibitor (e.g., carbidopa or benserazide) in order to prevent both the conversion to dopamine at the peripheral level, and side effects such as nausea and vomiting [64].

The optimal timing to undertake L-dopa therapy is determined by the appearance of an impairment of patient's daily activities or of walking disorders, determining an increased risk of falling.

Following a period of satisfactory pharmacological response, called "honeymoon," lasting several years, there are changes in the motor response to L-dopa. With the progression of the disease and neuronal degeneration, the therapeutic window is reduced and higher doses of the drug are necessary to alleviate the symptoms and the disability of patients.

> **Box 4: Music and Dancing Significantly Improve PD Symptoms**
> - Dance classes for PD improve both qualitative and quantitative assessments of disease symptoms.
> - Rhythmic motor training, a mechanism underlying dance training, impacts improvements in parkinsonian symptoms following a dance intervention.
> - Music empowers the ability of residual dopaminergic neurons to connect and synergize, to allow movements that are not possible without the neuronal synchronization of music.

However, as the dosage increases, side effects such as dyskinesias (involuntary movements corresponding to a plasma peak of levodopa) and "on-off" motor fluctuations (alternation of periods of response to L-dopa and periods of non-optimal or absent response) may appear. It is estimated that approximately 10% of patients/per year receiving L-dopa develop such invalidating effects [65].

More recent and advanced therapeutic techniques include apomorphine (dopamine receptor agonist, infused via subcutaneous pump, useful for unpredictable refractory fluctuations), duodopa (soluble formulation of levodopa, administered via gastro-jejunum-stoma, beneficial for periods of refractory fluctuations), and Deep Brain Stimulation (DBS) [3].

Other aspects that need attention in the therapeutic management of PD are physical exercise and nutrition [66]. In this regard, the patient is invited to perform FKT for rehabilitation purposes, while a low-protein diet is recommended in order to promote the absorption of L-dopa [64].

Non-medical therapies, like music and dance therapy (Box 4), and art therapy, deserve to be specially considered for their positive impact on mood, self-perception, emotional rewards, refreshed sense of hope, and positive impact of inner sense of worth as human being. In post-menopausal women, they can further improve the intimate sexual life, when combined with a well-tailored systemic MHT with a topical add of estradiol or prasterone, and testosterone cream, to prevent and cure the genitourinary syndrome of the menopause and its associate bladder, vulvovaginal, and sexual symptoms [66, 67].

6 Conclusions

PD has a more slowly progressive phenotype found in women. This could be related to a better striatal dopaminergic regulation, thanks to the protective effect of estrogens [43]. In fact, previous works have examined the relationship between estrogens and the risk of developing PD, identifying a protective role for estrogen [44].

Further evidence in favor of the beneficial effect of female sex hormones is given by the finding of a later onset of the disease in patients who have undergone hormone therapy (MHT) in the post-menopausal period, compared to patients who have not been undergoing MHT.

Therefore, the PD phenotype in females is less severe [41].

The key take-home messages for all the clinicians reading this chapter are as follows:

1. Seriously consider and serenely motivate women to use systemic MHT to reduce (also) their PD risk.
2. Inform patients that MHT can reduce PD aggressive progression once it has been diagnosed in post-menopausal women.
3. Be clear and proactive in clarifying that MHT, systemic or at least topical, improves menopausal symptoms that can worsen both the PD patient daily life, the sexual intimacy, and the clinical scenario.
4. Discuss with the patient the potential impact of women's body weight in modulating PD drug-related side effects.

Please read chapter on *"Sexuality across the lifespan III: women's vulnerabilities from early menopause to senescence"* to have a broader vision on how MHT can be tailored to increase symptom's control and patients' satisfaction, while definitely improving their sexual life with topical testosterone cream.

References

1. Post B, van den Heuvel L, van Ruissen TX, van de Warrenburg B, Nonnekes J. Young onset Parkinson's disease: a modern and tailored approach. J Parkinsons Dis. 2020;10:S29–36. https://doi.org/10.3233/JPD-202135.
2. Costa HN, Esteves AR, Empadinhas N, Cardoso SM. Parkinson's disease: a multisystem disorder. Neurosci Bull. 2023;39(1):113–24. https://doi.org/10.1007/s12264-022-00934-6.
3. Zhu B, Yin D, Zhao H, Zhang L. The immunology of Parkinson's disease. Semin Immunopathol. 2022;44(5):659–72. https://doi.org/10.1007/s00281-022-00947-3.
4. Marques Santa Rosa Malcher C, da Silva Gonçalves Oliveira KR, Coelho Fernandes Caldato M, Lopes dos Santos Lobato B, da Silva Pedroso J, de Tubino Scanavino M. Sexual disorders and quality of life in Parkinson's. Sex Med. 2021;9(1):100280. https://doi.org/10.1016/j.esxm.2020.10.008.
5. Van Overmeire R, Vesentini L, Vanclooster S, Bilsen J. Discussing sexual health among Flemish patients with Parkinson's disease. Acta Neurol Belg. 2023;123(2):497–505. https://doi.org/10.1007/s13760-022-02086-w.
6. Bronner G, Peleg-Nesher S, Manor Y, Rosenberg A, Naor S, Taichman T, Ezra A, Gurevich T. Sexual needs and sexual function of patients with Parkinson's disease. Neurol Sci. 2023;44(2):539–46. https://doi.org/10.1007/s10072-022-06467-0.
7. De Luca R, Bonanno M, Morini E, Marra A, Arcadi FA, Quartarone A, Calabrò RS. Sexual dysfunctions in females with Parkinson's disease: a cross-sectional study with a psycho-endocrinological perspective. Medicina (Kaunas). 2023;59(5):845. https://doi.org/10.3390/medicina59050845.
8. Haktanır D, Yılmaz SJ. Sexual dysfunction and related factors in patients with Parkinson's disease. Psychosoc Nurs Ment Health Serv. 2023;61(3):45–55. https://doi.org/10.3928/02793695-20220907-02.
9. Cong S, Xiang C, Zhang S, Zhang T, Wang H, Cong S. Prevalence and clinical aspects of depression in Parkinson's disease: a systematic review and meta analysis of 129 studies. Neurosci Biobehav Rev. 2022;141:104749. https://doi.org/10.1016/j.neubiorev.2022.104749.

10. Koza Z, Ayajuddin M, Das A, Chaurasia R, Phom L, Yenisetti SC. Sexual dysfunction precedes motor defects, dopaminergic neuronal degeneration, and impaired dopamine metabolism: insights from Drosophila model of Parkinson's disease. Front Neurosci. 2023;17:1143793. https://doi.org/10.3389/fnins.2023.1143793. eCollection 2023

11. Shahed J, Jankovic J. Motor symptoms in Parkinson's disease. Handb Clin Neurol. 2007;83:329–42. https://doi.org/10.1016/j.neubiorev.2016.07.010.

12. Abusrair AH, Elsekaily W, Bohlega S. Tremor in Parkinson's disease: from pathophysiology to advanced therapies. Tremor Other Hyperkinet Mov (N Y). 2022;12:29. https://doi.org/10.5334/tohm.712. eCollection 2022

13. Jankovic J. Parkinson's disease: clinical features and diagnosis. J Neurol Neurosurg Psychiatry. 2008;79:368–76.

14. Broussolle E, Krack P, Thobois S, Xie-Brustolin J, Pollak P, Goetz CG. Contribution of Jules Froment to the study of parkinsonian rigidity. Mov Disord. 2007;22:909–14.

15. Muzerengi S, Contrafatto D, Chaudhuri KR. Non-motor symptoms: identification and management. Parkinsonism Relat Disord. 2007;13:450–6.

16. Kempster PA, O'Sullivan SS, Holton JL, Revesz T, Lees AJ. Relationships between age and late progression of Parkinson's disease: a clinico-pathological study. Brain. 2010;133:1755–62.

17. Ragonese P, Salemi G, Aridon P, Gammino M, Epifanio A, Morgante L, Savettieri G. Risk of Parkinson disease in women effect of reproductive characteristics. Neurology. 2004;62:2010–4.

18. Echeverria V, Echeverria F, Barreto GE, Echeverría J, Mendoza C. Estrogenic plants: to prevent neurodegeneration and memory loss and other symptoms in women after menopause. Front Pharmacol. 2021;12:644103. https://doi.org/10.3389/fphar.2021.644103. eCollection 2021

19. Song Y-J, Li S-R, Li X-W, Chen X, Wei Z-X, Liu Q-S, Cheng Y. The effect of estrogen replacement therapy on Alzheimer's disease and Parkinson's disease in postmenopausal. Front Neurosci. 2020;14:157. https://doi.org/10.3389/fnins.2020.00157. eCollection 2020

20. Carrie N, Bennett T, Doody RS. Hormonal replacement therapy and risk of Parkinson's disease. Neurology. 2004;63(2):249–53.

21. Ferguson LW, Rajput AH, Rajput A. Early-onset vs. late-onset Parkinson's disease: a clinical-pathological study. Can J Neurol Sci. 2015;43:113–9.

22. Lau LM, Breteler M. Epidemiology of Parkinson's disease. Lancet Neurol. 2006;5:525–35.

23. Nalls MA, Blauwendraat C, Bandres-Ciga S, Leonard H, Faghri F, Gibbs JR, Hernandez DG, et al. Identification of novel risk loci, causal insights, and heritable risk for Parkinson's disease: a meta-analysis of genome-wide association studies. Lancet Neurol. 2019;18:1091–102.

24. Nicoletti A, Pugliese P, Nicoletti G, Arabia G, Annesi G, de Mari M, Lamberti P, Gallerini S, Marconi R, Epifanio A, Morgante L, Cozzolino PB, Torchia G, Quattrone A, Zappia M. The FRAGAMP study: environmental and genetic factors in Parkinson's disease, methods and clinical features. Neurol Sci. 2010;31:47–52.

25. Ascherio A, Schwarzschild MA. The epidemiology of Parkinson's disease: risk factors and prevention. Lancet Neurol. 2016;15:1257–72.

26. Belvisi D, Pellicciari R, Fabbrini A, Costanzo M, Ressa G, Pietracupa S, de Lucia M, Modugno N, Magrinelli F, Dallocchio C, Ercoli T, Nicoletti A, Zappia M, Solla P, Bologna M, Fabbrini G, Tinazzi M, Conte A, Berardelli A, Defazio G. Relationship between risk and protective factors and clinical features of Parkinson's disease. Parkinsonism Relat Disord. 2022;98:80–5.

27. Leodori G, de Bartolo MI, Belvisi D, Ciogli A, Fabbrini A, Costanzo M, Manetto S, Conte A, Villani C, Fabbrini G, Berardelli A. Salivary caffeine in Parkinson's disease. Sci Rep. 2021;11:9823.

28. Schepici G, Silvestro S, Bramanti P, Mazzon E. Caffeine: an overview of its beneficial effects in experimental models and clinical trials of Parkinson's disease. Int J Mol Sci. 2020;21:4766.

29. Neeper SA, Gdmez-Pinilla F, Choi J, Cotman CW. Physical activity increases MRNA for brain-derived neurotrophic factor and nerve growth factor in rat brain. Brain Res. 1996;726:49–56.

30. Cohen AD, Tillerson JL, Smith AD, Schallert T, Zigmond MJ. Neuroprotective effects of prior limb use in 6-hydroxydopamine-treated rats: possible role of GDNF. J Neurochem. 2003;85:299–305.

31. Lin TW, Kuo YM. Exercise benefits brain function: the monoamine connection. Brain Sci. 2013;3:39–53.
32. Zhang H, Wu X, Liang J, Kirberger M, Chen N. Irisin, an exercise-induced bioactive peptide beneficial for health promotion during aging process. Ageing Res Rev. 2022;80:101680. https://doi.org/10.1016/j.arr.2022.101680.
33. Kam TI, Park H, Chou SC, Van Vranken JG, Mittenbühler MJ, Kim H, Choi YR, Biswas D, Wang J, Shin Y, Loder A, Karuppagounder SS, Wrann CD, Dawson VL, Spiegelman BM, Dawson TM. Amelioration of pathologic α-synuclein-induced Parkinson's disease by irisin. Proc Natl Acad Sci USA. 2022;119(36):e2204835119.
34. Quik M, Perez XA, Bordia T. Nicotine as a potential neuroprotective agent for Parkinson's disease. Mov Disord. 2012;7:28.
35. Wee YV, Perry TL. Monoamine oxidase B, smoking, and Parkinson's disease. J Neurol Sci. 1986;72:265–72.
36. Mcgeer PL, Itagaki S, Boyes BE, Mcgeer EG. Reactive microglia are positive for HLA-DR in the Substantia Nigra of Parkinson's and Alzheimer's disease brains. Neurology. 1988;38:1285–91.
37. Hirsch EC, Hunot S. Neuroinflammation in Parkinson's disease: a target for neuroprotection? Lancet Neurol. 2009;8:382–97.
38. Reale C, Invernizzi F, Panteghini C, Garavaglia B. Genetics, sex, and gender. J Neurosci Res. 2023;101(5):553–62. https://doi.org/10.1002/jnr.24945.
39. Cerri S, Mus L, Blandini F. Parkinson's disease in women and men: What's the difference? J Parkinsons Dis. 2019;9:501–15.
40. Wickremaratchi MM, Perera D, O'Loghlen C, Sastry D, Morgan E, Jones A, Edwards P, Robertson NP, Butler C, Morris HR, Ben-Shlomo Y. Prevalence and age of onset of Parkinson's disease in Cardiff: a community based cross sectional study and meta-analysis. J Neurol Neurosurg Psychiatry. 2009;80:805–7.
41. Haaxma CA, Bloem BR, Borm GF, Oyen WJG, Leenders KL, Eshuis S, Booij J, Dluzen DE, Horstink MWIM. Gender differences in Parkinson's disease. J Neurol Neurosurg Psychiatry. 2007;78:819–24.
42. Lewis SJG, Foltynie T, Blackwell AD, Robbins TW, Owen AM, Barker RA. Heterogeneity of Parkinson's disease in the early clinical stages using a data driven approach. J Neurol Neurosurg Psychiatry. 2005;76:343–8.
43. Lavalaye J, Booij J, Reneman L, Habraken JB, van Royen EA. Effect of age and gender on dopamine transporter imaging with [123I]FP-CIT SPET in healthy volunteers. Eur J Nucl Med. 2000;27(7):867–9.
44. Benedetti MD, Maraganore DM, Bower JH, McDonnell SK, Peterson BJ, Ahlskog JE, Schaid DJ, Rocca WA. Hysterectomy, menopause, and estrogen use preceding Parkinson's disease: an exploratory case-control study. Mov Disord. 2001;16:830–7.
45. Miller IN, Cronin-Golomb A. Gender differences in Parkinson's disease: clinical characteristics and cognition. Mov Disord. 2010;25:2695–703.
46. Zappia M, Crescibene L, Arabia G, Nicoletti G, Bagalà A, Bastone L, Caracciolo M, Bonavita S, di Costanzo A, Scornaienchi M, Gambradella A, Quattrone A. Body weight influences pharmacokinetics of levodopa in Parkinson's disease. Clin Neuropharmacol. 2002;25:79–82.
47. Fabbrini G, Brotchie JM, Grandas F, Nomoto M, Goetz CG. Levodopa-induced dyskinesias. Mov Disord. 2007;22:1379–89.
48. Kumagai T, Nagayama H, Ota T, Nishiyama Y, Mishina M, Ueda M. Sex differences in the pharmacokinetics of levodopa in elderly patients with Parkinson disease. Clin Neuropharmacol. 2014;37:173–6.
49. Accolla E, Caputo E, Cogiamanian F, Tamma F, Mrakic-Sposta S, Marceglia S, Egidi M, Rampini P, Locatelli M, Priori A. Gender differences in patients with Parkinson's disease treated with subthalamic deep brain stimulation. Mov Disord. 2007;22:1150–6.
50. Yoritaka A, Ohizumi H, Tanaka S, Hattori N. Parkinson's disease with and without REM sleep behaviour disorder: are there any clinical differences? Eur Neurol. 2009;61:164–70.
51. Özekmekçi S, Apaydin H, Kiliç E. Clinical features of 35 patients with Parkinson's disease displaying REM behavior disorder. Clin Neurol Neurosurg. 2005;107:306–9.

52. Pals P, van Everbroeck B, Grubben B, Viaene MK, Rene'dom R, van der Linden C, Santens P, Martin JJ, Cras P. Case-control study of environmental risk factors for Parkinson's disease in Belgium. Eur J Epidemiol. 2003;18:1133–42.
53. Weintraub D, Claassen DO. Impulse control and related disorders in Parkinson's disease. Int Rev Neurobiol. 2017;133:679–717. https://doi.org/10.1016/bs.irn.2017.04.006.
54. Roediger J, Artusi CA, Romagnolo A, Boyne P, Zibetti M, Lopiano L, Espay AJ, Fasano A, Merola A. Effect of subthalamic deep brain stimulation on posture in Parkinson's disease: A blind computerized analysis. Parkinsonism Relat Disord. 2019;62:122–7.
55. Kalf JG, Munneke M, van den Engel-Hoek L, de Swart BJ, Borm GF, Bloem BR, Zwarts MJ. Pathophysiology of diurnal drooling in Parkinson's disease. Mov Disord. 2011;26:1270–6.
56. Göttgens I, Modderkolk L, Jansen C, Darweesh SKL, Bloem BR, Oertelt-Prigione S. The salience of gender in the illness experiences and care preferences of people with Parkinson's disease. Soc Sci Med. 2023;320:115757. https://doi.org/10.1016/j.socscimed.2023.115757.
57. Skogar Ö, Nilsson M, Lökk J. Gender differences in diagnostic tools, medication, time to medication, and nonmotor symptoms in Parkinsonian patients. Brain Circ. 2022;8(4):192–9. https://doi.org/10.4103/bc.bc_33_2210.4103. eCollection 2022 Oct-Dec
58. Poewe W. Clinical measures of progression in Parkinson's disease. Mov Disord. 2009;24:671–6.
59. Müller T. Drug therapy in patients with Parkinson's disease. Transl Neurodegener. 2012;1:10.
60. Leplow B, Renftle D, Thomas M, Michaelis K, Solbrig S, Maetzler W, Berg D, Liepelt-Scarfone I. Characteristics of behavioural addiction in Parkinson's disease patients with self-reported impulse control disorder and controls matched for levodopa equivalent dose: a matched case-control study. J Neural Transm (Vienna). 2023;130(2):125–33. https://doi.org/10.1007/s00702-023-02588-8.
61. Mata-Marín D, Pineda-Pardo JÁ, Michiels M, Pagge C, Ammann C, Martínez-Fernández R, Molina JA, Vela-Desojo L, Alonso-Frech F, Obeso I. A circuit-based approach to modulate hypersexuality in Parkinson's disease. Psychiatry Clin Neurosci. 2023;77(4):223–32. https://doi.org/10.1111/pcn.13523.
62. Bhattacharyya KB. The story of levodopa: a long and arduous journey. Ann Indian Acad Neurol. 2022;25(1):124–30. https://doi.org/10.4103/aian.aian_474_21.
63. Olanow CW, Watts RL, Koller WC. An algorithm (decision tree) for the management of Parkinson's disease 2001: treatment guidelines. Neurology. 2001;56:1–88.
64. Marsden CD, Parkes JD. Success and problems of long-term levodopa therapy in Parkinson's disease. Lancet. 1977;309:345–9.
65. Gaßner H, Trutt E, Seifferth S, Friedrich J, Zucker D, Salhani Z, Adler W, Winkler J, Jost WH. Treadmill training and physiotherapy similarly improve dual task gait performance: a randomized-controlled trial in Parkinson's disease. J Neural Transm (Vienna). 2022;129(9):1189–200. https://doi.org/10.1007/s00702-022-02514-4.
66. Graziottin A, Maseroli E, Vignozzi L. Female sexual dysfunctions: a clinical perspective on HSDD, FAD, PGAD, and FOD. In: Bettocchi C, Busetto GM, Carrieri G, Cormio L, editors. Practical clinical andrology. Springer Nature; 2022. p. 89–112.
67. Graziottin A, Maseroli E. Sexual pain disorders, vestibulodynia, and recurrent cystitis: the evil trio. A clinical conversation on the uroandrological perspective. In: Bettocchi C, Busetto GM, Carrieri G, Cormio L, editors. Practical clinical andrology. Springer Nature; 2022. p. 319–40.

Sexual Health in Individuals with Disabilities

Sara Laxe and Raquel Salinas

1   Introduction

Disability is a condition that can be defined as a physical, mental, cognitive, or developmental condition that significantly impairs an individual's ability to perform daily activities and participation in society [1]. According to the biopsychosocial model of disability adopted by the WHO (World Health Organization) with the International Classification of Functioning, Disability and Health (ICF), disability is the result of a problem in human functioning. Functioning is an umbrella term that represents the situation resulting from the interaction between the health condition (body or mind impairment) and the contextual factors influencing the participation of this individuals and can cause activities limitations and/or participation restrictions [2, 3]. Within this framework, functioning and disability may not necessarily be associated with a disease. Problems in functioning can appear after a disease but also after a developmental disorder such as cerebral palsy, a trauma (traumatic brain injury), or a health condition (pregnancy, aging, or transgender surgery). This last point is novel and unique since those mentioned conditions are not diseases, meaning that functioning does not always needs to be related to a disease or a trauma.

S. Laxe (✉)
Rehabilitation Service, Clinical Institute of Medical and Surgical Specialties, Hospital Clinic de Barcelona, Barcelona, Spain

WHOFIC Academic Collaborating Center, Universitat de Barcelona, Barcelona, Spain

Clinical Sexology Working Group, Hospital Clinic de Barcelona, Barcelona, Spain
e-mail: laxe@clinic.cat

R. Salinas
Rehabilitation Service, Clinical Institute of Medical and Surgical Specialties, Hospital Clinic de Barcelona, Barcelona, Spain
e-mail: rssalinas@clinic.cat

© The Author(s), under exclusive license to Springer Nature Switzerland AG 2024
C. Castelo-Branco, S. Anglès Acedo (eds.), *Medical Disorders and Sexual Health*, Trends in Andrology and Sexual Medicine,
https://doi.org/10.1007/978-3-031-55080-5_30

The impact of disability on sexuality and sexual health matters as WHO states that sexuality is a core aspect of human beings and highly linked with a better quality of life and self-esteem. Depending on the level of impairment and the individual's specific condition, sexual function and pleasure can be affected. In addition, individuals with disabilities may face discrimination or exclusion from sexual health education and resources, which can lead to feelings of isolation and shame.

WHO estimates that 1.3 billion people experience significant disability worldwide, this means that about 15% of the world's population live with some form of disability, of whom 2–4% experience significant difficulties in functioning [4]. Previous data from the 1970s, estimated a disability percentage of 10%, which means that there is an in crescendo number of people in the world suffering from some sort of problem in functioning. This number is expected to keep on rising due to impact of chronic diseases, population aging, global warming, and wars as reported by the WHO in the Rehab 2030 report [3].

One aspect that is important to highlight is that people with disability often are assumed to constitute a single group and neglect that they have diverse and varying needs including sexual health [5]. It is an important aspect of overall well-being that requires a positive and respectful approach to sexuality and sexual relationships.

Not in vain the WHO has a comprehensive research program specifically dedicated "Sexual and Reproductive Health and Research." [6] In order to have a good sexual health, people need to have access to good quality of information about sex and sexuality, they need to be aware of risks of sexuality such as sexually transmitted diseases, undesirable pregnancies, sexual misconduct, and violence.

In addition to informing about the risks, it is crucial to convey positive aspects related to sexuality to promote the autonomy of people with disabilities. Considering adaptations and accessibility as necessary, as well as empowering individuals to make informed decisions, are essential steps. Recognizing that people with disabilities can experience meaningful affective relationships and deserve to enjoy a healthy, equitable, and pleasurable sexuality is fundamental. Therefore, it is essential that both healthcare professionals and educators receive training on sexuality and disability, so they can provide appropriate and unbiased support to people with disabilities and their families.

These patients often face unique challenges in this area. The impact of disability on sexual health can vary widely, depending on the type and severity of disability but also with personal and social factors. Physical, psychological, and emotional changes that may result from a disability can affect sexual desire, function, and satisfaction with sexual life, both solo-sex and partnered-sex and therefore sexual health. If sexual health not considered in this populations is likely that there might be an unawareness of the risks of sexuality such as sexually transmitted diseases, undesirable pregnancies, sexual misconduct, and violence.

Through the lens of the ICF, healthcare providers can better understand the multidimensional nature of sexual health challenges in individuals with disabilities and develop comprehensive, patient-centered approaches to care.

This chapter aims to explore the challenges individuals with disabilities may face in relation to sexual health and how the ICF framework can be used to address these challenges. Additionally, we will discuss strategies for promoting sexual health and inclusion in individuals with disabilities. Through a multidisciplinary approach to care, individuals with disabilities can receive the support they need to achieve optimal sexual health and well-being.

2   Sexuality and Disability: An ICF Perspective

Sexuality is a complex concept that includes more than just anatomical and physiological functioning. It includes sexual knowledge, beliefs, behaviors, and values, as well as social gender roles, physical development, body image, social relationships, perceived social value, and feelings of physical attractiveness, as well as sharing of thoughts and emotions.

People with disabilities may face unique challenges related to their sexual health. On one hand due to the diseases or health condition can have problems in lubrication, erectile dysfunction, menopause but also scars, spasticity, amputations, use of stomas, joint limitation and retractions, pain, obesity, depression, anxiety.

These challenges may vary depending on the type, nature, and timing of disability. It has not the same impact on sexuality a person with a congenital disability than a person with an acquired one. In the case of an acquired disability, the impact on sexuality will depend on the nature of the disability, the age of onset of the disability as well as if the person has already been sexually active before. In the cases of conditions that lead to severe limitations in activities and participation such as traumatic brain injury, stroke, or spinal cord injury, the divorce rates tend to increase over time and the impact in the caregiver's sense of burden has an effect in the couple's psychosocial adjustment [7]. As an example, only 22% of the people who have sustained a brain injury are still sexually active 1 year after the lesion [8]. About 25% of women and 34% of men who suffered colon cancer and wear stoma reported having a sexual life [9].

If we use the International Classification of Functioning, Disability and Health (ICF) as a framework to describe health and health-related states in relation to a biopsychosocial model, sexual health in several areas can be identified (see Fig. 1).

2.1   Body Structures

The anatomical components of the body, including organs, limbs, and tissues, can be affected in ways that lead to reduced activity and limited participation. Patients facing structural issues in their genitals, such as penile amputation after cancer, female genital cancer, or breast cancer, as well as individuals dealing with mobility challenges due to upper or lower limb amputations, obesity, hip or knee replacements, spine surgery, hemiplegia, paraplegia, and conditions significantly impacting body image like head and neck cancer, facial palsy, or the use of artificial stomas, may experience consequences in their sexual health as a result [10–13].

Concept	
Disability (congenital – acquired)	
ICF perspective: framework to describe health and health-related states in relation to a biopsychosocial model	• <u>Body structures:</u> cancer, limb amputations, mobility challenges (wheel chair), brain injury, obesity, artificial stomas… • <u>Body functions:</u> sensory and motor functions, lack of lubrication, sexual desire, feeling of isolations, pain… • <u>Activities and participation:</u> communication, self care, mobility, moving around, domestic life, ability to mantain relationships or acquire new relationships… • <u>Environmental factors</u> (barriers or facilitators): products like medication or assistive devices, policys for people with disabilities, societal attitudes, professsional attitudes towards disability… • Personal factors: age, gender and sexual orientation

Patient-centered care.	• Holistic, collaborative and interdisciplinary approach
	    o Medical team, nurses, physioterapist, social workers, educator
	    o Sexual assistance,
	• Standards of care and guidelines to improve sexual health

Sexual rights	Empowerment, autonomy, consensual decision-making, awareness, advocacy
Inclusion	Positive education, dignity, support, inclusivity, non-discrimination, co-responsibility

Fig. 1 Sexual health and disability

2.2 Body Functions

These are physiological or psychological functions of the body, such as sensory and motor functions, mental functions, and cardiovascular and respiratory functions. Frequent conditions such as stroke, cerebral palsy, or spinal cord injury can impact sexual health by problems in erectile disfunction, lubrication, and body image. Also, the loss of bowel and bladder function, contractures, spasms, and weakness and lack of movement can impair sexual relations expectations. Pain in its different modalities, neuropathic, musculoskeletal, or chronic pain is another determinant of a poor sexual health [14, 15]. Most of the studies regarding sexual life after acquired disability highlight depression and anxiety as determinants of a sexual dysfunction [16].

2.3   Activities and Participation

These are the actions and tasks that a person performs in their daily life, such as self-care, mobility, communication, and social interaction. After suffering a serious illness or trauma, there are frequent changes in the couples' roles, decline in sexual desire, limited expression of affection (both verbally and physical) that can also impact sexual health perception [12].

It is relevant to highlight that people with disabilities who are single or not in a romantic relationship also experience the need for intimacy and affection [10]. The pursuit of emotional connection and feeling emotionally supported are fundamental aspects of their sexual well-being. This situation can influence how they perceive their sexual health, affecting their desire and ability to engage in intimate relationships. Additionally, feelings of isolation or lack of social support can also have a significant impact on their sexual experience and overall well-being [17].

When considering the impact of disability on activities and participation related to sexuality, various factors come into play. For individuals with physical disabilities, limitations in mobility or fine motor skills might affect their ability to engage in certain sexual activities. For those with communication or sensory impairments, expressing desires or boundaries could be challenging. Additionally, individuals with intellectual or developmental disabilities might face barriers in understanding consent or navigating relationships.

Addressing these concerns and providing a supportive and understanding environment are essential to promote a positive and fulfilling sexual experience, regardless of each individual's marital status or relationship situation.

2.4   Environmental Factors

This domain of the ICF refers to the physical, social, and attitudinal environment in which people live and conduct their lives. These factors can be either barriers to or facilitators of the person's functioning. Environmental factors constitute a broad spectrum of factors such as products design for personal use, physical geography, health professionals, and attitudes of people, societal norms, and policies.

It has been widely described that people with disabilities have less informal and formal opportunities to learn about health [18]. Sometimes due to the preconceived idea that they are already facing many problems with the body functions and the disease itself, but also due to difficulties in maintaining their partners or finding new ones, people with disabilities feel that they face difficulties in finding information about how to improve their sexual health. There are difficulties in assessing for preventive issues such as how to handle the use of a condom when you have problems in maintaining the erection or with impaired hand function or when to start having sex again after a stroke, a craniotomy, or a cerebrospinal shunt.

One of the domains covered by the area of environmental factors of ICF is that related to the support of professionals. Unfortunately, many healthcare professionals may have limited information about how their interventions can influence patients' sexual lives. Patient empowerment and education regarding post-operative expectations related to sexual activity are often low, highlighting a global need for research studies that assess the impact of various medical interventions on sexual health [15, 19–21].

For individuals with non-acquired disabilities, there have been more studies conducted. Many of these studies emphasize that their sexual aspirations are often restricted by societal attitudes, including those of friends, community members, service providers, professionals, funders, politicians, and educators. Numerous individuals in this group express the need for professionals with expertise in sexual health to assist them in navigating their unique experiences [16].

2.5   Personal Factors

Individual's age, gender, and sexual orientation are also important factors that influence sexual health and well-being. Additionally, there are many attitudinal factors such as a lack of access to sexual education, lack of sexual partners or difficulty forming relationships, negative attitudes toward their sexuality, and lack of information about sexual health resources. These challenges impact their ability to participate fully in society leading to social isolation, reduced employment opportunities, and a lower quality of life.

Despite common misconceptions that people with disabilities are asexual and do not engage in sexual activities, they are indeed sexually active. However, individuals with disabilities often encounter challenges with sexual activities and intimacy. Due to their disability, people with disabilities may feel that they are not sexually appealing. Research has shown that the severity of disability is linked to lower sexual esteem and satisfaction, increased sexual depression, and less frequent sexual activity [16, 22, 23].

3   Disability and Sexual Health Challenges

While rehabilitation for adults with acquired disabilities aims to help them adapt to new life circumstances, including changes to their sexuality, individuals with congenital disabilities have distinct needs that may require a developmental approach to explore their sexuality and intimate relationships. The disability sector and health research often prioritize impairments, daily living skills, and employment outcomes, while the needs related to sexuality and intimacy are frequently overlooked. Individuals with complex communication needs, who cannot use natural speech for everyday communication, may particularly benefit from augmentative and alternative communication systems, but these interventions and research tend to focus more on facilitating participation in education, employment, and family settings.

Physical barriers are a significant challenge for individuals with disabilities in terms of sexual health. It can include difficulties in finding accessible spaces and equipment for sexual activities or finding suitable products for contraception and sexual health care. In the case of congenital disabilities, lack of access to sexual education is another challenge. Many schools and institutions do not provide comprehensive sexual education programs that cater to their needs.

As a result, individuals with disabilities may not have access to the same information and resources regarding sexual health as their non-disabled peers. Additionally, they may have difficulties forming relationships or finding sexual partners due to negative attitudes toward their sexuality.

These negative attitudes toward disability and sexuality can make it challenging for individuals with disabilities to find partners or maintain healthy sexual relationships.

Lack of information about sexual health resources is another challenge, many sexual health resources and services are not designed or made accessible to individuals with disabilities. This lack of accessibility can create barriers to seeking and receiving sexual health care, including contraception, sexually transmitted infection (STI) testing and treatment, and counseling services.

It is important to recognize the diversity of experiences among individuals with disabilities, as well as the unique strengths and abilities that they possess. By promoting inclusivity, accessibility, and equal opportunities, we can work toward creating a more equitable and just society for all individuals, including them.

It appears that many of the things that help people with physical and communication disabilities in their sexual lives (such as strategies for alternative communication, mainstream technology, and support from friends and family) are also things that can make it harder for them (or act as barriers). Sometimes, family members and caregivers of people with disabilities can be overprotective and unintentionally limit opportunities or impose restraints, which can lead to a lack of privacy and result in the individuals expressing their sexual behaviors in public spaces because they are not given the opportunity to do so in private.

A decade ago, it was recognized that people with physical and communication disabilities lack opportunities to explore their sexuality and have poor access to sexual health services.

In addition, healthcare professionals may also face challenges when it comes to providing sexual health care to individuals with disabilities. Some of these challenges may include:

- Limited knowledge and training: may not have received adequate training on how to provide sexual health care for these patients, which can lead to a lack of confidence and uncertainty in their ability to provide appropriate care.
- Personal biases and attitudes which can contribute to stigmatization and lack of sensitivity in their doctor–patient relationship.
- Lack of accessible facilities and equipment can make it difficult for healthcare professionals to provide appropriate care.
- Communication barriers when attempting to understand the sexual health needs and concerns of individuals with disabilities, particularly if they require alternative forms of communication.

- Legal and ethical considerations: when providing sexual health care to individuals with disabilities, particularly about issues of consent, privacy, and abuse.

Addressing these challenges requires a commitment to ongoing education and training, as well as willingness to critically examine personal biases and attitudes. Additionally, healthcare facilities must be designed to accommodate individuals with disabilities, and appropriate communication strategies must be implemented to facilitate effective communication between healthcare professionals and their patients. Legal and ethical considerations must also be carefully navigated to ensure that the sexual health needs and rights of individuals with disabilities are respected and protected.

A multidisciplinary team can work together to develop comprehensive sexual health education programs that consider the unique needs and challenges faced by individuals with disabilities. This may involve developing alternative forms of communication for individuals with communication difficulties, providing education on sexual anatomy and function in accessible formats, and addressing issues related to relationships, intimacy, and consent. By working together, a multidisciplinary team can provide a holistic and integrated approach.

Standards of care and guidelines can be useful in guiding the assessment and management of sexual health issues in individuals with disabilities, while also allowing for individualized approaches. They provide a structured framework for healthcare professionals to provide effective and efficient care, ensuring consistency and quality of care for all individuals. Standards of care and guidelines are based on best practices and evidence-based recommendations, which can help healthcare professionals provide the most effective care possible. In addition, they can improve communication between healthcare professionals and individuals with disabilities, as well as increase efficiency by reducing the time and resources required to provide effective care. Ultimately, utilizing standards of care and guidelines can lead to better sexual health outcomes for individuals with disabilities.

4   Promoting Sexual Health and Inclusion in Disability

Since sexual health is a part of life and impacts quality of life, the United Nations Convention on the Rights of Persons with Disabilities in both article 23 and 25 focuses on the right of people with disability in having a family and participating in social relationships as well as have the right to access health care services which also include sexual health services.

As clinicians we have the obligation to help people with disabilities to avoid facing barriers in this area and increase participation.

There are some areas of development in sexual health that should be recommended to clinicians in order to improve their practice and care of people with disability:

(a) Increase awareness of the impact of diseases, trauma, and health conditions in sexual health. There is a need to improve knowledge about how health conditions impact sexual health and disease should not only be seen as a survival expectancy perspective but also as functioning and quality of life.

(b) Disability inclusive sexual education programs: Professionals have the duty to work and develop programs addressed to improve sexual health in people with disabilities, both acquired and not acquired. A person with a disability should have the opportunity to get more information about the consequences, treatment, and coping strategies to improve sexual health and minimize the impact of the disability. These programs should be accessible to all people with a certain health condition that is in a risk of impairing sexual health. At this moment, most of the studies conducted on the field report that patients or people that experience disability, get information regarding sexual health from friends, other patients, or internet resources.

(c) Advocacy and policy initiatives for improving sexual health: The different national, regional, and local governments must implement policies that are based both on the recognition of sexual health within the declaration of human rights by the United Nations but also within the section of sustainable development goals in the search for equality not only between men and women, between people with disabilities, and those who do not have it. One of the first identified issues is that sexual education continues to be a pending subject among the university programs in health professionals in countries across the world [24, 25].

(d) Increase awareness of risk of sexual violence in people with disability. People with disability are at an increased risk for suffering sexual violence; therefore, governments and institutions should promote social norms to protect against violence, invest in teaching skills to preventing sexual violence, and provide educational programs for those vulnerable groups such as people with disabilities. A correct monitoring of the extension of these problems and the evaluation of the result of the preventive strategies are important for surveillance.

The gender perspective emphasizes the importance of being aware of the context and system that reveal power dynamics and interdependence among individuals, influenced by historical and social conditions that affect relationships, language, family structure, and social structures at both micro and macro levels.

As health and education professionals, we understand that our observations, listening, and interventions with patients do not depend on our personal capabilities or private experiences but on our training, based on the theoretical tools acquired throughout our professional journey. The gender perspective requires theoretical training that allows us to question old theories and conceptualizations that conform to a cis-heteronormative world, rather than relying on professionals considering themselves respectful of gender diversity.

In the field of sexual and reproductive health, the gender perspective helps identify inequities between women and men, enabling us to carry out interventions that promote women's empowerment, equity, and consensual decision-making regarding their own and their partner's health. It also fosters men's co-responsibility during pregnancy and child-rearing, as well as their involvement in decisions regarding unplanned pregnancies without imposing pressure on women.

It is not about fragmenting rights or seeking privileges but about granting a broad significance to human rights in the exercise of sexuality. We advocate for the right to sexual life, equality, expression, free decision-making, and autonomy over one's own body, as well as the right to information, education, work, and freedom from discrimination. We recognize the right to pleasure and the practice of sexuality, regardless of its relation to reproduction.

From the perspectives of symbolic interactionism and structural functionalism, we understand that disability does not reside in the individual but in society itself, which is organized for non-disabled people. This social model of disability recognizes that limitations are not in the physical or individual elements of the subjects but in the interpretation of bodily or functional differences through social interactions, shaping how their capacity, competitiveness, and social productivity are perceived among human beings.

In this regard, individuals with disabilities are differentiated by social constructs in which they are immersed, leading to discriminatory attitudes toward them, whether they are men or women.

5 Collaborative Care and Multidisciplinary Approach

The subjective perception of good sexual health depends on various factors as discussed throughout this chapter. Therefore, implementing a multidimensional approach can enhance the subjective perception of improvement. A collaborative approach among different medical disciplines, including physical medicine and rehabilitation, urology, gynecology, neurology, and surgery, is essential. Additionally, the involvement of other healthcare professionals, such as nurses, occupational therapists, social workers, physiotherapists, and clinical sexologist, should be taken into account. This collaborative effort ensures a comprehensive and holistic approach to address the diverse aspects of sexual health.

A first step is to know the impact that different diseases, injuries, or health conditions have on the population. These will depend on external factors such as the type of society, the patient's environment, their age, and previous sexual experiences.

Professionals must coordinate with each other to understand how different diseases or health conditions affect their patients and try to create a climate of trust where the patient and their family can confidently express their doubts or even their fears. The scientific literature shows that there is a significant lack of knowledge on the part of health professionals about how diseases affect sexual health. This means that questions about sexual health are not asked in the interview and probably many of the patients consider that the question is perhaps not relevant taking into account that when they ask they do not get an answer that satisfies their concerns [20, 26].

Collaborating beyond hospital boundaries and incorporating the patient's perspective, values, environment, family, friends, and socioeconomic status can transform the traditional medical care model into a holistic, empathetic, and ultimately more equitable and effective approach. The combination of the social model of disability with a rights-based advocacy approach presents new challenges in ensuring the rights of individuals with disabilities. In this field, there have been some associations of patients who are advocating for the development of the so-called sexual assistance, that are professionals who intend to help people to experience a sexual life despite their limitations due to the disability [27].

The demand for sexual assistance originally arose from the field of physical disabilities, advocated by supporters of the social model of disability, and the independent living movement. However, this role requires debate and adaptation to the specific characteristics of countries, cultures, and the individuals with disabilities [28].

Sexual assistance is defined as "a service that provides sexual accompaniment for individuals with disabilities, offering educational services about sexual practices and support for sexual activity, with the aim of meeting sensual or sexual needs while considering the specific characteristics related to their disabilities." However, there are generally no widely accepted, agreed upon, or utilized models for providing sexual assistance services for individuals with intellectual disabilities [29–31].

Furthermore, it is recognized that this role lacks a specific professional definition, as theoretical models and professional practices vary between countries. For example, in Germany, the sexual assistant has been regulated under the Prostitute Protection Act since 2017. In Denmark, there are training programs lasting more than a year, certifying social workers as sexual advisors upon completion. Additionally, in the Netherlands, "sex care" is provided and subsidized in some cases for people with disabilities. Similarly, a growing number of private organizations in countries like Italy, Sweden, France, and Australia are training individuals to provide sexual accompaniment to people with disabilities.

6   Conclusions

Sexual health is a crucial aspect of our well-being, self-esteem, and overall quality of life. A decline in sexual activity, desire, or function can serve as an important indicator for potential adverse events and outcomes [32] particularly for individuals with disabilities, whether innate or acquired, who face higher risks compared to the general population. Health professionals must be cognizant of this fact, prompting a call to action to develop a comprehensive understanding of sexual health from a functional perspective. This knowledge will be a valuable addition to person-oriented medicine, aligning with the commitment to Sustainable Development Goals and contributing to a more equitable and inclusive society.

In conclusion, recognizing and respecting the significance of sexuality within the realm of disability are paramount for all individuals. People with disabilities deserve equal access to sexual education and information tailored to their unique needs, free from prejudice, or discrimination. Health and education professionals should be equipped with sensitivity and unbiased training to address sexuality within the context of disability.

Moreover, dismantling barriers that hinder access to sexual health information and services for people with disabilities is imperative. Cultivating a positive and empathetic outlook on sexuality within this context is pivotal in ensuring that everyone can enjoy a fulfilling and satisfying sexual life, devoid of any fear of exclusion or discrimination.

References

1. Global estimates of the need for rehabilitation based on the Global Burden of Disease study 2019: a systematic analysis for the Global Burden of Disease Study 2019. https://pubmed.ncbi.nlm.nih.gov/33275908/. Accessed 1 May 2023.
2. Laxe S, Cieza A, Castaño-Monsalve B. Rehabilitation of traumatic brain injury in the light of the ICF. NeuroRehabilitation. 2015;36(1):37–43. https://doi.org/10.3233/NRE-141189.
3. Wade DT, Halligan PW. The biopsychosocial model of illness: a model whose time has come. Clin Rehabil. 2017;31(8):995–1004. https://doi.org/10.1177/0269215517709890.
4. World Report on Disability. https://www.who.int/teams/noncommunicable-diseases/sensory-functions-disability-and-rehabilitation/world-report-on-disability. Accessed 1 May 2023.
5. Seidu AA, Malau-Aduli BS, McBain-Rigg K, Malau-Aduli AEO, Emeto TI. "Sex should not be part of the lives of persons with disabilities, but they are human beings too": perceptions of healthcare providers and factors affecting service delivery in Ghana. Healthc Basel Switz. 2023;11(7):1041. https://doi.org/10.3390/healthcare11071041.
6. Defining sexual health. https://www.who.int/teams/sexual-and-reproductive-health-and-research/key-areas-of-work/sexual-health/defining-sexual-health. Accessed 1 May 2023.
7. Wilson CS, DeDios-Stern S, Bocage C, Gray AA, Crudup BM, Russell HF. A systematic review of how spinal cord injury impacts families. Rehabil Psychol. 2022;67(3):273–303. https://doi.org/10.1037/rep0000431.
8. Ek AS, Holmström C, Elmerstig E. Sexuality >1 year after brain injury rehabilitation: a cross-sectional study in Sweden. Brain Inj. 2023;37(1):34–46. https://doi.org/10.1080/02699052.2022.2145358.
9. Paszyńska W, Zborowska K, Czajkowska M, Skrzypulec-Plinta V. Quality of sex life in intestinal stoma patients-a literature review. Int J Environ Res Public Health. 2023;20(3):2660. https://doi.org/10.3390/ijerph20032660.
10. Woods L, Hevey D, Ryall N, O'Keeffe F. Sex after amputation: the relationships between sexual functioning, body image, mood and anxiety in persons with a lower limb amputation. Disabil Rehabil. 2018;40(14):1663–70. https://doi.org/10.1080/09638288.2017.1306585.
11. Henderson AW, Turner AP, Williams RM, Norvell DC, Hakimi KN, Czerniecki JM. Sexual activity after dysvascular lower extremity amputation. Rehabil Psychol. 2016;61(3):260–8. https://doi.org/10.1037/rep0000087.
12. Zizzo J, Gater DR, Hough S, Ibrahim E. Sexuality, intimacy, and reproductive health after spinal cord injury. J Pers Med. 2022;12(12):1985. https://doi.org/10.3390/jpm12121985.
13. Hanks RA, Sander AM, Millis SR, Hammond FM, Maestas KL. Changes in sexual functioning from 6 to 12 months following traumatic brain injury: a prospective TBI model system multicenter study. J Head Trauma Rehabil. 2013;28(3):179–85. https://doi.org/10.1097/HTR.0b013e31828b4fae.
14. Ferrari S, Vanti C, Giagio S, et al. Low back pain and sexual disability from the patient's perspective: a qualitative study. Disabil Rehabil. 2022;44(10):2011–9. https://doi.org/10.1080/09638288.2020.1817161.
15. Hauer G, Sadoghi P, Smolle M, et al. Sexual activity after short-stem total hip arthroplasty. Does stem size matter? Arch Orthop Trauma Surg. 2022;23:696. https://doi.org/10.1007/s00402-022-04614-y.
16. Coulter D, Lynch C, Joosten AV. Exploring the perspectives of young adults with developmental disabilities about sexuality and sexual health education. Aust Occup Ther J. 2023;70(3):380–91. https://doi.org/10.1111/1440-1630.12862.
17. Khan N, Ryan NP, Crossley L, Hearps SJC, Catroppa C, Anderson V. Associations between peer relationships and self-esteem after childhood traumatic brain injury: exploring the mediating role of loneliness. J Neurotraumaonline. 2023;40(19-20):2100–9. https://doi.org/10.1089/neu.2022.0420.
18. Matin BK, Williamson HJ, Karyani AK, Rezaei S, Soofi M, Soltani S. Barriers in access to healthcare for women with disabilities: a systematic review in qualitative studies. BMC Womens Health. 2021;21:44. https://doi.org/10.1186/s12905-021-01189-5.

19. Hwang JHA, Fraser EE, Downing MG, Ponsford JL. A qualitative study on the attitudes and approaches of Australian clinicians in addressing sexuality after acquired brain injury. Disabil Rehabil. 2022;44(26):8294–302. https://doi.org/10.1080/09638288.2021.2012605.

20. Neonakis EM, Perna F, Traina F, et al. Total hip arthroplasty and sexual activity: a systematic review. Musculoskelet Surg. 2020;104(1):17–24. https://doi.org/10.1007/s12306-020-00645-z.

21. Mülkoğlu C, Ayhan F, Erel S. Sexual functions and quality of life in patients developing lymphedema after total mastectomy: a pilot study. Lymphat Res Biol. 2022;20(2):220–7. https://doi.org/10.1089/lrb.2020.0053.

22. Deierlein AL, Sun Y, Prado G, Stein CR. Socioeconomic characteristics, lifestyle behaviors, and health conditions among males of reproductive age with and without disabilities, NHANES 2013-2018. Am J Mens Health. 2023;17(4):15579883221138190. https://doi.org/10.1177/15579883221138190.

23. Addlakha R, Price J, Heidari S. Disability and sexuality: claiming sexual and reproductive rights. Reprod Health Matters. 2017;25(50):4–9. https://doi.org/10.1080/09688080.2017.1336375.

24. Jiménez-Ríos FJ, González-Gijón G, Martínez-Heredia N, Amaro AA. Sex education and comprehensive health education in the future of educational professionals. Int J Environ Res Public Health. 2023;20(4):3296. https://doi.org/10.3390/ijerph20043296.

25. Endler M, Al-Haidari T, Benedetto C, et al. Are sexual and reproductive health and rights taught in medical school? Results from a global survey. Int J Gynaecol Obstet. 2022;159(3):735–42. https://doi.org/10.1002/ijgo.14339.

26. Walton AB, Leinwand GZ, Raheem O, Hellstrom WJG, Brandes SB, Benson CR. Female sexual dysfunction after pelvic fracture: a comprehensive review of the literature. J Sex Med. 2021;18(3):467–73. https://doi.org/10.1016/j.jsxm.2020.12.014.

27. Benoit C, Mellor A, Premji Z. Access to sexual rights for people living with disabilities: assumptions, evidence, and policy outcomes. Arch Sex Behav. 2022;52:3201–55. https://doi.org/10.1007/s10508-022-02372-x.

28. What Sexual Assistants Want and Need: Creating a Toolkit and New Solutions to Help Them Better Perform Their Work with Individuals with Disabilities | SpringerLink. https://link.springer.com/article/10.1007/s11195-019-09614-2. Accessed 24 July 2023.

29. Limoncin E, Galli D, Ciocca G, et al. The psychosexual profile of sexual assistants: an internet-based explorative study. PLoS One. 2014;9(2):e98413. https://doi.org/10.1371/journal.pone.0098413.

30. Sexual Professionalism: For Whom? The case of sexual facilitation in Swedish personal assistance services: Disability & Society: Vol 30, No 5. https://www.tandfonline.com/doi/abs/10.1080/09687599.2015.1021761?journalCode=cdso20. Accessed 24 July 2023.

31. Sexual Assistance in Italy: An Explorative Study on the Opinions of People with Disabilities and Would-Be Assistants | SpringerLink. https://link.springer.com/article/10.1007/s11195-016-9435-y. Accessed 24 July 2023.

32. Jackson SE, Yang L, Koyanagi A, Stubbs B, Veronese N, Smith L. Declines in sexual activity and function predict incident health problems in older adults: prospective findings from the English longitudinal study of ageing. Arch Sex Behav. 2020;49(3):929–40. https://doi.org/10.1007/s10508-019-1443-4.

Sexual Activity After Total Hip Replacement

Jenaro A. Fernández-Valencia, Ferran Fillat,
and Ernesto Muñoz-Mahamud

1   Introduction

Hip osteoarthritis can provoke limited motion and pain; for cases not responding to conservative treatments, hip arthroplasty is an excellent solution with outstanding results. After hip arthroplasty implantation, patients can resume progressively their life activities, including their sexual aspect. The present chapter deals about how hip osteoarthritis can affect sexual function, what recommendations can we provide, and how surgical approach could be key in diminishing the time to resume normal activities. Also, we are going to explore the research on patient–doctor communication about this specific subject and what can be improved.

2   Hip Osteoarthritis and Sexual Function Impairment

Osteoarthritis (OA) is a prevalent joint disorder that is commonly recognized as "wear-and-tear" arthritis, age-related arthritis, or degenerative joint disease. The classification of hip OA into primary and secondary types is consistent with OA from other joints. In primary hip OA, the etiology is idiopathic, and it often involves

J. A. Fernández-Valencia (✉) · E. Muñoz-Mahamud
Hip Unit, Department of Orthopedic Surgery and Traumatology, Clinical Institute of Medical and Surgical Specialties, Hospital Clinic de Barcelona, Barcelona, Spain

Surgery and Medical-Surgical Specialties, Faculty of Medicine and Health Sciences, Universitat de Barcelona (UB), Barcelona, Spain
e-mail: jenarofv@clinic.cat; emunoz@clinic.cat

F. Fillat
Hip Unit, Department of Orthopedic Surgery and Traumatology, Clinical Institute of Medical and Surgical Specialties, Hospital Clínic de Barcelona, Barcelona, Spain
e-mail: fillat@clinic.cat

C. Castelo-Branco, S. Anglès Acedo (eds.), *Medical Disorders and Sexual Health*, Trends in Andrology and Sexual Medicine,
https://doi.org/10.1007/978-3-031-55080-5_31

multiple joints, with a higher incidence in the elderly population. In contrast, secondary OA is a monoarticular condition that results from a specific disorder affecting the joint articular surface. Secondary hip OA can be attributed to various factors including avascular necrosis of the hip with subsequent collapse of the femoral head surface or sequelae from trauma.

Hip OA typically presents with pain in the hip joint, with the most common location being the groin area, although it can also be found in the trochanteric area or, less commonly, in the buttock. The pain can have an acute onset, but it usually develops gradually and worsens over time. Morning stiffness and stiffness after resting or sitting can also occur, but typically lasts for only a few minutes and subsides within 30 min. Physical activity and exercise that help to mobilize the joint generally improve OA symptoms.

With the progression of the disease, painful symptoms tend to increase and can also occur during rest [1]. Patients commonly report that certain activities or positions exacerbate hip pain, including prolonged inactivity, hip abduction, external and internal rotation, bending the hip, and entering or exiting a car, as well as sustained physical activity. This condition is particularly notable for its impact on the ability of younger patients to carry out sportive activities [2]. Pain and stiffness can also affect other aspects of a patient's life, including sexual activity. In some cases, patients may find it challenging to engage in sexual activity due to their hip pain and stiffness [3, 4].

When conservative treatments, such as lifestyle modifications, medications, and physical therapy, have failed to provide adequate relief for pain and disability associated with hip osteoarthritis, total hip arthroplasty (THA) is indicated. The decision to proceed with THA also considers the individual's age, general health status, and the extent of joint damage. In general, total hip replacement is recommended for patients with advanced hip osteoarthritis, severe pain, and significant functional limitations that affect their quality of life. Regarding sexual activity, it has been estimated that between 65% and 80% of individuals with hip OA who undergo arthroplasty surgery experience impaired sexual health [5, 6], and the effect of the surgery has a direct translation into the quality and frequency of sexual activity [7, 8].

3 Sexual Activity After Total Hip Replacement

Following a THA surgery, as with any major surgery, a fatigue can be expected. This fatigue could influence in appealing to resume sexual activity. Moreover, special situations such as the indication of implantation because of oncological disease or trauma (i.e., accident with multiple other victims), the patient might need a psychological support and sexual activity turns to be less of the preoccupation in that situation. On the other hand, inflammation and post-surgical pain can also limit the need for sexual relation or its duration. Patients may experience pain and be concerned about the risk of implant dislocation associated with certain hip joint positions during sexual activity. Dislocation is a painful condition, and the patient will need to go to a medical center to get the joint back into position under anesthesia (Fig. 1). While this can be solved in this way, some patients will have this as a recurring problem, and that could lead to need further surgeries exchanging implant

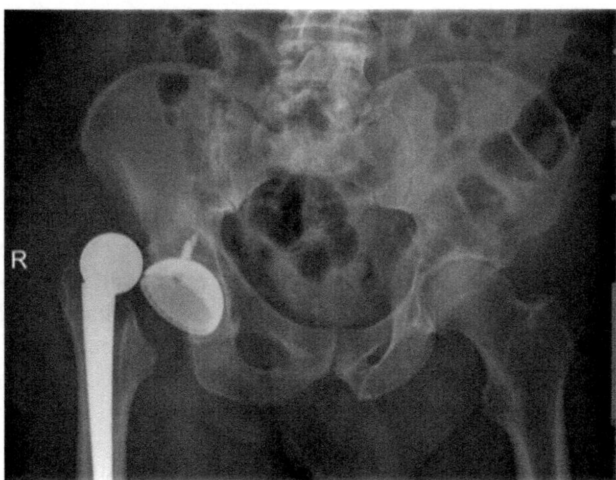

Fig. 1 Radiology depicting a dislocation of a right total hip replacement. Extreme positions during sexual activity could increase the risk for this event. While this complication is one the most feared after a total hip replacement, its occurrence has decreased over the years due to the improvement of tribology (implants with bigger prosthetic heads or dual mobility joints) and to the improvement of the technique of the surgical approach

components to improve the stability of the joint. Despite hip arthroplasty dislocation is the main fear that justifies the delay of resuming sexual activity after surgery, just few cases of dislocation occurred during sexual activity after THA have been reported [8, 9], and in those reports, the position that provoked dislocation was not specified (Navas). Moreover, recent improvements in surgical techniques and implants have decreased the chances for this complication [11]. But most important, dislocation can be prevented especially by the proper positioning of the components of the total hip arthroplasty, and this implies a careful preoperative planning and surgical execution, considering the biomechanics of the joint to be replaced [12].

The positions to avoid during sexual activity are derived from those positions that create a risk for dislocation in the postoperative period. While this is relevant for patients and doctors, just few of the recommendations is founded on studies dealing about this subject focusing on the intercourse during sexual activity. But it is not common to evaluate the risk regarding other possible factors such as the type of implant, or the performed surgical approach, which could play a major role in joint stability. Most of the recommendations are assumptions or conclusions based on the experience of experts, but there is not, to our best knowledge a consensus by a panel of experts, as it occurs with the resuming of sports practice after total hip replacement. If we look to the opinion of doctors regarding sports, for instance, from the consensus of the European Hip Society, there is not a uniform statement to when to resume and to what level of intensity, especially regarding high impact sports [13]. We could assume the same regarding resuming sexual activity. Moreover, regarding the type of THA, some designs are inherently more stable. Resurfacing total hip arthroplasty has the biggest possible femoral head, and it shows outstanding results in preventing dislocation, as well as THA using dual mobility. This resurfacing THA, popularized by the famous tennis player Andy Williams, is based on a metal-on-metal bearing; the surfaces facing both sides of the joint are made of cobalt and chrome. It has some limitations and inherent risks, and not every patient is suitable for resurfacing, especially women and patients with femoral components with diameter inferior to 48 mm, since the release of the ions of this metal from the joint can provoke reaction in the surrounding tissues. It is now under research the evolution of hip resurfacing to a new bearing based on ceramics and without cobalt and chrome, which could have better tolerance for the body, but still those implants are under preclinical research. On the other hand, dual mobility total hip arthroplasty shows excellent properties to prevent dislocation, also because provides a bigger than average effective diameter for the prosthetic joint. While this type of implant is gaining popularity for revision total hip arthroplasty, its use in primary THA is controversial due to a potential increased cost but also because of concerns of wear and specific complications with this implant that are beyond the focus of this book chapter. But as a resume, these two types of prosthesis for the hip, resurfacing, and dual mobility THA provide more stability but the recommendations for sexual activity after total hip replacement surprisingly do not differ for this subset of patients, possibly indicating a subject for future research.

Moreover, there is a misconception about sexual activity, since sometimes it is just intercourse what is assumed in the conversation but there is more than that in sexual activity specially for the older adult. As stated by Steckenrider, it is mistakenly believed that the word "sex" solely pertains to sexual activity with a partner involving intercourse and this is not the case for numerous older individuals who must adjust their sexual behaviors due to issues such as erectile dysfunction, vaginal dryness, arthritis, mobility limitations, medication effects, or serious health conditions [14]. This misconception is translated to most of the research related to sexual activity after total hip replacement, since those studies are focused on sexual intercourse and avoid addressing other expressions of sexuality that involve physical and emotional intimacy as part of what it is considered as having sex [15]. Other forms of sexual activity beyond penetrative sex, such as oral sex, kissing, fondling, and solo sex (masturbation) are not the focus of the research since possibly do not pose the joint of the hip at any special risk. These could be areas for further research.

Among the different studies evaluating what are the recommended postures and what are the most dangerous for a hip with a total hip replacement, a relevant study by Charbonnier et al. was performed by using motion capture data. They evaluated different common positions during sexual activity [16] and the risk for dislocation due to the position of the joint or to the risk of internal impingement between structures that could potentially dislocate the artificial joint. A resume is accessible in YouTube as per March 2023 in the link https://www.youtube.com/watch?v=lys45y1iTmQ. Interestingly, during the writing of this chapter, the video was 9 years on the internet, and received 19 million of visits, while other videos related to health information for joints pathology and treatment do barely surpass the half of millions of visits. This study is very explicit regarding the postures that are allowed and the differences of risk depending on the position for man and

Representation of several positions for sexual activity with penetrative sex after total hip replacement

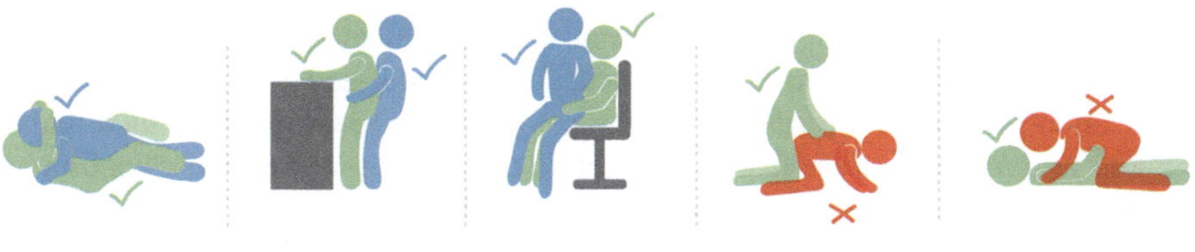

Fig. 2 Several positions during sexual intercourse. Safe positions are marked with a "V." Positions at risk for dislocation are marked with an "X," and the subject is colored in red

woman. While that video can be visited, we provide a figure including several positions that are safe and some other that are at risk during intercourse. If we carefully observe the positions that are at risk, commonly there is an extreme flexion of the joint in those cases (Fig. 2).

It can be assumed, as for many other aspects of resuming with normal life activities after THA, that 6 weeks provides a safe period of time for tissues to heal in order to prevent dislocation in extreme positions of the hip. While this is accepted both for men and women, possible man could resume before the activity since men sexual positions require less mobility and are considered safer [10].

4   Could Surgical Approach Play a Role in the Recovery of Sexual Function?

The direct anterior approach has emerged as a revolutionary technique for total hip arthroplasty (THA) implantation. This approach is characterized by its intermuscular and internervous nature, which allows patients to resume normal activities with less pain and a lower risk of dislocation. Moreover, the overall risk for revision is lower compared to the other surgical approaches, both for dislocation and for any other cause, as shown in a study of the Duch registry evaluating a 9-year period of time [17]. As a result of these advantages, the direct anterior approach has become increasingly popular in recent years as a preferred method for THA implantation. While the number of patients suffering a dislocation has decreased during the years to <2%, and occasionally <1%, with any approach, thanks to the improvement of the surgical technique, and the design and manufacture of implants, direct anterior approach is the safest regarding dislocation according to multiple studies, decreasing the risk for dislocation to just a 0.3% of patients.

A widely accepted notion suggests that the position which poses a risk to patients, not only during sexual intercourse but also during routine daily activities, is when patients flex their hip, bring their knee across the midline of their body, and rotate it internally. This is a commonly repeated message to protect patients from dislocation, but this is a specific recommendation only for patients operated by posterior approach. Patients operated by anterior approach do not need to follow these restrictions since the joint is inherently more stable and are allowed to move freely the joint if it is not provoking pain or discomfort.

While direct anterior approach has a translation into decreasing hospital stay and increased patient satisfaction regarding pain control and speed of recovery, its direct implication into resuming sexual activity has not been extensively studied and it remains as a future possible line of research to be clarified, and possible the time to resume sexual activity can be as short as the patient feels like to it but not regarding a specific time for tissues to heal. However, to the opinion of the authors of this chapter, it makes sense to be cautious and avoid any extenuating or extreme activity for the very first weeks after THA.

5   A Topic That Is Infrequently Addressed

Discussing sexual activity impairment related to hip disease can be challenging due to the personal and sensitive nature of this topic, as well as the intimate and unique aspects of sexual activity. Patients are typically provided with information on various aspects of the postoperative period, such as wound care, proper use of crutches, and warning signs to watch for during recovery. However, discussions about resuming sexual activity can be challenging for both patients and physicians, and therefore such advice is often not provided. This fact has been documented in the study by Ugwuoke et al. [18]. In this study, questionnaires were given to clinicians and patients to evaluate the topic of sexual activity after hip replacement. The clinicians' questionnaire focused on their approach to addressing this issue, being all the patients under the age of 80. They were asked about their experience and suggestions for improvement. All 17 clinicians responded to the questionnaire, and none reported using printed materials or routinely discussing sexual activity with patients. Of the 340 patients who responded, 244 indicated a desire for their surgeon to discuss sexual activity after total hip replacement with them, and over 90% expressed willingness to be directly asked about the subject.

Wall et al., in a survey of 83 surgeons, found that only 39% provided written information about sexual activity following surgery. In addition, only 25% of surgeons explicitly advised patients about when it was safe to resume sexual activities [19]. In addition, Dahm et al. in a survey among members of the American Association of Hip and Knee Surgeons, found that greater than 90% of surgeons surveyed, 233 out of 254, rarely or never had a discussion about sex with their patients before or after undergoing THA.

Interesting to notice, it is a common situation not only affecting orthopedic surgeons but also doctors from many other specialties. This has been related to many factors such as that sexual history was not included in a traditional medical history, doctors do have tittle teaching about sexuality and sexual difficulties in medical school, worries about offending the patient, or stereotyping the patient since the doctor thinks that patient is too old, sick, or disabled for sex [20].

6 Conclusions

The resumption of sexual activity following total hip replacement can occur once the patient feels comfortable doing so. Although a widely held belief recommends a 6-week waiting period before engaging in sexual intercourse, this recommendation is primarily based on expert opinion and largely pertains to hips operated on using the posterior approach. To guide patients toward the safest postures during intercourse, figures are available. Sexual activities not involving the hip joint may be resumed as soon as the patient feels ready. For patients who have undergone an anterior approach procedure, it may be possible to resume sexual activity earlier and without the restrictions on range of motion typically described; however, more research is needed in this area. Despite being of interest to patients, sexual activity after total hip replacement is not typically discussed with patients and is a topic worthy of further attention to improve patient outcomes.

References

1. Lespasio MJ, Sultan AA, Piuzzi NS, et al. Hip osteoarthritis: a primer. Perm J. 2018;22:17–084. https://doi.org/10.7812/TPP/17-084.
2. Gallart X, Riba J, Fernández-Valencia JA, Bori G, Muñoz-Mahamud E, Combalia A. Hip prostheses in young adults. Surface prostheses and short-stem prostheses. Rev Esp Cir Ortop Traumatol (Engl Ed). 2018;62(2):142–52.
3. Yoon BH, Lee KH, Noh S, et al. Sexual activity after total hip replacement in Korean patients: how they do, what they want, and how to improve. Clin Orthop Surg. 2013;5(4):269.
4. Meiri R, Rosenbaum TY, Kalichman L. Sexual function before and after total hip replacement: narrative review. Sex Med. 2014;2(4):159.
5. Harmsen RTE, den Oudsten BL, Putter H, Leichtenberg CS, Elzevier HW, Nelissen R. Patient expectations of sexual activity after Total hip arthroplasty: a prospective multicenter cohort study. JBJS Open Access. 2018;3(4):e0031.
6. Lavernia CJ, Villa JM. High rates of interest in sex in patients with hip arthritis. Clin Orthop Relat Res. 2016;474(2):293–9.
7. Laffosse JM, Tricoire JL, Chiron P, Puget J. Sexual function before and after primary total hip arthroplasty. Joint Bone Spine. 2008;75(2):189–94. https://doi.org/10.1016/j.jbspin.2007.05.006.
8. Stern SH, Fuchs MD, Ganz SB, Classi P, Sculco TP, Salvati EA. Sexual function after total hip arthroplasty. Clin Orthop Relat Res. 1991;269:228–35.
9. Dahm DL, Jacofsky D, Lewallen DG. Surgeons rarely discuss sexual activity with patients after THA: a survey of members of the American association of hip and knee surgeons. Clin Orthop Relat Res. 2004;428:237–40.
10. Navas L, Hauschild M, Miehlke W, Schmidt S, Streit M, Kinkel S, Zimmerer A. Length doesn't play a role - sexual activity in men after short stem total hip arthroplasty. BMC Musculoskelet Disord. 2022;23(1):696.
11. Wright-Chisem J, Elbuluk AM, Mayman DJ, Jerabek SA, Sculco PK, Vigdorchik JM. The journey to preventing dislocation after total hip arthroplasty: how did we get here? Bone Joint J. 2022;104-B(1):8–11.
12. Gallart X, Daccach JJ, Fernández-Valencia JÁ, García S, Bori G, Rios J, Riba J. Estudio de la concordancia de un sistema de planificación preoperatoria digital en artroplastia total de cadera [study of the consistency of a system for preoperative planning digital in total arthroplasty of the hip]. Rev Esp Cir Ortop Traumatol. 2012;56(6):471–7.

13. Thaler M, Khosravi I, Putzer D, Siebenrock KA, Zagra L. Return to sports after total hip arthroplasty: a survey among members of the European hip society. J Arthroplast. 2021;36(5):1645–54. https://doi.org/10.1016/j.arth.2020.11.009. Epub 2020 Nov 11
14. Steckenrider J. Sexual activity of older adults: let's talk about it. Lancet Healthy Longev. 2023;4(3):e96–7. https://doi.org/10.1016/S2666-7568(23)00003-X. Epub 2023 Feb 2
15. Gore-Gorszewska G. "What do you mean by sex?" a qualitative analysis of traditional versus evolved meanings of sexual activity among older women and men. J Sex Res. 2021;58:1035–49.
16. Charbonnier C, Chagué S, Ponzoni M, Bernardoni M, Hoffmeyer P, Christofilopoulos P. Sexual activity after total hip arthroplasty: a motion capture study. J Arthroplast. 2014;29(3):640–7. https://doi.org/10.1016/j.arth.2013.07.043. Epub 2013 Sep 7
17. van Steenbergen LN, de Reus IM, Hannink G, Vehmeijer SB, Schreurs BW, Zijlstra WP. Femoral head size and surgical approach affect dislocation and overall revision rates in total hip arthroplasty: up to 9-year follow-up data of 269,280 procedures in the Dutch arthroplasty register (LROI). Hip Int. 2023;33(6):1056–62.
18. Ugwuoke A, Syed F, Hefny M, Robertson T, Young S. Discussing sexual activities after total hip arthroplasty. J Orthop Sci. 2020;25(4):595–8. https://doi.org/10.1016/j.jos.2019.06.010. Epub 2019 Jul 5
19. Wall PD, Hossain M, Ganapathi M, Andrew JG. Sexual activity and total hip arthroplasty: a survey of patients' and surgeons' perspectives. Hip Int. 2011;21(2):199–205. https://doi.org/10.5301/HIP.2011.6518. Epub 2011 Apr 5
20. Goodwach R. Let' talk about sex. Aust Fam Physician. 2017;46(1):14–8.

Sexual Activity After Hip Preservation Surgery: Hip Arthroscopy for Femoroacetabular Impingement and Periacetabular Osteotomy

Luis J. Ramirez Núñez, Alfonso Alias, and Adria Serra Trullas

1   Introduction

Sexual activity plays a critical role in an individual's overall well-being, encompassing both physical and emotional aspects of life. Despite this, patients who undergo hip preservation surgery, such as hip arthroscopy and periacetabular osteotomy, often express concerns about how these procedures might affect their sexual function. While the primary goal of these surgeries is to address hip joint conditions and enhance patient outcomes, the potential impact on sexual activity and associated patient-reported outcomes has not been extensively studied.

Recent studies have begun to address this important topic, evaluating the impact of hip preservation surgery on sexual function and quality of life [1, 2]. To address this deficiency, this chapter delves into the presence and significance of sexual difficulties experienced by patients with chronic hip pain both before and after hip arthroscopic surgery for symptomatic femoroacetabular Impingement (FAI). In doing so, it aims to provide a more comprehensive understanding of the issue and identify areas where further research is needed.

L. J. Ramirez Núñez (✉)
Hip Unit, Clinical Institute of Medical and Surgical Specialties, Hospital Clinic de Barcelona, Barcelona, Spain
e-mail: ljramirez@clinic.cat

A. Alias
Hip Unit, Department of Orthopedic Surgery and Traumatology, Clinical Institute of Medical and Surgical Specialties, Hospital Clínic de Barcelona, Barcelona, Spain
e-mail: alias@clinic.cat

A. Serra Trullas
Department of Orthopaedic Surgery, Clinical Institute of Medical and Surgical Specialties, Hospital Clínic de Barcelona, Barcelona, Spain
e-mail: serra@clinic.cat

Sexual activity in patients with hip pain can be limited by various factors, including pain and restricted range of motion. Extended periods of inactivity due to pain can lead to weakened pelvic floor and hip girdle muscles, resulting in increased discomfort in both the affected and unaffected hips.

Following hip preservation surgery, it is essential for patients to adhere to specific motion and position restrictions to avoid damaging repaired structures such as the labrum and capsule. A compromised capsular integrity post-primary hip arthroscopy has been linked to poor patient-reported outcomes and the need for revision surgery. Similarly, labral reinjury or deficiency can also result in suboptimal outcomes and further surgical intervention. Consequently, preserving the integrity of the capsule and labrum is crucial for achieving the best possible post-arthroscopic outcomes.

To assist healthcare providers in addressing patient concerns and optimizing postoperative care, this chapter offers a comprehensive overview of the existing literature on sexual activity following hip preservation surgery. By focusing on procedures such as hip arthroscopy, periacetabular osteotomy, surgical hip dislocation, core decompression, and proximal femoral osteotomy, the chapter highlights the importance of understanding the relationship between these surgical procedures and sexual function. Furthermore, it emphasizes the need for continued research in this area, with the ultimate goal of improving patient care and education regarding sexual activity after hip preservation surgery.

2 Hip Arthroscopy

Hip arthroscopy is a minimally invasive surgical procedure that can be used to treat a variety of hip conditions, mainly femoroacetabular impingement (FAI) and instability of the femoroacetabular joint. Usually, the procedure involves the use of a perineal post and traction to create the necessary distraction force for accessing the coxofemoral joint. However, complications related to perineal compression or soft tissue traction, such as pudendal neuralgia or neurapraxia, can occur as a result of excessive traction force and exceeded time.

Pudendal neurapraxia impacts the perineal region, which includes the genitalia and rectum, and can induce a range of symptoms. These manifestations may extend from numbness to sexual dysfunction, incorporating conditions such as erectile dysfunction, decreased libido, dyspareunia, and vulvodynia. The incidence of pudendal neurapraxia after hip arthroscopy varies widely, with studies reporting rates ranging from 1.8% to 27.6% [3]. The complexity and duration of the procedure are directly related to the reported rates of pudendal nerve injury.

To minimize the risk of complications related to traction, it is recommended that tractions exceeding 2 h or more than 23 kg be avoided [4]. Advancements in surgical techniques that eliminate the need for a perineal post have significantly reduced the incidence of these complications. Patients should also be educated on the signs and symptoms of perineal post-related nerve injuries and advised to report any discomfort or pain after the procedure.

Hip arthroscopic surgery for symptomatic FAI has been shown to improve sexual function, with patients able to return to pain-free sexual activity on average 48 days after the operation [5].

Female and older patients reported worse sexual difficulties as compared with male or younger patients after hip arthroscopic surgery. Despite this, discussions about sexual difficulties in the preoperative and postoperative period were infrequent. Patients are desired and may benefit from additional discussion or information specific to this issue. Healthcare providers should be more proactive in discussing sexual function with their patients to identify and address any concerns related to sexual activity after hip arthroscopy [6].

Postoperative protocols play a crucial role in ensuring the best possible outcomes for patients. The goal of postoperative protocols is to avoid extension, abduction, and external rotation early to avoid instability. Patients should also avoid positions that cause excessive deep flexion, adduction, external rotation, or abduction, as this can disrupt the capsule and labrum. Active hip flexion, including active iliopsoas firing, should also be avoided as it may disrupt both the capsule and labrum due to its location and anterior stabilization effect on the capsule and femoroacetabular articulation.

3 Resuming Sexual Activity After Hip Arthroscopy

A study aimed to determine the safety of sexual activity after hip arthroscopy in relation to hip instability and impingement risk [5]. Twelve common sexual positions were assessed for both male and female patients to determine potential risk. The study found that most male and female sexual positions caused either instability or impingement, with only four positions for each gender deemed safe. This information is important to consider when counseling patients pre- and postoperatively regarding sexual activity.

Taking the above information into consideration, and understanding penetrative sex as an extended sexual behavior regardless gender and sexual orientation, our team identify safety positions for sexual activity with penetrative sex after total hip replacement versus four risky sexual positions (see Fig. 2 of chapter "Sexual Activity After Total Hip Replacement"). All positions that require hip flexion beyond 90 degrees in the sex-receiving subject may potentially be detrimental in the initial postoperative weeks and should thus be avoided.

4 Periacetabular Osteotomy

Developmental Dysplasia of the Hip (DDH) involves a range of anatomical abnormalities, with the most significant issue being insufficient acetabular coverage. This problem leads to an uneven distribution of forces on the hip joint. Consequently, the pressure on the articular cartilage increases, causing instability and a higher likelihood of soft tissue damage, damage to periarticular structures, and eventually, the possibility of coxarthrosis [7, 8].

Young (15–40 years) and active patients who have symptoms and show this acetabular coverage alteration in radiological studies are considered suitable candidates for surgical treatment, provided there is no articular cartilage degeneration. The primary goal of surgery is to enhance the patient's clinical-functional status and, as much as possible, prevent severe degenerative changes from developing.

Periacetabular osteotomy (PAO), also referred to as Ganz osteotomy or Bernese osteotomy, is a leading therapeutic approach for skeletally mature patients. This method has gained recognition due to its proven results and high survival rate [9]. PAO involves an osteotomy, or surgical cutting of the bone, around the acetabulum, using polygonal cuts to allow its reorientation. This process achieves the following:

- Even distribution of forces on the femoral head.
- Improved acetabular coverage across all planes.
- Preservation of contact between the acetabular hyaline cartilage and the femoral cartilage.

Ganz et al. [7] first detailed this technique in 1988, utilizing a modified Smith-Petersen approach. This method involved detaching and reattaching the muscles of the anterosuperior iliac spine and the rectus anterior to expose the acetabulum adequately.

5 Impact on Sexual Activity After Periacetabular Osteotomy

Sexual activity plays a crucial role in an individual's overall well-being, encompassing both physical and emotional aspects of life. Patients who undergo hip preservation surgeries, such as periacetabular osteotomy (PAO), often express concerns about how these procedures might affect their sexual function and satisfaction.

While there is limited scientific literature specifically addressing the impact of PAO on sexual activity, some studies have begun to explore the long-term effects of this surgery on patients' sex lives. Klit et al. [1] indicated that both men and women experienced improvements in their sex life for 9–12 years after undergoing PAO surgery. Interestingly, the improvements observed in women were statistically significant, while the improvements in men did not reach the same level of statistical significance.

Valenzuela et al. [10] conducted a study examining the impact of periacetabular osteotomy (PAO) on the sex lives of patients. The findings revealed that 25–40% of female patients experienced positive changes in their sexual function and satisfaction following the surgery. This significant proportion of women who reported improvements after undergoing PAO highlights the potential benefits of this procedure in addressing hip-related issues that may have been negatively affecting their sexual well-being.

These positive changes in sexual function might be attributed to several factors, such as reduced pain, increased mobility, and overall improvements in hip joint function. As a result, these women may have found it easier to engage in and enjoy sexual activities, leading to an enhanced quality of life.

In conclusion, while the available scientific literature on the impact of PAO on sexual activity is limited, there is evidence to suggest that improvements in hip function and pain relief may lead to a better sex life for patients who undergo this procedure. Despite the increased recognition of sexual health's significance in overall quality of life, our understanding of the impact of Periacetabular Osteotomy (PAO) on sexual function remains limited. Notably absent from existing literature are comprehensive studies exploring sexual activity in the context of sexual and gender minority populations. The development of robust, evidence-based guidelines for healthcare providers to address postoperative sexual concerns is contingent upon a more in-depth examination of these relationships. Future research is needed to broaden our understanding and to inform optimal postoperative patient care strategies.

6   Resuming Sexual Activity After Periacetabular Osteotomy

Postoperative recovery from PAO is a crucial period, and patients should be provided with clear instructions and expectations regarding resuming sexual activity. According to the limited literature available on this subject, the general recommendation is that patients may resume sexual activity approximately 6–8 weeks following surgery. However, this timeline can vary depending on individual factors such as healing progress, overall health, and the presence of any postoperative complications.

When advising patients on resuming sexual activity, it is essential to emphasize the importance of gradual reintroduction and open communication with their partner. Patients should be encouraged to listen to their bodies and avoid positions that may place excessive stress on the hip joint, particularly during the initial stages of resuming sexual activity.

In some instances, patients may benefit from seeking the guidance of a physical therapist or sex therapist, who can provide specific techniques and exercises to facilitate a smooth transition back to a healthy sex life. This interdisciplinary approach may be particularly beneficial for patients experiencing ongoing difficulties or concerns related to sexual activity following PAO.

It is crucial to acknowledge the variability in patient experiences and the influence of factors such as the severity of the hip condition, overall health, and surgical success. As clinicians and researchers in the field of hip preservation, our responsibility is to continue expanding our understanding of the relationship between PAO and sexual function, providing evidence-based guidance for optimizing patient care and outcomes.

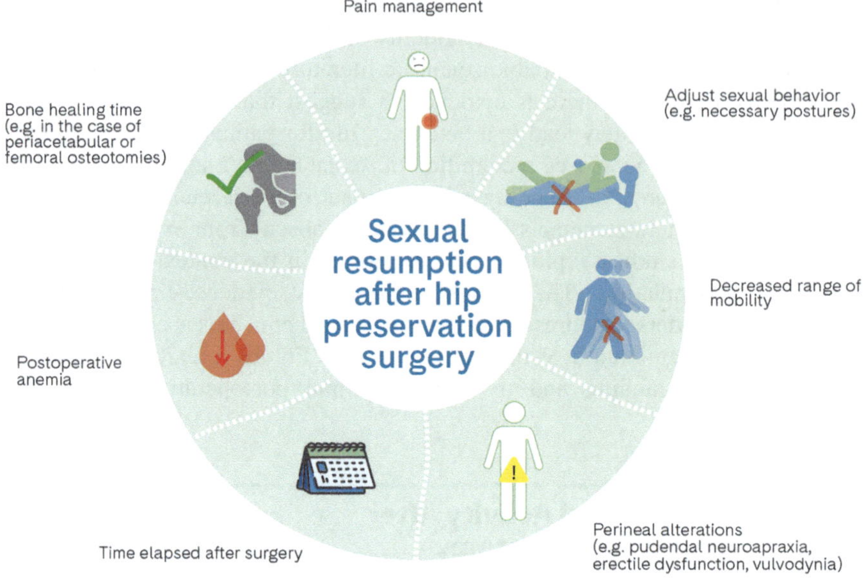

Fig. 1 Sexual resumption after hip preservation surgery

7 Factors Influencing Return to Sexual Activity

Several factors can influence the return to sexual activity after hip preservation procedures, and these factors can be patient-related, surgery-related, or environmental-related (Fig. 1). Postoperative pain levels can significantly affect a patient's ability to resume sexual activity, making pain management crucial in the early stages of recovery. As pain decreases, patients may feel more comfortable engaging in sexual activities.

Hip preservation procedures often lead to temporary limitations in hip range of motion, and as patients regain their range of motion through rehabilitation, they will likely find it easier to resume sexual activity without discomfort. Different hip preservation procedures, such as hip arthroscopy, periacetabular osteotomy, and surgical hip dislocation, may have different recovery timelines and impact on sexual function. The surgical approach and technique can also affect recovery and the ability to resume sexual activities.

Surgeons may impose specific movement and position restrictions following hip preservation surgery to protect the repaired structures. Adhering to these restrictions may temporarily limit the range of sexual positions that are safe and comfortable for patients. Engaging in a structured rehabilitation program can help patients regain strength and mobility in the hip joint, and as they progress through their rehabilitation, they may experience increased confidence and ability to engage in sexual activities.

Anxiety, depression, or concerns about reinjury can influence a patient's readiness to resume sexual activity. Addressing these psychological factors through counseling or reassurance from healthcare providers may help patients feel more comfortable returning to sexual activities. A patient's overall health and the presence of other medical conditions can also impact their ability to resume sexual activity. Patients with better overall health and fewer comorbidities may recover more quickly and feel more comfortable engaging in sexual activities sooner.

Considering these factors on an individual basis is essential, as each patient's experience and recovery may vary. Open communication between patients and healthcare providers can help address concerns and guide patients through the process of resuming sexual activity safely and comfortably.

8   Management of Sexual Concerns

Addressing common concerns related to hip preservation procedures is paramount for both patients and healthcare providers to ensure optimal postoperative care and recovery. Primary patient concern after surgery lies in adequate pain management, and healthcare providers should have detailed discussions about various pain relief options to enhance patient comfort and promote successful rehabilitation. The rehabilitation process might also spark concern, as patients frequently inquire about the duration and intensity of their recovery. Offering clear, personalized guidelines and regular follow-up appointments can help patients understand the process and successfully reach their rehabilitation milestones.

Resumption of sexual activity is an additional significant concern for patients. It is critical for healthcare providers to provide specific guidelines for safe and gradually progressive sexual activities during the recovery period. Initiating with more comfortable practices such as self-stimulation, mutual masturbation, and receiving oral sex can help ease the patients into their sexual routine. Over time, patients can progressively move toward less comfortable practices, such as performing oral sex, vaginal sex, and anal sex. Open communication and reassurance can help mitigate patient anxiety and facilitate a smooth transition back to sexual activity.

Managing sexual concerns post-hip preservation surgery is crucial for ensuring a smooth recovery and return to a satisfying sex life. Various strategies, including physical therapy, pain management, and assistive devices, can be employed to address these concerns.

A structured rehabilitation program under the supervision of a physical therapist can help patients regain strength, flexibility, and hip joint range of motion, facilitating a more comfortable return to sexual activity. Specific exercises targeting hip and pelvic muscles can enhance stability and reduce discomfort during intercourse. Additionally, a physical therapist can recommend safe sexual positions and techniques to minimize stress on the healing hip joint and to reintroduce sexual activities gradually.

Effective pain management is pivotal in enabling patients to resume sexual activity without discomfort. Healthcare providers should discuss various pain relief options, like over-the-counter medications, prescription drugs, and alternative therapies such as acupuncture or massage. A tailored pain management plan can alleviate pain during sexual activities and promote a positive experience.

The use of assistive devices, such as pillows or cushions, might benefit some patients by supporting their body and minimizing hip joint stress during sexual activities. These devices can be particularly helpful during early recovery stages when patients are still regaining strength and mobility. Moreover, using a pillow to elevate the pelvis or support the affected hip can assist patients in finding more comfortable intercourse positions.

Emotional and psychological factors can also impact a patient's return to sexual activity. Anxiety, depression, and the fear of reinjury can hinder comfort and confidence during sexual activities. Addressing these concerns through counseling or reassurance from healthcare providers can bolster patients' security in their recovery and comfort in resuming sexual activities.

Promoting open communication between patients and their partners is essential for managing sexual concerns. Encouraging patients to discuss their feelings, limitations, and any discomfort with their partners fosters an open dialogue. This mutual understanding can help both parties accommodate the patient's recovery, leading to effective solutions.

9 Conclusion

In conclusion, sexual activity is a vital aspect of an individual's overall well-being, and understanding its relationship with hip preservation procedures is critical for optimizing patient care. Recent studies have started to explore the impact of various hip preservation surgeries, such as hip arthroscopy, periacetabular osteotomy, surgical hip dislocation, core decompression, and proximal femoral osteotomy, on sexual function and satisfaction. These studies suggest that improvements in hip function and pain relief may lead to enhanced sexual experiences for patients. However, more research is needed to provide definitive information on this relationship and establish evidence-based guidelines for healthcare providers.

Addressing patients' concerns regarding pain management, rehabilitation, resuming daily activities, and potential complications is essential for facilitating a smooth postoperative recovery. By providing personalized guidelines and fostering open communication, healthcare providers can help patients navigate the challenges of returning to sexual activity and alleviate anxiety.

References

1. Klit J, Hartig-Andreasen C, Jacobsen S, Søballe K, Troelsen A. Periacetabular osteotomy: sporting, social and sexual activity 9-12 years post-surgery. Hip Int. 2014;24(1):27–31.

 2. Clohisy JC, Ackerman J, Baca G, Baty J, Beaule PE, Kim YJ, et al. Patient-reported outcomes of periacetabular osteotomy from the prospective ANCHOR cohort study. J Bone Joint Surg. 2017;99:33–41.
 3. Jean PO, Simunovic N, Duong A, Heels-Ansdell D, Ayeni OR. Sexual and urinary function post-surgical treatment of femoroacetabular impingement: experience from the FIRST trial and embedded cohort study. J Hip Preserv Surg. 2022;9(1):28–34.
 4. Kern MJ, Murray RS, Sherman TI, Postma WF. Incidence of nerve injury after hip arthroscopy. J Am Acad Orthop Surg. 2018;26(21):773–8.
 5. Morehouse H, Sochacki KR, Nho SJ, Harris JD. Gender-specific sexual activity after hip arthroscopy for femoroacetabular impingement syndrome: position matters. J Sex Med. 2020;17(4):658–64.
 6. Lee S, Frank RM, Harris J, Song SH, Bush-Joseph CA, Salata MJ, et al. Evaluation of sexual function before and after hip arthroscopic surgery for symptomatic femoroacetabular impingement. Am J Sports Med. 2015;43(8):1850–6.
 7. Ganz R, Klaue K, Vinh TS, Mast JW. A new periacetabular osteotomy for the treatment of hip dysplasias. Clin Orthop Relat Res. 1988;232:26–36.
 8. Ramírez-Núñez L, Payo-Ollero J, Comas M, Cárdenas C, Bellotti V, Astarita E, et al. Periacetabular osteotomy for hip dysplasia treatment through a mini-invasive technique. Our results at mid-term in 131 cases. Rev Esp Cir Ortop Traumatol. 2020;64(3):151–9.
 9. Steppacher SD, Tannast M, Ganz R, Siebenrock KA. Mean 20-year follow-up of Bernese periacetabular osteotomy. Clin Orthop Relat Res. 2008;466(7):1633–44.
10. Valenzuela RG, Cabanela ME, Trousdale RT. Sexual activity, pregnancy, and childbirth after periacetabular osteotomy. Clin Orthop Relat Res. 2004;418:146–52.

Sexual Health and Chronic Dermatosis

Irene Fuertes and Josep Riera

1   Introduction

The skin is the largest organ of the human body. It is a dynamic and complex organ that plays several essential roles. The skin acts as a barrier that protects the rest of the organs and also allows the relationship with the outside, collecting information through different types of receptors. It is sensitive to pain, temperature changes, and touch, from a gentle caress to aggression. It is an organ with an important social and relational function, as it determines to a significant extent our physical appearance and therefore acts as a "letter of introduction" to the environment.

Today's society exposes our bodies, including our skin, to the scrutiny and judgment, often severe, of others. We can modify our skin intentionally (piercing, tattoos...) often with the intention of expressing or claiming part of our convictions, ideals, etc.but the skin can also be affected or modified by different pathologies. In this context, skin modifications of pathological origin express negative attributes and emotions and this has an important impact on patients affecting various spheres of their QoL. Some chronic inflammatory skin diseases with a high incidence in general population, such as psoriasis, atopic dermatitis, or hidradenitis suppurativa, may have a significant impact on the QoL [1], affecting social, psychological, and sexual aspects.

I. Fuertes (✉)
Dermatology and Venereology Unit, Clinical Institute of Medicine and Dermatology, Hospital Clínic de Barcelona, Barcelona, Spain

Clinical Sexology Working Group, Hospital Clinic de Barcelona, Barcelona, Spain
e-mail: ifuertes@clinic.cat

J. Riera
Dermatology and Venereology Unit, Clinical Institute of Medicine and Dermatology, Barcelona, Spain
e-mail: jriera@clinic.cat

© The Author(s), under exclusive license to Springer Nature Switzerland AG 2024
C. Castelo-Branco, S. Anglès Acedo (eds.), *Medical Disorders and Sexual Health*, Trends in Andrology and Sexual Medicine,
https://doi.org/10.1007/978-3-031-55080-5_33

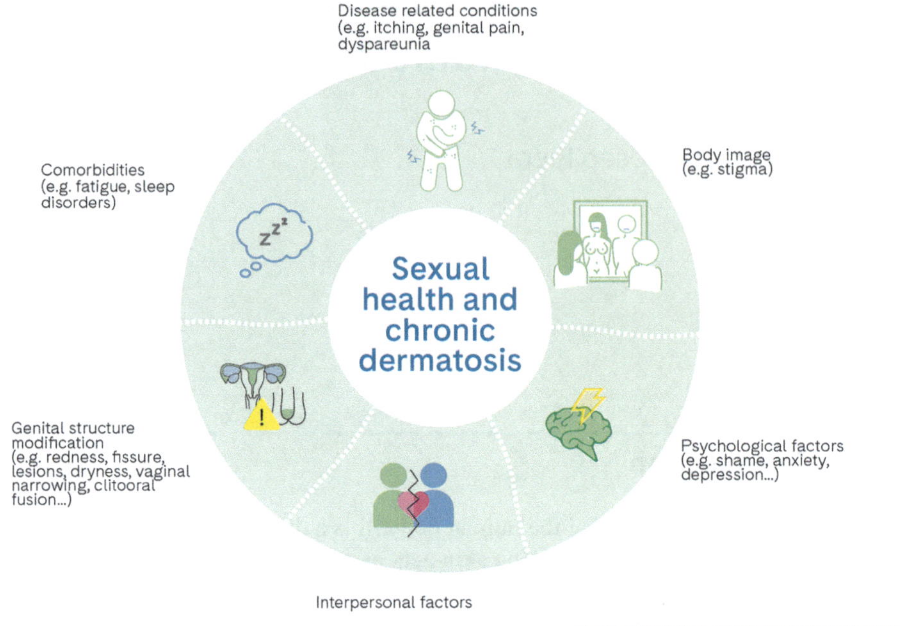

Fig. 1 Different factors related to the impact of chronic dermatoses on sexual function

Presenting skin lesions in visible areas and even in areas that are usually covered has been associated with feelings of stigmatization, isolation, low self-esteem, and alexithymia [2, 3]. This whole spectrum of negative emotions will indeed have an effect on the patient's sexual sphere.

Furthermore, the presence of lesions or changes in the skin and mucous membranes, especially when located in the genital or perianal area, can have a direct impact on sexual relations. Thus, some patients may present pain, itching, or impossibility for some practices due to these lesions, which will directly affect their sexual health (Fig. 1).

The aim of this chapter is to compile the available evidence on the impact that the main chronic dermatoses have on the sexual health of patients.

2 Hidradenitis Suppurativa and Sexual Health

Hidradenitis Suppurativa (HS) is a chronic, relapsing, and debilitating inflammatory disease with a high prevalence (estimated between 0.5 and 4%) in western countries [4]. It specifically affects the hair follicle complex, especially in areas with apocrine sweat glands such as the genitals, perianal area, groin, and armpits. It usually debuts in the second and third decades of life, presenting the highest incidence between 20 and 50 years of age. HS lesions cause pain due to the associated inflammation, which can be intense and difficult to manage. Furthermore, these skin lesions often secrete foul-smelling material that conditions for many patients the way they dress, avoiding numerous outfits that either by their shape, color, or texture can make a spot of purulent material more evident. In addition, HS lesions can became fibrotic and develop into chronic hypertrophic scars or fistulous tracts that respond poorly to medical treatment (in some cases requiring aggressive surgical treatment) and can lead to functional impairment in addition to significant cosmetic deterioration.

Patients with HS often experience a sense of shame and a high level of distress in relation to the active lesions and scars they present. Psychological disorders, such as substance abuse, depression, anxiety, sleep disorders, or impaired body image perception are common comorbidities [5–7] that typically lead to reclusion and alienation from society. On the other hand, pain, fever, and fatigue can prevent individuals with HS from performing even the most common daily tasks and, of course, they may have a negative effect on patients' work capacity and their leisure and socialization activities.

In fact, HS has been defined by several studies as the skin dermatosis that causes the greatest impairment in the QoL [7–9] compared to other chronic skin dermatoses. The impact of HS is particularly relevant in the sexual sphere [9–11].

The site of HS lesions, the associated signs and symptoms, as well as the age of onset and increased activity of this disease lead to an impairment of the sexual function (SF) in the majority of patients. In this regard, several studies have confirmed the impact of HS on sexuality [12–14] in both men and women.

In 2016, in a cross-sectional study about the impact on sexual health of various skin pathologies, 3485 patients from 13 European countries were assessed [11]. The authors used question number 9 of the Dermatology Life Quality Index (DLQI) survey as a basis for assessing sexual health (DLQI question 9: During the last 7 days, have your skin problems interfered with your sex life?). They observed that the greatest deterioration in patients' sexual health was associated with hidradenitis suppurativa. The impact on SF/health was associated with the presence of depression, anxiety, and suicidal ideation. Overall, the impairment of sexual health was more frequent in younger patients and it was positively correlated with clinical severity and pruritus.

In 2012, Kurek et al. [12] conducted a study on the impact of HS on patients' sexuality using a self-administered questionnaire to 44 patients volunteers and 41 controls including the following data: Female Sexual Function Index (FSFI), the International Index of Erectile Function (IIEF), and the Frankfurt Sexuality Self-Concept Scale. They observed that patients with HS had greater sexual dysfunction than their age-, sex-, and body mass index-matched controls. In particular, women reported significantly greater sexual distress and lower QoL than men at equal disease severity which could be due to the difference in age of onset (younger in women), breast affectation, or even socio-cultural reasons regarding impact of disfigurement in women.

Janse et al. [13] in a multicenter, survey-based cross-sectional study involving 300 patients with HS found a prevalence of sexual dysfunction of 62% in women and 52% in men with this skin condition. This group concludes that late age of onset and disease activity are risk factors for sexual dysfunction in women with HS. They also found a correlation between sexual dysfunction and poor QoL in women but not in men.

Furthermore, a cross-sectional observational study of 50 patients with HS and 50 healthy volunteers concluded that male patients with HS experienced greater sexual dysfunction and lower sexual QoL of life, while women with HS had greater sexual distress, compared to the control groups [8]. Authors observed an impact of sexual dysfunction on QoL in both males and females with HS regardless of the presence of genital lesions.

A recent cross-sectional study [15]using an online questionnaire circulated among 393 HS patients found that 51% of women presented sexual dysfunction and 60% of men had erectile dysfunction. The data reflect that, in women, educational level, disease activity, pain, odor, and absence of a stable partner were factors associated with sexual dysfunction while for men, the main factors associated with erectile dysfunction were age, presence of active lesions in the genital area, and number of areas with active lesions. In this study, authors used two different tools in order to assess sexual dysfunction: i) the Female Sexual Function Index-6 (FSFI-6), a validated questionnaire that explores the 6 domains of FSFI (desire, excitation, lubrication, orgasm, global satisfaction, and pain) and ii) the International Index of Erectile Function-5 (IIEF-5), a validated questionnaire with 5 questions about erectile function.

A recent systematic review [14] showed that both females and males with HS have worsening SF compared to controls of the same sex. According to this meta-analysis, the overall impairment is greater in women with HS despite the fact that this disease may more directly affect sexual functioning in men.

In light of all these data, it seems evident to claim the need to specifically address the problems affecting SF in patients with HS and to treat them adequately and early.

3   Psoriasis and Sexual Health

Psoriasis is an immune-mediated inflammatory skin disease, affecting between 2 and 3% of worldwide population [1]. Typical plaque psoriasis, which is the most frequent presentation of psoriasis, consists of red and scale plaques located on extensor extremities such as knees and elbows. However, there are other forms such as intertriginous or inverted, which affects folds such as armpits, under breast. Psoriasis is considered moderate or severe (up to 1/3 of cases) when more than 10% of body surface area is compromised, is accompanied by psoriatic arthritis, and/or affects one or more of the considered special locations (genital, palmoplantar, face, and scalp) [2]. Psoriasis may have a high impact on quality of life, which correlates with the severity of the disease. Psoriasis itself has been linked to a higher risk of anxiety and depression. The impact of psoriasis on sexual health is linked to several factors, such as lack of self-esteem, perception of body image, stigmatization, the impact of psoriatic lesions in terms of itch, scaling, fissures, anxiety, and depression among others.

In a systematic review, 12–42% patients were found to have genital psoriasis on the day of the examination. The prevalence of genital psoriasis through past history was 33–63% of patients [3].

Genital psoriasis is more frequent in patients with younger age of onset, male sex, disease severity, and other special locations involvement (scalp, nail, and inframammary in women) [4]. Symptoms of genital psoriasis may include redness, itching, and soreness in the affected areas [2]. In contrast to plaque psoriasis, it may not have scaling. Moreover, genital psoriasis may present greater pruritus and fissure formation in folds. In an observational study which included 354 male and female patients with genital psoriasis, 39% of them reported pain, 42% dyspareunia, 32% a worsening of their genital psoriasis after sexual intercourse, and 43% a decreased frequency of sexual intercourse [4]. In fact, the presence of genital psoriasis compared to those psoriasis patients without genital involvement portended a poorer prognosis in sexual function, sexual frequency, and fear of sexual relations. Moreover, patient with current genital involvement had a more severe impairment of Quality of Life measured by DLQI (Dermatology Life Quality Index score) and Center for Epidemiological Studies Depression Scale [4].

In women with psoriasis, several studies have been conducted to evaluate the prevalence of sexual dysfunction. Using the Female Sexual Function Index questionnaire (FSFI), the prevalence of female sexual dysfunction was estimated to be 48.7% [5]. Of all FSFI domains, which include desire, arousal, lubrication, orgasm, satisfaction, and pain, all are affected except for lubrication and pain [6]. As a consequence, it has been shown by González-Cantero et al. that the fertility age-standardized rate among women of childbearing age with moderate-to-severe psoriasis was lower than half the fertility rate for women of the same age in the Spanish population [7].

In the case of men, rejection because of the presence of psoriasis is experienced by 44.7% patients [8]. Male erectile dysfunction is frequently caused by pelvic atherosclerosis and is considered a marker for future cardiovascular events. Patients with psoriasis also have a higher risk of developing major cardiovascular events, as well as metabolic syndrome [5 > 7]. Using the validated five-item version of the International Index of Erectile Function (IIEF-5), Boulding and colleagues carried out a cross-sectional study in which patients with psoriasis had an age-adjusted odds ratio of 2.0 of suffering erectile dysfunction [6 > 8]. As expected, increasing age and hypertension were risk factors for erectile dysfunction.

Treatment options for genital psoriasis include topical and systemic medications. Topical corticosteroids and calcineurin inhibitors are commonly used as first-line therapies for genital psoriasis. However, in patients with severe disease, this may not be enough to achieve disease control. Biologic agents, such as TNF-α inhibitors, IL-23 inhibitors, and IL-17 inhibitors, have also been shown to be effective in treating psoriasis, including genital psoriasis. Disease control can minimize and even restore sexual dysfunction and quality of life [9]. For example, treatment with ustekinumab in patients with moderate-severe showed a reduction in sexual dysfunction from 22.4% to 2.7% [10]. In the specific case of genital psoriasis, ixekizumab proved in a randomized controlled trial to control genital psoriasis after 12 weeks of treatment in 73% of patients compared to 3% in the placebo group.

4   Atopic Dermatitis and Sexual Health

Atopic dermatitis (AD) is a chronic dermatosis with a very high prevalence (up to 10% of the world population if we consider pediatric patients and around 1–5% in the adult population) affecting all ages. The main manifestations of this chronic dermatosis are dryness, itching, and the presence of eczematous lesions (erythema, vesicles, exudate, crusts, etc.).

Numerous studies agree that AD has a great physical and psychological impact on patients (and often on their families as well). This impact has been observed to be related to the severity of the disease [7]. Clinical pruritus, itching, and visible lesions limit activities of daily living in most patients, especially those with more severe or worse controlled forms. Actually, up to 17% of patients with AD report any grade of dissatisfaction with their life [16].

According to the literature, psychiatric and psychosocial processes are present in more than 30% of AD patients [17]. They also present an increased risk of anxiety, depression, suicidal ideation, as well as sleep disturbances [18].

Regarding the evidence of the impact of this cutaneous disease on sexual life, we have some studies and a recent systematic review.

A cross-sectional study [19] on 266 patients with atopic dermatitis in which patients and their partners were assessed by a series of questionnaires asking about their general health and QoL [Short Form 12, Epworth, DLQI] and completed an idiosyncratic measure asking about their sexual functioning. A decrease in sexual desire due to AD was noted in 57.5% of patients. The QoL of partners did not appear to be particularly impaired, but 36.5% reported that the appearance of eczema had an impact on their sex life.

The same group published [20] recently a multicentre prospective transversal study in patients with AD including 1024 patients. Severity of AD, sites involved, and treatment type was found to negatively impact the sexual desire of patients and their partners. In addition, the involvement of the genital and visible areas was associated with a higher burden and more significant alterations in QoL.

A recent systematic review achieved data from 8088 patients with AD from five articles. Tools used to assess SD were variable between these studies, most of them including DLQI. Prevalence of SD ranged from 6.7% to 57.9%. In one study (Sampogna et al), the highest prevalence of SD was observed between 40 and 59 years of age. These authors also concluded that sexual impairment was related to young age, high severity of AD, anxiety, and depression. AD patients presented higher prevalence of SD compared to healthy subjects, though impact on sexual health seems to be lower compared to other chronic pathologies such as psoriasis. One of the studies from this review only refer to male population. Authors assess erectile dysfunction in patients with AD and report a significant association between ED and prior diagnosis of AD.

In conclusión, AD, even though its influence may be lower than other chronic dermatosis as psoriasis or HS, seems to have its own impact on SD of patients independently of other frequently associated pathologies (anxiety, depression...). More studies in this field are needed that assess sexual health in patients with AD in both sexes and in regard to severity of AD and comorbidities.

5   Lichen Sclerosus and Sexual Health

Lichen sclerosus (LS) is a chronic inflammatory dermatosis of autoimmune origin that predominantly affects the vulva and vagina.

Patients with LS may present with burning and itching in the affected areas related to skin inflammation as well as the eventual presence of erosions and fissures. Furthermore, the anatomical changes due to chronic inflammation and consequent fibrosis that leads to a loss of the labia minora, clitoral fusion, and a progressive narrowing of the vaginal introitus are some of the manifestations that may have the greatest impact on QoL.

In addition, LS has an estimated risk of progression to squamous cell carcinoma of about 2% [21].

The incidence of LS has increased during recent years. It is higher in perimenopausal and postmenopausal women but it can also occur in prepuberal girls and young women. Different studies have shown incidences of 14.6–22/100000 woman years [22, 23].

No definitive treatment for LS is currently available. Topical corticosteroids are the first line of management, and their chronic use helps to control discomfort, structural changes and even reduce the risk of malignancy. However, diagnostic delay and inherent failures of adherence to topical treatments often represent a management challenge.

LS is therefore associated with several factors that impact the QoL and more specifically on the sexual health of women who suffer from it.

Vulvar discomfort in the form of itching and pain may be increased when having sexual contact. Moreover, dissatisfaction with the cosmetic appearance of the genitalia as well as physical architectural problems of the vulva can definitely compromise some aspects of the sexual function of patients.

Several studies and a recent systematic review [24] on the impact of LS on patients' sexuality have provided valuable information on this topic that, on the whole, points to a significant and prevalent impact of LS on the sexual health of patients.

Dalziel et al., published in 1995 [25] a study based on data collected prospectively through an anonymous survey at a vulvar dermatosis clinic in England. Based on 45 women's responses, the authors concluded that the majority of women, regardless of age, associated LS with a detrimental effect on sexual function, with problems such as dyspareunia, apareunia, and difficulty reaching orgasm.

More recently, other studies have confirmed this connection between LS and sexual dysfunction.

In a retrospective study involving 222 patients with vulvar lichen sclerosus [26], 83% of the participants complained of vulvar itching and pain, which most of them considered severe and of at least 1 year's duration. Of all, 22% of patients presented an impact on sexual health such as dyspareunia and apareunia.

Yang et al presented in 2018 a retrospective study [27] on 129 Chinese women diagnosed with LS according to the 2015 Guidelines on LS. Based on their data, pruritus was the most frequent symptom presented in up to 94% of patients. In addition, one-third of the patients reported vulvar pain and dryness. These signs and symptoms conditioned in up to 55% of the cases the presence of dyspareunia and impaired sexual function.

A pilot study [17] conducted in Spain on 20 women with LS, 65% of whom were postmenopausal, used the FSFI in order to collect information on the sexual function of the patients. Interestingly, 30% of the participants scored the lowest possible score (2) on the FSFI and up to 70% of them scored below 26 (the cut-off point considered for female sexual dysfunction).

In addition, a retrospective study [28] of 177 patients with LS showed that, among patients who reported sexual activity, 56.7% complained of dyspareunia, which was more frequent and severe among patients who had not previously been treated with topical steroids and correlated with higher scores of vulvar pruritus and burning. The authors also concluded that pruritus proved to be the most difficult symptom to control, early treatment was associated with an improvement in the incidence and severity of dyspareunia.

A Danish cross-sectional study [29] on 158 participants with LS who were assessed by using three questionaries: FSFI, DLQI, and WHO Well-Being Index-5 concluded that women with LS presented a low score on all FSFI scales, with a mean score of 13.83. Subgroup assessment scored for desire 2.32, arousal 2.23, lubrication 2.39, orgasm 2.28, satisfaction 3.02, and pain 1.59. Furthermore, DLQI results revealed a mean score of 7.88, showing an impact on women's daily lives. Finally, the scores obtained on WHO-5 (mean score 56.66), suggested that 40% of these patients presented signs of depression.

The same group of authors has published the results of the effect on QoL and sexuality of a psychosexual intervention performed on these patients. This randomized controlled study [30] included 158 women with newly diagnosed LS who were randomized in a 1:1 ratio to topical treatment with steroids and emollients or to an intervention group receiving in addition up to 8 individual consultations with a sexual counseling specialist. Women completed the FSFI, the DLQI, and the WHO Well-Being Index-5 at the beginning of the study and after 6 months. Authors observed significant effect of psychosexual counseling on sexuality, QoL, and well-being. However, they also pointed out that most of the participants scored less than 26.55 on the FSFI, suggesting that they still have a need for sexual treatment.

Finally, a meta-analysis published in 2022 [24] on LS and SD including 23 studies with 486 cumulative patients concludes that the prevalence of sexual dysfunction among LS patients is very high (approximately 59%). Patients' scores on the FSFI were lower than those of healthy controls while they were higher on the FSDS. This indicates that LS is associated with lower sexual function and higher sexual distress. QoL was also deteriorated in SL patients mainly because of SD. As for the possibility of improvement with treatment, it was observed that patients with vulvar adhesions improved their sexual function after surgery.

In conclusion, there is ample evidence associating SD with LS. This association is justified by several factors including pain, pruritus, alteration of the genital structure, and psycho-emotional impact due to the possibility of oncologic sequelae. It is therefore crucial that health care providers caring for patients with LS pay attention to this important aspect of their lives.

6 Conclusion

As we show in this chapter, there is now substantial evidence that several highly prevalent cutaneous dermatoses can have a significant impact on the sexual quality and function of the patients who present with them and their sexual partners.

We consider it highly important that the healthcare personnel who treat these patients keep their attention on this point. This means including the assessment of the impact that the disease has on the sexual function of our patients and having tools and resources to offer them, keeping in mind that they may often require multidisciplinary management to improve or preserve their sexual function.

References

1. Augustin M, et al. Unveiling the true costs and societal impacts of moderate-to-severe atopic dermatitis in Europe. J Eur Acad Dermatol Venereol. 2022;36(Suppl 7):3–16.
2. Hrehorów E, Salomon J, Matusiak L, Reich A, Szepietowski JC. Patients with psoriasis feel stigmatized. Acta Derm Venereol. 2012;92:67–72.
3. Schmid-Ott G, et al. Significance of the stigmatization experience of psoriasis patients: a 1-year follow-up of the illness and its psychosocial consequences in men and women. Acta Derm Venereol. 2005;85:27–32.
4. Ingram JR, et al. Population-based clinical practice research datalink study using algorithm modelling to identify the true burden of hidradenitis suppurativa. Br J Dermatol. 2018;178:917–24.
5. Machado MO, et al. Depression and anxiety in adults with hidradenitis suppurativa: a systematic review and meta-analysis. JAMA Dermatol. 2019;155:939–45.
6. Schneider-Burrus S, et al. Association of hidradenitis suppurativa with body image. JAMA Dermatol. 2018;154:447–51.
7. Onderdijk AJ, et al. Depression in patients with hidradenitis suppurativa. J Eur Acad Dermatol Venereol. 2013;27:473–8.
8. Alavi A, Farzanfar D, Rogalska T, Lowes MA, Chavoshi S. Quality of life and sexual health in patients with hidradenitis suppurativa. Int J Women's Dermatol. 2018;4:74–9.
9. Wolkenstein P, Loundou A, Barrau K, Auquier P, Revuz J. Quality of life impairment in hidradenitis suppurativa: a study of 61 cases. J Am Acad Dermatol. 2007;56:621–3.
10. Von Der Werth JM, Jemec GBE. Morbidity in patients with hidradenitis suppurativa. Br J Dermatol. 2001;144:809–13.
11. Sampogna F, et al. Impairment of sexual life in 3,485 dermatological outpatients from a multicentre study in 13 European countries. Acta Derm Venereol. 2017;97:478–82.
12. Kurek A, et al. Profound disturbances of sexual health in patients with acne inversa. J Am Acad Dermatol. 2012;67:422.
13. Janse IC, et al. Sexual health and quality of life are impaired in hidradenitis suppurativa: a multicentre cross-sectional study. Br J Dermatol. 2017;176:1042–7.
14. Varney P, et al. A systematic review and meta-analysis of sexual dysfunction in patients with hidradenitis suppurativa. Int J Dermatol. 2022;62(6):737–46. https://doi.org/10.1111/IJD.16328.
15. Cuenca-Barrales C, Molina-Leyva A. Risk factors of sexual dysfunction in patients with hidradenitis suppurativa: a cross-sectional study. Dermatology. 2020;236:37–45.
16. Silverberg JI, et al. Patient burden and quality of life in atopic dermatitis in US adults: a population-based cross-sectional study. Ann Allergy Asthma Immunol. 2018;121:340–7.
17. Gutierrez-Ontalvilla P, et al. The female sexual function index to assess patients with moderate to severe vulvar lichen sclerosus. Eur J Dermatol. 2019;29:430–1.

18. Misery L, Seneschal J, Reguiai Z, Merhand S, Héas S, Huet F, Taïeb C, Ezzedine K. Patient Burden is Associated with Alterations in Quality of Life in Adult Patients with Atopic Dermatitis: Results from the ECLA Study. Acta Derm Venereol. 2018;98(7):713–4. https://doi.org/10.2340/00015555-2940. PMID: 29648674.

19. Misery L, et al. Atopic dermatitis: impact on the quality of life of patients and their partners. Dermatology. 2007;215:123–9.

20. Misery L, et al. The impact of atopic dermatitis on sexual health. J Eur Acad Dermatol Venereol. 2019;33:428–32.

21. Vieira-Baptista P, et al. Risk of development of vulvar cancer in women with lichen sclerosus or lichen planus: a systematic review. J Low Genit Tract Dis. 2022;26:250–7.

22. Bleeker MCG, Visser PJ, Overbeek LIH, Van Beurden M, Berkhof J. Lichen sclerosus: incidence and risk of vulvar squamous cell carcinoma. Cancer Epidemiol Biomarkers Prev. 2016;25:1224–30.

23. Halonen P, Jakobsson M, Heikinheimo O, Gissler M, Pukkala E. Incidence of lichen sclerosus and subsequent causes of death: a nationwide Finnish register study. BJOG. 2020;127:814–9.

24. Pope R, et al. Lichen Sclerosus and sexual dysfunction: a systematic review and meta-analysis. J Sex Med. 2022;19:1616–24.

25. Dalziel KL. Effect of lichen sclerosus on sexual function and parturition. J Reprod Med. 1995;40(5):351–4.

26. Simpkin S, Oakley A. Clinical review of 202 patients with vulval lichen sclerosus: A possible association with psoriasis. Australas J Dermatol. 2007;48(1):28–31. https://doi.org/10.1111/j.1440-0960.2007.00322.x. PMID: 17222298.

27. Yang M, Wen W, Chang J. Vulvar lichen sclerosus: a single-center retrospective study in China. J Dermatol. 2018;45:1101–4.

28. Corazza M, Virgili A, Minghetti S, Borghi A. Dyspareunia in vulvar lichen sclerosus: an overview of a distressing symptom. G Ital Dermatol Venereol. 2020;155:299–305.

29. Vittrup G, et al. Quality of life and sexuality in women with lichen sclerosus: a cross-sectional study. Clin Exp Dermatol. 2022;47:343–50.

30. Vittrup G, et al. The impact of psychosexual counseling in women with lichen sclerosus: a randomized controlled trial. J Low Genit Tract Dis. 2022;26:258–64.

STI and Sexuality

Pere Fusté and Irene Fuertes

The association between sexual behavior and sexually transmitted infections (STI) can be approached from two assumptions. On the one hand, analyzing how sexual behaviors increase sexually transmitted infections. And secondly, considering how sexually transmitted infections can alter one's own sexual behavior, beyond the prevention measures associated with the treatment of the infection itself.

1 Scope of the Problem

1.1 Introduction

STIs have a deep impact on sexual and reproductive health worldwide through stigmatization, infertility, cancers, and pregnancy complications. In addition, having an STI may increase the risk of transmitting and contracting the human immunodeficiency virus (HIV) in unprotected sexual intercourse.

The website of the World Health Organization (WHO) remarks [1]:

More than 1 million STIs are acquired every day. In 2020, WHO estimated 374 million new infections with 1 of 4 STIs: chlamydia (129 million), gonorrhea (82 million), syphilis (7.1 million), and trichomoniasis (156 million). More than

The original version of the chapter has been revised. A correction to this chapter can be found at
https://doi.org/10.1007/978-3-031-55080-5_36

P. Fusté (✉)
Gynecological Department, Clinical Institute of Gynecology, Obstetrics and Neonatology, Hospital Clinic de Barcelona, Barcelona, Spain
e-mail: pfuste@clinic.cat

I. Fuertes
Dermatology and Venereology Unit, Clinical Institute of Medicine and Dermatology, Hospital Clínic de Barcelona, Barcelona, Spain

Clinical Sexology Working Group, Hospital Clinic de Barcelona, Barcelona, Spain
e-mail: ifuertes@clinic.cat

C. Castelo-Branco, S. Anglès Acedo (eds.), *Medical Disorders and Sexual Health*, Trends in Andrology and Sexual Medicine,
https://doi.org/10.1007/978-3-031-55080-5_34

490 million people were estimated to be living with genital herpes in 2016, and an estimated 300 million women have a human papillomavirus (HPV) infection, the primary cause of cervical cancer in women and anal cancer. An estimated 296 million people are living with chronic hepatitis B globally.

STIs can have serious consequences beyond the immediate impact of the infection itself.

- Ulcerative and suppurative STIs increase the risk of HIV acquisition.
- Mother-to-child transmission of STIs can result in stillbirth, neonatal death, low-birth weight and prematurity, sepsis, neonatal conjunctivitis, and congenital deformities.
- HPV infection causes cervical and other anogenital and head and neck cancers.
- Hepatitis B resulted in an estimated 820,000 deaths in 2019, mostly from cirrhosis and hepatocellular carcinoma.
- STIs such as gonorrhea and chlamydia are major causes of pelvic inflammatory disease and infertility in women.

Though most STI are asymptomatic, when they are symptomatic, they present with vaginal or urethral discharge, genital or perianal ulcers, mucocutaneous lesions in the anogenital area, and lower abdominal pain. It is easy to imagine that the presence of mucocutaneous lesions, pain or discharge in the anogenital area may have an impact on the sexual function of the patient and his or her sexual partners. The most prevalent, curable STIs are *Trichomonas vaginalis*, *Chlamydia* spp., gonorrhea, and syphilis. Both bacterial STIs and trichomoniasis are considered an important public health problem (mainly due to the frequency of asymptomatic cases), which happily have a simple treatment in most cases (with the exception of the antimicrobial resistance problems presented by gonococcus and *Mycoplasma genitalium*).

On the other hand, most viral STIs including HIV, genital herpes simplex virus (HSV), viral hepatitis B (VHB), and HPV lack or have limited treatment options. Vaccines are available for VHB to prevent this infection that can lead to liver cancer and for HPV to prevent cervical cancer. Actually, HPV vaccines have decreased the incidence of HPV-related lesions in populations with high rates of vaccination coverage [2]. However, HIV and HSV are lifelong infections for which primary prevention is not available.

1.2 A Growing Problem

Though there are differences according to the infection considered, geographical area, degree of development, age, gender, sexual risk behaviors and other variables [3–8], and high incidence and prevalence rates of have been widely documented worldwide, both in developed and developing countries during the last decades. The increase is more evident among viral infections.

2   Risk Groups

2.1   Adolescence

Adolescence should be considered as a special group at risk not only for STIs but also for sexual abuse and exploitation and therefore should be treated with special care.

The burden of STIs in adolescent and young people in the United States is high. In 2018, almost half of incident STIs occurred in persons aged 15– 24. This year, there were an estimated 67.6 (Q1, 66.6; Q3, 68.7) million prevalent and 26.2 (Q1, 24.0; Q3, 28.7) million incident STIs in the United States. Chlamydia, trichomoniasis, genital herpes, and HPV composed 97.6% of all prevalent and 93.1% of all incident STIs. Persons aged 15–24 years composed 18.6% (12.6 million) of all prevalent infections; however, they composed 45.5% (11.9 million) of all incident infections. Focusing STI prevention efforts on the 15- to 24-year-old population may be key to lowering the STI burden [9].

Adolescents are growing up in a highly sexualized society exposed to content that is frequently not validated, especially on the Internet. Different factors may play a role in the increased incidence of STIs among these groups of population. Adolescents and young adults have been related to some risky sexual behavior as having multiple or simultaneous partners, greater substance abuse, less use of protective measures, either due to lack of information or in relation to their socioeconomic status and for multiple reasons, greater difficulty in accessing quality health care.

A key aspect regarding the management of these patients, especially when it comes to STIs, is confidentiality. Adolescents and young adults have the right to participate in their health care and to receive information appropriate to their age, maturity, and understanding.

Some interesting strategies for the control of STIs in young people and adolescents should be directed to:

- Empowering them through education on safe and pleasurable sex, sexual risk behaviors, STIs, prevention.
- Facilitate the access of adolescents and young people to sexual health services.
- Ensure confidentiality in patient care.

2.2   Other High-Risk Groups

Other groups at risk of acquiring STIs are sex workers and their clients, people who use recreational drugs during sex (chemsex users), men who have sex with men (MSM) who engage in risky sexual practices, people from countries with a higher prevalence of STIs, and adolescents who engage in risky sexual practices. Each of these groups requires specific actions on the part of health care providers. Therefore, information on STI prevention, STI screening and treatment, epidemiological surveillance, and preventive measures should be tailored to the characteristics of each group. It is worth clarifying that it is a person's sexual practices, not their membership of a group, that determine their individual risk of STIs.

3 Prevention

3.1 Specific Preventive Measures

3.1.1 Risk Groups

As a result of the increase in the incidence of HIV and STIs in worldwide risk groups, actions aimed at reducing this risk are essential. These measures will depend on the risk groups involved. Among these measures, we can list the use of physical protection barriers (condoms), lower-risk sexual practices, rapid diagnostic tests, post-exposure treatments, a test of cure, partner notification, and structured measures for education and information on STIs. The effectiveness of each of these measures is not fully established [4, 10–16].

A recent assay carried out among gay and bisexual men (GBM) to provide initial evidence of efficacy for a 10-session integrated cognitive-behavioral therapy for social anxiety, substance use management in sexual situations, and HIV sexual risk reduction for HIV-negative GBM. Data of this open trial showed a 50% reduction in engagement in HIV/STI sexual risk behavior at 6-month follow-up. A large uncontrolled treatment effect was also observed in social anxiety disorder and problematic alcohol use. These preliminary findings suggest that integrated cognitive-behavioral therapy may offer an efficient way of concurrently reducing social anxiety, problematic alcohol use, and the risky sexual behaviors as CAS (condomless anal sex) among HIV-negative GBM [17].

3.1.2 Partner Notification

Partner notification (PN) is an essential element of STI prevention and control programs. The rate of use of public health services that facilitate PN may be affected by variables such as the degree of anxiety, socioeconomic status, substance abuse, HIV infection, sexual gender, or type of sexual practice, among others. Unfortunately, the efficacy of PN is suboptimal. In this regard, efforts should be increased. New tools such as the internet and social networks can be promising [12, 18–22].

3.1.3 Condom Use

The use of condoms is one of the most encouraging prevention measures. However, there are difficulties with its use in some populations at risk, such as adolescents. Recently, a decrease in the use of condoms has been verified in some surveys [10, 23].

3.1.4 Vaccines

HPV and hepatitis B vaccines have been implemented in health care for years. Others are under investigation, such as vaccines for the herpes virus and HIV.

The efficacy and effectiveness of HPV vaccines are high among young women who were HPV seronegative before vaccination. HPV vaccination has led to a dramatic decline in anogenital warts incidence in populations that have achieved high vaccination rates. Likewise, a decrease in the incidence of HPV-related intraepithelial lesions has been verified. However, the vaccines' effectiveness in reducing the incidence of and mortality rates from HPV-related cancers should be observed in long term [2, 24–27].

3.1.5 Telling Partner About STI

One of the aspects that can affect sexual and affective behavior in couples is how we communicate the infection of an STI to couples.

It's normal to be nervous about telling a partner about STDs. Here are some ideas for handling the conversation [28]:

- Imagine that your roles are reversed.
- It's best to be direct.
- It's best to be honest.
- Let the conversation proceed naturally.
- Don't push your partner to make decision.
- Encourage your partner to ask questions.

One study aimed to investigate psychological functioning, relationship factors, stigma perception, disclosure outcomes, and regret for the disclosure decision in people receiving treatment for anogenital warts, comparing disclosers, and non-disclosers. In terms of individual characteristics, only anxiety was significantly different in disclosers and non-disclosers. Perceptions of stigma and expected outcomes of disclosure were not significantly different in the two groups. Interestingly, partner response was significantly more supportive than disclosers expected and disclosers expressed significantly less regret about their disclosure decision than did non-disclosers [29].

4   Repercussions on Sexual Behavior and Mental Health

Fear or worry about acquiring an STI is associated with an increased risk of decreased quality of life in the emotional-affective-social sphere, and in sexual behavior in particular. The impact of STIs on sexual behavior depends on many factors: generic fear of contracting an STI, being in contact with a partner with an STI, having suffered from an STI, other health conditions (physical and mental), age, reproductive desires, previous knowledge about STIs, habitual use of protection measures, habitual sexual practices, number of partners, etc.

The association between psychological symptoms and sexual risk behaviors highlights the importance of holistic assessment of patients' needs by both general and sexual health clinicians. The AURAH (*Attitudes to and Understanding of Risk of Acquisition of HIV*) study carried out on non-HIV heterosexual men and women population, observed an association between psychological symptoms and sexual risk behaviors among women (not among men) in which direction of causality cannot be inferred [30]. However, we don't currently have much data on how STIs impact mental health. Most of the knowledge about impact of STI on mental health is obtained from STI clinics users. Even though, mental health issues are often difficult to detect and address these clinics [31].

In a study among 938 STI clinic patients, psychological problems were reported by 20.4% of users [32]. Anxiety is one of the most frequent symptoms in patients attending an STI clinic, and it is associated with issues concerning stigma, embarrassment, isolation, and shame. Fear of HIV acquisition and pregnancy and factors related to medical care increase the degree of anxiety. Current research should focus on education and empowering women to prevent STI and mental health problems [17, 33–36].

Men who have sex with men (MSM) constitute a group of risk for STIs, including HIV. In a study among 155 high-risk MSM, psychosocial and addiction-related problems were alarmingly high [37].

Unfortunately, being a "sexual or gender minority" today undeniably implies a series of difficulties in terms of development and social integration that may vary greatly depending on the socio-cultural environment, but is certainly related to the high prevalence of psycho-affective disorders and the high rate of drug use in these population groups. As expected, sexual health is also affected in this context. Some data on mental health problems in at-risk minorities are available. At one publicly funded STI clinic, among 1115 respondents, 65% of whom were sexual minorities, 39% reported a recent need for MHSU-related care, most frequently concerning anxiety (29%), depression (26%), substance use (10%), or suicide ideation (7%). Seventy-two percent of this group had not yet talked to a health care provider about their concern. Common barriers included shame (26%) and inability to afford the service (24%) [33]. Similar problems, including suicidal behavior, have been observed among female sex workers [38].

As mentioned above, one of the greatest challenges in the management of STIs is the control of chronic viral infections. Given that most sexually transmitted bacterial infections are relatively easy to treat, it is reasonable to assume that the greatest burden of problems in the sexual sphere in patients with STIs is attributable to patients with chronic viral STIs.

4.1 HIV

Prior to the introduction of highly active antiretroviral therapy (HAART), sexual dysfunction (SD) was frequent in PLWHIV, and it was attributed to opportunistic infections and debilitating illnesses. Results from an intercohort analysis study among 612 PLWHIV based on a self-administered anonymous 16-item questionnaire showed that 21% of participants reported some degree of SD while 6%

reported "moderate" or severe impairment of their sexuality. Interestingly SD was associated with suboptimal HAART adherence [39]. A cross-sectional, observational study on the frequency of screening positive for SD on self-report measures in a cohort of PLWHIV who have been in treatment with HAART for a significant amount of time has been published. Authors observed that the chance of screening positive for ED was 49.7%, premature ejaculation 16.9%, female SD 27.4%, and hypoactive desire in women 45.1%. Lower testosterone and prolactin levels were associated with ED in heterosexual men; lower levels of estradiol and higher levels of follicle stimulating hormone were associated with female SD and hypoactive desire in female women. Furthermore previous studies have pointed to depression and anxiety, both highly prevalent among PLWHIV, as playing an important role in SD in HIV-infected patients [40].

Despite the enormous progress in the efficacy of HAART, increased occurrence of SD among patients undergoing these treatments has been reported. On the other hand, SD impacts the quality of life and may lead individuals to engage in risky behaviors, such as low adherence to HAART and unprotected sex [41].

In a study on sexual health in men on HAART, [42] a 10% rate of ED was observed in HIV-uninfected patients compared to 25% in patients on HAART, while low libido problems were reported in 2% to 48%, respectively. The prevalence of both problems was 26% in HIV-infected MSM not taking HAART. The authors conclude that decreased libido and ED are more common in HIV-infected men and that HAART is associated with a higher prevalence of low sexual desire and elevated serum estradiol levels. A recent meta-analysis [43] on prevalence of ED in men living with HIV involving 4252 participants reported that all studies showed a significant association between HIV infection and increased prevalence of ED (relative risk = 2.32, 95% confidence interval). Authors observed factors classically associated with ED in the general population have a minor impact on men with HIV while other factors like the own infection and its treatment were the strongest predictors of ED. Furthermore, the increase in patient survival also has increased HIV-related comorbidities. In this regard, hypogonadism is a common endocrinological problem in men living with HIV, and it is also associated with SD, specifically ED and low sexual desire [42, 44]. Chronic androgen supplementation may be indicated in these patients. An Australian study on SD and depression among MSM attending a STI clinic observed that sexual problems in HIV-negative MSM were associated with poorer general health and interpersonal isolation, whereas sexual problems in HIV-infected MSM were associated with the adoption of avoidance strategies to cope with daily stress, risky sexual behaviors, and the use of antidepressants [45].

We have much less evidence on the sexual health problems of HIV-infected women. In this regard, a questionnaire-based cross-sectional survey [46]conducted among women attending the HIV clinic in Nigeria observed that among 370 participants, SD was as high as 89.2%. The overall median Female Sexual Function Index Scoring (FSFI) score was 19.2. Satisfactory health and history of alcohol use were independently associated with female SD.

Regarding the factors that are related to SD in PLWHIV (men and women), a recent systematic review [41]concluded that older age, general physical health, depression, body image, and psychological distress have been reported as the most relevant factors, while different studies have not found evidence of an association between SD and CD4, viral load, HIV symptom severity, HIV disease progression, and time since diagnosis.

4.2   HPV

HPV causes benign lesions in the form of genital warts but is also the cause of some anogenital neoplasms with significant prevalence as cervical, vulvar, or anal cancer.

A recent systematic review focused on SD in women with genital warts including 19 articles [47] showed that the prevalence of sexual health problems in women with condylomas ranged from 41.4% to 82.8%. The problems interfering with the sexual health of patients with condylomata can have a variety of causes as presenting pain during intercourse, fear of transmitting the disease, fear of being judged by others, fear of rejection, sense of guilt, and dissatisfaction with the appearance of the genitalia.

The main affected areas of sexual health according to these studies were sexual desire, arousal, orgasm, sexual pain, lubrication, and sexual satisfaction. Being decreased libido the most prevalent of these problems [48]. The authors highlight significant differences in the results obtained in these studies according to the different cultural and social backgrounds of the participants.

The effect of genital warts on the sexual function of their partners has also been studied [47], and it has been observed that, in contrast to the high percentage of women with genital warts who suffered SD, the sexual function of their partners was not affected in most cases.

Most studies on the subject note that genital warts have a negative impact on the psychosocial sphere of patients, whether they are male or female. However, some studies suggest that this impact is greater in women [49, 50]. In this regard, Piñeros et al [49] reported a 90% decrease in self-esteem levels in women compared to a 62% decrease in men after diagnosis of genital warts. In the same way, these authors observed that genital warts have a negative effect on sex life in 77% of women compared to 44% of men.

A cross-sectional study [51]on 105 men with genital warts in Iran reported that SD was present in 35.2% of all participants. Data were collected using International Index of Erectile Function (IIEF) and Sexual Quality of Life-Men (SQOL-M). The highest disorder rate was related to ED and the lowest was related to the desire domain. The main score for SQOL-M was 38.36.

A hospital-based survey [50] conducted China in 2008 on patients who had a recent diagnosis of genital warts revealed these patients experienced heavier psychosocial burdens than general population does. "Self Image" and "sexual impact" were the two domains that affected patients the most. Authors also observed that females experienced significant heavier burdens than males affecting specifically the domain of "Worries and Concerns" while males presented higher psychosocial burdens in the domains of "Sexual Impact" and "Interactions with Doctors."

HPV virus causes genital warts but also cancer. In most resourceful countries, women are screened for cervical cancer prevention, this screening test increasingly includes, in addition to cytology, a cervical HPV test. Being aware of having high-risk HPV in the cervix can have an impact on patients' quality of life and sexual function. A systematic review on psychosexual impact of testing positive for high-risk cervical HPV that included 25 studies concluded that receiving an abnormal cervical cytology result can have a negative impact on sexual health, specifically affecting frequency of sex, interest in sex, and satisfaction with sex [52, 53].

Woman may feel a high level of stress. When the test result is HPV positive, she may feel fear, shame, guilt, and other feelings. These emotions can have an impact on whether the woman adheres to the referral for diagnostic and treatment services. Testing positive for HPV has been associated with a range of negative emotional consequences including distress, anxiety, fear, anger, and feelings of self-blame and can impact adversely on a woman's sexual relationships. A review on the possible impact of the introduction of primary HPV screening protocols in organized screening programs highlighted that communication of HPV positivity may increase anxiety and suggested that this effect may vary socio-economically [54].

The qualitative literature suggested that psychosexual concerns are raised by some women who test HPV+ and that these concerns cover a broad range of aspects relating to their current and past relationships, both interpersonal and sexual. One review found that most studies reported changes in women's sexual relationships following a HPV diagnosis and the other [55] found no conclusive evidence regarding the psychosexual consequences of an HPV diagnosis.

4.3 HSV

Genital herpes is a prevalent, chronic, recurrent, ulcerative STI. When primoinfection is symptomatic, it may be severe but, fortunately, recurrences are usually short-lasting and mild.

Several studies have described significant psychosexual morbidity associated with genital herpes infection, especially in patients with frequent and severe recurrent episodes.

Indeed, some case reports suggest that genital herpes-associated psychosexual morbidity may be more severe and long-lasting than that associated with other STIs and that these problems may act, on their own, as a trigger for new recurrences. However, this association has not been demonstrated in prospective studies.

Patients with genital herpes are advised not to have sex when they have symptoms of recurrence in order to protect their partners. In addition, some people may experience pain of neuropathic origin that can affect the anogenital area and may persist beyond outbreaks of virus activity. These factors can of course have an impact on the sexual health of genital herpes patients.

Furthermore, individuals with recurrent genital herpes may experience a range of emotional responses to the infection, including depression, anguish, distress, anger, reduction of self-esteem and confidence, and hostility toward the person they believe was the source of infection.

Suppressive treatment with antiviral drugs in long regimens is effective in reducing or eliminating recurrences of genital herpes [56], and several studies point to a positive effect of the use of suppressive treatment on psychosexual morbidity in these patients [57].

5   STIs Clinics Attendance and Global Health Services

Health services specifically designed to provide comprehensive care to patients with STIs should be promoted. In many settings, STI services are often neglected and underfunded.

In 2016, WHO launched the Global Health Sector Strategy on STIs, 2016–2021 (GHSS) to provide guidance and benchmarks for country achievement by 2020 and four global targets for achievement by 2030. The results of a recent global survey show the challenge of implementing this project. In this regard, for example, only 59% (65/110) of countries reported the inclusion of the HPV vaccine for young women in the national immunization schedule. Furthermore, stockouts of STI medicines, primarily benzathine penicillin, were reported by 34% (37/110) of countries in the previous 4 years [58].

STI patient care clinics must be staffed by qualified personnel who are skilled in dealing with users, trust, intimacy, and affection must prevail. In addition, they must have rapid diagnostic tests, be able to administer treatment on site and carry out follow-up of patients and contacts.

For some at-risk groups, such as adolescents, STI clinics can be the first place of contact with health services, so they are a great opportunity to inform them about general aspects of preventive health. In addition, these centers should promote informative actions for patients and the community.

Comprehensive sexual health care for patients should include specific interventions to assess and improve sexuality from a biopsychosocial and inclusive point of view, promoting safe and pleasurable sexuality, considering the diversity of sexual identities, orientations, and behaviors of the people who come to the consultation, without stigmatizing or prejudging.

References

1. WHO.		https://www.who.int/health-topics/sexually-transmitted-infections#tab=tab_1. Accessed 13 Jan 2023.
2. Kamolratanakul S, Pitisuttithum P. Human papillomavirus vaccine efficacy and effectiveness against cancer. Vaccine. 2021;9(12):1413. https://doi.org/10.3390/VACCINES9121413.
3. Rowley J, Vander HS, Korenromp E, et al. Chlamydia, gonorrhoea, trichomoniasis and syphilis: global prevalence and incidence estimates, 2016. Bull World Health Organ. 2019;97(8):548. https://doi.org/10.2471/BLT.18.228486.

4. Tsuboi M, Evans J, Davies EP, et al. Prevalence of syphilis among men who have sex with men: a global systematic review and meta-analysis from 2000–20. Lancet Glob Heal. 2021;9(8):e1110–8. https://doi.org/10.1016/S2214-109X(21)00221-7.

5. James C, Harfouche M, Welton NJ, et al. Herpes simplex virus: global infection prevalence and incidence estimates, 2016. Bull World Health Organ. 2020;98(5):315. https://doi.org/10.2471/BLT.19.237149.

6. Kissinger PJ, Gaydos CA, Seña AC, et al. Diagnosis and management of trichomonas vaginalis: summary of evidence reviewed for the 2021 centers for disease control and prevention sexually transmitted infections treatment guidelines. Clin Infect Dis. 2022;74(Supplement_2):S152–61. https://doi.org/10.1093/cid/ciac030.

7. Ngangro NN, Viriot D, Fournet N, et al. Bacterial sexually transmitted infections in France: recent trends and characteristics in 2015. Bull Epidemiol Hebd. 2016;2016(41-42):738–44.

8. Shaw SY, Elliott LJ, Nowicki DL, et al. Comparing the ecological niches of chlamydial and gonococcal infections in Winnipeg, Canada: 2007–2016. Sex Transm Dis. 2021;48(11):837–43. https://doi.org/10.1097/OLQ.0000000000001446.

9. Kreisel KM, Spicknall IH, Gargano JW, et al. Sexually transmitted infections among US women and men: prevalence and incidence estimates, 2018. Sex Transm Dis. 2021;48(4):208–14. https://doi.org/10.1097/OLQ.0000000000001355.

10. Beksinska M, Wong R, Smit J. Male and female condoms: their key role in pregnancy and STI/HIV prevention. Best Pract Res Clin Obstet Gynaecol. 2020;66:55–67. https://doi.org/10.1016/j.bpobgyn.2019.12.001.

11. Berg R. The effectiveness of behavioural and psychosocial HIV/STI prevention interventions for MSM in Europe: a systematic review. Euro Surveill. 2009;14(48):19430. https://doi.org/10.2807/ese.14.48.19430-en.

12. Brookmeyer KA, Hogben M, Kinsey J. The role of behavioral counseling in STD prevention program settings. Sex Transm Dis. 2016;43(0 0 1):S102. https://doi.org/10.1097/OLQ.0000000000000327.

13. DiClemente RJ. Behavioral counseling associated with STI prevention. J Pediatr. 2021;228:310–3. https://doi.org/10.1016/j.jpeds.2020.10.067.

14. Henderson JT, Senger CA, Henninger M, Bean SI, Redmond N, O'Connor EA. Behavioral counseling interventions to prevent sexually transmitted infections: updated evidence report and systematic review for the US preventive services task force. JAMA J Am Med Assoc. 2020;324(7):674–81. https://doi.org/10.1001/jama.2020.10371.

15. Slurink IAL, Van Benthem BHB, Van Rooijen MS, Achterbergh RCA, Van Aar F. Original research: latent classes of sexual risk and corresponding STI and HIV positivity among MSM attending centres for sexual health in The Netherlands. Sex Transm Infect. 2020;96(1):33. https://doi.org/10.1136/SEXTRANS-2019-053977.

16. Tran J, Fairley CK, Bowesman H, Aung ET, Ong JJ, Chow EPF. Non-conventional interventions to prevent gonorrhea or syphilis among men who have sex with men: a scoping review. Front Med. 2022;9:952476. https://doi.org/10.3389/FMED.2022.952476/FULL.

17. Hart TA, Noor SW, Vernon JRG, Antony MM, Gardner S, O'Cleirigh C. Integrated cognitive-behavioral therapy for social anxiety and HIV/STI prevention for gay and bisexual men: a pilot intervention trial. Behav Ther. 2020;51(3):503–17. https://doi.org/10.1016/J.BETH.2019.09.001.

18. Clark JL, Segura ER, Oldenburg CE, et al. Traditional and web-based technologies to improve partner notification following syphilis diagnosis among men who have sex with men in Lima, Peru: pilot randomized controlled trial. J Med Internet Res. 2018;20(7):e232. https://doi.org/10.2196/jmir.9821.

19. Ferreira A, Young T, Mathews C, Zunza M, Low N. Strategies for partner notification for sexually transmitted infections, including HIV. Cochrane Database Syst Rev. 2013;2013(10):CD002843. https://doi.org/10.1002/14651858.CD002843.pub2.

20. Marcus U, Jonas K, Berg R, et al. Association of internalised homonegativity with partner notification after diagnosis of syphilis or gonorrhoea among men having sex with men in 49 countries across four continents. BMC Public Health. 2023;23(1):8. https://doi.org/10.1186/S12889-022-14891-2.

21. Mimiaga MJ, Reisner SL, Tetu AM, et al. Psychosocial and behavioral predictors of partner notification after HIV and STI exposure and infection among MSM. AIDS Behav. 2009;13(4):738–45. https://doi.org/10.1007/S10461-008-9424-Y/TABLES/3.

22. Hogben M, Collins D, Hoots B, O'Connor K. Partner services in sexually transmitted disease prevention programs: a review. Sex Transm Dis. 2016;43(2):S53–62. https://doi.org/10.1097/OLQ.0000000000000328.

23. Katz DA, Copen CE, Haderxhanaj LT, et al. Changes in sexual behaviors with opposite-sex partners and sexually transmitted infection outcomes among females and males ages 15–44 years in the USA: National Survey of Family Growth, 2008–2019. Arch Sex Behav. 2022;52:809–21. https://doi.org/10.1007/S10508-022-02485-3.

24. Bergman H, Buckley BS, Villanueva G, et al. Comparison of different human papillomavirus (HPV) vaccine types and dose schedules for prevention of HPV-related disease in females and males. Cochrane Database Syst Rev. 2019;2019(11) https://doi.org/10.1002/14651858.CD013479.

25. Drolet M, Bénard É, Pérez N, et al. Population-level impact and herd effects following the introduction of human papillomavirus vaccination programmes: updated systematic review and meta-analysis. Lancet (London, England). 2019;394(10197):497. https://doi.org/10.1016/S0140-6736(19)30298-3.

26. Tyros G, Mastraftsi S, Gregoriou S, Nicolaidou E. Incidence of anogenital warts: epidemiological risk factors and real-life impact of human papillomavirus vaccination. Int J STD AIDS. 2020;32(1):4–13. https://doi.org/10.1177/0956462420958577.

27. Arbyn M, Xu L, Simoens C, Martin-Hirsch PPL. Prophylactic vaccination against human papillomaviruses to prevent cervical cancer and its precursors. Cochrane Database Syst Rev. 2018;2018(5):CD009069. https://doi.org/10.1002/14651858.CD009069.PUB3.

28. Gavin M. KidsHealth. 2019. https://kidshealth.org/en/teens/stds-talk.html. Accessed 13 Jan 2023.

29. Scrivener L, Green J, Hetherton J, Brook G. Disclosure of anogenital warts to sexual partners. Sex Transm Infect. 2008;84(3):179–82. https://doi.org/10.1136/sti.2007.029116.

30. Coyle R, Miltz A, Sewell J, et al. Symptoms of depression and anxiety and sexual health and behaviour among heterosexual men and women attending genitourinary medicine (GUM) clinics in England. HIV Med. 2018;19(Supplement 2):S62.

31. Black S, Salway T, Dove N, Shoveller J, Gilbert M. From silos to buckets: a qualitative study of how sexual health clinics address their clients' mental health needs. Can J Public Health. 2020;111(2):220. https://doi.org/10.17269/S41997-019-00273-6.

32. Osborn DPJ, King MB, Weir M. Psychiatric health in a sexually transmitted infections clinic effect on reattendance. J Psychosom Res. 2002;52(4):267. https://doi.org/10.1016/S0022-3999(01)00299-9.

33. Salway T, Ferlatte O, Shoveller J, et al. The need and desire for mental health and substance use-related services among clients of publicly funded sexually transmitted infection clinics in Vancouver, Canada. J Public Heal Manag Pract. 2019;25(3):E1–E10. https://doi.org/10.1097/PHH.0000000000000904.

34. Arkell J, Osborn DPJ, Ivens D, King MB. Factors associated with anxiety in patients attending a sexually transmitted infection clinic: qualitative survey. Int J STD AIDS. 2006;17(5):299. https://doi.org/10.1258/095646206776790097.

35. Coyle RM, Lampe FC, Miltz AR, et al. Associations of depression and anxiety symptoms with sexual behaviour in women and heterosexual men attending sexual health clinics: a cross-sectional study. Sex Transm Infect. 2019;95(4):254. https://doi.org/10.1136/sextrans-2018-053689.

36. Bondade S, Hosthota A, Karthik KN, Raj R. Intimate partner violence, anxiety, and depression in women with sexually transmitted infections—a hospital-based case control study. J Psychosexual Heal. 2021;3(1):65. https://doi.org/10.1177/2631831821992656.

37. Achterbergh RCA, van Rooijen MS, de Vries HJC. High prevalence of psychosocial problems in a syndemic based intervention to facilitate psychosocial care for high risk MSM in

Amsterdam: the SYN.BAS.IN randomized controlled trial—preliminary results. IUSTI 2018 World Congress 2018.

38. Beksinska A, Jama Z, Kabuti R, et al. Prevalence and correlates of common mental health problems and recent suicidal behaviour among female sex workers in Nairobi, Kenya: findings from the Maisha Fiti study. BJPsych Open. 2021;7(S1):S238. https://doi.org/10.1192/bjo.2021.637.

39. Trotta MP, Ammassari A, Murri R, et al. Self-reported sexual dysfunction is frequent among HIV-infected persons and is associated with suboptimal adherence to antiretrovirals. AIDS Patient Care STDs. 2008;22(4):291–9. https://doi.org/10.1089/APC.2007.0061.

40. Schuster R, Bornovalova M, Hunt E. The influence of depression on the progression of HIV: direct and indirect effects. Behav Modif. 2012;36(2):123–45. https://doi.org/10.1177/0145445511425231.

41. Huntingdon B, Muscat DM, de Wit J, Duracinsky M, Juraskova I. Factors associated with general sexual functioning and sexual satisfaction among people living with HIV: a systematic review. J Sex Res. 2020;57(7):824–35. https://doi.org/10.1080/00224499.2019.1689379.

42. Lamba H, Goldmeier D, Mackie NE, Scullard G. Antiretroviral therapy is associated with sexual dysfunction and with increased serum oestradiol levels in men. Int J STD AIDS. 2004;15(4):234–7. https://doi.org/10.1258/095646204773557749.

43. Luo L, Deng T, Zhao S, et al. Association between HIV infection and prevalence of erectile dysfunction: a systematic review and meta-analysis. J Sex Med. 2017;14(9):1125–32. https://doi.org/10.1016/J.JSXM.2017.07.001.

44. Richardson D, Goldmeier D, Frize G, et al. Letrozole versus testosterone. A single-center pilot study of HIV-infected men who have sex with men on highly active anti-retroviral therapy (HAART) with hypoactive sexual desire disorder and raised estradiol levels. J Sex Med. 2007;4(2):502–8. https://doi.org/10.1111/J.1743-6109.2007.00451.X.

45. Mao L, Newman CE, Kidd MR, Saltman DC, Rogers GD, Kippax SC. Self-reported sexual difficulties and their association with depression and other factors among gay men attending high HIV-caseload general practices in Australia. J Sex Med. 2009;6(5):1378–85. https://doi.org/10.1111/J.1743-6109.2008.01160.X.

46. Agaba PA, Meloni ST, Sule HM, Agaba EI, Idoko JA, Kanki PJ. Sexual dysfunction and its determinants among women infected with HIV. Int J Gynaecol Obstet. 2017;137(3):301–8. https://doi.org/10.1002/IJGO.12140.

47. Adeli M, Moghaddam-Banaem L, Shahali S. Sexual dysfunction in women with genital warts: a systematic review. BMC Womens Health. 2022;22(1):516. https://doi.org/10.1186/S12905-022-02073-6.

48. Nahidi M, Nahidi Y, Kardan G, et al. Evaluation of sexual life and marital satisfaction in patients with anogenital wart. Actas Dermosifiliogr. 2019;110(7):521–5. https://doi.org/10.1016/J.AD.2018.08.005.

49. Piñeros M, Hernández-Suárez G, Orjuela L, Vargas JC, Pérez G. HPV knowledge and impact of genital warts on self esteem and sexual life in Colombian patients. BMC Public Heal. 2013;13:272. https://doi.org/10.1186/1471-2458-13-272.

50. Qi S-Z, Wang S-M, Shi J-F, et al. Human papillomavirus-related psychosocial impact of patients with genital warts in China: a hospital-based cross-sectional study. BMC Public Heal. 2014;14:739. https://doi.org/10.1186/1471-2458-14-739.

51. Nia MH, Rahmanian F, Ghahartars M, Janghorban R. Sexual function and sexual quality of life in men with genital warts: a cross-sectional study. Reprod Heal RH. 2022;19(1):102. https://doi.org/10.1186/s12978-022-01403-z.

52. Bennett KF, Waller J, Ryan M, Bailey JV, Marlow LAV. The psychosexual impact of testing positive for high-risk cervical human papillomavirus (HPV): a systematic review. Psychooncology. 2019;28(10):1959–70. https://doi.org/10.1002/PON.5198.

53. Bennett KF, Waller J, McBride E, et al. Psychosexual distress following routine primary human papillomavirus testing: a longitudinal evaluation within the English cervical screening programme. BJOG An Int J Obstet Gynaecol. 2021;128(4):745–54. https://doi.org/10.1111/1471-0528.16460.

54. O'Connor M, O'Leary E, Waller J, et al. Socio-economic variations in anticipated adverse reactions to testing HPV positive: implications for the introduction of primary HPV-based cervical screening. Prev Med. 2018;115:90–6. https://doi.org/10.1016/j.ypmed.2018.08.017.
55. Bennett KF, Waller J, Ryan M, Bailey JV, Marlow LA V. The psychosexual impact of testing positive for high-risk cervical human papillomavirus (HPV): a systematic review. Psycho-Oncology. 2019;28(10):1959–70. https://doi.org/10.1002/pon.5198.
56. Mindel A, Marks C. Psychological symptoms associated with genital herpes virus infections: epidemiology and approaches to management. CNS Drugs. 2005;19(4):303–12. https://doi.org/10.2165/00023210-200519040-00003.
57. Mindel A. Long-term clinical and psychological management of genital herpes. J Med Virol. 1993;Suppl 1(1 S):39–44. https://doi.org/10.1002/JMV.1890410509.
58. Taylor MM, Wi T, Gerbase A, et al. Assessment of country implementation of the WHO global health sector strategy on sexually transmitted infections (2016-2021). PLoS One. 2022;17(5):e0263550. https://doi.org/10.1371/JOURNAL.PONE.0263550.

Correction to: Pelvic Floor Disorders and Sexuality 1: Urinary Incontinence

Sònia Anglès Acedo, Lorena López Frías, and Cristina Ros Cerro

---

Correction to:
Chapter 6 in: C. Castelo-Branco, S. Anglès Acedo (eds.),
Medical Disorders and Sexual Health,
Trends in Andrology and Sexual Medicine,
https://doi.org/10.1007/978-3-031-55080-5_6

The book was inadvertently published with an error in Chapter 6 title and has been corrected as below.

    It appeared: Pelvic Floor Disorders and Sexuality 1: Urinary Caution

    Instead of: Pelvic Floor Disorders and Sexuality 1: Urinary Incontinence

---

The updated version of this chapter can be found at
https://doi.org/10.1007/978-3-031-55080-5_6

Correction to: STI and Sexuality

Pere Fusté and Irene Fuertes

Correction to:
Chapter 34 in: C. Castelo-Branco, S. Anglès Acedo (eds.),
Medical Disorders and Sexual Health,
Trends in Andrology and Sexual Medicine,
https://doi.org/10.1007/978-3-031-55080-5_34

This book was inadvertently published with an error on page 501, in Chapter 34. The header "4.3 VHS" has been changed to "4.3 HSV."

The updated version of this chapter can be found at
https://doi.org/10.1007/978-3-031-55080-5_34